Fundamentals
of Drug Metabolism
and Drug Disposition

Fundamentals of Drug Metabolism and Drug Disposition

EDITED BY

Bert N. La Du, M.D., Ph.D.

Professor and Chairman, Department of Pharmacology,
New York University Medical School, New York

H. George Mandel, Ph.D.

Professor and Chairman, Department of Pharmacology,
The George Washington University School of Medicine, Washington, D.C.

E. Leong Way, Ph.D.

Professor of Pharmacology and Toxicology,
University of California School of Medicine, San Francisco

BALTIMORE

The Williams & Wilkins Company

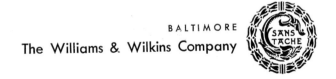

Library of Congress Catalog Card Number 71-163118
SBN 683-04812-0

Reprinted 1972

Composed and printed at the
WAVERLY PRESS, INC.
Mt. Royal and Guilford Aves.
Baltimore, Md. 21202, U.S.A.

Preface

The aim of this book is to present a general introduction to the current principles and methods for studying the metabolic transformation and physiological disposition of drugs and other chemicals of pharmacological and toxicological interest.

The book, although updated, follows the format of the lecture topics and laboratory experiments presented in three teaching workshops on drug metabolism held in 1966 at New York University Medical School, in 1967 at the George Washington University Medical School and in 1968 at the University of California San Francisco Medical Center. The workshops were sponsored by the Committee on Problems of Drug Safety of the Drug Research Board of the National Academy of Sciences-National Research Council. The Committee on Problems of Drug Safety initiated the teaching workshop programs and encouraged the three workshop directors to act as coeditors of the present volume.

The coeditors are indebted to many workshop faculty members for their valuable contributions. In particular, we wish to thank the instructors who organized the laboratory experiments in all three workshops. They have submitted laboratory exercises which illustrate both the principles and practical application of experimental methods used in drug metabolism research. We also thank the Pharmaceutical Manufacturers Association Foundation, Inc. for its support of the workshops and its generous grant to help meet the publication expenses of this book.

B. N. L.
H. G. M.
E. L. W.

List of Contributors

Joseph H. Asling, M.D., Department of Anesthesia, University of California Medical Center, San Francisco

Bernard B. Brodie, Ph.D., Chief, Laboratory of Chemical Pharmacology, National Heart and Lung Institute, National Institutes of Health, Bethesda, Md.

John J. Burns, Ph.D., Vice President for Research, Hoffmann-La Roche, Inc., Nutley, N. J.

Thomas C. Butler, M.D., Professor of Pharmacology, University of North Carolina, Chapel Hill

Edward J. Cafruny, M.D., Ph.D., Professor and Chairman, Department of Pharmacology and Therapeutics, Medical College of Ohio, Toledo

Victor H. Cohn, Ph.D., Professor, Department of Pharmacology, The George Washington University School of Medicine, Washington, D. C.

Allan H. Conney, Ph.D., Director, Department of Biochemistry and Drug Metabolism, Hoffmann-La Roche, Inc., Nutley, N. J.

Clarke Davison, Ph.D., Senior Research Biochemist and Section Head, Metabolic Chemistry, Sterling Winthrop Research Institute, Sterling Winthrop Co., Rensselaer, N. Y.

Edmond I. Eger, II, M.D., Professor, Department of Anesthesia, University of California, San Francisco Medical Center, San Francisco

Henry M. Fales, Ph.D., Chief, Laboratory of Chemistry, National Heart and Lung Institute, National Institutes of Health, Bethesda, Md.

Harry V. Gelboin, Ph.D., Chief, Chemistry Branch, National Center Institute, National Institutes of Health, Bethesda, Md.

James R. Gillette, Ph.D., Head, Section on Drug Metabolism, Laboratory of Chemical Pharmacology, National Heart and Lung Institute, National Institutes of Health, Bethesda, Md.

Ronald G. Kuntzman, Ph.D., Associate Director, Department of Biochemistry and Drug Metabolism, Hoffmann-La Roche, Inc., Nutley, N. J.

Bert N. La Du, Jr., M.D., Ph.D., Professor and Chairman, Department of Pharmacology, New York University School of Medicine, New York

H. George Mandel, Ph.D., Professor and Chairman, Department of Pharmacology, The George Washington University School of Medicine, Washington, D. C.

Gilbert J. Mannering, Ph.D., Professor, Department of Pharmacology, University of Minnesota School of Medicine, Minneapolis

Paul Mazel, Ph.D., Professor, Department of Pharmacology, The George Washington University School of Medicine, Washington, D. C.

Edwin S. Munson, M.D., Associate Professor, Department of Anesthesiology, University of California School of Medicine, Davis

Gabriel L. Plaa, Ph.D., Professor and Chairman, Department of Pharmacology, Faculty of Medicine, University of Montreal, Montreal, Quebec, Canada

David P. Rall, M.D., Ph.D., Associate Scientific Director for Experimental Therapeutics, National Cancer Institute, National Institutes of Health, Bethesda, M.D.

Watson D. Reid, M.D., Head, Section on Drug-Tissue Interaction, Laboratory of Chemical Pharmacology, National Heart and Lung Institute, National Institutes of Health, Bethesda, Md.

Malcolm Rowland, Ph.D., Assistant Professor, School of Pharmacy, University of California Medical Center, San Francisco

Lewis S. Schanker, Ph.D., Professor of Pharmacology, School of Pharmacy and School of Dentistry, University of Missouri-Kansas City, Kansas City, Mo.

Elwood O. Titus, Ph.D., Head, Section on Organic Chemistry, National Heart and Lung Institute, National Institutes of Health, Bethesda, Md.

Thomas N. Tozer, Ph.D., Assistant Professor of Pharmacy and Pharmaceutical Chemistry, School of Pharmacy, University of California San Francisco Medical Center, San Francisco

Anthony J. Trevor, Ph.D., Assistant Professor, Department of Pharmacology, University of California San Francisco Medical Center, San Francisco

William J. Waddell, M.D., Professor of Oral Biology and Pharmacology, Dental Research Center and Department of Pharmacology, The University of North Carolina, Chapel Hill

E. Leong Way, Ph.D., Professor of Pharmacology and Toxicology, University of California San Francisco Medical Center, San Francisco

Grant R. Wilkinson, Ph.D., Assistant Professor, Department of Pharmacology, Vanderbilt University, Nashville, Tenn.

R. Tecwyn Williams, Ph.D., Professor and Head, Department of Biochemistry, St. Mary's Hospital Medical School, University of London, London, England

Vincent G. Zannoni, Ph.D., Associate Professor, Department of Pharmacology, New York, University School of Medicine, New York

Contents

4. Protein Binding   C. DAVIDSON

5. Drug Entry into Brain and Cerebrospinal Fluid   D. RALL

6. Placental Transfer of Drugs   J. ASLING and E. L. WAY

7. Pulmonary Disposition of Drugs

E. MUNSON and E. EGER

8. Renal Excretion of Drugs

E. J. CAFRUNY

9. Extrarenal Excretion of Drugs

G. L. PLAA

PART TWO

DRUG BIOTRANSFORMATION: ENVIRONMENTAL AND GENETIC FACTORS WHICH MODIFY DRUG METABOLISM

10. Pathways of Drug Biotransformation: Biochemical Conjugations

H. G. MANDEL

15. Genetic Factors Modifying Drug Metabolism and Drug Response
B. N. LA DU

16. The Value of Determining the Plasma Concentration of Drugs in Animals and Man
B. B. BRODIE and W. D. REID

17. Application of Metabolic and Disposition Studies in the Development and Evaluation of Drugs
J. J. BURNS

PART THREE

TECHNIQUES FOR STUDYING DRUG BIOTRANSFORMATION

18. Techniques for Studying Drug Disposition In Vivo
A. TREVOR, M. ROWLAND and E. L. WAY

19. Techniques for Studying Drug Metabolism In Vitro   J. R. GILLETTE

20. Isolation Procedures—Liquid Extraction and Isolation Techniques
E. O. TITUS

21. Isolation and Identification Procedures—Spectral Methods
H. M. FALES

22. Qualitative and Quantitative Applications of Thin-Layer, Gas-Liquid, and Column Chromatography   G. R. WILKINSON

23. Applications of Tracer Techniques in Drug Metabolism Studies   R. KUNTZMAN

24. Autoradiography in Drug Disposition Studies   W. WADDELL

25. Application of Computers in Drug Metabolism Studies T. N. TOZER

PART FOUR

LABORATORY EXPERIMENTS IN THE STUDY OF DRUG METABOLISM AND DRUG DISPOSITION

26. General Principles and Procedures for Drug Metabolism In Vitro
P. MAZEL

27. Experiments Illustrating Drug Metabolism In Vitro   P. MAZEL

28. Experiments Illustrating Drug Distribution and Excretion

V. G. ZANNONI

29. Correlation of Drug Disposition with Pharmacologic Actions

A. TREVOR

PART One

PHYSICAL PROPERTIES OF DRUGS, DISTRIBUTION AND EXCRETION

1

Transmembrane Movement of Drug Molecules

VICTOR H. COHN

I. INTRODUCTION

A drug introduced into the body must cross several cellular and subcellular membrane structures when it is distributed to its sites of action, storage, metabolism, and excretion. This process is schematically represented in Figure 1.1. In this chapter I shall attempt to relate the physicochemical properties of a drug with those of the membrane which together control or modify transmembrane movement. In addition, the forces available to effect this movement will be discussed.

II. PHYSICOCHEMICAL PROPERTIES OF DRUG MOLECULES

There are three properties of a drug molecule that are of principal concern: its lipid solubility, the extent to which it is ionized, and its molecular size. Together these properties determine whether a molecule will move from one biologic compartment to another separated by a membranous structure, and provide some bases for predicting the rate and extent of such transmembrane intercompartment movement.

A. Lipid Solubility

As will be discussed in detail later, biologic membranes are lipoid in nature. For a molecule to cross a membrane it may have to initially "dissolve" in the membrane. The extent to which this dissolution can take place depends on the lipid solubility of the molecule. Lipid solubility is determined by the presence of lipophilic (hydrophobic) or non-polar groups in the structure of the drug molecule. Alkyl groups are non-polar, and this property increases with the length of the alkyl group; thus, the lipophilic properties increase in the series CH_3- $< CH_3CH_2- < CH_3CH_2CH_2- < CH_3(CH_2)_n-$. An aromatic phenyl group is approximately equivalent in lipophilic properties to an n-propyl group; a naphthyl group is equivalent to an n-hexyl group. The increase in lipophilic properties brought about by insertion of an alkyl group into a molecule is manifest whether the substitution occurs on carbon, nitrogen, oxygen, or sulfur. Replacement of oxygen by sulfur often produces a marked increase in the lipophilic properties of a molecule. Addition of a halogen likewise tends to increase lipid solubility.

Table 1.1 illustrates some of these effects in the barbiturate series. Replace-

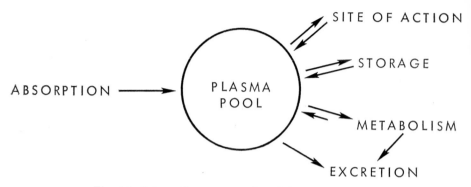

Fig. 1.1. Schematic representation of drug distribution

TABLE 1.1

Lipid solubility of some barbiturates

	"Lipid Solubility"[a]
Barbital	0.072
Phenobarbital	0.40
N-Methylphenobarbital	18.0
Thiophenobarbital	14.1

[a] Defined as the partition ratio of the un-ionized molecule between butyl chloride and an aqueous phase. See Section V, A for experimental details of determining lipid solubility. Data kindly supplied by Dr. Paul Mazel.

ment of one ethyl group of barbital with a phenyl group to form phenobarbital increases the lipid solubility more than five times. N-Methylation of phenobarbital results in a further 45-fold increase; conversion of phenobarbital to thiophenobarbital produces a comparable increase.

When a molecule contains structural elements that allow for hydrogen bonding with water, the lipophilic properties of the molecule are decreased and the hydrophilic or polar properties of the molecule are increased. Polarity is high for ionized molecules, including the ionized form of a dissociable molecule. Thus, many functional groups increase hydrophilic properties: OH, $-CO_2H$, $-NH_2$, $-NR_3^+$, $-SO_2H$, $-SO_2NH_2$, and to a lesser extent, $-CO_2CH_3$, $-CONH_2$ and $-OCH_3$.

The relative lipophilic/hydrophilic properties ("lipid solubility") of the entire molecule appear to determine whether the molecule will readily cross a biological membrane by a passive process. In general, the greater the lipid solubility, the greater the rate of its transmembrane movement.

B. Ionization

Most drugs are weak acids or weak bases and have one or more functional groups capable of ionizing. The extent to which this ionization takes place is dependent on the pK_a of the drug and the pH of the solution in which the drug is dissolved. Biologic membranes are permeable to the un-ionized form of a drug molecule if it is sufficiently lipid soluble; they are relatively impermeable to the ionized species.

The ionization of a weak acidic drug proceeds as

(1) $$[HA] \rightleftharpoons [H^+] + [A^-]$$

where [HA] is the concentration (or more properly, the activity) of the un-ionized species, $[A^-]$ the concentration of the ionized species, and $[H^+]$ the concentration of hydrogen ions. The relationship between this ionization, the pK_a of the drug, and the pH of its solution is described by the Henderson-Hasselbalch equation:

(2) $$pH = pK_a + \log \frac{[A^+]}{[HA]}$$

If (2) is rearranged to

(3) $$\frac{[A^-]}{[HA]} = 10^{pH-pK_a}$$

one can readily deduce that a small change in pH near the pK_a can effect a large change in the extent of ionization. This is shown in Figure 1.2.

Figure 1.3 presents the range of pK_a values for some frequently encountered ionizable groups in drug molecules, and Figure 1.4 lists pK_a values for some representative drugs. Experimental techniques for the determination of ionization constants are outlined in Section V,B.

C. Molecular Size and Shape

The influence of molecular size and shape on transmembrane movement is discussed in Sections III and IV.

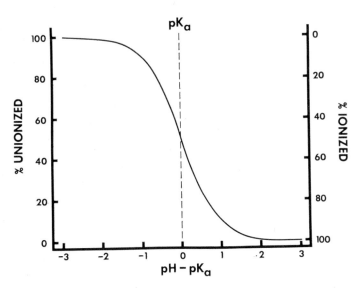

Fig. 1.2. The effect of pH on the ionization of a weak acid. The acid is 50% ionized at a pH = pK_a. At higher pH values it becomes increasingly more ionized; at lower pH values it becomes increasingly more un-ionized. The rate of change of ionization is greatest at pH values near the pK_a.

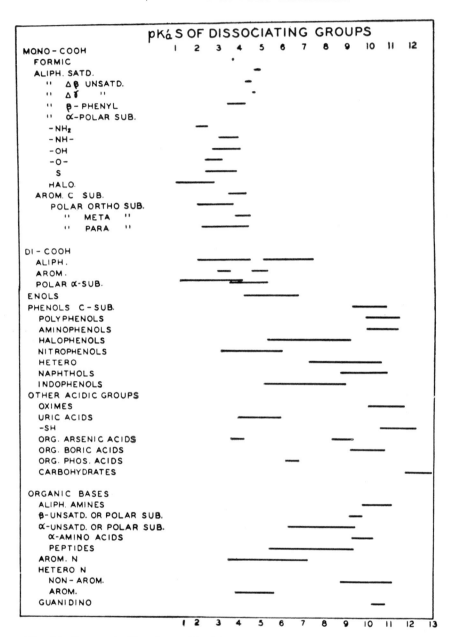

Fig. 1.3. Range of pK$_a$ values of ionizing groups (from Parke and Davis, 1954)

III. PROPERTIES OF CELLULAR MEMBRANES

The concept of a lipoid membrane had its origin in the classic studies of Overton in the 1890's. In an extensive series of experiments involving the penetration of organic compounds into both plant and animal cells, Overton observed that whereas ethers, esters, aldehydes, and ketones penetrate the cells very rapidly, more polar compounds, such as urea, polyhydric alcohols (glycerol and sugars), and amino acids, enter much more slowly. This initial correlation between rate

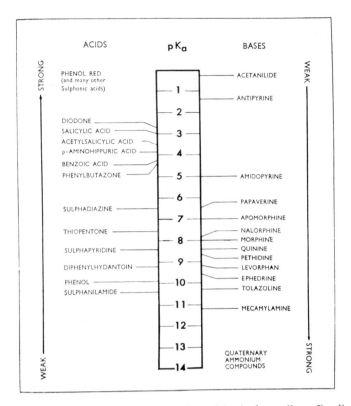

Fig. 1.4. pK$_a$ values for some typical acidic and basic drugs (from Brodie, 1964)

of penetration and lipid solubility led Overton (1895) to suggest that the chemical composition of the plasma membrane included a component with selective (lipid) dissolving properties.

These observations were confirmed and extended by Collander and Bärlund (1933), who correlated the cell permeability of compounds with their olive oil/water partition coefficients, as a measure of lipid solubility (Fig. 1.5). Some apparent discrepancies with the lipoid-theory were noted. For example, several molecules had permeabilities greater than would be expected from their lipid solubilities. For these compounds, permeability appeared to be inversely correlated with molecular volume. Thus, the plasma membrane seemed capable of acting as a molecular sieve whose pore size determined the rate of passage for these small, un-ionized but polar molecules. Table 1.2 contains some illustrative data. In the series shown, there is a *decrease* in permeability with increasing lipid solubility, but an increase in permeability with decreasing molecular volume. From these studies emerged the concept formulated by Collander and Bärlund (1933) of a lipoid-sieve plasma membrane. This general concept for the permeation of plasma membranes by un-ionized organic molecules is still valid.

The lipoid nature of membranes has been confirmed by chemical analysis. Various cellular and subcellular membranes have been shown to contain large amounts of phospholipids, cholesterol, and neutral lipids, in association with protein. Rat liver plasma membrane, for example, contains approximately 40% lipids, over half of which are phospholipids, and approximately 60% protein

(Bendetti and Emmelot, 1968). Other plasma membranes and the membranes associated with mitochondria and endoplasmic reticulum have characteristic amounts and kinds of lipids and proteins (Rouser *et al.*, 1968; Korn, 1969).

The precise structural arrangement of these components in the membrane is not known, although several models have been proposed. Gortner and Grendel's

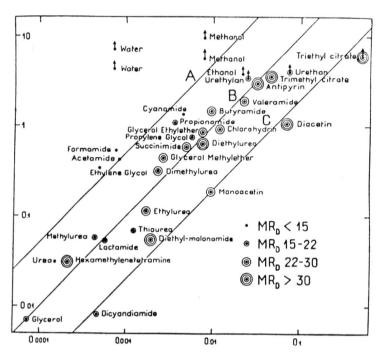

Fig. 1.5. The permeability of *Chara ceratophylla* cells to organic nonelectrolytes of different lipid solubility and molecular volume. The ordinate: P × M.W.⁴ (P expressed as cm/hr); the abscissa: the olive oil/water partition coefficient. MR$_D$ (molar refraction) is related to molecular volume (see Table 1.2). (From Collander, 1949.)

TABLE 1.2

Relationship between permeability and molecular volume for small polar molecules[a]

	Relative Permeability[b]	Molecular Volume[c]	Lipid Solubility[d]
Urea	0.35	13.67	0.0005
Methyl urea	0.01	18.47	0.0012
Dimethyl urea	0.005	23.43	0.0116
Diethyl urea	0.003	32.66	0.0185

[a] Data of Ruhland and Hoffmann (1925) for the sulfur algae, *Beggiatoa mirabilis*.
[b] Experimentally determined as the plasmolytic threshold concentration (moles/liter). Greater penetrating power is associated with higher plasmolytic threshold concentration.
[c] Expressed in terms of molecular refraction, which has dimensions of volume:

$$MR = \frac{n^2 - 1}{n^2 - 1} \cdot \frac{M.W.}{\rho}$$ Where n = refraction index of the substance and ρ = density of

the substance
[d] Ether/water partition ratio.

(1925) original proposal for a bimolecular lipid membrane was elaborated in subsequent years by Davson and Danielli (1952). The latter model, now classic, proposes that the membrane is composed of a double layer of lipid molecules, each oriented perpendicularly to the cell surface. The polar ends of the lipid molecules are directed outwards, and this lipid core is covered on each side with a layer of protein bound to the lipids by ionic forces. This model (Fig. 1.6) was deduced from studies of membrane permeability, electrical properties, x-ray diffraction patterns and other physicochemical measurements. It seemed to be confirmed by electron microscopy, which revealed a triple-layered structure having two electron-dense regions separated by a light, intermediate zone (Fig. 1.7). It was further proposed that all cellular membranes had identical structures (Robertson, 1960).

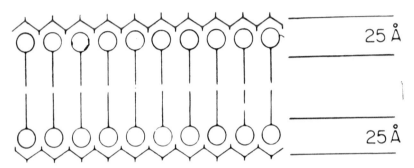

Fig. 1.6. Schematic drawing of the Davson-Danielli model for the structure of the plasma membrane. The lipid molecules are indicated by circles for the hydrophilic (polar) ends, and rods for the lipophilic (hydrophobic) ends. The zigzag lines represent the protein layers covering the lipid leaflet. (Modified from Sjöstrand, 1968.)

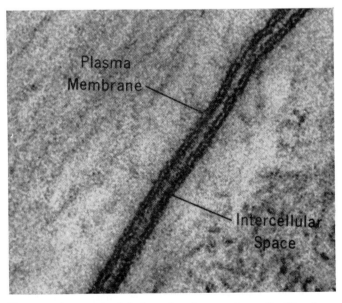

Fig. 1.7. Electron micrograph of the boundary between two cells. The plasma membrane of each appears as two dense lines separated by a less dense intermediate layer. Note the suggestion of some substructure in the electron-dense areas. (From Fawcett, 1966.)

Recently, reinvestigation and reinterpretation of physicochemical data and electron micrographs, and the utilization of newer techniques, have suggested to some that the "unit membrane" concept outlined above is an over-simplification. As suggested above, cellular membranes differ significantly in their chemical composition. It is possible that they also differ in structure, depending on their chemical composition and physiologic function. For example, the orientation of lipids may be a globular or micellar substructure embedded in protein, rather than a bilayer. Moreover, some recent models place increased emphasis on the protein or lipoprotein nature of the membrane and stress the importance of protein-protein (rather than lipid-lipid) interactions as the basis for membrane structure (Korn, 1969; Bendetti and Emmelot, 1968). Whatever the eventual architecture of the membrane may be, it is probable that the membrane's lipid content accounts for its relative permeability to lipid-soluble solutes; the membrane proteins are involved not only in membrane structure but are associated with the specialized specific transport mechanisms (see below).

IV. FORCES OPERATING TO INDUCE TRANSMEMBRANE MOVEMENT OF DRUG MOLECULES

A. Diffusion

The most important force effecting transmembrane movement of most drugs results from a difference in concentration of the drug across the membrane. The random motion of solute molecules brings about a movement of the molecules from a region of higher to one of lower concentration. This process is called *diffusion*. The rate of diffusion (dQ/dt), as defined by Fick, depends on the magnitude of the concentration gradient across the membrane (Δc), the area of the membrane (A) through which the solute molecules pass, the thickness of the membrane (Δx), and the partition (R) of the molecule between the membrane and aqueous phase:

$$(4) \qquad -\frac{dQ}{dt} = \frac{DRA\Delta c}{\Delta x}$$

The diffusion coefficient, D, is defined as the number of moles of drug that diffuse across a membrane of unit area in unit time when the concentration *gradient* across the membrane is unity; its dimensions are area per unit time, e.g., cm²/sec. The diffusion coefficient is difficult to evaluate because of the uncertainty in estimating R and Δx. A permeability coefficient (P) is therefore defined as:

$$(5) \qquad P \equiv \frac{DR}{\Delta x}$$

Although the permeability coefficient depends on the diffusivity of the molecule through the membrane, the membrane/aqueous phase partition for the molecule, and the thickness of the membrane at the site of diffusion, it is directly measurable as the number of moles of drug that cross a membrane of unit area in unit time when the concentration *difference* across the membrane is unity. The dimensions of the permeability coefficient are distance per unit time, e.g., cm/sec.; thus, it is clearly a rate. Fick's law, in terms of permeability, is then:

$$(6) \qquad \frac{dQ}{dt} = -PA\Delta c.$$

The diffusion coefficient for a drug is dependent on a number of factors. Molecular size influences the coefficient. For small molecules diffusing in water, the diffusion coefficients are inversely related to the square roots of their molecular weights (i.e., $(M.W.)^{\frac{1}{2}} \times D$ = constant). For large molecules, the diffusion coefficients in water are inversely related to the cube roots of their molecular weights (Fig. 1.8). The principal resistance to diffusion of molecules in water results from the interaction (friction) of the solute molecules with the solvent molecules. As molecular size (volume) increases, this frictional resistance becomes increasingly important. In addition, the interaction is influenced by the shape of the molecule. The diffusion coefficient for a spherical molecule is greater than that for a non-spherically shaped molecule of identical volume. Frictional resistance is similarly a function of the viscosity of the drug solution.

The interposition of a membrane impedes diffusion by several orders of magnitude. In order to enter the membrane, the solute must first overcome its tendency to associate with water molecules by hydrogen bonding, and "dissolve" in the lipoid areas of the membrane. The molecule must then cross the membrane and re-enter the aqueous phase on the other side of the membrane. The first step, namely the acquisition of sufficient energy to overcome the hydrogen bonding of the solute molecules to water molecules, may be the major determinant of the transmembrane permeability. Figure 1.9 (Stein, 1967) shows the data of Collander and Bärlund replotted to relate solute permeability to the number of hydrogen bond forming groups in the solute molecule. Clearly, the

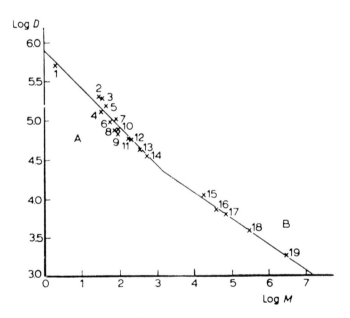

Fig. 1.8. The diffusion coefficient (D) as a function of molecular weight (M). In the portion of the curve labeled A, the relation $DM^{\frac{1}{2}}$ is constant; in the portion labeled B, the relation $DM^{\frac{1}{3}}$ is constant. All values were obtained at or near 20°C. Diffusing molecules as follows: 1, hydrogen; 2, nitrogen; 3, oxygen; 4, methanol; 5, carbon dioxide; 6, acetamide; 7, urea; 8, n-butanol; 9, n-amyl alcohol; 10, glycerol; 11, chloral hydrate; 12, glucose; 13, lactose; 14, raffinose; 15, myoglobin; 16, lactoglobulin; 17, hemoglobin; 18, edestin; 19, erythrocruorin. (From Stein, 1962.)

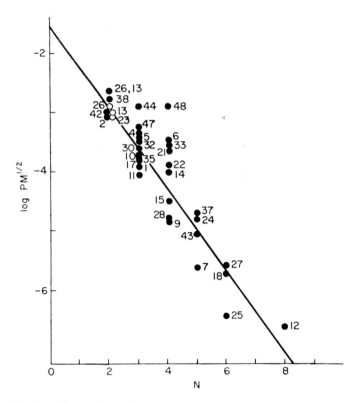

Fig. 1.9. The dependence of membrane permeability ($PM^{\frac{1}{2}}$) on the number of hydrogen bond-forming groups (N) in a molecule. The permeants are the same as those shown in Figure 1.5 and have been assigned the following numbers: 1, acetamide; 2, antipyrin; 3, butanol; 4, butyramide; 5, cyanamide; 6, diacetin; 7, dicyandiamide; 8, diethylene glycol; 9, diethyl malonamide; 10, diethyl urea; 11, dimethyl urea; 12, erythritol; 13, ethanol; 14, ethylene glycol; 15, ethyl urea; 16, ethyl urethane; 17, formamide; 18, glycerol; 19, glycerol + CO_2; 20, glycerol + Cu^{2+}; 21, glycerol ethyl ether; 22, glycerol methyl ether; 23, isopropanol; 24, lactamide; 25, malonamide; 26, methanol; 27, methylol urea; 28, methyl urea; 29, monoacetin; 30, monochlorohydrin; 31, propanol; 32, propionamide; 33, (α,β)-propylene glycol; 34, (α,γ)-propylene glycol; 35, succinimide; 36, tetraethylene glycol; 37, thiourea; 38, triethyl citrate; 39, triethylene glycol; 40, trihydroxybutane; 41, trihydroxybutane + Cu^{2+}; 42, trimethyl citrate; 43, urea; 44, urethane; 45, urethylan; 46, urotropin; 47, valeramide; 48, water; 49, 2,3-butylene glycol. (From Stein, 1967.)

highest permeability is associated with molecules with the fewest hydrogen bonding moieties.

Since the driving force for diffusion is a concentration gradient, one would expect no further net transmembrane movement when the drug attains the same concentration on each side of the membrane. This can be demonstrated experimentally for un-ionized molecules. However, for drugs that ionize it is possible under certain conditions to find at equilibrium *unequal* concentrations of the drug on either side of the membrane. Only the un-ionized molecules readily cross the membrane and achieve the same equilibrium concentrated on either side of the membrane; the ionized molecules are virtually excluded from transmembrane diffusion. If a pH gradient exists across the membrane, the drug will ionize to a different extent on each side of the membrane and, as a result, there will be an unequal *total* concentration (ionized plus un-ionized) of the drug on each side of the membrane. The theoretical equilibrium concentration ratio may be calculated. We can rearrange equation (3) (Section II,B) to obtain an expression for $[A^-]$ in terms of $[HA]$:

$$(7) \qquad\qquad [A^-] = [HA] \cdot 10^{pH-pK_a}$$

The total concentration of drug on one side of the membrane (c_1) will be the sum of the un-ionized and ionized molecules on that side:

$$(8) \qquad c_1 = [HA_1] + [A_1^-] = [HA_1] + [HA_1] \cdot 10^{pH_1-pK_a}$$

Similarly, on the other side of the membrane:

$$(9) \qquad c_2 = [HA_2] + [A_2^-] = [HA_2] + [HA_2] \cdot 10^{pH_2-pK_a}$$

At equilibrium, the ratio of the concentrations across the membrane (R) will be:

$$(10) \qquad R = \frac{c_1}{c_2} = \frac{[HA_1] + [HA_1] \cdot 10^{pH_1-pK_a}}{[HA_2] + [HA_2] \cdot 10^{pH_2-pK_a}}$$

Since the membrane is freely permeable to the un-ionized molecules, at equilibrium $[HA_1] = [HA_2]$ and equation (10) may be simplified to:

$$(11) \qquad\qquad R = \frac{1 + 10^{pH_1-pK_a}}{1 + 10^{pH_1-pK_a}}$$

For a weak base the corresponding equation is:

$$(12) \qquad\qquad R_{base} = \frac{1 + 10^{pK_a-pH_1}}{1 + 10^{pK_a-pH_2}}$$

For both weak acids and bases the total concentration of drug is greater in the compartment where it is more highly ionized.

Figure 1.10 is an example of the effect of a pH gradient on the theoretical gastric juice/plasma concentration gradient for probenecid, a weak acid with a pK_a of approximately 3.4. This drug is almost totally un-ionized at the pH of gastric juice and almost completely ionized at the pH of plasma. The calculated value for $R_{GJ/Pl}$ is approximately 10^{-4}. One would predict that, if sufficient time to attain equilibrium were available, probenecid should be very well absorbed from the stomach.

An analogous situation obtains with a weak base. Figure 1.11 illustrates the urine/plasma partition of quinine, a weak base with a pK_a of approximately 8.4. In this case, the drug is more highly ionized in the acidic urine, and the theoretical value for $R_{Ur/Pl}$ is approximately 10^2. The prediction that acidifying the urine should increase the excretion of a weak basic drug such as quinine is borne out in practice.

Additional implications of this pH partition to drug absorption, distribution, and excretion will be discussed in subsequent chapters.

An unequal distribution of drug across the cell membrane can also exist at equilibrium if there is a difference in the extent of protein (or other macromolecule) binding on each side of the membrane. Protein-bound drug molecules, like ionized molecules, cannot permeate cellular membranes. Thus, at equilibrium there will be a larger *total* concentration of drug on the side of the membrane

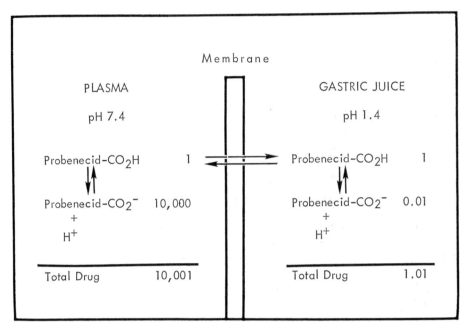

Fig. 1.10. The pH dependent distribution of probenecid between plasma and gastric juice at equilibrium. Probenecid is a weak acid with a $pK_a = 3.4$. It is assumed that the membrane is freely permeable to the un-ionized form, but impermeable to the ionized form of the drug.

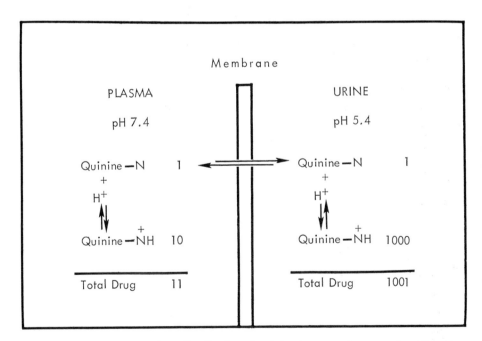

Fig. 1.11. The pH dependent distribution of quinine between plasma and acidic urine. Quinine is a weak base with a $pK_a = 8.4$. It is assumed that the membrane is freely permeable to the un-ionized form, but impermeable to the ionized form of the drug.

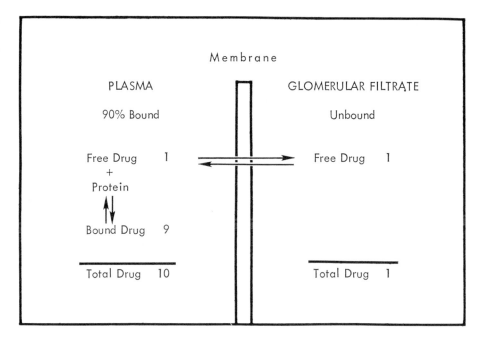

Fig. 1.12. The distribution of phenylbutazone between plasma and the glomerular filtrate. Phenylbutazone is highly bound to plasma proteins, but there is little or no binding in the relatively protein-free glomerular filtrate.

where the greater extent of binding occurs. Figure 1.12 is illustrative. Phenylbutazone is highly bound to plasma proteins. The portion that is bound is not available for glomerular filtration, and essentially no binding takes place in the relatively protein-free glomerular filtrate. Thus, at equilibrium one would predict a plasma/filtrate gradient of 10.

B. Movement Through Aqueous Channels

As was discussed in Section III, the permeability of membranes to water, urea, methanol, and other small, non-lipid soluble molecules seems to depend on the presence of aqueous channels or pores penetrating the membrane. If pores are large, the diffusion of small solute molecules through these aqueous channels in the membrane will be reduced only in proportion to the reduction in area available for diffusion. As pore size is reduced and approaches the size of the diffusing solute molecule, increasing interaction (frictional resistance) takes place between the solute and the membrane that further restricts diffusion. If a hydrostatic pressure or an osmotic gradient is imposed across the cell membrane, bulk flow (filtration) of water takes place through the aqueous channels, and solutes small enough to pass through the pores will be carried along by this additional driving force.

The apparent diameter of these aqueous channels has been estimated for several membranes. Some examples are shown in Table 1.3. Considerable variation is found to exist in the estimated pore size of various membranes and, correspondingly, the size molecule that can pass through these pores. Thus, molecules up to about the size of albumin (M.W. = 69,000; major axis = 150Å: minor

TABLE 1.3
Apparent pore size of some biological membranes[a]

	Apparent Pore Diameter Å
Erythrocyte (human)	8[b]
Capillary—muscle (cat)	60[c]
—glomerulus (dog)	70–80[d]
Arachnoid villi (monkey)	40–120[e]

[a] Calculated from data on restricted diffusion of solute molecules of different sizes. [b] Goldstein and Solomon, 1960. [c] Pappenheimer, *et al.*, 1951. [d] Pappenheimer, 1955. [e] Welch and Friedman, 1960.

axis = 35Å) can appear in the glomerular filtrate, but molecules larger than 4Å radius are excluded from the erythrocyte. While membrane permeability behavior suggests the presence of these aqueous channels, electron microscopic confirmation of their presence is lacking, except for the arachnoid villi.

Drug permeation through aqueous channels is of importance in renal excretion, removal of drugs from the cerebral spinal fluid, and entry of drugs into the liver. This will be discussed further in subsequent chapters.

C. Carrier Mediated Transport

In addition to the mechanisms discussed so far, some biologic membranes are capable of facilitating the transfer of large, lipid-insoluble, or ionized molecules by specialized processes. These processes deviate in several important aspects from Fick's diffusion equation. For the specialized processes, the rate of permeation is faster than would be predicted by $(M.W.)^{\frac{1}{2}} \times D$; moreover, the rate reaches an upper limit as the concentration gradient is increased. The specialized processes display a high degree of selectivity; for example, optical enantiomorphs may be distinguished and permeate at different rates. Another characteristic is that structural analogs of the permeating molecule frequently competitively inhibit its transmembrane movement.

The mechanism for this type of facilitated permeation is thought to involve a component of the membrane (carrier) that can bind the solute molecule non-covalently. This carrier-solute complex diffuses from one side of the membrane to the other where it dissociates and discharges the solute molecule. The carrier returns to its original site to complete the cycle, and to accept another solute molecule. This hypothetical carrier is available only in limited amounts in the cell membrane and is capable of displaying a high degree of structural specificity with respect to the molecules that can complex with it. There are apparently a large number of specific carrier systems available to each cell.

Two types of carrier mediated transport may be distinguished. *Facilitated diffusion* is the term applied to a carrier mediated transport system that operates along a concentration gradient of the permeating solute. At equilibrium the solute will attain the same concentration on either side of the membrane as in simple diffusion. No apparent energy expenditure is involved in facilitated diffusion: it is not inhibited by metabolic poisons that interfere with energy production. Facilitated diffusion has been demonstrated to operate for the movement of sugars into erythrocytes (LeFevre, 1961) and for sugars, amino acids and nucleosides in various other cells and tissues (Wilbrandt and Rosenberg, 1961; Stein, 1967). There has been no clear demonstration of facilitated diffusion playing an important role in the transmembrane movement of drug molecules.

Active transport has all of the characteristics of a carrier mediated transport outlined above, but, in addition, active transport processes are capable of moving a solute molecule against a concentration gradient. Consequently, active transport requires the expenditure of energy and is inhibited by metabolic poisons that interfere with energy production. Active transport processes are important in the membrane permeation of drug molecules. As will be discussed in detail in subsequent chapters, active transport figures prominently in renal and biliary excretion of many drugs and their metabolites; in the removal of some drugs from the central nervous system at the choroid plexus and ciliary body; and, to a lesser extent, in the intestinal absorption of some drugs structurally related to normal dietary constituents.

Thus, there are several forces and processes that can effect the transmembrane movement of a drug molecule. Other mechanisms are known for natural substrates, but their involvement for drugs has yet to be demonstrated. The precise architecture of cellular membranes is still unknown. Similarly, the molecular basis for transmembrane permeation is still largely conjectural. Despite this, it does appear that membranes behave as though lipoid in nature, allowing lipid soluble molecules to penetrate at rates related to their lipid solubility. Lipid insoluble molecules and ionized molecules must depend largely on specialized transfer process for membrane permeation. Water and very small lipid insoluble molecules may traverse aqueous channels, but bulk flow and ultrafiltration are important processes for the translocation of drugs only at sites where the plasma membrane has been specially modified to facilitate these processes. Subsequent chapters will illustrate the application of these general phenomena to specific processes involving drugs.

V. EXPERIMENTAL PROCEDURES

A. Determination of Lipid Solubility

Lipid solubility is determined experimentally by measuring the partition of the drug between an aqueous phase and any of several organic, immiscible, lipophilic solvents, for example, chloroform, heptane, diethyl ether, butyl chloride and olive oil. A quantity of the drug is dissolved in a buffered aqueous solution which is then shaken with the selected solvent until equilibrium is attained. The drug concentration is determined in each phase and the solvent/aqueous concentration ratio is calculated. While none of these lipophilic solvents is an entirely satisfactory model for the membrane, the partition coefficients determined with them allow for some reasonable predictions. For a drug that can ionize, the observed partition will be dependent on the extent of ionization of the drug, and thus the pH of the aqueous phase. The partition of the un-ionized species is independent of pH, however, and can be calculated from the relationship described by Butler (1953):

$$\log \left(\frac{C_a}{C_o} - 1 \right) = pH - pK_a$$

where C_a is the partition coefficient of the un-ionized moiety and C_o, the observed partition ratio. If the pK_a of the drug is not known, determination of the partition coefficient at two different pH values will allow solution of two simultaneous equations for both C_a and pK_a.

B. Determination of the pK_a for a Weak Acid or Weak Base

In addition to the technique described in Section V,A the pK_a of a drug can be determined by either titration or spectrophotometry.

1. Determination of pK_a by Titration. In the procedure recommended by Albert and Serjeant (1962), an accurately weighed sample of desiccated drug is dissolved in sufficient CO_2-free distilled water to yield a 0.01 M solution. Five ml of the drug solution is placed in a beaker and the pH is determined precisely. Using a microburet, the titrant (either 1.00 N HCl or 1.00 N KOH) is added in equal portions, each one-tenth of the calculated total required volume for one ionizing group. After each addition, the pH is again determined precisely. Utilizing the procedure outlined in Table 1.4, the concentrations of ionized and un-ionized species after each addition are calculated. From these and the corresponding pH values, nine estimates of the pK_a may be computed and then averaged.

In the procedure utilized by Parke and Davis (1954), approximately 5 mg of the drug dissolved in 3 ml of distilled water is titrated with 2 N HCl or 2 N KOH. After each addition of titrant the pH is determined. A curve of volume of titrant plotted against pH is made for the drug solution and for an equal volume of water similarly titrated. The curve for the titration of solvent is subtracted from that for the titration of the drug. The resultant difference-curve represents the hydrogen binding capacity of the drug as a function of pH. The midpoint of each inflection occurring in this difference-curve represents the pK_a of an ionizing

TABLE 1.4

Determination of the pK_a for tromethamine ("Tris")

1	2	3	4	5	6	7
Titrant N-HCl ml.	pH	Stoichiometric concentrations*		$\dfrac{[BH^+]}{[B]}$	log of column 5	pK_a (= pH + column 6)
		[BH+]	[B]			
0	10.12	0	0.010			
0.05	9.12	0.001	0.009	1/9	−0.95	8.17
0.10	8.78	0.002	0.008	2/8	−0.60	8.18
0.15	8.55	0.003	0.007	3/7	−0.37	8.18
0.20	8.36	0.004	0.006	4/6	−0.18	8.18
0.25	8.19	0.005	0.005	5/5	0.00	8.19
0.30	8.01	0.006	0.004	6/4	+0.18	8.19
0.35	7.81	0.007	0.003	7/3	+0.37	8.18
0.40	7.57	0.008	0.002	8/2	+0.60	8.17
0.45	7.21	0.009	0.001	9/1	+0.95	8.16
0.50	4.32	0.010	0			

Tromethamine, (2-amino-2-hydroxymethyl-1,3-propanediol),/(60.6 mg), dried in air at 110°, was dissolved in 50 ml of deionized water (0.01 M) and titrated at 20° under a nitrogen atmosphere (to exclude CO_2). The titrant was 1.00 N HCl. [B] is the concentration of the un-ionized base, and [BH+] the concentration of the ionized base. The pK_a was calculated after each addition of titrant from $pK_a = pH + \log ([BH^+]/[B])$. The average $pK_a = 8.18 \pm 0.02$. (From Albert and Serjeant, 1962.)

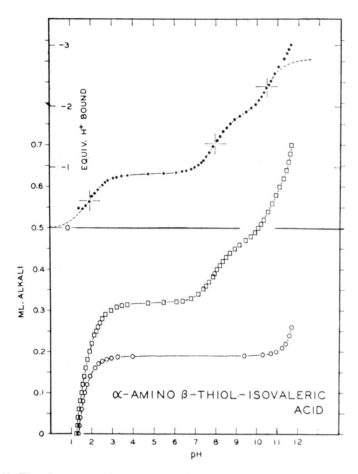

Fig. 1.13. Titration curves for α-amino-β-thiol-isovaleric acid. The open squares are the curve for the titration of the acid. The open circles are the curve for the titration of solvent. When the solvent-titration curve is subtracted from the acid-titration curve, a third curve (solid circles) results. This curve represents the equivalents of H^+ bound as a function of pH; three ionizing groups are apparent with pK_a values of approximately 2.0, 8.0, and 10.5. (From Parke and Davis, 1954.)

group. This graphical procedure, illustrated in Figure 1.13, gives approximate values for the pK_a.

2. Spectrophotometric Determination of pK_a. The absorption spectrum of many compounds is dependent on pH, and advantage may be taken of this to determine the pK_a. For an acid:

$$(13) \qquad pK_a = pH + \log \frac{E_A - E}{E - E_{HA}}$$

where E_A is the extinction coefficient of the ionized molecule, E_{HA} the extinction of the un-ionized molecule at the same wavelength, and E the extinction coefficient of a mixture of both at the same wavelength and at the given pH. (If identical concentrations of a drug are used throughout, optical densities may be substituted for extinction coefficients in the calculation.) A solution of the drug (approximately 10^{-4} N) is made in 0.1 N HCl and 0.1 N KOH, and the spectra

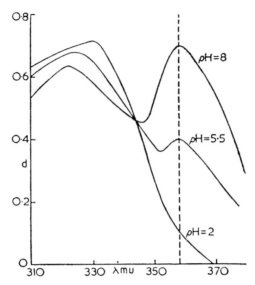

Fig. 1.14. Determination of the pK$_a$ of an acid by spectrophotometry. The spectra for the completely ionized form (pH 8), the completely un-ionized form (pH 2), and a mixture of both forms (pH 5.5) are shown. At 358 mμ the optical densities are 0.700, 0.105, and 0.395, respectively, from which the pK$_a$ = 5.52 was calculated. (From Albert and Serjeant, 1962.)

are recorded using a solution identical in composition except for drug in the reference cell. A wavelength is selected at which the two spectra differ most in optical density. The optical density is then determined at this wavelength for the completely ionized and the completely un-ionized species. Another solution of the drug is prepared buffered to a pH which will yield a mixture of ionized and un-ionized species, and the optical density of this solution is obtained at the same wavelength. The pK$_a$ value is then calculated from the above equation. To d 'termine the pK$_a$ more exactly, drug solutions are prepared that are buffered to a pH equivalent to the approximate pK$_a$ ± 0.2, ±0.4, and ±0.6. The optical densities are again determined and a set of pK$_a$ values calculated. Figure 1.14 shows the spectra of a weak acid at pH 2 (completely un-ionized), pH 8 (completely ionized), and pH 5.5 (mixture of ionized and un-ionized species) from which the pK$_a$ can be calculated.

Acknowledgments

The preparation of this chapter was supported in part by USPHS research grant GM 13749 and training grant GM 26 from the National Institute of General Medical Sciences, NIH, Bethesda, Md.

REFERENCES

Albert, A. and Serjeant, E. D.: *Ionization Constants of Acids and Bases. A Laboratory Manual.* New York, Wiley, 1962.

Bendetti, E. L. and Emmelot, P.: Structure and function of plasma membranes isolated from liver. In *The Membranes* (A. J. Dalton and F. Haguenau, Eds.), New York, Academic Press, 1968, pp. 33–120.

Brodie, B. B.: Physico-chemical factors in drug absorption. In *Absorption and Distribution of Drugs* (T. B. Binns, Ed.), Baltimore, Williams & Wilkins, 1964, pp. 16–48.

Butler, T. C.: Quantitative studies of the demethylation of N-methyl barbital. J. Pharmacol. Exp. Therap. *108:* 474-480, 1953.

Collander, R.: The permeability of plant

protoplasts to small molecules. Physiol. Plantarum *2:* 300–311, 1949.

Collander, R. and Bärlund, H.: Permeabilitäts-studien an *Chara ceratopylla.* Acta Botan. Fennica *11:* 1–14, 1933.

Davson, H. and Danielli, J. F.: *Permeability of Natural Membranes.* New York, Cambridge Univ. Press, 1952.

Fawcett, D. W.: *An Atlas of Fine Structure. The Cell.* Philadelphia, W. B. Saunders, 1966, p. 346.

Goldstein, D. A. and Solomon, A. K.: Determination of equivalent pore radius for human red cells by osmotic pressure measurement. J. Gen. Physiol. *4:* 11–17, 1960.

Gortner, E. and Grendel, F.: On biomolecular layers of lipoids on the chromocytes of the blood. J. Exp. Med. *41:* 439, 1925.

Kedem, O. and Katchalsky, A.: Thermodynamic analyses of the permeability of biological membranes to non-electrolytes. Biochim. Biophys. Acta *27:* 229–246, 1958.

Korn, E. D.: Current concepts of membrane structure and function. Fed. Proc. *28:* 6–11, 1969.

LeFevre, P. G.: Sugar transport in the red blood cell. Pharmacol. Rev. *13:* 39–70, 1961.

Milne, M. D., Scribner, B. H., and Crawford, M. A.: Non-ionic diffusion and the excretion of weak acids and bases. Amer. J. Med. *24:* 709–729, 1958.

Overton, E.: Über die osmotischen Eigenschaften der lebenden Pflanzen- und Tierzelle. Vierteljahrschr. Naturforsch. Ges. Zürich *40:* 159, 1895.

Overton, E.: Beitrage zur allgemeinen Muskel- und Nervenphysiologie. Arch. ges. Physiol. *92:* 115, 1902.

Pappenheimer, J. R.: Über die Permeabilität der Glomerulummembranen in der Niere. Klin. Wochschr. *33:* 362–5, 1955.

Pappenheimer, J. R., Rankin, E. M., and Borrero, L. M.: Filtration, diffusion, and molecular sieving through peripheral capillary membranes. Amer. J. Physiol. *167:* 13–46, 1951.

Parke, T. V. and Davis, W. W.: Use of apparent dissociation constants in qualitative organic analysis. Anal. Chem. *26:* 642–645, 1954.

Robertson, J. D.: The molecular structure and contact relationship of cell membranes. Prog. Biophys. Chem. *10:* 343–408, 1960.

Rouser, G., Nelson, G. J., Fleischer, S., and Simon, G.: Lipid composition of animal cell membranes, organelles, and organs. In *Biological Membranes* (D. Chapman, Ed.), New York, Academic Press, 1968, pp. 5–69.

Ruhland, W. and Hoffmann, C.: Die Permeabilität von *Beggiatoa mirabilis.* Ein Beitrag zur Ultrafiltertheorie des Plasmas. Planta *1:* 1–13, 1925.

Schanker, L. S.: Passage of drugs across body membranes. Pharmacol. Rev. *14:* 501–530, 1962.

Sjöstrand, F. S.: Ultrastructure and functions of cellular membranes. In *The Membranes* (A. S. Dalton and F. Haguenau, Eds.), New York, Academic Press, 1968, pp. 151–210.

Stein, W. D.: Diffusion and osmosis. In *Comprehensive Biochemistry* (M. Florkin and E. H. Stotz, Eds.), New York, Elsevier, 1962, v. 2, pp. 283–310.

Stein, W. D.: *The Movement of Molecules Across Cell Membranes.* New York, Academic Press, 1967.

Welch, K. and Friedman, V.: The cerebrospinal fluid valves. Brain *83:* 454–469, 1960.

Wilbrandt, W. and Rosenberg, T.: The concept of carrier transport and its corollaries in pharmacology. Pharmacol. Rev. *13:* 109–183, 1961.

2

Drug Absorption

LEWIS S. SCHANKER

I. INTRODUCTION

Drug absorption is usually defined as the passage of a drug from its site of administration into the circulation. Accordingly, we are concerned with absorption whenever a medicinal is given orally, by inhalation, or by any route outside the vascular system. Drugs may be administered orally in a variety of dosage forms, which include capsules, tablets, solutions, emulsions and suspensions; they are administered sublingually as tablets; rectally as suppositories or solutions; topically as ointments, liniments, lotions, creams or solutions; by inhalation as gases, vapors, aerosols or dusts; and by injection as solutions or suspensions. The rate of absorption from these sites will be determined by the physicochemical properties of the drug, the dosage form of the drug, and by a number of physiological and anatomical factors.

Ordinarily when a drug is administered for systemic action, a rapid rate of absorption is desired. On the other hand, a slow rate of absorption may be advantageous when there is a need for prolonged pharmacologic action from a single dose of drug. In addition, a slow rate of absorption is a definite requirement for medicinals applied to skin or mucous membranes for local action.

II. ABSORPTION FROM THE ALIMENTARY CANAL

A. Methods of Study

For many years, absorption from the gastrointestinal tract was assessed simply on the basis of whether a drug was effective or not when administered by the oral route. Later, this method was improved by comparing the pharmacologic response seen after oral administration with that obtained after intravenous injection. With the advent of specific chemical methods for estimating drugs in biological material, the study of drug absorption was put on a quantitative basis. Rates of absorption could be measured accurately, and the mechanism of absorption could be investigated by obtaining detailed kinetic data. Moreover, it became possible to determine whether poor absorption was due to an inability of drug molecules to penetrate gastrointestinal membranes or to destruction of the drug by gastric acid or intestinal enzymes.

In keeping with the definition of drug absorption, the most direct way of demonstrating that absorption has occurred would be to detect the drug in blood or urine after administration into the alimentary tract. Unfortunately, except under special circumstances, such a method is not quantitative. It gives no idea of the rate or completeness of absorption. Moreover, the relative rates of absorption of two or more drugs cannot be assessed because of differences in metabolism, distribution and excretion of drugs. Sometimes it is possible to make the method quantitative by obtaining a detailed kinetic comparison of blood or urinary levels of drug after both oral and intravenous administration (Nelson, 1961; Wagner, 1961; Wagner and Nelson, 1963). However, if a drug is rapidly metabolized by the liver, its blood levels will differ after oral and intravenous administration, because drug absorbed from the intestine goes directly to the liver before becoming distributed in the body. The main applications of the method are in studies on the human and in studies in which it is important to know the blood levels of drug achieved with various doses and dosage forms.

Another direct method of assessing absorption involves measurement of the amount of drug in the entire body and collected excreta after removal of the gastrointestinal tract. This method is limited to small animals—those that will fit into a homogenizer. In addition, the method would be quantitative only in the rare instance of a drug that is not metabolized. On the other hand, by using a radioactive labelled drug and measuring the isotope in expired air as well as in the body and excreta, it is possible to overcome the problem with drugs that are metabolized (Schanker and Tocco, 1960).

The most useful quantitative methods of measuring absorption are indirect in that they involve estimation of the amount of drug that has disappeared from the gastrointestinal canal. Of course before disappearance can be equated with absorption, it must be proven that the drug is not destroyed within the lumen of the canal. Numerous variations on this method have been applied in studies of the absorption of drugs, sugars, amino acids, lipids, and inorganic ions (Höber, 1945; Schanker, 1962; Wilson, 1962; Wiseman, 1964). In the most physiologic type of experiment, a drug is administered orally to unanesthetized animals, the animals are killed after various times, and the entire gastrointestinal tract and its contents are removed and assayed for remaining drug. If only the luminal contents and washings are assayed, it must be proven that drug did not disappear through binding or adsorption to gastrointestinal tissue. Although this type of experiment is highly physiological, it has the drawback of high variability. Because of variations in the rate of gastric emptying, a drug will remain in the stomach for unknown lengths of time. Different degrees of intestinal motility will result in various rates of drug movement along the intestinal canal as well as different degrees of drug mixing and exposure to the absorbing surface. In addition, unless the animals have been fasted, the amount and type of food and its state of digestion will influence the absorption of a drug, since many drugs become bound to food components and the sheer bulk of the food will interfere with drug mixing.

To eliminate many of the above-described variables, most investigators have turned to less physiologic experimental conditions. To study gastric absorption, drugs are introduced into the stomach, which is ligated at the pyloric and cardiac ends. Or drugs are placed in a surgically prepared portion of the stomach, such as a Heidenhain or Pavlov gastric pouch. In the small intestine, drugs may be placed in a segment of intestine isolated by ligatures; or in surgically prepared intestinal loops, such as the Thiry and Vella loops, which open to the exterior of the animal to facilitate repeated introduction and withdrawal of drug solutions.

To further reduce variability, drug solutions may be passed at a constant rate through intestinal segments or loops. With these perfusion methods, it is possible to reduce the variability of motility and to maintain a constant hydrostatic pressure and constant fluid volume within the lumen of the segment. The perfusion techniques provide the highest degree of reproducibility of all the absorption methods.

A radically different approach to the study of absorption involves measurement of the passage of a substance across the entire wall of the intestine *in vitro*; that is, movement from the mucosal side to the serosal side (Wilson, 1962). By definition, such movement does not constitute absorption, since there is no blood supply in the tissue. In one type of experiment, a segment of intestine is perfused with oxygenated saline-buffer solution containing the substance to be studied; and the outer surface of the segment is bathed in a similar solution that does not contain the substance. The rate of passage of the substance from one solution to the other is readily measurable. By far the most popular of the *in vitro* preparations is the everted sac of rat or hamster small intestine, in which a short segment of everted gut is filled with solution, ligated at both ends, and suspended in a beaker containing a similar solution (Wilson and Wiseman, 1954). With the mucosa on the outside, oxygenation of this sensitive tissue is improved. Moreover, movement of a substance from mucosa to serosa brings the substance into the interior of the sac in which it is readily detected because of the small fluid volume and the accordingly small degree of dilution.

An important drawback to the use of *in vitro* preparations of the intestine is the leakiness of the tissue. A polysaccharide such as inulin (molecular weight (m.w.) 5,000), which is hardly absorbed at all from the intestine *in vivo*, diffuses across the wall of the everted intestinal sac at a slow but significant rate. Moreover a number of organic ions cross the wall of the everted sac quite readily, whereas their rates of absorption *in vivo* are very slow. Because of this unusual degree of permeability, rates of drug "absorption" determined from studies with the intestine *in vitro* bear no meaningful relation to rates of absorption as measured *in vivo*.

The main value of the *in vitro* preparations of intestine is their usefulness in studying the mechanism of active transport of substances such as monosaccharides, amino acids and pyrimidines. Even though diffusion of the substances is exaggerated by the leakiness of the tissue, it is possible to demonstrate uphill transport—that is, transport from a mucosal solution of low concentration to a serosal solution of higher concentration. In addition, it is an easy matter to expose the *in vitro* preparation to metabolic poisons, anaerobic conditions or competitive inhibitors of transport to determine the qualitative nature of the transport process.

B. Nature of the Gastrointestinal-Blood Boundary

Two cellular boundaries separate the gastrointestinal canal from the bloodstream: the epithelial lining of the canal; and the wall of the blood capillary. Since the capillary endothelium is a highly porous structure that is readily penetrated by most drugs and other crystalloids (Pappenheimer, 1953; Schou, 1961), the gastrointestinal epithelium must constitute the main barrier to absorption.

The various ways in which drugs might cross an epithelial membrane (see

Chapter 1) include: simple diffusion through lipoid regions or through pores of the membrane; filtration through membrane pores; carrier-transport, such as active transport or facilitated diffusion (Wilbrandt anu ... berg, 1961); and vesicular transport, such as pinocytosis (Fawcett, 1965).

Early studies on the intestinal absorption of some foreign organic non-electrolytes in the rat (Höber and Höber, 1937) suggested a lipoid-pore structure for the intestinal epithelium. Mannitol, erythritol and glycerol were shown to be absorbed at rates roughly proportional to the size of the molecules. Moreover, a similar relationship was shown for three aliphatic acid amides, succinimide, lactamide and acetamide. However, it was noted that with both classes of compounds the rates of absorption could just as well be related to the relative lipid-to-water partition coefficients as to molecular size. Although it could not be proven which of the two properties governed the rate of absorption, it was felt that molecular size was the more important characteristic, since the lipid solubilities were so small. Later evidence for the presence of membrane pores was provided by the finding that small, lipid-insoluble molecules like D_2O and urea are absorbed from the rat intestine much more rapidly than are larger lipid-insoluble molecules such as mannitol and inulin (Schanker et al., 1958).

One of the first definite indications of a lipoid character for the intestinal boundary was supplied by additional studies with non-electrolytes in the rat (Höber and Höber, 1937). Valeramide, with an oil-to-water partition ratio forty times that of lactamide, was shown to be absorbed more rapidly than the latter compound despite the larger molecular weight of valeramide. Moreover, succinimide and malonamide, compounds of similar molecular size, were shown to be absorbed at widely different rates in accordance with their relative lipid-solubilities.

C. Absorption from the Stomach

Evidence that the gastric epithelium is more permeable to the non-ionized form of a drug than to the ionized form was first provided by a study of gastric absorption of some alkaloids in the cat (Travell, 1940). It was noted that large doses of strychnine and several other weak organic bases, administered into the pyloric-ligated stomach, produced no toxic effects when the gastric contents were highly acidic. When the stomach contents were made alkaline, however, the drugs were readily absorbed and the animals killed. From a careful study of strychnine absorption over a wide range of gastric pH values, it was concluded that the rate of absorption was dependent on the concentration of the non-ionized drug molecule.

The results of the above investigation support the idea of a lipid-like character for the gastric epithelium, since the non-ionized form of a weak base or weak acid is usually much more lipid soluble than the ionized form (see Chapter 1).

More definite evidence for the preferential permeability of the gastric epithelium to uncharged drug molecules was supplied by a study of the distribution of drugs between gastric juice and plasma (Shore et al., 1957). Acidic and basic drugs were administered intravenously to dogs with Heidenhain gastric pouches, and the concentration of drug in gastric juice and plasma was measured after a steady state had been achieved. A number of organic bases, partly to almost completely non-ionized in plasma, entered the gastric lumen to the extent that the gastric juice-to-plasma concentration ratios ranged from 1 to 40. In constrast, acidic compounds, which were highly ionized in plasma, gave ratios of 0 to 0.6. The results were shown to be consistent with a model system in which the gastric juice is separated from plasma by a boundary permeable only to the non-ionized form of a weak acid or base (Fig. 2.1). The steady-state distribution of a weak electrolyte across such a boundary is given by the following equations:

for an acid,
$$\frac{C_{GJ}}{C_{PL}} = \frac{1 + 10^{(pH_{GJ}-pK_a)}}{1 + 10^{(pH_{PL}-pK_a)}}$$

and for a base,
$$\frac{C_{GJ}}{C_{PL}} = \frac{1 + 10^{(pK_a-pH_{GJ})}}{1 + 10^{(pK_a-pH_{PL})}}$$

where C_{GJ} is the concentration of drug in gastric juice, C_{PL} is that in plasma (corrected for protein binding), and pK_a is the negative logarithm of the acidic dissociation constant of the weak acid or base. From these equations, it can be readily calculated that a basic drug will be concentrated in gastric juice, but an acidic drug will be concentrated in plasma.

The concentration ratios observed in this study were generally in close agreement with the calculated ratios; however a maximum ratio of 40, observed for a number of basic compounds, was considerably less than the calculated value. This apparent inconsistency was resolved when it was shown that a gastric juice-to-plasma concentration ratio of 40 represented a limiting value imposed by the rate of gastric mucosal blood flow. In other words, the amount of drug transferred from plasma into gastric juice is limited by the rate at which drug is delivered to the gastric mucosa.

The observation that the gastric epithelium is permeable to uncharged drug molecules but relatively impermeable to ions led to a detailed study of the absorption of drugs from the rat stomach (Schanker et al., 1957). A variety of compounds, dissolved in 0.1 N hydrochloric acid solution, were introduced into the

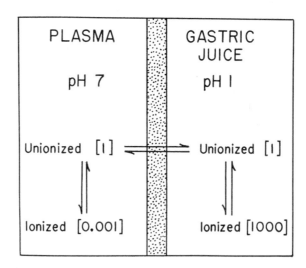

Fig. 2.1. Distribution of a weak base, pK_a 4, between plasma and gastric juice, assuming that the fluids are separated by a barrier that is permeable only to the non-ionized (unionized) form of the weak base.

stomach, which was ligated at both the pyloric and cardiac ends. The degree of absorption was estimated from the amount of drug remaining in the stomach after one hour. Since weak acids are non-ionized in the acid gastric contents, and most weak bases are highly ionized, only the acidic compounds would be expected to be absorbed. In accord with this view, ready absorption was observed for all the acidic drugs except the strong sulfonic acids, which are ionized even in solutions of low pH (Table 2.1 and Fig. 2.2). Thus salicylic acid, aspirin, benzoic acid, thiopental, secobarbital and phenol (pK_a 3–10) were readily absorbed; whereas phenolsulfonphthalein and sulfosalicylate ($pK_a < 1$) were not measurably absorbed. Furthermore, none of the basic compounds were absorbed except those so weakly basic that they are partly non-ionized in an acidic solution. Thus aniline, aminopyrine, quinine and other alkaloids, and quaternary ammonium compounds (pK_a 4.6– > 13) were very poorly absorbed, whereas acetanilide, caffeine and antipyrine (pK_a 0.3–1.4) were absorbed to a significant extent.

TABLE 2.1

Effect of drug pK_a and gastric pH on absorption of drugs from the rat stomach[a]

Drug	pK$_a$	% Absorbed in 1 Hour	
		0.1 N HCl	NaHCO₃, pH 8
Acid			
5-Sulfosalicylic	(strong)	0	0
Phenolsulfonphthalein	(strong)	2	2
5-Nitrosalicylic	2.3	52	16
Salicylic	3.0	61	13
Acetylsalicylic	3.5	35	—
Benzoic	4.2	55	—
Thiopental	7.6	46	34
p-Hydroxypropiophenone	7.8	55	—
Barbital	7.8	4	—
Secobarbital	7.9	30	—
Phenol	9.9	40	40
Base			
Acetanilide	0.3	36	—
Caffeine	0.8	24	—
Antipyrine	1.4	14	—
m-Nitroaniline	2.5	17	—
Aniline	4.6	6	56
Aminopyrine	5.0	2	—
p-Toluidine	5.3	0	47
α-Acetylmethadol	8.3	0	—
Quinine	8.4	0	18
Dextrorphan	9.2	0	16
Ephedrine	9.6	3	—
Tolazoline	10.3	7	—
Mecamylamine	11.2	0	—
Darstine	(strong)	0	—
Procaine amide ethobromide	(strong)	0	5
Tetraethylammonium	(strong)	0	—

[a] Five ml of a solution of a drug was placed in the stomach, which was ligated at both ends, and the degree of absorption measured after 1 hour (Schanker *et al.*, 1957).

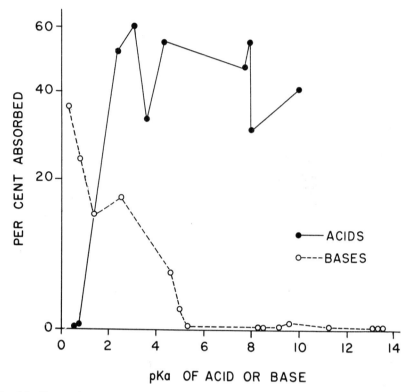

Fig. 2.2. Comparison between gastric absorption of drugs in the rat and the pK$_a$ value of drugs. Five ml of a 0.1 N HCl solution of a drug was placed in the stomach, which was ligated at both ends, and the degree of absorption measured after 1 hour (Schanker et al., 1957).

It was also shown in this study that the rate of gastric absorption of a drug could be altered by changing its degree of ionization. For example on raising the pH of the gastric contents to a value of 8 with sodium bicarbonate, basic drugs became more non-ionized and showed a more rapid absorption rate. Acidic compounds, which became more highly ionized at the alkaline pH, showed a decrease in absorption rate (Table 2.1).

The importance of lipid-solubility in determining the rate of gastric absorption was shown clearly in a study of three barbiturates of similar pK$_a$ value (Table 2.2). The compounds were absorbed from the rat stomach at rates roughly pro-

TABLE 2.2

Comparison between gastric absorption of barbiturates in the rat and lipid-to-water partition coefficient (K) of the non-ionized form of the barbiturates[a]

Barbiturate	pK$_a$	% Absorbed from 0.1 N HCl	K (chloroform)	K (heptane)
Barbital	7.8	4	0.7	<0.001
Secobarbital	7.9	30	23.3	0.10
Thiopental	7.6	46	>100.0	3.30

[a] Partition coefficients were determined after distributing the drugs between equal volumes of 0.1 N HCl and an organic solvent (Schanker et al., 1957).

portional to the organic solvent-to-water partition ratio of the non-ionized drug molecules: thiopental > secobarbital > barbital.

In a subsequent study of the gastric absorption of drugs in man, it was found that the pattern of absorption was the same as that observed in the rat (Hogben *et al.*, 1957). Acidic drugs, such as salicylate, aspirin, thiopental and secobarbital, were readily absorbed; basic compounds, such as quinine, ephedrine and aminopyrine, were not absorbed.

D. Intestinal Absorption of Weak Electrolytes

The understandable manner in which drugs cross the gastric epithelium raises the question of whether the principles that govern gastric absorption can be applied to the absorption of drugs from the small intestine. That the degree of ionization and lipid solubility of weak electrolytes do indeed determine their rates of intestinal absorption has been revealed in studies of the transfer and distribution of drugs across the rat intestine (Hogben *et al.*, 1959; Schanker *et al.*, 1958). For example, when solutions of various drugs were passed through the small intestine, a relation between the degree of ionization and rate of absorption of the compounds was revealed (Table 2.3 and Fig. 2.3): many weak acids and bases, including salicylates, barbiturates, phenols, xanthines, antipyrine, aminopyrine, various plant alkaloids, and a number of aniline derivatives, were readily absorbed; stronger, more highly ionized acids and bases such as *o*-nitrobenzoic acid, tolazoline, and mecamylamine were less readily absorbed; and completely ionized compounds like phenol red, sulfosalicylic acid, tetraethylammonium, edrophonium, and mepiperphenidol were very slowly absorbed.

Another indication that weak electrolytes cross the intestinal boundary mainly in their non-ionized form was provided by the change in the rate of absorption that resulted from a change in pH of the intestinal contents. For instance, raising the intestinal pH increased the absorption of bases such as quinine and aminopyrine, and decreased the absorption of acids such as benzoate and salicylate (Table 2.4).

On investigating the steady-state distribution of drugs between the intestinal contents and plasma, these investigators noted that the observed intestine-to-plasma concentration ratios (corrected for plasma binding) agreed only roughly with the ratios calculated from the equations described earlier in this chapter. For example, when the measured pH value of the gut solution (6.6) and that of plasma (7.4) were substituted in the equations, the resulting ratios for acidic drugs were greater than the observed values, and those of basic drugs lower than the observed values. This suggested that the pH of the intestinal contents might not be the same as the effective pH at the site of absorption. From the observed concentration ratios and the above-mentioned equations, it was possible to calculate a hypothetical or "virtual" intestinal pH; a value of 5.3 was obtained. An effective pH of 5.3, possibly located at the surface of the intestinal epithelial boundary, would explain the observations that the lowest pK_a of an acidic drug consistent with very rapid absorption was about 3, while the corresponding highest pK_a for a basic drug was about 8 (see Fig. 2.3). Assuming an effective pH of 5.3, the ratio of non-ionized to ionized drug necessary for very rapid absorption is 1:300 for both an acid of pK_a 2.8 and a base of pK_a 7.8. On the other hand, if the intestinal pH is accepted as 6.6, the necessary proportion of

TABLE 2.3

Relation between drug pK_a and absorption of drugs from the rat small intestine[a]

Drug	pK$_a$	% Absorbed
Acid		
5-Sulfosalicylic	(strong)	<2
Phenol red	(strong)	<2
Bromphenol blue	(strong)	<2
o-Nitrobenzoic	2.2	5
5-Nitrosalicylic	2.3	9
Tromexan	2.9	35
Salicylic	3.0	60
m-Nitrobenzoic	3.4	53
Acetylsalicyclic	3.5	20
Benzoic	4.2	51
Phenylbutazone	4.4	65
Acetic	4.7	42
Thiopental	7.6	55
Barbital	7.8	30
p-Hydroxypropiophenone	7.8	61
Phenol	9.9	51
Base		
Acetanilide	0.3	42
Theophylline	0.7	29
p-Nitroaniline	1.0	68
Antipyrine	1.4	32
m-Nitroaniline	2.5	77
Aniline	4.6	54
Aminopyrine	5.0	33
p-Toluidine	5.3	59
Quinine	8.4	15
Ephedrine	9.6	7
Tolazoline	10.3	6
Mecamylamine	11.2	<2
Darstine	(strong)	<2
Procaine amide ethobromide	(strong)	<2
Tetraethylammonium	(strong)	<2
Tensilon	(strong)	<2

[a] The entire small intestine of the anesthetized rat was perfused with a drug solution (1.5 ml/min) and the extent of absorption estimated from the difference in the concentration entering and leaving the intestine (Schanker *et al.*, 1958).

non-ionized to ionized drug is 1:6000 for acids and 1:16 for bases—an unlikely circumstance if the lipoid membrane concept is valid.

That many drugs cross the intestinal boundary by a process of simple diffusion is evident from the direct proportionality between the concentration of drug in the intestine and the amount of drug absorbed over a wide range of concentrations (Schanker *et al.*, 1958; Schedl and Clifton, 1960). An additional indication of a simple, nonsaturable process is seen in the failure of one drug to compete with another for transfer. For example, when solutions of various combinations of drugs were passed through the rat intestine, each compound was absorbed at its usual rate as though it were present alone (Schanker *et al.*, 1958).

Evidence that lipid solubility is the physical property that dictates the speed of passage of non-ionized molecules across the intestinal epithelium was furnished

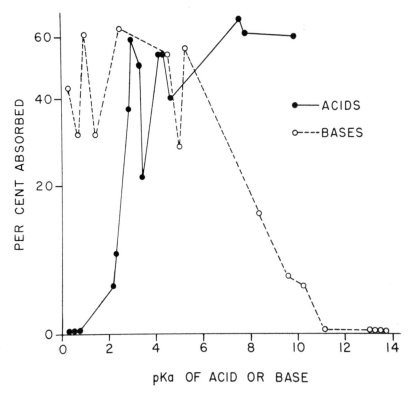

Fig. 2.3. Comparison between intestinal absorption of drugs in the rat and the pK_a value of drugs. The entire small intestine of the anesthetized rat was perfused with a drug solution (1.5 ml/min) and the extent of absorption estimated from the difference in the concentration entering and leaving the intestine (Schanker et al., 1958).

when Hogben et al. (1959) demonstrated a rough parallelism between the rates of absorption of various weak electrolytes and the lipid-to-water partition ratios of their non-ionized form (Table 2.5). Moreover, in a study of the intestinal absorption of steroid compounds in the rat, Schedl and Clifton (1961) showed that the absorption rates paralleled roughly the lipid solubilities of the compounds.

Recent reports indicate that it is possible to enhance markedly the intestinal absorption of certain therapeutic agents by increasing their lipid solubility by making minor structural changes in the molecule. For example, acetylation of the hydroxyl groups of psicofuranine, a lipid-insoluble compound that is very poorly absorbed in man, resulted in a lipid-soluble tetraacetate derivative that was well absorbed (Hoeksema et al., 1961). Moreover, acetylation of the hydroxyl groups of 6-azauridine resulted in a compound (2′,3′,5′-triacetyl-6-azauridine) which was much more readily absorbed than the parent compound (Handschumacher et al., 1962).

E. Intestinal Absorption of Organic Ions

While the intestinal absorption of most weak organic acids and bases is explainable in terms of diffusion of non-ionized molecules across a lipid-like boundary, the question remains how organic ions are absorbed. It is clear that organic

TABLE 2.4

Effect of intestinal pH and drug pK_a on absorption of drugs from the rat small intestine[a]

Drug	pK_a	% Absorbed			
		pH of Intestinal Solution			
		3.6–4.3	4.7–5.0	7.2–7.1	8.0–7.8
Base					
Aniline	4.6	40	48	58	61
Aminopyrine	5.0	21	35	48	52
p-Toluidine	5.3	30	42	65	64
Quinine	8.4	9	11	41	54
Acid					
5-Nitrosalicylic	2.3	40	27	<2	<2
Salicylic	3.0	64	35	30	1C
Acetylsalicylic	3.5	41	27	—	—
Benzoic	4.2	62	36	35	5
p-Hydroxypropiophenone	7.8	61	52	67	60

[a] Data from Hogben *et al.*, 1959.

anions and cations cross the intestinal epithelium much more slowly than do lipid-soluble, uncharged molecules. Nevertheless, it is well known that ions such as the quaternary ammonium compounds are absorbed to a significant extent when administered therapeutically. For example, it has been estimated that 5 to 10% of an oral dose of tetraethylammonium or hexamethonium is absorbed in man.

In a study of the absorption of a quaternary amine, benzomethamine, from the rat intestine, Levine and Pelikan (1961) demonstrated a rough proportionality between the amount of drug administered and the amount absorbed over a wide range of doses. This relation suggested that absorption occurs by simple diffusion. However, deviations from proportionality over a portion of the dosage range led the authors to suggest that a second process might have a role in the absorption of this drug. On the assumption that benzomethamine is absorbed in part as a complex with some endogenous substance, Levine and Spencer (1961) investigated the effect of a crude "phosphatidopeptide" extract of intestinal tissue on the absorption of the compound in the rat. They showed that the tissue extract increased the extent of absorption of benzomethamine, and that the degree of enhancement was roughly related to the amount of extract administered. Evidence was obtained *in vitro* that the phosphatidopeptide material can form a complex with the quaternary amine.

Tetracycline, which exists largely as a zwitterion at neutral pH, is another example of a highly ionized, poorly lipid-soluble drug that is incompletely absorbed from the gastrointestinal tract when administered therapeutically. In a study of the absorption of tetracycline from loops of the dog small intestine, Pindell *et al.*, (1959) showed that only about 3% of an administered dose of the drug was absorbed in 1.5 hours. Since the rate of absorption remained constant throughout this period, and the amount of drug absorbed was directly proportional to the concentration over a ten-fold range, it was concluded that absorption occurs by passive diffusion.

TABLE 2.5

Comparison between intestinal absorption of weak organic acids and bases in the rat and lipid-to-water partition coefficient (K) of the non-ionized form of the compounds[a]

Drug	% Absorbed	K(heptane)	K(chloroform)
Rapid rate of absorption			
Phenylbutazone	54	>100	>100
Thiopental	67	3.30	>100
p-Toluidine	56	3.26	97.5
Aniline	54	1.10	26.4
m-Nitroaniline	63	0.24	39.2
Benzoic acid	54	0.19	2.9
Phenol	60	0.15	2.3
p-Nitroaniline	61	0.13	19.8
p-Hydroxypropiophenone	61	0.12	5.1
Salicylic acid	60	0.12	2.9
m-Nitrobenzoic acid	50	0.06	2.6
Moderate rate of absorption			
Aminopyrine	27	0.21	>100
Acetylsalicylic acid	21	0.03	2.0
Acetanilide	43	0.02	7.6
Theophylline	30	0.02	0.3
Antipyrine	30	0.005	21.2
Barbital	25	<0.002	0.7
Theobromine	22	<0.002	0.4
Sulfanilamide	24	<0.002	0.03
p-Hydroxybenzoic acid	23	<0.002	0.01
Slow rate of absorption			
Barbituric acid	5	<0.002	0.008
Sulfaguanidine	<2	<0.002	<0.002
Mannitol	<2	<0.002	<0.002

[a] Partition coefficients were determined after distributing the drugs between an organic solvent and an aqueous phase, the pH of which was such that the drug was largely in the non-ionized form (Hogben *et al.*, 1959).

F. Intestinal Absorption of Macromolecules

Very little is known about the processes by which trace amounts of proteins and other macromolecules are absorbed from the intestine. Familiar examples of the absorption of protein molecules include the allergic response to ingested proteins of food, and the toxicity of ingested bacterial exotoxins. It has been shown that the diphtheria, tetanus and botulinus toxins are absorbed to a slight extent from the alimentary canal of mice; the oral LD_{50} values of the toxins are hundreds of thousands of times greater than the intraperitoneal LD_{50} values (Lamanna, 1960). The absorption of these substances may possibly be accounted for by pinocytosis, diffusion through imperfections in the epithelium, or phagocytosis by macrophages with subsequent migration of these cells between the intestinal epithelial cells.

G. Active Transport Across the Intestinal Epithelium

While most drugs and other foreign organic compounds appear to cross the intestinal boundary by a process of simple diffusion, there is evidence that a drug can be absorbed by a specialized active transport process if its chemical structure is similar enough to that of the substrate naturally transported. For example the anti-tumor agents 5-fluorouracil and 5-bromouracil are actively transported across the rat intestinal epithelium by the process which transports the natural pyrimidines uracil and thymine (Schanker and Jeffrey, 1961, 1962). This process differs from simple diffusion in a number of ways: transport of the solute occurs against a concentration gradient; the transport mechanism becomes saturated when the concentration of the pyrimidine is raised high enough; the process shows specificity for a certain molecular structure; and one pyrimidine may depress the absorption of another by competing with it for the transport mechanism.

As seen in Figure 2.4, thymine is rapidly absorbed when its concentration in the intestine is low; but on raising the concentration, the proportion absorbed declines markedly as a result of saturation of the transport mechanism. At the higher concentrations of the pyrimidine, the percentage absorption is constant, indicating that passive diffusion has become the predominant mode of absorption. With uracil, there is a similar relation between concentration and rate of absorption. As would be expected, the rates of passive absorption of thymine and uracil correlate with the relative lipid solubilities of the two pyrimidines, thymine having the higher absorption rate and the greater lipid-to-water partition coefficient (Schanker and Tocco, 1960).

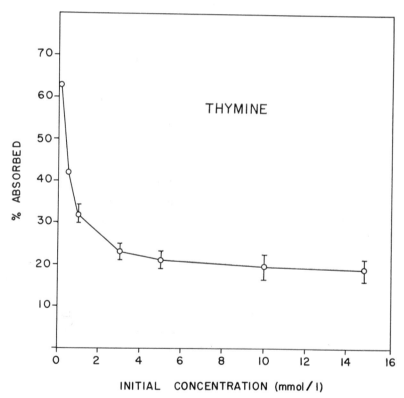

Fig. 2.4. Absorption of thymine from solutions of various concentrations. Fifty ml of a solution of thymine was continuously circulated through the entire small intestine of the anesthetized rat and the extent of absorption measured after 1 hour (Schanker and Tocco, 1960).

A number of pyrimidines of closely related chemical structure compete for the active transport process. For example, the absorption of uracil is inhibited by thymine, 5-bromouracil, 5-fluorouracil, 5-aminouracil, dithiothymine, and dithiouracil (Schanker and Jeffrey, 1962; Schanker and Tocco, 1962).

The most definitive characteristic of an active transport process, the ability to transfer a substance from a solution of low concentration to one of higher concentration, is readily demonstrated for the pyrimidine transport process. Thus uracil, thymine, fluorouracil, and bromouracil are transported from the mucosal to the serosal side of the intestinal wall *in vitro* against substantial concentration gradients (Table 2.6).

An additional example of active intestinal transport of foreign compounds is the active absorption of several foreign sugars that are structurally similar to glucose. These compounds utilize the monosaccharide transport process of the small intestine (Wilson and Landau, 1960).

H. Effect of EDTA on Drug Absorption from the Intestine

Although one substance may affect the intestinal absorption of another when the mechanism of absorption is active transport, the same is not ordinarily true when absorption occurs by passive diffusion. It has been shown that many drugs, administered in true solution to eliminate the variables of dosage form, rate of dissolution, and particle size, are absorbed from the intestine at rates which are not influenced by the presence of other drugs (O'Reilly and Nelson, 1961; Schanker et al., 1957, 1958). An exception to this generalization is seen in the increased absorption of drugs that occurs in the presence of the chelating agent ethylenediaminetetraacetic acid (EDTA). When given orally in sufficient amounts (100–500 mg/kg in rats), the chelator increases markedly the rates of absorption of heparin, sulfopolyglucin (Windsor and Cronheim, 1961), mannitol, inulin, decamethonium, sulfanilic acid, and EDTA-2-C[14] (Schanker and Johnson, 1961), and phenol red (Cassidy and Tidball, 1967), all lipid-insoluble substances which ordinarily are poorly absorbed from the gastrointestinal tract. The wide variety of the chemical structures of these compounds suggests that the chelating agent is acting in a nonspecific way and is not affecting the physical or chemical state of the compounds within the intestine. Direct evidence that EDTA acts by increasing the permeability of the intestinal epithelium was provided by the marked increase in the rate at which intravenously-administered inulin passes from the bloodstream into the intestinal lumen when the lumen contains the

TABLE 2.6

Active transport of pyrimidines across the wall of the everted rat small intestine in vitro[a]

Pyrimidine	Serosal-to-Mucosal Concentration Ratio	
	Initial	After Incubation at 37°C for 1 Hour
Uracil	1	4.7
Thymine	1	3.1
5-Fluorouracil	1	4.5
5-Bromouracil	1	3.0

[a] Data from Schanker (1963).

chelator (Schanker and Johnson, 1961). Perhaps EDTA alters permeability by increasing the size of the membrane pores or by widening the spaces between the epithelial cells through the removal of calcium ions (Cassidy and Tidball, 1967). In any case, until more is known, it might be wise to consider the action of this agent as potentially dangerous to the organism, since it might promote the absorption of ingested allergens and also that of toxic substances normally produced within the intestinal contents.

Perhaps any chemical agent that can alter the cellular structure of the intestine is capable of producing changes in the rate of drug absorption. Thus, caustic substances, irritants, protoplasmic poisons and surfactants may have this potential. Moreover, diseases of the intestine may well have an influence on the rates at which drugs are absorbed.

I. Absorption from the Colon

A study of the absorption of drugs from the rat colon (Schanker, 1959) has revealed an absorption pattern very similar to that of the small intestine. Weak acids and bases are in general readily absorbed; stronger, more highly ionized acids and bases are less readily absorbed; and completely ionized compounds are very slowly absorbed. Furthermore, the amount of drug absorbed is directly proportional to its concentration within the colon, and absorption is favored by changes in the colonic pH which increase the proportion of drug in the non-ionized form.

The rough proportionality between the rate of absorption of a number of barbiturates and the lipid-to-water partition coefficient of their non-ionized forms (Fig. 2.5) emphasizes the importance of lipid solubility in determining the rate of passage of drug molecules across the colonic epithelium.

J. Absorption from the Rectum

What has been said about the mechanism of drug absorption in the small intestine and colon appears to apply equally well to the passage of medicinals across the rectal mucosa. It has been shown in the rat that aminopyrine, aniline and a number of sulfonamides are absorbed by simple diffusion at rates related to the degree of ionization and lipid-to-water partition coefficient of the compounds (Kakemi et al., 1965).

K. Absorption from the Oral Cavity

The epithelial lining of the mouth, like that of the rest of the alimentary canal, behaves as a lipid-like barrier to the passage of drugs. It has been shown in dogs that cocaine, atropine, strychnine and a number of opium alkaloids are absorbed from the oral cavity at rates roughly parallel to the oil-to-water partition ratios of the compounds (Walton, 1935, 1944). Moreover Beckett and Triggs (1967) have reported that a large number of basic compounds are absorbed from the mouth of humans by a process of simple diffusion of the non-ionized form of the compounds. Small amounts of enzymes, insulin and other large molecules may be absorbed when administered sublingually (Gibaldi and Kanig, 1965).

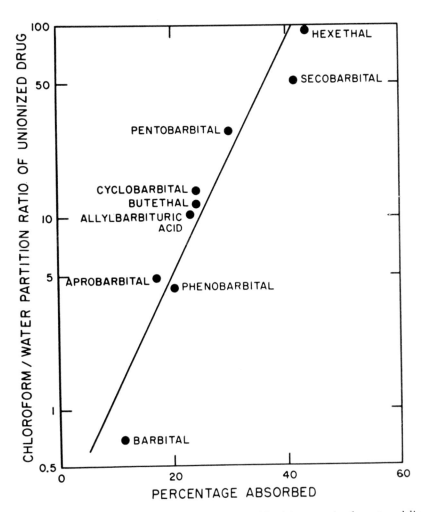

Fig. 2.5. Comparison between colonic absorption of barbiturates in the rat and lipid-to-water partition coefficient of the non-ionized form of the barbiturates. The entire colon of the anesthetized rat was perfused with a drug solution (0.2 ml/min) and the extent of absorption estimated from the difference in the concentration entering and leaving the colon (Schanker, 1959).

L. Physiological Factors and Dosage Forms of Drugs as Related to Absorption from the Alimentary Canal

Although the oral route of administration is the most convenient, safest and most economical of the various routes, it has certain disadvantages: (1) destruction of some drugs by gastric acid or digestive enzymes; (2) precipitation or insolubility of some drugs in gastrointestinal fluids; (3) formation of non-absorbable complexes between drugs and food materials; (4) variable rates of absorption resulting from physiological factors such as gastric emptying time, gastrointestinal motility and mixing; (5) too slow an absorption rate for effectiveness in an emergency situation; and (6) irritation to the gastric mucosa with resultant nausea or vomiting.

Some of these disadvantages can be overcome by modifying the dosage form of a drug. For example, gastric irritation as well as the destruction, precipitation or complexing of drugs in the stomach, can be avoided by the use of an enteric coated tablet or capsule; the coating, composed of shellac or other materials, resists gastric acid but dissolves in the higher pH range of the intestine or in the presence of intestinal enzymes. In some instances, gastric irritation can be minimized simply by administering a drug immediately after a meal. The food will dilute the drug, protect the gastric mucosa from contact with drug, and possibly bind some of the drug reversibly; of course the rate of absorption will be slowed. Conversely, for rapid absorption, a drug should be taken with the stomach empty; and a glass of water should accompany the dose to dissolve the drug and wash it into the intestine. Even though some drugs are absorbed directly from the stomach, they are absorbed more rapidly from the intestine because of the much greater area of epithelial surface.

The time that a drug remains in the stomach after oral administration can vary widely. Gastric emptying time depends on many factors including the pH, volume, consistency, chemical composition and osmolar concentration of the food present. Water, taken on an empty stomach, begins to leave the stomach almost immediately. Solid foods, on the other hand, do not normally leave until they are reduced to a fluid-like consistency. A carbohydrate meal enters the ntestine more rapidly than a meal high in protein or fat; and a fatty meal remains in the stomach for a relatively long time.

The prolonged-action dosage forms of drugs for oral administration have been developed with the aim of supplying in one dose all the drug that will be needed over a period of many hours. These dosage forms have been prepared in many ways. For instance, a tablet might consist of several layers of drug with each layer dissolving at a different rate; or a capsule might contain numerous small pellets of drug with varying thicknesses of coating which delay their rate of dissolving. Prolonged action may also be obtained with liquid preparations such as emulsions or suspensions of slowly dissolving forms of the drug (Lazarus and Cooper, 1959). A major obstacle to the use of these dosage forms is the high variability of physiological factors in patients. If the dosage form is propelled too rapidly through the gastrointestinal tract, only a portion of the intended dose may be released, or the doses may be released at the wrong place and at the wrong time. If the multiple doses are released too rapidly, there is a danger of toxicity.

A point to be emphasized in considering absorption after oral administration is that a drug must be dissolved before it can be absorbed. Although a compound may penetrate the intestinal epithelium very rapidly when administered in aqueous solution, the same compound administered in solid form will be absorbed at a rate limited by the speed with which it dissolves in the intestinal contents. A number of factors influence the rate of solution, or the "dissolution rate" as it is sometimes called; these include: (1) solubility, particle size, crystalline form and salt form of the drug; (2) the rate of disintegration of the solid dosage form in the gastrointestinal lumen; and (3) gastrointestinal pH, motility and food content (Levy, 1968).

III. ABSORPTION FROM OTHER SITES

A. Absorption from the Lungs

Drugs administered as gases penetrate the respiratory tract epithelium with great rapidity. These substances have small molecular sizes and high lipid-to-water partition coefficients (see Chapter 7).

Very little quantitative information is available concerning the pulmonary absorption of organic crystalloids. Although many drugs and other chemicals appear to be absorbed readily when inhaled as sprays, aerosols or dusts, the observations are based on the appearance of pharmacologic action or appearance of drug in blood or urine; consequently rates of absorption and relative rates of absorption are unknown (Dautrebande, 1962).

An indication of a lipid-like character for the pulmonary membrane has been supplied by a quantitative study with the isolated, perfused dog lung (Taylor et al., 1965). It was shown that the lipid-soluble compound dinitrophenol crosses the pulmonary epithelium more than one hundred times faster than a lipid-insoluble substance such as glucose.

A preliminary report on quantitative studies with the rat lung in vivo (Enna and Schanker, 1969) suggests a lipoid-pore nature for the pulmonary membrane. In this work, 0.1 ml of drug solution was administered to anesthetized rats through a tracheal cannula. After various times, the lungs and trachea were removed and assayed for remaining drug. Although lipid-insoluble substances such as p-aminohippurate and sucrose were absorbed fairly readily, much more rapid rates of absorption were seen with lipid-soluble compounds such as aniline and procaine amide. A suggestion of the presence of membrane pores was provided by the observation that inulin, a large, lipid-insoluble molecule (m.w. 5,000), was absorbed at a significant rate, and the smaller sucrose molecule was absorbed even more readily.

B. Absorption from the Skin

The skin is not ordinarily used as a site of absorption for drugs, although accidental poisonings and deaths have resulted from exposure of the skin to organic solvents, organophosphate insecticides, and nicotine-containing insecticides.

Results of numerous studies have indicated that drugs penetrate the skin predominantly by passing through a lipid-like barrier. This conclusion is based on many isolated observations that lipid-soluble molecules are absorbed much more readily than lipid-insoluble molecules and ions (Calvery et al., 1946; Rothman, 1954; Malkinson, 1956; Gemmell and Morrison, 1957; Wilson, 1961), and on a study by Treherne (1956) of the passage of non-electrolytes across the excised rabbit skin. The latter investigator showed that various alcohols and urea derivatives diffuse across whole skin at rates roughly proportional to the ether-to-water partition coefficients of the compounds. It was concluded that the lipoid barrier of the skin is located within the epidermal layer, since the dermis is freely permeable to many solutes, and displays the characteristics of a highly porous membrane.

For some time, there was no general agreement among investigators as to the main pathway by which drugs traverse mammalian skin. Some authors stressed the importance of the epidermal route, while others contended that the appendageal route—through hair follicles, sweat glands and sebaceous glands—was predominant. In later work, Tregear (1961) developed a technique whereby drug penetration could be assessed using small areas of skin which contain either a desired number of hair follicles or none at all. Studying in this way the absorption of tri-*n*-butyl phosphate from the skin of living pigs, he showed that the hair follicle is no more penetrable than an equivalent area of epidermis; in fact, regions of the skin devoid of hair follicles were penetrated slightly more rapidly than regions containing these structures.

Because of the relatively great thickness of the skin, drugs penetrate this boundary much more slowly than they do most other body membranes. However the percutaneous absorption of ionized drugs can be enhanced by the method of iontophoresis, in which drug solution in contact with an electrode is placed against the skin and a galvanic current applied to both the drug electrode and another electrode placed elsewhere on the body. Absorption through the skin can also be enhanced by dissolving a drug in oil, an ointment base or other organic solvent and rubbing it into the skin. The unusual solvent dimethyl sulfoxide (DMSO), which is miscible with water as well as with many organic solvents, also enhances the percutaneous absorption of certain drugs (Stoughton and Fritsch, 1964; Weyer, 1967).

C. Absorption from Subcutaneous and Intramuscular Sites

Absorption of drugs from aqueous solutions injected subcutaneously or intramuscularly depends mainly on the ease of penetration of the capillary wall, the area over which the solution has spread, and the rate of blood flow through the area (Schou, 1961; Sund and Schou, 1964a, 1964b).

Most drugs traverse the capillary wall by a combination of two processes, diffusion and filtration (hydrodynamic flow) (Pappenheimer, 1953; Renkin, 1952). Diffusion is the predominant mode of transfer for lipid-soluble molecules as well as for small, lipid-insoluble molecules and ions. Filtration, on the other hand, predominates for large, lipid-insoluble molecules whose rates of diffusion across the capillary wall are relatively slow. Lipid-soluble compounds penetrate readily at rates related to their lipid-to-water partition coefficients, and lipid-insoluble substances penetrate less readily at rates related to their molecular sizes. While the latter substances appear to pass through aqueous pores whose total area comprises less than 0.2% of the capillary surface, lipid-soluble molecules appear to penetrate through the entire surface. The slow passage of macromolecules across the capillary wall may be explained in part by pinocytosis.

Most drugs, whether lipid-soluble or not, cross the capillary wall at rates which are extremely rapid in comparison with their rates of passage across many other body membranes. Thus, the supply of drugs to the various tissues may be limited more by the rate of blood flow than by the restraint imposed by the capillary endothelium.

After subcutaneous or intramuscular injection of an aqueous solution of drug, the rate of drug absorption can be influenced by a number of procedures (Schou, 1961; Sund and Schou, 1965). Absorption can be hastened by massage or application of heat to increase blood flow to the injected area; or by including the enzyme hyaluronidase in the injection solution. The enzyme breaks down hyaluronic acid of the connective tissue matrix thereby allowing the drug solution to spread over a wider area. Absorption can be slowed by reducing circulation to the injected area, for example by local cooling or by inclusion of a vasoconstrictor agent in the drug solution.

To obtain a slow, continuous rate of absorption from a subcutaneous site, drugs may be injected as a suspension of poorly soluble crystals, or implanted under the skin in the form of a compressed pellet. The rate of absorption is determined primarily by the solubility of the drug and the surface area of the crystals or pellet; secondarily absorption is determined by the factors mentioned above for solutions. Similarly in muscle, aqueous or oil suspensions of poorly soluble salts of drugs may be injected to obtain a prolonged pharmacologic action.

REFERENCES

Beckett, A. H. and Triggs, E. J.: Buccal absorption of basic drugs and its application as an in vivo model of passive drug transfer through lipid membranes. J. Pharm. Pharmacol. 19 (Suppl.): 31S–41S, 1967.

Calvery, H. O., Draize, J. H. and Laug, E. P.: The metabolism and permeability of normal skin. Physiol. Rev. 26: 495–540, 1946.

Cassidy, M. M. and Tidball, C. S.: Cellular mechanism of intestinal permeability alterations produced by chelation depletion. J. Cell Biol. 32: 685–698, 1967.

Dautrebande, L.: Microaerosols, New York, Academic Press, 1962.

Enna, S. J. and Schanker, L. S.: Drug absorption from the lung. Fed. Proc. 28: 359, 1969.

Fawcett, D. W.: Surface specializations of absorbing cells. J. Histochem. Cytochem. 13: 75–91, 1965.

Gemmell, D. H. O. and Morrison, J. C.: The release of medicinal substances from topical applications and their passage through the skin. J. Pharm. Pharmacol. 9: 641–656, 1957.

Gibaldi, M. and Kanig, J. L.: Absorption of drugs through the oral mucosa. J. Oral Ther. Pharmacol. 1: 440–450, 1965.

Handschumacher, R. E., Creasey, W. A., Fink, M. E., Calabresi, P. and Welch, A. D.: Pharmacological and clinical studies with triacetyl 6-azauridine. Cancer Chemother. Rep. 16: 267–269, 1962.

Höber, R.: Physical Chemistry of Cells and Tissues, Philadelphia, Blakiston Co., 1945.

Höber, R. and Höber, J.: Experiments on the absorption of organic solutes in the small intestine of rats. J. Cell. Comp. Physiol. 10: 401–422, 1937.

Hoeksema, H., Whitfield, G. B. and Rhuland, L. E.: Effect of selective acylation on the oral absorption of a nucleoside by humans. Biochem. Biophys. Res. Commun. 6: 213–216, 1961.

Hogben, C. A. M., Schanker, L. S., Tocco, D. J. and Brodie, B. B.: Absorption of drugs from the stomach. II. The human. J. Pharmacol. Exp. Ther. 120: 540–545, 1957.

Hogben, C. A. M., Tocco, D. J., Brodie, B. B. and Schanker, L. S.: On the mechanism of intestinal absorption of drugs. J. Pharmacol. Exp. Ther. 125: 275–282, 1959.

Kakemi, K., Arita, T. and Muranishi, S.: Absorption and excretion of drugs. XXV. On the mechanism of rectal absorption of sulfonamides. Chem. Pharm. Bull. (Tokyo) 13: 861–869, 1965.

Lamanna, C.: Toxicity of bacterial exotoxins by the oral route. Science (Washington) 131: 1100–1101, 1960.

Lazarus, J. and Cooper, J.: Oral prolonged action medicaments: Their pharmaceutical control and therapeutic aspects. J. Pharm. Pharmacol. 11: 257–290, 1959.

Levine, R. R. and Pelikan, E. W.: The influence of experimental procedures and dose on the intestinal absorption of an onium compound, benzomethamine. J. Pharmacol. Exp. Ther. 131: 319–327, 1961.

Levine, R. R. and Spencer, A. F.: Effect of a phosphatidopeptide fraction of intestinal tissue on the intestinal absorption of a quaternary ammonium compound. Biochem. Pharmacol. 8: 248–250, 1961.

Levy, G.: Kinetics and implications of dissolution rate limited gastrointestinal absorption of drugs. In Physico-Chemical Aspects of Drug Actions, Proceedings of the Third International Pharmacological Meeting (E. J. Ariens, ed.) Vol. 7, pp. 33–62, Oxford, Pergamon Press, 1968.

Malkinson, F. D.: Radioisotope techniques in the study of percutaneous absorption. J. Soc. Cosmet. Chem. 7: 109–122, 1956.

Nelson, E.: Kinetics of drug absorption, distribution, metabolism, and excretion. J. Pharm. Sci. 50: 181–192, 1961.

O'Reilly, I. and Nelson, E.: Urinary excretion kinetics for evaluation of drug absorption IV. Studies with tetracycline absorption enhancement factors. J. Pharm. Sci. *50:* 413–416, 1961.

Pappenheimer, J. R.: Passage of molecules through capillary walls. Physiol. Rev. *33:* 387–423, 1953.

Pindell, M. H., Cull, K. M., Doran, K. M. and Dickison, H. L.: Absorption and excretion studies on tetracycline. J. Pharmacol. Exp. Ther. *125:* 287–294, 1959.

Renkin, E. M.: Capillary permeability to lipid-soluble molecules. Amer. J. Physiol. *168:* 538–545, 1952.

Rothman, S.: *Physiology and Biochemistry of the Skin*, Chicago, University of Chicago Press, 1954.

Schanker, L. S.: Absorption of drugs from the rat colon. J. Pharmacol. Exp. Ther. *126:* 283–290, 1959.

Schanker, L. S.: Passage of drugs across body membranes. Pharmacol. Rev. *14:* 501–530, 1962.

Schanker, L. S.: Passage of drugs across the gastrointestinal epithelium, In *Proceedings of the First International Pharmacological Meeting* (C. A. M. Hogben, ed.), vol. 4, pp. 120–130, London, Pergamon Press, 1963.

Schanker, L. S. and Jeffrey, J. J.: Active transport of foreign pyrimidines across the intestinal epithelium. Nature (London) *190:* 727–728, 1961.

Schanker, L. S. and Jeffrey, J. J.: Structural specificity of the pyrimidine transport process of the small intestine. Biochem. Pharmacol. *11:* 961–966, 1962.

Schanker, L. S. and Johnson, J. M.: Increased intestinal absorption of foreign organic compounds in the presence of ethylenediaminetetraacetic acid (EDTA). Biochem. Pharmacol. *8:* 421–422, 1961.

Schanker, L. S., Shore, P. A., Brodie, B. B. and Hogben, C. A. M.: Absorption of drugs from the stomach. I. The rat. J. Pharmacol. Exp. Ther. *120:* 528–539, 1957.

Schanker, L. S. and Tocco, D. J.: Active transport of some pyrimidines across the rat intestinal epithelium. J. Pharmacol. Exp. Ther. *128:* 115–121, 1960.

Schanker, L. S. and Tocco, D. J.: Some characteristics of the pyrimidine transport process of the small intestine. Biochim. Biophys. Acta *56:* 469–473, 1962.

Schanker, L. S., Tocco, D. J., Brodie, B. B. and Hogben, C. A. M.: Absorption of drugs from the rat small intestine. J. Pharmacol. Exp. Ther. *123:* 81–88, 1958.

Schedl, H. P. and Clifton, J. A.: Small intestinal absorption of steroids, In *Advance Abstracts of Short Communications, First International Congress of Endocrinology* (F. Fuchs, ed.), p. 741, Copenhagen, Periodica Copenhagen, 1960.

Schedl, H. P. and Clifton, J. A.: Small intestinal absorption of steroids. Gastroent. *41:* 491–499, 1961.

Schou, J.: Absorption of drugs from subcutaneous connective tissue. Pharmacol. Rev. *13:* 441–464, 1961.

Shore, P. A., Brodie, B. B. and Hogben, C. A. M.: The gastric secretion of drugs: a pH partition hypothesis. J. Pharmacol. Exp. Ther. *119:* 361–369, 1957.

Stoughton, R. B. and Fritsch, W. C.: Influence of dimethylsulfoxide (DMSO) on human percutaneous absorption. Arch. Dermatol. *90:* 512–517, 1964.

Sund, R. B. and Schou, J.: The determination of absorption rates from rat muscles: an experimental approach to kinetic descriptions. Acta Pharmacol. Toxicol. *21:* 313–325, 1964a.

Sund, R. B. and Schou, J.: Absorption of atropine: anticholinergic agents as inhibitors of absorption from muscles. Acta Pharmacol. Toxicol. *21:* 339–346, 1964b.

Sund, R. B. and Schou, J.: Hyaluronidase as an accelerator of muscular absorption of water and water-soluble compounds. Acta Pharmacol. Toxicol. *23:* 194–204, 1965.

Taylor, A. E., Guyton, A. C. and Bishop, V. S.: Permeability of the alveolar membrane to solutes. Circ. Res. *16:* 353–362, 1965.

Travell, J.: The influence of the hydrogen ion concentration on the absorption of alkaloids from the stomach. J. Pharmacol. Exp. Ther. *69:* 21–33, 1940.

Tregear, R. T.: Relative penetrability of hair follicles and epidermis. J. Physiol. (London) *156:* 307–313, 1961.

Treherne, J. E.: The permeability of skin to some nonelectrolytes. J. Physiol. (London) *133:* 171–180, 1956.

Wagner, J. G.: Biopharmaceutics: absorption aspects. J. Pharm. Sci. *50:* 359–387, 1961.

Wagner, J. G. and Nelson, E.: Per cent absorbed time plots derived from blood level and/or urinary excretion data. J. Pharm. Sci. *52:* 610–611, 1963.

Walton, R. P.: Absorption of drugs through the oral mucosa. II. Proc. Soc. Exp. Biol. Med. *32:* 1486–1488, 1935.

Walton, R. P.: Sublingual administration of drugs. J.A.M.A. *124:* 138–143, 1944.

Weyer, E. M. (ed.): Biological actions of dimethyl sulfoxide. Ann. N. Y. Acad. Sci. *141:* 1–671, 1967.

Wilbrandt, W. and Rosenberg, T.: The concept of carrier transport and its corollaries in pharmacology. Pharmacol. Rev. *13:* 109–183, 1961.

Wilson, K.: New methods for the study of percutaneous absorption. Drug Cosmet. Ind. *88:* 444–529, 1961.

Wilson, T. H.: *Intestinal Absorption*, Philadelphia, W. B. Saunders Co., 1962.

Wilson, T. H. and Landau, B. R.: Specificity of sugar transport by the intestine of the hamster. Amer. J. Physiol. *198:* 99–102, 1960.

Wilson, T. H. and Wiseman, G.: The use of sacs of everted small intestine for the study of the transference of substances from the mucosal to the serosal surface. J. Physiol. (London) *123:* 116–125, 1954.

Windsor, E. and Cronheim, G. E.: Gastrointestinal absorption of heparin and synthetic heparinoids. Nature (London) *190:* 263–264, 1961.

Wiseman, G.: *Absorption from the Intestine*, London, Academic Press 1964.

3

The Distribution of Drugs

THOMAS C. BUTLER

I. INTRODUCTION

The ultimate and perhaps the most intellectually attractive goal in pharmacology is an understanding of the molecular interaction between a drug and the so-called "receptors" of a cell that brings about the alteration of cellular function finally manifest in a grossly observable pharmacological effect. Preoccupation with this goal, laudable as it is, should not cause us to lose sight of the fact that drugs also interact with normal constituents of the body other than receptors. With most drugs, only a very small proportion of the total amount in the body is at any time in direct interaction with the receptors producing the pharmacological action. Usually a very high proportion of the total drug in the body is localized in parts of the body remote from the site of action. Yet it is this bulk of the drug remote from the site of action that governs the kinetics of the movements of the drug through the tissues of the body and its ultimate disappearance from the body and thus determines the temporal course of the intensity of the pharmacological effect. These are factors that determine such practical matters as dosage schedules and even the field of useful clinical application of a drug.

This discussion will be largely concerned with distribution patterns that result from forces of passive diffusion and reversible interactions with the normal constituents of the body. It will not deal with the rather unusual instances of drugs that are almost completely localized at specific receptor sites. No more than this passing mention will be devoted to processes of active transport and secretion and phagocytosis as they may affect drug distribution. Such processes, when they result in the concentration of a preponderant amount of a substance in a specific organ, may be exploited in diagnostic procedures. There may be cited the uptake of iodide by the thyroid, drugs excreted in urine and bile used in radiological examination of the urinary and biliary systems, and the radioactive colloidal materials phagocytized by the reticuloendothelial cells used for scanning of the liver.

The viewpoint of this review is to be that of human therapeutics. It will deal with mammalian pharmacology; and unless otherwise stated, all considerations are applicable to man.

Interest in the concentrations of drugs in blood and tissues dates to the middle of the last century. In the year after the introduction of ether as an anesthetic, Lassaigne (1847) measured the tension of ether in the blood of a dog anesthetized

44

with that agent, and from this calculated the concentration of ether in the blood. In the following year Snow (1848) calculated the concentrations of ether and chloroform in the blood during anesthesia. He clearly realized that quantitative knowledge of the concentrations of these drugs in blood was needed as a basis for their proper use in medical practice.

The role of Rudolf Buchheim in the recognition of the potential value of quantitative chemistry in understanding of pharmacological action is worthy of examination, since it was from his efforts in initiating a new science of pharmacology that much of the development of that discipline in its modern form can be directly traced. Between the years of 1847 and 1867, when he was at the University of Dorpat (now Tartu), Buchheim directed the research of numerous candidates for the degree of Doctor of Medicine. He recognized that a theoretical understanding of the mechanism of action of a drug often can be arrived at only through quantitative knowledge of the concentrations in the various parts of the body. Much of the work of Buchheim's students appeared only in the doctoral dissertations, many of them in Latin. The subjects of these dissertations, which have been listed and abstracted by Schmiedeberg (1911), give an insight into Buchheim's efforts to apply the chemistry of his day to pharmacological problems. Several of the dissertations, one as early as 1852, concerned alcohol and made use of quantitative analytical methods. Oswald Schmiedeberg, who was to become the most illustrious and influential of Buchheim's students, wrote his dissertation in 1866 on the subject of the quantitative determination of chloroform in blood. Of the dissertation problems on alcohol and chloroform, that of Schulinus (1866) on the distribution of alcohol in the body and that of Schmiedeberg (1867) on chloroform were published in the Archiv der Heilkunde.

In the past the lack of adequate analytical methods was an insuperable obstacle to knowledge of the distribution of most drugs. As recently as 40 years ago there was little knowledge of the concentrations in blood or tissues of drugs other than some of the inhalation anesthetics and alcohol. These are drugs that can occur in the body in such high concentrations that analytical methods of relatively low sensitivity and specificity suffice for their determination. The revolutionary developments in instrumentation and analytical methodology that have taken place in the past three decades have progressively increased the potentialities for analytical determination of drugs in the concentrations in which they occur in the body. Knowledge of the distribution of drugs in the body has consequently been increasing rapidly in recent years. It is the feeling of some workers in this field that with the instruments and techniques available today it should be possible to develop an analytical method for almost any drug in the concentrations occurring in the body.

There has long been a particular interest in the concentrations of drugs in blood. Blood is the only tissue that can be repeatedly sampled without undue trauma or physiological disturbance. In human studies it is usually the only tissue that can be sampled. Furthermore, since blood circulates through all tissues, some approximation of equilibrium can be expected between the concentration of a drug in blood plasma and its concentrations in tissues. It can often be justifiably assumed that the concentration of a drug in plasma is proportional to its concentration at the site of action, even though this site may be unknown, and that the plasma concentration furnishes a better index of therapeutic action than does dosage. This assumption can be misleading if the concentration in plasma is very low relative to that in tissues. For instance, the antimalarial activity of quinacrine in ducks was found to be better correlated with dosage than with plasma concentration (Marshall and Dearborn, 1946).

Because of the particular interest in concentrations of drugs in plasma, much of the succeeding discussion will be concerned with the information about drug distribution that can be derived from analysis of plasma alone.

II. THE APPARENT VOLUME OF DISTRIBUTION

The apparent volume of distribution is a concept that has been found useful in the study of drugs. Through the use of this calculated quantity, analytical measurements that may perforce be limited to those that can be carried out on plasma can permit at least some tentative inferences as to the distribution of a drug in the body and can aid an understanding of the kinetics of the disposition of the drug in the body.

A. Definition

The apparent volume of distribution of a drug is the volume in which the total amount of drug in the body would be uniformly distributed to give the observed plasma concentration.

$$V_d = Q/c$$

where V_d = apparent volume of distribution
Q = total amount of drug in body
c = concentration of drug in plasma

If Q were expressed in mg and c in mg/l, V_d would be expressed in liters. A common if loose usage is to equate the corresponding metric units of mass and volume. Thus, for instance, Q might be expressed in mg/kg and c in mg/l. V_d would then be a dimensionless ratio that can be considered a proportion of the body weight.

B. Significance

The apparent volume of distribution is a mathematical ratio that may or may not have a literal anatomical meaning in that it corresponds to an actual compartment of the body to which the drug is confined. Some substances are distributed approximately in the actual anatomical spaces represented by plasma water, extracellular water, or total body water. Such a substance will have an apparent volume of distribution equal to the real space in which it is distributed. Measurements of the volumes of distribution of appropriate substances of known distribution have been used for the purpose of measuring the volumes of plasma water, extracellular water, and total body water. If the apparent volume of distribution of a drug under investigation proves to have a value corresponding approximately to one of these water compartments, the tentative inference is permissible that the drug is actually distributed in the corresponding compartment. However, the apparent volume of distribution as derived from plasma concentrations alone is not of itself sufficient proof that a drug is actually uniformly distributed in an anatomical compartment of a volume equal to that volume of distribution. Substantiation by analysis of tissues would be required for conclusive establishment of the distribution.

Many drugs are bound in part to plasma albumin. Some comment is in order concerning the plasma concentration of such drugs to be used in calculating the apparent volume of distribution. Although the volume of distribution calculated from the total plasma concentration may be of use for some purposes, only the volume calculated from the unbound plasma concentration should ever be used in drawing any inferences as to the anatomical distribution of a drug. Consider, for instance, a hypothetical drug that is bound to albumin to the extent that 70 % of the total in plasma is bound and 30 % is free. The drug is otherwise distributed in total body water in a concentration equal to the unbound plasma concentration. If the apparent volume of distribution were calculated from the total plasma concentration, a value would be obtained approximating the volume of extracellular water and the inference might be reached that the drug was confined to the extracellular space. Erroneous conclusions of this nature have found their way into the literature.

The most obvious examples to illustrate the fact that the apparent volume of distribution as defined above as a mathematical ratio does not necessarily signify literally a real anatomical volume are to be found with drugs that are extensively localized anywhere outside the plasma. With such a drug, the value c in the equation above may be so small relative to Q that V_d may exceed the body weight. For instance, for quinacrine the value of V_d is of the order of 1000 times the body weight. A value of V_d exceeding the volume of the total body water indicates localization of the drug somewhere other than in simple physical solution in body water. The higher the value of V_d, the more extensive the localization in sites other than plasma water, but the value of V_d alone as it is derived from plasma concentrations can of course give no information as to the localization of the sites of concentration.

Implicit in the concept of volume of distribution is the assumption that its value remains approximately constant as the values of Q and c vary over wide ranges. This is more likely to be true if the distribution of a drug corresponds to one of the water compartments than if a high proportion of the drug is localized outside plasma water owing to strong interactions with, for instance, proteins or nucleic acids. As will be discussed below, the apparent volumes of distribution of acidic and basic drugs are influenced by metabolic and respiratory acidosis and alkalosis and may change quickly to significant degrees in response to changes in extracellular or intracellular pH. In quinacrine we find an example of a drug with a very high apparent volume of distribution that shows a wide range of not altogether predictable variability. Since the total amount of quinacrine in the plasma is a very small proportion of the total in the body, it is not surprising that tissue/plasma distribution ratios for quinacrine are highly variable (Dearborn, 1947). The total amount of quinacrine in the liver is of the order of at least a thousand times the total amount in the plasma. A minute proportional change in the amount of quinacrine in the liver brought about by uptake from or release into the plasma would cause a large proportional change in the plasma concentration. It has been found (Jailer et al., 1948), as might be predicted for a basic drug, that hypercapnia causes an increase in the plasma concentration of quinacrine, but there are probably unrecognized factors aside from pH gradients that could cause shifts of quinacrine between plasma and cells such as to bring about the conspicuous variabilities in plasma concentrations observed in patients on the same dosage schedule. For drugs having such high apparent volumes of distribution as quinacrine, the concept of the volume of distribution is of principal value simply to indicate a high degree of localization outside the plasma.

The relationship of the volume of distribution to the kinetics of the elimination of drugs from the body is of interest. The factors of interaction between drugs and the normal constituents of the body that determine the volume of distribution also play a role in influencing the rate at which a drug is eliminated from the body. Whatever the route or process of elimination, the rate is in general at least roughly proportional to the concentration of drug reaching the site of elimination. For processes of enzymatic destruction, the rate is usually proportional to the concentrations of drug at the enzymatic site because drug concentrations are generally low relative to the Michaelis constants of the enzymes metabolizing them and the availability of cofactors is not rate-limiting. In the process of pulmonary elimination, the rate is proportional to the concentration of drug in whole blood reaching the lung, this being a reflection of the fact that blood/air partition ratios of many substances are nearly constant over wide ranges of concentration. Owing to the variation of albumin binding with concentration and owing to the complexity of the processes of tubular reabsorption and secretion, the rate of renal excretion cannot be expected to be a simple function of plasma concentration. Nevertheless, it is a fact that the renal clearances of many drugs do not change greatly with change of plasma concentration; that is, the rate of renal elimination does not deviate to an important degree from proportionality to plasma concentration. The interactions of drugs with the normal constituents of the body that result in extensive localization outside the plasma remove a high proportion of the drug from accessibility to the processes of excretion and destruction. It is to be expected that high volumes of distribution, which reflect such localization outside the plasma, would be associated with slow disappearance of drugs from the body.

As will appear in the discussion below, the actual calculation of an apparent volume of distribution is of necessity based on assumptions that embody some elements of uncertainty. These uncertainties are of such nature that it is not to be expected that they can be altogether eliminated through refinement and elaboration of technique. The apparent volume of distribution cannot accordingly be regarded as a quantity susceptible to measurement with a high degree of precision. However, despite limitations to precision of measurement and limitations to scope of interpretation, the concept of the apparent volume of distribution and the estimates of its magnitude as arrived at experimentally can be helpful in understanding the disposition of drugs in the body and in devising the optimal methods of using drugs in practical therapeutics.

C. Experimental Determination

It is generally desired to measure the apparent volume of distribution under conditions in which an approximation to equilibrium between plasma and tissues has been attained. If a drug is leaving the body at a rate unequal to that at which it is entering, as is usually the case, there will be no true equilibrium. However, unless the processes of elimination of the drug are very rapid, conditions can be found in which equilibrium is approximated sufficiently closely for practical purposes. Whether the drug is given intravenously or by a route of slow absorption, some time must elapse between the time of administration and the time of approximate equilibrium when the volume of distribution is to be measured. During this elapsed time there will be loss of the drug from the body. This loss must be evaluated in order that it may be subtracted from the administered dose to arrive at the total amount, Q, present in the body at the time when the volume of distribution is to be calculated.

In the following discussion it will be assumed that Q cannot be determined by direct analysis of the whole body and that only blood, urine, and expired air are accessible for analysis, the conditions imposed in nearly all studies in man and many studies in laboratory animals. It is furthermore assumed that we are dealing with a drug disappearing from the body at a rate approximately proportional to the plasma concentration.

After there is an approximation to equilibrium,

$$dc/dt = -kc$$

$$c = c_0 e^{-kt}$$

$$\ln c = \ln c_0 - kt$$

If $\ln c$ is plotted as a function of time, a linear relationship between $\ln c$ and t will be approached as equilibration between plasma and tissues progresses after an intravenous injection. If the drug has been given by a route of slow absorption, the linear relationship will be attained after absorption is complete. The slope of this linear segment of the curve is $-k$. If the plot is made with a scale of logarithms to the base 10 rather than to the base e, as is usually done, the slope is multiplied by the factor 2.30 to arrive at the value of k. (It may be noted that k^{-1} is the time required for c to decline to a value of $1/e$ times c_0. As with other exponential processes of decay, the half-life, $t_{\frac{1}{2}}$, is sometimes used in relation to drug disappearance. It is the time required for the amount of drug in the body to decline to half the amount originally present. The relationship of $t_{\frac{1}{2}}$ to k is $t_{\frac{1}{2}} = k^{-1} \ln 2$. The half-life may be a convenient means of comparing closely related drugs. However, it should be kept in mind that it is not a measure of the duration of action of a drug. The time at which the amount of drug in the body has diminished to the extent that the action of the drug is no longer of practical consequence may be a time much shorter or much longer than the half-life.)

If the drug is known not to be metabolized but to be eliminated entirely unchanged in the urine or in the expired air, the amount lost from the body up to any time can be ascertained by direct analytical measurement.

Most drugs are at least in part metabolized in the body, and the amount remaining at an interval after administration must be arrived at indirectly. A simple means of estimating the apparent volume of distribution is to extrapolate the linear segment of the logarithmic curve to zero time to find the hypothetical concentration, c_0, that would have been obtained if equilibration of the administered dose had been attained instantaneously. Division of the administered dose by c_0 gives the apparent volume of distribution. The assumption is being made that the loss before the time of equilibration is the same as if the plasma concentration had actually declined along the extrapolated line at the early times. If the drug were given intravenously, the early plasma concentrations would be above the extrapolated line and the actual loss would be greater than that estimated. Likewise, if the drug had been given by a route of slow absorption, the early plasma concentrations would be below the extrapolated line and the actual loss less than that estimated. While this method of estimating the apparent volume of distribution by simple extrapolation obviously entails assumptions that are to some degree erroneous, the value so obtained is often satisfactory for the purposes to which it is to be put.

Account can be taken of the actual temporal course of the plasma concentration to attempt a more refined assessment of the loss of drug from the body. For a drug that is disappearing from the body (by the summation of all processes of excretion and metabolism) at a rate proportional to the plasma concentration, the rate of loss at any time is $kV_d c$.

The amount lost between the times t_1 and t_2 is

$$kV_d \int_{t_1}^{t_2} c \, dt$$

The integral is the area under the curve of c plotted as the ordinate (on an arithmetic, not a logarithmic scale) against t as the abscissa. If the integration is performed between the limits of 0 and ∞, that is, if the area of the entire curve is measured to the time when c becomes zero, the total amount of drug that has entered the body has been lost. If the drug has been administered by a route known to give complete absorption, the loss can be equated with the administered dose. Then

$$Dose = kV_d \cdot Area$$

$$V_d = Dose/k \cdot Area$$

The value of k can be assessed from the logarithmic plot as described above, and all the quantities are known necessary for the calculation of V_d .

If V_d has already been measured in some other way, the relationship between loss and area under the concentration-time curve can be put to other uses. For instance, if a drug is given by mouth and absorption is incomplete, the value of $kV_d \cdot Area$ will be less than the administered dose, and the ratio of this value to the administered dose is the proportion absorbed. Also, it is sometimes desired to estimate the amount of drug disappearing between certain time limits, as for example to evaluate what proportion of a drug that has disappeared can be accounted for by the production of a metabolite.

It may be noted that the method outlined above also entails assumptions that may be erroneous. One is that V_d is constant over the entire period. Actually V_d can be expected to be nearly constant only at such times as there is approximate equilibrium between plasma and tissues. There might not be serious deviation from this condition if the drug is slowly absorbed. However, in the period immediately following a rapid intravenous injection, a drug is distributed in a smaller volume than later after penetration of tissues has progressed.

Furthermore, the assumption is made that no large loss of drug has occurred between the site at which the drug enters the body and that at which plasma is sampled. If this condition is not fulfilled, a serious error could be introduced by assuming that the area under the concentration-time curve is proportional to the absorbed dose. For instance, if ethanol is being absorbed from the intestine at a rate below that at which complete metabolism occurs in one passage through the liver, large total amounts of ethanol could be absorbed without a measurable concentration being attained in peripheral blood. When chloral hydrate is given by mouth in therapeutic doses, the unchanged drug does not appear in detectable concentrations in peripheral blood (Marshall and Owens, 1954). Yet absorption has occurred, as evidenced by the presence of the metabolites, trichloroethanol and trichloroacetic acid.

III. DISTRIBUTION AS AFFECTED BY MEMBRANE BARRIERS

After a drug has entered the blood either by direct injection into the blood or by absorption through any of the various routes used to introduce drugs into the body, there are membranes that must be traversed before the drug can penetrate into body cells. Capillary membranes are generally freely permeable to small molecules. Except for the substances of high molecular weight used as plasma expanders, nearly all of the compounds we consider as drugs are of a molecular size that permits ready permeation of capillary membranes. Most drugs will gain access to the extracellular interstitial spaces of most tissues in a rather short time. The magnitude of the extracellular space of brain, or indeed whether it exists, has been a matter of controversy. If this space is of the magnitude proposed by some recent workers (Rall et al., 1962; Bourke et al., 1965; Korobkin et al., 1968), it is clear that drugs that readily enter extracellular spaces of other tissues are excluded from that of the brain. This is true also of cerebrospinal fluid and the aqueous humor of the eye. The physical properties of drugs requisite for penetration into these water compartments are the same as those favoring penetration of cellular membranes, which will be discussed below. This is because a drug molecule must traverse cellular membranes to pass from blood into these spaces.

If a drug is reversibly bound to plasma albumin, that portion so bound has only the very limited filterability of albumin itself.

The plasma membranes surrounding cells constitute barriers to penetration of drugs quite different from the capillary membranes. A drug that diffuses readily through capillary membranes into the extracellular interstitial spaces may penetrate cellular membranes very slowly or scarcely at all. The physical properties that determine the facility with which a drug penetrates cellular membranes are in a general way recognized. Yet they cannot be so precisely formulated as to permit reliable predictions based on physical measurements. The factors most important in determining penetration of cellular membranes appear to be molecular size, relative strengths of interaction with water and lipids, and ionization.

High affinity for lipid relative to water is particularly important in penetration of drugs into the brain. A compound such as urea, which penetrates other cells rapidly, enters the brain only very slowly (Schoolar et al., 1960; Waddell, 1968). Anesthetic activity, like penetration of membranes, is correlated with affinity for lipid relative to that for water. Most drugs used as anesthetics, whether inhalation or intravenous, come to a rapid equilibrium between brain and blood. As will be discussed below, this is an important attribute of a drug to be used as a general surgical anesthetic. Some drugs that are anesthetic, such as barbital, penetrate the brain slowly (Butler, 1950) and would for that reason (as well as others) be unsuitable for intravenous anesthetics in man.

IV. DISTRIBUTION IN THE WATER COMPARTMENTS

The capillary walls and the cellular membranes are barriers to such large general classes of substances that the plasma water, the total extracellular water, and the total body water are compartments of special interest in studies of drug distribution. There are classes of drugs the distribution of which corresponds approximately to these spaces. This is not to imply that either extracellular water or total body water behaves as a homogeneous space free of barriers, a space into which a drug will become rapidly and uniformly distributed. Even those drugs approximating these distributions do not among themselves have exactly the same volumes of distribution, nor do they approach these volumes of distribution with the same rapidity.

A. Plasma Water

Substances of high molecular weight or substances almost completely bound to plasma albumin will disappear only slowly from the vascular spaces and will have apparent volumes of distribution approximating the plasma water, which is about 4% of the body weight. Except for substances such as dextran used as plasma expanders, a substance confined to plasma is not useful as a drug. There are a number of substances that have been used to measure the volume of plasma water. These include ^{131}I-albumin and dyes that are almost completely bound to albumin.

B. Extracellular Water

Substances having an apparent volume of distribution corresponding to total extracellular water, which is about 20% of the body weight, are those substances that penetrate capillary membranes but do not penetrate cellular membranes. These include some inorganic ions and organic compounds lacking those physical properties discussed above as necessary for penetration of lipid membranes. Among the normal constituents of the body, the sodium and the chloride ions are largely, although not entirely, extracellular. A number of substances have been used for measurement of extracellular water in the whole body, in tissue samples, and in cellular suspensions. These include the sodium, chloride, bromide, thiocyanate, and sulfate ions, inulin, sucrose, and mannitol. The apparent volumes of distribution of these various substances are not exactly equal, either in the whole body or in individual tissues. The chloride ion, for instance, while present in low concentration in the cells constituting the bulk of the body, is present in high concentration in some cells. Probably none of the substances used for measurement of extracellular water is excluded completely from all cells. On the other hand, some of them are excluded from water compartments that might be considered part of the extracellular water, such as cerebrospinal fluid, the aqueous humor, and the water in the lumen of the gastrointestinal tract. The long and extensive experience with inulin for measurement of extracellular water has generally validated the concept that this compound does not penetrate any cellular membranes except perhaps very slowly. A radioactive derivative of inulin, inulin-carboxyl-^{14}C, has been prepared by reaction of inulin with ^{14}C-cyanide and hydrolysis of the product. This compound, while it differs from inulin in that it contains an ionizing group, appears to behave like the parent compound with regard to its distribution. It has been found useful for measurement of extracellular water, particularly in preparations of tissues and cells *in vitro*.

C. Total Body Water

If a drug penetrates cellular membranes and if the strength of its interaction with water predominates over that of its interactions with other normal constituents of the body, it will be distributed with approximately equal concentration in all water compartments of the body, intracellular and extracellular. The measurement of its apparent volume of distribution will give a value equal to the total body water, which is about 60% of the body weight. Except for small molecules, the penetration of cellular membranes by organic molecules is favored by high affinity for lipid relative to that for water. If the fat/water partition coefficient of a drug is very high, significant concentration of the drug in depot fat will take place. Thus, it may be expected that some drugs that can penetrate to reach intracellular water will also be concentrated in fat to such an extent that the apparent volume of distribution will be significantly higher than the total body water.

Among the various substances the distributions of which approximate total body water, there are some differences in the patterns of distribution and in the rapidity with which equilibration with different tissues occurs. Some substances that are distributed approximately in total body water are ethanol, urea, sulfanilamide, antipyrine, and N-acetyl-4-aminoantipyrine. Some of these have been used for measurement of total body water. As might be expected, the isotopic forms of water, deuterium oxide and tritium oxide, distribute uniformly with ordinary water and can be used to measure total water.

V. DISTRIBUTION AS AFFECTED BY INTERACTION WITH FAT

Drugs will be distributed between depot fat and extracellular water in accordance with their fat/water partition coefficients, which are the resultants of the relative strengths of the interactions of the drug molecules with fat and with water. Owing to the paucity of the blood supply to fat, equilibration between fat and blood proceeds slowly, and concentration ratios approximating the equilibrium fat/water partition coefficient may not be attained during the sojourn of the drug in the body. If the fat/water partition coefficient of a drug is high, the proportion of a drug localized in fat may be high, and this will be reflected in a high apparent volume of distribution. The expected association of a high volume of distribution with persistence of action has been commented upon above. A high volume of distribution of methoxyflurane consequent to concentration in fat, as well as its high blood/air partition coefficient, contribute to the conspicuous persistence of this inhalation anesthetic in the body (Chenoweth *et al.*, 1962; Eger and Shargel, 1963). Concentration of chlorophenothane in depot fat creates stores of the compound that remain in the body for prolonged periods (Hayes *et al.*, 1956). A high proportion of the intravenous anesthetic, thiopental, is ultimately localized in fat (Brodie *et al.*, 1950; Brodie *et al.*, 1952). Passage of the drug out of the brain and into fat is a part of the redistribution process terminating the anesthetic action, but redistribution into tissues other than fat may be more important at the early times (Goldstein and Aronow, 1960).

VI. DISTRIBUTION AS AFFECTED BY INTERACTION WITH PLASMA ALBUMIN

Plasma albumin is unique among proteins in its capacity to undergo strong reversible interaction with a large number of compounds of low molecular weight of the most diverse chemical structures. Most organic compounds used as drugs interact to significant degrees with albumin. Many drugs that are extensively bound to albumin are not bound to a significant extent to other plasma proteins or to intracellular proteins.

It is of interest to consider the proportion of the total drug in the body that is bound to plasma albumin. Table 3.1 shows calculations for some hypothetical drugs that are assumed to be partially bound to plasma albumin and otherwise distributed in total body water in a uniform concentration equal to the unbound concentration in plasma. The plasma water is assumed to be 4% of the body weight and the total body water 60% of the body weight. In the first column is the percentage of the drug in plasma that is bound. In the second column is the percentage of the total in the body that is in the bound form in plasma. As this table shows, it is only when the extent of binding is very high, really only above 90%, that any very high proportion of the total in the body is bound in plasma.

Although the apparent volume of distribution, as calculated from unbound plasma concentrations, is not increased to a major degree by binding except at the very high levels of binding, even a moderate degree of binding can affect the persistence of the drug in the body. The drug bound to albumin is not filterable in the renal glomerulus, and if excretion by filtration is the major mode of elimination of the drug, binding can decrease the rate of elimination to an important extent. Binding to albumin is responsible for some extraordinary examples of drug persistence. Suramin is so slowly eliminated that a single dose is protective against trypanosomiasis for three months (Hawking, 1940). The x-ray contrast medium, iophenoxic acid, is so extensively bound in low concentrations that it disappears with a half-life of 2.5 years (Astwood, 1957).

There are numerous examples of competition between drugs for binding sites on albumin. If a patient is being treated with one drug that is bound to albumin, and a second drug that is also bound is administered, the second drug may in part displace the first from albumin. The consequences of this displacement de-

TABLE 3.1

Proportion of total drug in body bound to plasma albumin

Hypothetical substances distributed uniformly throughout total body water in the concentration unbound in plasma water. Plasma water is assumed to be 4% and total water 60% of the body weight.

% in plasma in the bound form	% of total in body bound in plasma
50	6
60	9
70	13
80	21
90	38
95	56
98	76
99	87

pend upon the extent to which the drug was originally bound. As shown by the calculations of Table 3.1, displacement of a drug that is 50 % bound would cause a decrease in the total plasma concentration that might appear impressive but would be accompanied by little increase in the concentration elsewhere.

It is only when substances are bound in plasma to the extent of about 90 % or more that it can be expected that displacement from binding would release amounts of drug that on distribution into other parts of the body would cause serious increase in concentration in tissues. An example of practical importance is the displacement of unconjugated bilirubin by drugs such as sulfonamides and salicylates. Unconjugated bilirubin is normally almost completely bound to albumin. In the condition of kernicterus in newborn infants there is an excessive level of unconjugated bilirubin. If the binding capacity of albumin is exceeded, bilirubin enters tissues and exerts serious toxic effects on the brain. Administration to a hyperbilirubinemic infant of a drug that displaces bilirubin from albumin can greatly increase the entrance of bilirubin into the brain.

An experiment of Schmid et al. (1965) in a strain of rat with a hereditary deficiency of the enyzme conjugating bilirubin illustrates well the effect of salicylate in displacing bilirubin from albumin. Administration of salicylate caused a striking fall of the serum bilirubin as bilirubin was displaced from albumin and entered tissues. Later administration intravenously of human albumin, which has a greater binding capacity for bilirubin than does rat albumin, brought bilirubin back into the plasma.

VII. DISTRIBUTION AS AFFECTED BY INTERACTION WITH NUCLEIC ACIDS

Numerous drugs of different chemical classes have been shown to interact with DNA, and there is evidence that some of these interactions involve intercalation of the drug between adjacent base-pairs of the double helix. There has understandably been more interest in the distortions of structure of DNA and consequent disturbances of its function as possible mechanisms of pharmacological action of drugs than there has been in the effect of these interactions on the patterns of distribution of the drugs in the body. With drugs such as quinacrine and chloroquine that are very highly localized within cells and that have been demonstrated to interact strongly with DNA (Parker and Irvin, 1952; Kurnick et al., 1962; Hahn et al., 1966), it may be presumed that this interaction is a factor in their intracellular concentration.

VIII. DISTRIBUTION AS AFFECTED BY INTERACTION WITH MELANIN

A number of polycyclic aromatic compounds have been shown to interact strongly in vitro with melanin in uveal pigment granules and with synthetic melanin made by oxidation of dihydroxyphenylalanine (Potts, 1964). Attention was directed to this interaction by the discovery that phenothiazines (Potts, 1962) and chloroquine (Bernstein et al., 1963) are concentrated to very high degrees in the uveal tracts of pigmented experimental animals but not of albino animals. The high concentrations of chloroquine and phenothiazines accumulating in the melanin-containing tissues of the eye suggest a relationship to the retinopathies produced by those drugs. The analog of chloroquine in which Cl is replaced by ^{125}I has been used to visualize melanomas (Beierwaltes *et al.*, 1968). Whether interaction with the melanin in skin causes sufficient localization of any drug in skin as to influence the pattern of distribution to a degree of practical importance is a question that appears not to have attracted attention.

IX. DISTRIBUTION OF PARTIALLY IONIZED DRUGS

A large proportion of the compounds used in medicine as drugs are weak organic acids and bases that are partially ionized at physiological pH. Because of the impermeability of cellular membranes to organic ions, which is discussed in Chapter 1, the distribution of a partially ionized drug between intracellular water and extracellular water is a function of the pH values in both phases. Change of either intracellular pH or extracellular pH will be accompanied by a shift of the drug between intracellular and extracellular water.

In skeletal muscle, which constitutes a large part of the bulk of the body, it has been found that changes of extracellular pH at constant pCO_2 have little effect on intracellular pH and that changes of pCO_2 change intracellular pH but to a lesser extent than they change extracellular pH (Waddell and Butler, 1959). Production of either metabolic or respiratory acidosis causes a fall of the plasma concentration of an acidic drug consequent to a shift from extracellular to intracellular water. Production of either metabolic or respiratory alkalosis causes a rise in the plasma concentration of an acidic drug consequent to a shift from intracellular to extracellular water. The shifts in the distribution of a basic drug produced by acidosis and alkalosis are in the opposite directions to those of an acidic drug.

Shifts of distribution with acidosis and alkalosis have been observed with a number of acidic and basic drugs. One such drug that has been studied is phenobarbital, an acid with a pK' such that important shifts might be expected (Waddell and Butler, 1957). In experiments in dogs in which blood pH was altered by CO_2 inhalation, overventilation, or intravenous $NaHCO_3$ infusion, the plasma concentration of phenobarbital changed in the same direction as the blood pH. Analysis of tissues showed that for brain, fat, liver, and muscle, the tissue/plasma concentration ratios varied in a direction opposite to that of blood pH.

An example of a valuable therapeutic application of the shifts in distribution between intracellular and extracellular water that can be effected by manipulalation of extracellular pH is to be found in the treatment of phenobarbital poisoning. The shift of phenobarbital out of brain into extracellular water that can be produced by intravenous infusion of $NaHCO_3$ lightens anesthesia. This can be observed in dogs and can be more conclusively demonstrated by measurement in mice of the median anesthetic dose of phenobarbital, which can be raised to the extent of 20% by $NaHCO_3$ treatment (Waddell and Butler, 1957). In patients poisoned with phenobarbital, it has been the impression that intravenous $NaHCO_3$ causes a prompt lightening of depression. This is a benefit of $NaHCO_3$ in addition to the increase in the rate of renal excretion of phenobarbital that it also produces.

The dependence of the intracellular/extracellular concentration ratio of an acid on the pH gradient across the cellular membrane has been made use of for the purpose of measuring intracellular pH. If the concentration of an acid or base can be measured on both sides of a membrane and the pH measured directly on one side, the pH on the other side can be calculated.

The assumptions on which this calculation of intracellular pH are based and the evidence for the validity of the experimentally determined values have been reviewed by Butler *et al.* (1967). The principle was first utilized by E. J. Warburg (1922), who calculated the pH of the erythrocyte from the intracellular/extracellular distribution of CO_2. Subsequently a number of other workers used the distribution of CO_2 to measure intracellular pH of various tissues *in vivo* and *in vitro*. The method is based on the fact that cellular membranes are freely permeable to CO_2 but not to the bicarbonate ion. Waddell and Butler (1959) suggested that the weak acid, 5,5-dimethyl-2,4-oxazolidinedione (DMO), which is the product of demethylation of trimethadione, has the attributes to be desired in a compound for measurement of intracellular pH. There have now been numerous studies in which DMO has been used for measurement of intracellular pH in various tissues and cells. In general there has been rather close agreement between the results obtained with DMO and with CO_2. One important advantage of DMO over CO_2 is that, being a non-volatile, non-metabolized foreign compound, DMO labeled with ^{14}C can be used. This permits the development of simple, specific methods of great sensitivity for measurement of DMO. The use of DMO-^{14}C in conjunction with inulin-carboxyl-^{14}C for measurement of extracellular water is particularly useful for *in vitro* investigations. Methods for the determination of these two radioactive compounds in the presence of each other were described in a study of Ehrlich ascites tumor cells (Poole *et al.*, 1964).

X. NON-EQUILIBRIUM DISTRIBUTIONS

If a drug equilibrates between plasma and the various tissues at different rates, a rapid change in the plasma concentration will result in a change in the pattern of distribution of the drug that may cause changes in drug concentration at an effector site disproportionate to changes in the total amount of drug in the body. There are large differences in the rates at which drugs equilibrate between plasma and various tissues. These differences may reflect the presence of special types of diffusion barriers, such as the barrier to free diffusion of certain substances from plasma to brain, cerebrospinal fluid, and aqueous humor. A more general source of difference in equilibration rates is the large disparity in blood flow to different tissues. Table 3.2 shows a compilation of some approximate values for blood flow to various human tissues. It is notable that about three-fourths of the cardiac output is delivered to tissues that comprise less than one-tenth of the body weight. Some small organs receive blood flows more than 100 times as great as those of some of the bulkier tissues. In the absence of specific barriers to diffusion, it may be expected that a drug will equilibrate more rapidly between plasma and a tissue with a high blood flow than between plasma and a tissue with a low blood flow. When the plasma concentration of a drug is undergoing rapid change, it is in the organs with high blood flow that one might expect to see the most rapid changes in drug concentration and the most rapid changes in the intensity of any pharmacological effect that may be exerted by the drug within the organ. Of the organs with high blood flow, the brain is the one in which rapid changes in intensity of pharmacological effect are most readily observable. It is in the brain that redistribution phenomena consequent to rapid equilibration between plasma

TABLE 3.2*

Blood flow to human tissues

Tissue	% Body weight	% Cardiac output	Blood Flow
			ml./100 g. tissue per min.
Adrenals	0.02	1	550
Kidneys	0.4	24	450
Thyroid	0.04	2	400
Liver hepatic	2	5	20
portal		20	75
Portal-drained viscera	2	20	75
Heart (basal)	0.4	4	70
Brain	2	15	55
Skin	7	5	5
Muscle (basal)	40	15	3
Connective tissue	7	1	1
Fat	15	2	1

Adapted for the most part from data from Spector, W. S. (Editor), *Handbook of Biological Data*, Table 273 (Saunders, Philadelphia, 1956), and Jones, H. B., Respiratory system: nitrogen elimination, in Glasser, O. (Editor); *Medical Physics*, Vol. II, p. 855 (Year Book Publishers, Chicago, 1950). The data from which the values in this table were derived came from many sources and have been adjusted somewhat in the interests of consistency. The values are to be considered only as approximations.

* From Butler, T. C.: Proc. First International Pharmacological Meeting, Vol. 6, p. 197 (Pergamon Press, 1962).

and the tissue are of practical importance both in intravenous and in inhalation anesthesia.

In the initial period after a rapid intravenous injection the proportion of the drug confined to plasma is higher than after equilibration with tissues is more closely approached. The drug is leaving the plasma not only by elimination from the body but also by passage into tissues. In the rapid fall of plasma concentration in the period soon after the injection, passage of the drug from plasma to tissues is a more important factor than elimination of the drug from the body.

If a tissue equilibrates rapidly with plasma, the concentration of drug in that tissue will rise to high levels soon after the injection when the plasma concentration is high. It will then fall rapidly when the plasma concentration is falling rapidly. The rapid disappearance of drug from the tissue during this early period is due in large part to the physical withdrawal of the drug from that tissue and its redistribution into other tissues that equilibrate more slowly with plasma. The time required for the concentration in the rapidly equilibrating tissue to decline from its maximal value to half that value may be much less than the half-life for the body as a whole.

The ultra-short action of intravenous anesthetics such as thiopental is now recognized as being the result of a more rapid rate of equilibration between plasma and brain than between plasma and the other tissues in which a large proportion of the drug will ultimately be localized. Brodie *et al.* (1950, 1952) showed that most of a dose of thiopental eventually becomes localized in fat depots and concluded that redistribution into fat accounts in large part for the termination of action. Goldstein and Aronow (1960) presented evidence that accumulation of thiopental in fat is a slow process and that redistribution into other sites is more important in the early events.

Drugs such as thiopental behave as ultra-short acting agents only if rapidly introduced into the blood steam and only if the body tissues do not already contain large amounts of drug. In the mouse a rapid intravenous dose of 20 mg/kg of thiopental produces deep anesthesia of only about 1 or 2 minutes duration. If the drug is administered subcutaneously, a dose of about 100 mg/kg is required to anesthetize, and anesthesia persists for over an hour. When successive doses of an intravenous anesthetic are administered to maintain anesthesia, the effect becomes progressively more persistent and the anesthesia less controllable.

These effects are readily demonstrated with electrical models in which networks of capacity and resistance represent analogies to compartmental models of the body (Butler, 1962).

Figure 3.1 shows electrical simulation of brain concentrations of a drug after rapid intravenous injection and after injection into a site from which absorption is slow. Curve A simulates the intravenous injection. The peak occurs rapidly and the concentration falls rapidly as the drug passes into more slowly equilibrating bulky body compartments. Curve B simulates injection of the same dose into a site of slow absorption. The maximum is only a quarter that of Curve A and occurs much later. Curve C simulates injection into the site of slow absorption of a dose 4 times that used for A and B. The peak is now equal to that in Curve A but it occurs later, and the time required for decline from the peak value to half that value is over twice as long for Curve C as for Curve A.

Figure 3.2 shows electrical simulation of repeated intravenous injections. Curve A is analogous to brain concentration and Curve B to concentration in composite bulky tissues of the body. When the analogue of brain concentration had fallen to half its original peak value, injection of a smaller dose was simulated. The simulation of injection of the same smaller dose was performed four additional times. With each successive injection, the brain concentration declined more slowly. This illustrates by analogy the situation in which an intravenous anesthetic is injected repeatedly to maintain anesthesia. As the drug accumulates in extracerebral tissues, the gradient between brain and these tissues diminishes and the amount removed from brain by redistribution into other tissues decreases.

The phenomenon of redistribution within the body is probably of more importance than is generally realized in affecting the course of action of intravenously administered drugs other than anesthetics.

The suddenly rising, transiently high concentrations of some drugs in brain that can be produced by rapid intravenous injection bring about psychological effects that have been valued by drug addicts. The intravenous route of administration of addictive drugs has had particular attractions and has led to patterns of addiction peculiar to that route. Despite the rapid deacetylation of heroin, addicts can distinguish heroin from morphine on intravenous injection, and often prefer heroin (Martin and Fraser, 1961). Intravenous injection of cocaine or amphetamine and its congeners produces orgasmic psychological effects of a sort not experienced on oral administration. Compulsive repetition of the injection of such drugs at frequent intervals constitutes a particularly rapidly destructive form of drug abuse (Kramer et al., 1967).

If a gas or volatile liquid has been administered by way of the lungs until the

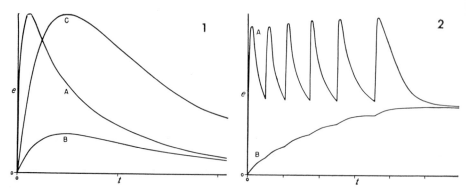

Fig. 1 (*left*). Electrical simulation of brain concentrations of a drug after rapid intra-venous injection and after injection into a site from which absorption is slow. Curve A: simulation of rapid intravenous injection. Curve B: simulation of injection of the same dose into a site of slow absorption. Curve C: simulation of injection of 4 times as high a dose into the site of slow absorption. (From Butler, *Proc. First International Pharmacological Meeting*, Vol. 6, p. 201, Pergamon Press, 1962.)

Fig. 2 (*right*). Electrical simulation of repeated intravenous injection of a drug. Curve A is analogous to concentration in brain and Curve B to concentration in composite bulky tissues of the body. The simulation is of an initial injection followed by repeated injection of a smaller dose each time the brain concentration had fallen to half the value of the first peak. (From Butler, *Proc. First International Pharmacological Meeting*, Vol. 6, p. 201, Pergamon Press, 1962.)

body is equilibrated with the concentration of drug in the inspired air and if the drug is then withdrawn, the concentration of drug in the blood leaving the lungs drops very rapidly. The ratio of the concentration in systemic arterial blood just after withdrawal to that before withdrawal is approximately $C_P/(\lambda C_P + V_P)$, in which λ is the partition coefficient between whole blood and air, C_P is the pulmonary circulation in liters per minute, and V_P is the effective pulmonary ventilation in liters per minute. If the value of λ is low, the concentration in arterial blood very rapidly falls to a small fraction of its initial value. Because of the abundant blood supply to the brain and the rapid equilibration of most anesthetics between blood and brain, the concentration of an inhalation anesthetic in brain will follow the concentration in arterial blood more closely than will the average concentration for other tissues of the body. If the value of λ is low, the concentration of drug in brain will fall to half its initial value in much less time than the half-life for the body as a whole. For inhalation anesthetics with low values of λ, the initial stage of recovery is very rapid and is affected only to a slight extent by the pattern of distribution in tissues other than the brain.

For instance, with values of C_P of 4 l/min and V_P of 6 l/min, the concentration of nitrous oxide ($\lambda = 0.5$) will fall in arterial blood immediately after withdrawal to $\frac{1}{4}$ that prevailing immediately before. Thus recovery from nitrous oxide anesthesia will progress well toward completion before the total amount of anesthetic in the body has diminished by any large proportion.

The extreme examples of unequal distribution of drugs to different tissues are observed when a drug is administered by such a route that it reaches one region exclusively or in much higher concentration than others. Regional perfusion has been used for carcinolytic agents too toxic to be used systemically. Intra-arterial injection, creating a transient high concentration of drug in the tissues supplied by that vessel, can sometimes be used to localize the site of action of a drug. An elegant example is the localization of action of respiratory stimulants acting on the chemoreceptors of the carotid body. If a drug has its site of action in these chemoreceptors, a much smaller dose will stimulate respiration when injected into the carotid artery than when injected into the vertebral artery or any other vessel.

Acknowledgment

Public Health Service Research Career Program Award 4 K06 GM 19,429 from the National Institute of General Medical Sciences.

REFERENCES

Astwood, E. B.: Occurrence in the sera of certain patients of large amounts of a newly isolated iodine compound. Trans. Ass. Am. Physicians *70:* 183–191, 1957.

Beierwaltes, W. H., Lieberman, L. M., Varma, V. M., and Counsell, R. E.: Visualizing human malignant melanoma and metastases. Use of chloroquine analog tagged with iodine 125. J.A.M.A. *206:* 97–102, 1968.

Bernstein, H., Zvaifler, N., Rubin, M., and Mansour, A. M.: The ocular deposition of chloroquine. Invest. Ophthalmol. *2:* 384–392, 1963.

Bourke, R. S., Greenberg, E. S., and Tower, D. B.: Variation of cerebral cortex fluid spaces in vivo as a function of species brain size. Am. J. Physiol. *208:* 682–692, 1965.

Brodie, B. B., Mark, L. C., Papper, E. M., Lief, E. B., Bernstein, E., and Rovenstine, E. A.: The fate of thiopental in man and a method for its estimation in biological material. J. Pharmacol. Exp. Ther. *98:* 85–96, 1950.

Brodie, B. B., Bernstein, E., and Mark, L. C.: The role of body fat in limiting the duration of action of thiopental. J. Pharmacol. Exp. Ther. *105:* 421–426, 1952.

Butler, T. C.: Duration of action of drugs as affected by tissue distribution. *Proc. First International Pharmacological Meeting,* Vol. 6, pp. 193–205, Pergamon Press, 1962.

Butler, T. C.: The rate of penetration of barbituric acid derivatives into the brain. J. Pharmacol. Exp. Ther. *100:* 219–226, 1950.

Butler, T. C., Waddell, W. J., and Poole, D. T.: Intracellular pH based on the distribution of weak electrolytes. Fed. Proc. Fed. Am. Socs. Exp. Biol. *26:* 1327–1332, 1967.

Chenoweth, M. B., Robertson, D. N., Erley, D. S., and Golhke, R.: Blood and tissue levels of ether, chloroform, halothane and methoxyflurane in dogs. Anesthesiology *23:* 101–106, 1962.

Dearborn, E. H.: The distribution of quin-

acrine in dogs and in rabbits. J. Pharmacol. Exp. Ther. *91:* 174–177, 1947.

Eger, E. I., and Shargel, R.: The solubility of methoxyflurane in human blood and tissue homogenates. Anesthesiology *24:* 625–627, 1963.

Goldstein, A., and Aronow, L.: The duration of action of thiopental and pentobarbital. J. Pharmacol. Exp. Ther. *128:* 1–6, 1960.

Hahn, F. E., O'Brien, R. L., Ciak, J., Allison, J. L., and Olenick, J. G.: Studies on modes of action of chloroquine, quinacrine, and quinine and on chloroquine resistance. Military Medicine *131:* 1071–1089, 1966.

Hawking, F.: Concentration of Bayer 205 (Germanin) in human blood and cerebrospinal fluid after treatment. Trans. R. Soc. Trop. Med. Hyg. *34:* 37–52, 1940.

Hayes, W. J., Jr., Durham. W. F., and Creto, C., Jr.: The effect of known repeated oral doses of chlorophenothane (DDT) in man. J.A.M.A. *162:* 890–897, 1956.

Jailer, J. W., Zubrod, C. G., Rosenfeld, M., and Shannon, J. A.: Effect of acidosis and anoxia on the concentration of quinacrine and chloroquine in blood. J. Pharmacol. Exp. Ther. *92:* 345–351, 1948.

Korobkin, R. K., Lorenzo, A. V., and Cutler, R. W. P.: Distribution of C^{14}-sucrose and I^{125}-iodide in the central nervous system of the cat after various routes of injection into the cerebrospinal fluid. J. Pharmacol. Exp. Ther. *164:* 412–420, 1968.

Kramer, J. C., Fischman, V. S., and Littlefield, D. C.: Amphetamine abuse. Pattern and effects of high doses taken intravenously. J.A.M.A. *201:* 305–309, 1967.

Kurnick, N. B., and Radcliffe, I. E.: Reaction between DNA and quinacrine and other antimalarials. J. Lab. Clin. Med. *60:* 669–688, 1962.

Lassaigne: Résultats obtenus en examinant, sous le point de vue chimique, le sang veineux d'un animal avant et après l'inhalation de l'air chargé de vapeurs d'éther. C. R. Acad. Sci. *24:* 359–360, 1847.

62 DRUGS, DISTRIBUTION AND EXCRETION

Marshall, E. K., Jr., and Dearborn, E. H.: The relation of the plasma concentration of quinacrine to its antimalarial activity. J. Pharmacol. Exp. Ther. *88:* 142–153, 1946.

Marshall, E. K., Jr., and Owens, A. H., Jr., Absorption, excretion and metabolic fate of chloral hydrate and trichloroethanol. Bull. Johns Hopkins Hosp. *95:* 1–18, 1954.

Martin, W. R., and Fraser, H. F.: A comparative study of physiological and subjective effects of heroin and morphine administered intravenously in postaddicts. J. Pharmacol. Exp. Ther. *133:* 388–399, 1961.

Parker, F. S., and Irvin, J. L.: The interaction of chloroquine with nucleic acids and nucleoproteins. J. Biol. Chem. *199:* 897–909, 1952.

Poole, D. T., Butler, T. C., and Waddell, W. J.: Intracellular pH of the Ehrlich ascites tumor cell. J. Nat. Cancer Inst. *32:* 939–946, 1964.

Potts, A. M.: The concentration of phenothiazines in the eye of experimental animals. Invest. Ophthalmol. *1:* 522–530, 1962.

Potts, A. M.: The reaction of uveal pigment in vitro with polycyclic compounds. Invest. Ophthalmol. *3:* 405–416, 1964.

Rall, D. P., Oppelt, W. W., and Potlak, C. S.: Extracellular space of brain as determined by diffusion of inulin from the ventricular system. Life Sci. *1:* 43–48, 1962.

Schmid, R., Diamond, I., Hammaker, L. and Gundersen, C. B.: Interaction of bilirubin with albumin. Nature *206:* 1041–1043, 1965.

Schmiedeberg, O.: Ueber die quantitative Bestimmung des Chloroforms im Blute und sein Verhalten gegen dasselbe. Arch. d. Heilk. *8:* 273–320, 1867.

Schmiedeberg, O.: Rudolf Buchheim, sein Leben und seine Bedeutung für die Begründung der wissenschaftlichen Arzneimittellehre und Pharmakologie. Arch. Exp. Path. Pharmak. *67:* 1–54, 1911.

Schoolar, J. C., Barlow, C. F., and Roth, L. J.: The penetration of carbon-14 urea into cerebrospinal fluid and various areas of the cat brain. J. Neuropath. Exp. Neurol. *19:* 216–227, 1960.

Schulinus, H.: Untersuchungen über die Vertheilung des Weingeistes im thierischen Organismus. Arch. d. Heilk. *7:* 97–128, 1866.

Snow, J.: On narcotism by the inhalation of vapors. London Med. Gaz. *6* (n.s.): 850–854, 893–895, 1848.

Waddell, W. J.: Distribution of urea-^{14}C in pregnant mice studied by whole-body autoradiography. J. Appl. Physiol. *24:* 828–831, 1968.

Waddell, W. J., and Butler, T. C.: The distribution and excretion of phenobarbital. J. Clin. Invest. *36:* 1217–1226, 1957.

Waddell, W. J., and Butler, T. C.: Calculation of intracellular pH from the distribution of 5,5-dimethyl-2,4-oxazolidinedione (DMO). Application to skeletal muscle of the dog. J. Clin. Invest. *38:* 720–729, 1959.

Warburg, E. J.: Studies on carbonic acid compounds and hydrogen ion activities in blood and salt solutions. Biochem. J. *16:* 153–340, 1922.

4

Protein Binding

CLARKE DAVISON

I. DEFINITION AND SIGNIFICANCE

Binding is a *reversible* interaction between a small molecule and a protein or other macromolecule. It is analogous to the enzyme-substrate interaction except that the complex does not decompose to yield new products; it is also analogous to most drug-receptor complexes unless they involve covalent bonding.

Because of the relative ease of the experiments, most binding is measured in plasma or with purified plasma proteins. However, as noted in Chapter 3, while plasma bound drug is usually thought of as a depot, it only becomes significant in reducing drug available to the tissues when its extent is quite large.

The bound drug is of high molecular weight and is unavailable for membrane transport as such. However, if the complex is rapidly dissociable, this should not necessarily affect rate of transport since the free drug passing a membrane could be immediately replaced by newly dissociating drug. Froese, *et al.* (1962) noted that an azo dye dissociated from albumin with a half-life of about 20 milliseconds. However, even such a short half-life for dissociation might alter transport across a glomerulus or renal tubule, and certainly many drugs which are extensively protein bound are rather slowly excreted, i.e., suramin and iophenoxic acid persist in the body for months, and sulfamethoxypyridazine has a duration of action several times that of early weakly bound "sulfa" drugs. It may also be that not all dissociations are so rapid; as noted in Section III, many protein-bound compounds may be successfully separated by chromatography or electrophoresis. In any case, the importance of drug binding lies in several areas.

1. Drug excretion may be delayed by prevention of glomerular filtration or of tubular secretion.

2. Tissue distribution may be markedly modified, e.g. plasma-red cell, plasma-extracellular and extracellular-intracellular transport, and even intracellular distribution may be changed.

3. Binding may be modified in disease state, due to changes in nature or amount of protein, dehydration or alteration of pH.

4. Binding may be modified in the presence of other substances, as in combination drug therapy.

II. PRESENTATION OF BINDING DATA

A. Percentage of Drug Bound

Table 4.1 and Figure 4.1A present hypothetical data for free and total drug concentration in a 10^{-4} M protein solution from which can be calculated the per-

TABLE 4.1

Values used for plotting binding data by various techniques

[D]* Molar	[D] + [PD†] Molar	Percentage Drug Bound	r‡	1/r	1/[D]	r/[D]
10^{-5}	1.99×10^{-5}	50	0.099	10	10^5	10^4
10^{-4}	1.9×10^{-4}	47	0.9	1.1	10^4	9×10^3
10^{-3}	1.5×10^{-3}	33	5.0	0.2	10^3	5×10^3
10^{-2}	1.09×10^{-2}	8	9.0	0.11	10^2	9×10^2
10^{-1}	1.0099×10^{-1}	1	9.9	0.1	10^1	9.9×10

* Hypothetical free drug concentration attained after equilibrium is reached with protein.

† Hypothetical total drug concentration attained after equilibrium is reached with protein.

‡ Moles of drug bound per mole of protein, assuming protein concentration is 10^{-4} M.

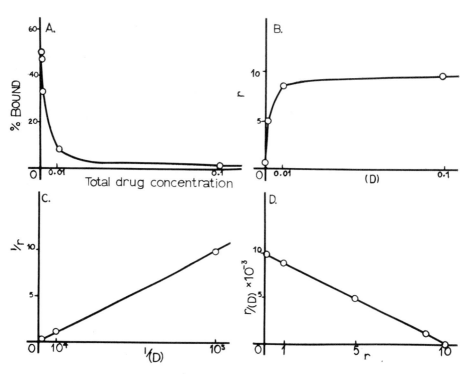

Fig. 4.1. Various plots for hypothetical binding data of Table 4.1. See text for discussion.

centage bound of the total. Such a plot merely shows that more drug is bound at lower concentrations, and may be suitable if a poorly described protein solution such as plasma is employed. However, if an accurate concentration of a pure protein can be prepared, and measurements are made at several concentrations of drug, more meaningful treatments can be employed to determine:

1. The number of classes of identical binding sites.
2. The number of binding sites of each class, N_1, N_2, etc.
3. The association constants for each class, K_1, K_2, etc.

B. Mass Action Treatment

More commonly binding is considered as a simple reversible reaction.

$$[P] + [D] \rightleftarrows [PD] \quad \text{where} \quad [P] = \text{free protein concentration}$$
$$[D] = \text{free drug concentration}$$
$$[PD] = \text{drug-protein complex concentration}$$

which at equilibrium will have the *association* constant:

(1)
$$K_A = \frac{[PD]}{[P][D]}$$

Therefore $[PD] = K_A[P][D]$, and the quantity r may be defined as

(2) $\quad r = \dfrac{\text{moles drug bound}}{\text{total moles protein}} = \dfrac{[PD]}{[PD] + [P]} = \dfrac{K_A[P][D]}{K_A[P][D] + [P]} = \dfrac{K_A[D]}{1 + K_A[D]}$

The similarity of these derivations to enzyme kinetic calculations is apparent. If there are a number (N) of identical *independent* sites, a series of independent equations can be written and summated:

(3)
$$r_1 + r_2 + \cdots r_N = r_{(total)} = \frac{NK_A[D]}{1 + K_A[D]}$$

There is often more than one type of site on a given protein, each with its own association constant, so that a more general form of equation (3) is:

(4)
$$r(total) = \frac{N_1K_1[D]}{1 + K_1[D]} + \frac{N_2K_2[D]}{1 + K_2[D]} + \cdots \frac{N_1K_1[D]}{1 + K_1[D]}$$

This is the equation for a hyperbola; the value of [D] may be measured and r(total) calculated from the free and total drug concentration and protein concentration. The data may then be plotted in several ways so as to determine the values of N and K. The example of Table 4.1 was set up as a simple, one class, type of binding with 10 sites, each exhibiting an association constant of 1000.

1. Direct plot, r vs [D], Figure 4.1B. This is a hyperbolic plot which is difficult to fit. $r = N$ at the plateau; at $r = N/2$, $[D] = 1/K$, in analogy to the Michaelis-Menten plot.

2. Reciprocal plot, 1/r vs 1/[D], Figure 4.1C. This is a straight line plot, which can be fitted by usual statistical techniques. It has the disadvantage of spreading the low values of 1/r poorly, so that some of the points are not utilized. It is analogous to the Lineweaver-Burk plot and is obtained by inverting equation (3).

(5)
$$\frac{1}{r} = \frac{1 + K[D]}{NK[D]} = \frac{1}{NK[D]} + \frac{1}{N}$$

In this plot the y intercept $= 1/N$, the slope $= 1/KN$. A similar plot, with the same limitations, has been used in which [D]/r is plotted vs $=$[D].

3. r/[D] vs r (Scatchard, 1949), Figure 4.1D. This is a straight line plot, which spreads the data well. This is the most used manner of plotting binding data and calculating the values of N and K. By rewriting (3)

(6a)
$$r + rK[D] = NK[D]$$

and by rearranging

(6b)
$$r/[D] = NK - rK$$

Here the y intercept $= NK$, slope $= K$ and x intercept $= N$

While with certain substances, such as inorganic ions, straight line plots have been obtained, curvilinear plots are generally seen with organic substances. This indicates that there are at least two classes of binding sites; in some cases three or more classes are found. Such curves may be fitted as the summation of two or more straight lines each due to a different class of binding site. Figure 4.2 presents the experimental points for interaction of salicylic acid with bovine albumin. The trial and error substitution of various values for N_1, N_2, K_1 and

$$r = \frac{N_1 K_1[D]}{1 + K_1[D]} + \frac{N_2 K_2[D]}{1 + K_2[D]}$$

K_2 in the above equation results in the theoretical curve (I and II) which is the sum of the lines (I, II) represented by the two classes.

Recently, a procedure has been published for the computer analysis of macro-molecule-ligand binding studies (Fletcher and Spector, 1968). Such procedures

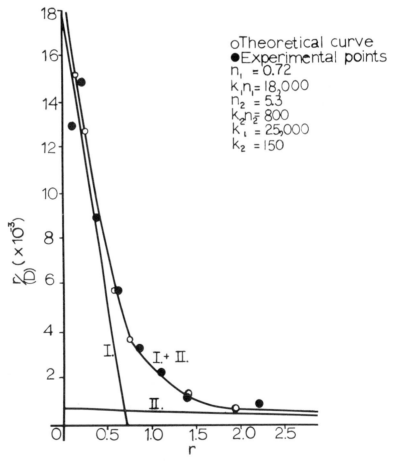

Fig. 4.2. Binding curves for salicylic acid to crystalline bovine serum albumin. Curve I, plot for one class, $N_1 = 0.72$, $K_1 = 25000$. Curve II, plot for second class, $N_2 = 5.3$, $K_2 = 150$. Curve I + II, plot for both binding sites, sum of the above.

permit a statistical evaluation of the uncertainties associated with the choice of number of classes of binding site, as well as the association coefficients.

C. Problems in the Mathematic Treatment

1. Interactions Between Groups. The above derivations assume that binding sites of a given class are independent of each other and that binding of the first molecule does not affect that of subsequent molecules. While this appears to be generally true there are recognized examples, such as the binding of oxygen to hemoglobin, where pronounced interactions do occur. Mathematical aspects of such interactions have been discussed (Nozaki *et al.*, 1957).

2. Electrostatic, Osmotic and Competition effects. It is obvious that the binding of a charged molecule alters the over-all electrostatic environment of the macromolecule, which increases the difficulty of adding another similar ion. Values can be corrected for such electrostatic interaction factors by using a rather complex equation (Scatchard *et al.*, 1950). However, most authors report uncorrected data and the association coefficients are, therefore, only apparent values. Moreover, if experiments are carried out in buffer, the bound substance may be only displacing buffer ions, and electrostatic corrections may not be indicated. However, the competition between drug and buffer ion for the same site may produce much greater changes in degree of association. Fortunately, simple anions, such as acetate (Table 4.2), are usually bound rather weakly. An alteration in pH will also affect the over-all charge on the protein, as well as the charge on individual amino acids and on the drug, and thereby affect the drug interaction.

Binding experiments in distilled water avoid the competition problem, but if a dialysis technique is employed this will introduce osmotic effects which change the concentration of the protein and will also bring the Donnan equilibrium into play. The latter can also be corrected mathematically. Nevertheless, while the measurement of binding in distilled water is theoretically easier to handle, it certainly bears little relationship to the physiological situation.

III. TECHNIQUES OF MEASUREMENT OF BINDING

A. Equilibrium Dialysis.

This commonly used procedure (Klotz *et al.*, 1946) involves equilibration of a given volume of protein solution within a dialysis bag with a known volume of a solution of the drug. Once equilibrium has been attained, measurement of the free drug concentration outside the bag will permit calculation of the amount of drug which has been taken up by the protein, subject to the reservations in Section II, C. If the protein is a single entity of known molecular weight, the molecules of drug taken up per molecule of protein (r) may be calculated and the mathematical derivation of N and K values can be carried out. The equilibrium dialysis technique is very simple and convenient for multiple samples. Drawbacks include the period of 12 hours or more required to attain equilibrium, which may permit time for decomposition of unstable compounds or for growth of bacteria. While these problems may be minimized by carrying out experiments at lower temperatures, binding will thereby be altered. Often compounds will bind not only to the glass of the containers, but also, to a greater degree, to the dialysis bag. Appropriate controls without protein should be run to detect such problems.

TABLE 4.2

Representative binding data for a number of compounds

Substance	Protein	Class I		Reference
		N_1	$K_1 (\times 10^{-4})$	
Warfarin	Human serum albumin	1	6.8	A
6-hydroxy warfarin	Human serum albumin	1	1.0	A
7-hydroxy warfarin	Human serum albumin	1	0.4	A
8-hydroxy warfarin	Human serum albumin	1	0.8	A
Octanol	Bovine serum albumin	4–5	0.3	B
Dodecanol	Bovine serum albumin	4–5	15	B
Octanoate	Bovine serum albumin	4–5	5	B
Dodecanoate	Bovine serum albumin	6–7	23	B
Octyl sulfate	Bovine serum albumin	4–5	60	B
Dodecyl sulfate	Bovine serum albumin	8–9	120	B
Laurate	Human serum albumin	2	160	C
Myristate	Human serum albumin	2	400	C
Palmitate	Human serum albumin	2	6000	C
Stearate	Human serum albumin	2	8000	C
Oleate	Human serum albumin	2	11000	C
Acetate	Bovine serum albumin	5	.008	D
Valerate	Bovine serum albumin	5	.042	D
Caproate	Bovine serum albumin	4.5	.055	D
Heptanoate	Bovine serum albumin	4.7	.155	D
Caprylate	Bovine serum albumin	4.2	.645	D
Phenol	Bovine serum albumin	Negligible		E
Benzoate	Bovine serum albumin	0.3	1.5	E
2-hydroxy benzoate	Bovine serum albumin	0.4	3.0	E
3-hydroxy benzoate	Bovine serum albumin	0.4	1.5	E
4-hydroxy benzoate	Bovine serum albumin	0.4	0.8	E
2-hydroxy-3-t-butylben-zoate	Bovine serum albumin	0.8	11	E
2-hydroxy benzamide	Bovine serum albumin	Negligible		E
2-ethoxybenzamide	Bovine serum albumin	Negligible		E

A. O'Reilly (1968). B. Reynolds *et al.* (1968). C. Goodman (1958). D. Teresi and Luck (1952). E. Davison and Smith (1961).

B. Ultrafiltration

If a solution of drug and protein is exposed under pressure to a dialysis membrane, a protein-free filtrate containing free drug only will collect beyond the membrane (Rehberg, 1943). Knowledge of the initial concentration of drug present, and of that in the ultrafiltrate, will permit calculation of the appropriate values of N and K. Pressure may be exerted by a column of mercury, or by centrifugation for 30 minutes or more. Various types of commercial apparatus are available for pressure or centrifugal dialysis. An easy technique is to centrifuge a dialysis bag containing the solution in a tube partially filled with glass beads. Ultrafiltration is faster than equilibrium dialysis since the drug is initially in direct contact with the protein, but is perhaps not so readily adapted for large numbers of samples, and uses somewhat more expensive and complicated apparatus. An important reservation is that a portion of the aqueous phase is forced away from the protein and the latter solution becomes more concentrated, thereby tending to increase binding. If the amount of solution removed by filtration is a relatively small portion of the whole, such concentration effects are quite small. A recent technique, *diafiltration*, involves a more elaborate ultrafiltration cell, in which the lost volume is replaced, thereby avoiding concentration changes.

C. Gel Filtration

A very popular technique for measuring binding is that of passing a solution of drug and protein through a column containing a dextran molecular exclusion gel to separate the protein-bound drug in a fraction emerging before the free drug peak. If the equilibrium between bound and free drug is rapidly reversible, this simple approach would not be appropriate. One would expect that the molecules of bound drug should dissociate as the protein-drug complex begins to separate from the free drug and that the drug should emerge from the column as a smear rather than discrete peaks. Nevertheless, in certain cases, as of salicylate binding (Potter and Guy, 1964) the method does succeed. This suggests that either the drug molecules slowly dissociate in some cases, or that the association constant is so great that the small amounts of drug which do dissociate are not readily detectable.

A theoretically satisfactory manner of using gel filtration is to elute the protein solution, not with water or buffer, but with a solution of the drug (Hummel and Dreyer, 1962). In this case the protein is exposed to a constant concentration of drug, and any complex should not dissociate. Analysis of eluted fractions for the drug will show a peak where the protein-drug complex emerges, followed by a dip in concentration which also measures the amount of drug taken up by the protein. A batch method using molecular exclusion gels has also been used.

D. Differential Spectrophotometry

Often the bound form of a drug will exhibit an absorption spectrum which is unlike that of the free drug. The magnitude of such an absorption peak can be used as a measure of drug binding. Alternatively, one may use displacement of another drug exhibiting a specific spectrum when protein-bound.

E. Changes in Physical Properties of Drug Solutions

Changes in EMF, conductivity, vapor pressure, boiling point, freezing point and osmotic pressure which occur when substances interact with protein have been used in determining the degree of binding. Even the solubility of drugs may be markedly altered; the administration of insoluble drugs, such as steroids, in albumin solution or in plasma is occasionally used in the research laboratory.

F. Bioassay

Generally only the unbound form of a drug can exert antibacterial or other biological action. Differences in the activity of a drug in the presence or absence of protein therefore provide a basis for measuring binding.

G. Electrophoresis and Crossing Electrophoresis

If drugs are strongly bound the drug-protein complex may be separated from free drug and/or protein by usual electrophoretic techniques, and measured by color reagents, bioautography or the use of radioactive drugs. Tata *et al.* (1961) used such an approach to show that at low concentrations labelled thyroxine was found largely in a specific thyroxine-binding globulin with high association constant but low total capacity, but that as the concentration was increased this protein became saturated and greater percentages of drug were found in the serum albumin and prealbumin.

If drugs exhibit weak affinity for protein, one would anticipate that dissociation would occur as the proteins undergo separation in the field. In the technique called *crossing electrophoresis* (Bickel and Bovet, 1962), a stripe of the free drug solution is laid perpendicularly to the protein strip. As the protein moves that portion which is continually exposed to drug binds the compound, its net charge is altered and a change in mobility is exhibited as an acceleration or deceleration of that particular area. This approach is useful for a rapid qualitative evaluation of the binding potential of a series of drugs.

IV. FACTORS AFFECTING BINDING

A. Type of Compound

Virtually every type of chemical compound, ranging from inorganic ions to organic acids and bases, dyes, vitamins, carbohydrates, steroids, proteins and even neutral hydrocarbons has been shown to undergo measurable binding. Goldstein (1949) assembled an extensive list of such compounds. At that time, most of the compounds were studied using plasma or serum as the protein, and little attempt to derive detailed information about number of sites and strength of binding was made. Many recent papers measure these parameters but the systems studied are often artificial and not related to the physiological situation.

B. Type of Protein

1. *Plasma.* Most studies have been performed with plasma, serum, or crystalline serum albumin. The latter seems to be uniquely adapted for binding. Surprisingly, many anions are bound even though it has a considerable negative charge at physiological pH. Klotz (1949) points out that albumin has a large number of alcoholic groups of serine which would be available for hydrogen bonding within the protein molecule and that the binding energy of the $RCOO^-$—OH hydrogen bond (6 kcal/mole) is considerably greater than that of the RNH_2^+—OH bond (2.5 kcal/mole). He suggests therefore that the anionic portion of the protein is effectively bound internally, leaving the cations available for external binding of anionic substances. Due to its great affinity, lack of specificity and to its high concentration in plasma, albumin is probably responsible for the major portion of plasma binding of most drugs.

Certain compounds, notably natural products, are specifically bound by other plasma proteins. A thyroxine-binding beta-globulin has been recently isolated in a high state of purity as has a thyroxine binding prealbumin. An iron binding globulin has long been recognized, as well as specific proteins reacting with vitamin D and vitamin B-12. Corticosteroid, testosterone and estrogen binding proteins are also known in plasma and tissues. A method for the measurement of progestational hormones in plasma depends upon the displacement of labelled corticosterone from a protein by the hormone-containing extract.

2. *Tissue proteins.* A variety of tissue constituents bind drugs and contribute to the localization of certain compounds. For example, cardiac glycosides and procaine bind to cardiac proteins, thyroxine to microsomes of liver and muscle, estradiol is taken up by the cytoplasmic and nuclear fraction of the endometrium, etc. Most of such studies are relatively crude measures of the uptake of compounds to tissue homogenates, or to centrifugal fractions. Tissue proteins are generally too insoluble and too poorly understood for more definitive studies.

As noted in Chapter 3, other macromolecules, such as nucleic acids or melanin, can also react reversibly with specific compounds.

C. Physiological and Pathological Conditions

Differences in thyroxine binding in patients exhibiting obesity, thyrotoxicosis, hypothyroidism, and severe illness, all have been reported by various investigators. Changes in the vitamin B-12 binding proteins have been seen in patients with polycythemia vera and leukemia, and in cortisol binding in stress conditions (postoperative, infections, burns) but not in Cushing's nor in Addison's syndromes. Differences in binding between the fetus or newborn and the adult have been frequently reported. In one study, Ganshorn and Kurz (1968) showed with 16 of 17 drugs that the plasma free drug concentrations were 1.2 to 2.4 times as great in the newborn as in the adult. Differences in blood-brain barrier, kidney function and drug metabolizing enzymes are also conspicuous in the newborn—this over-all picture must explain the increased drug sensitivity and toxicity frequently seen in the very young.

D. Species and Genetic Variation

A number of studies have compared the affinity of specific drugs for plasma, serum or crystalline albumin in various species. Differences may be quite dramatic—Sturman and Smith (1967) found that the monkey, rabbit and guinea pig, like man, bound salicylate to plasma to the extent of 50 to 90% depending on the drug concentration; while 7 other species bound this drug less than 20%. Borga *et al.* (1968) found equally large differences among 5 species in the binding of the basic drug, desipramine.

Of more immediate clinical significance may be genetic differences which may exist in the human. It has been reported that the protein bound iodine in Negro pre-adolescent children significantly exceeds that of white children (Starr *et al.*, 1967). Differences in the thyroxine binding globulin, total gamma globulin and albumin concentrations, but not in the thyroxine binding prealbumin, were seen. Genetic albumin variants which exhibit differences in thyroxine, bromphenol blue and barbiturate affinity, have also been reported in various American Indian tribes.

V. APPROACHES TO INVESTIGATING THE NATURE OF THE INTERACTION BETWEEN DRUG AND MACROMOLECULE

A. Structure of Drug

Forces which may be involved in binding of drugs include ion-ion interactions, hydrogen bonding, dipole-dipole interactions and van der Waals-London forces.

Some idea of the relative importance of the various forces may be inferred by comparing binding of various related structures (Table 4.2), although few comprehensive studies have been made.

1. *Major interacting group.* The presence of an ionizing group seems to confer the greatest affinity (largest association constant). Table 4.2 shows that benzoic acid binds more strongly than does phenol, or two benzamide derivatives, and that the long chain carboxylic acids and sulfates have greater affinities than comparable alcohols.

2. *Nature and position of substituents.* Polar substituents such as the hydroxyl group can contribute to interaction. In the benzoic acid series (Table 4.2), hydroxyl groups increase the association constants but not the apparent number of binding sites. *Ortho* hydroxyl or amino substituted compounds are more strongly bound than corresponding *meta* or *para* substituted derivatives. Klotz *et al.* (1948) has suggested that such ortho substituted compounds undergo hydrogen bonding within the drug molecule, whereas the meta and para isomers can exhibit more interaction with water molecules which tends to prevent binding to protein. In contrast, O'Reilly (1968, Table 4.2) has demonstrated reduced affinities of three hydroxylated warfarin molecules for albumin, and correlates this finding with the observation that only warfarin is found in plasma while only its hydroxy-metabolites are found in urine.

As noted in the table, non-polar alkyl chains, either as substituents on aromatic acids or in straight chain alcohols, acids and sulfates also increase binding markedly. Such enhancement is due to the lipophilic portions of both the protein and the bound substance, rather than to hydrogen bonding. The correlation between association constant and alkyl chain length in the fatty acid series was also seen in the second class of binding (Teresi and Luck, 1952). In binding studies with crystalline albumin, one must carefully remove by extensive dialysis or charcoal treatment the fatty acids which remain bound during the purification process, otherwise there will be extensive competition effects with other anions.

3. *Aromatic rings.* Such rings have "pi" electrons which can contribute to lipophilic attraction.

4. *Optical and geometric isomerism.* It is not surprising that proteins possessing optically active amino acids should show specificity for optical or geometric isomers, e.g., McMenamy and Oncley (1958) noted that D tryptophan showed no appreciable binding to mercaptalbumin, while the L-isomer was extensively bound.

B. Use of Chemically Modified Proteins

The nature of the binding group on the protein may be studied by reacting the protein with a series of "covering" groups. Salicylate and methyl orange binding to bovine serum albumin was not significantly affected by procedures such as iodination of tyrosine moieties, methylation of carboxyl groups, oxidation of sulfhydryl groups or guanidination of lysine moieties, but was totally abolished by acetylation of the amino groups (Davison and Smith, 1961; Klotz, 1949). This suggests that such anions interact predominantly with the positively charged amino groups of albumin. Other protein modifying reagents which have been used include carbobenzoxy chloride, dinitrofluorobenzene, nitrous acid, phenyl isocyanate and urea.

C. Acidity of the Protein Solution

The effect of pH on binding may afford some clues as to the site of binding. For example, since the histidine residues in albumin ionize over the range of pH 5 to 6, a substance interacting with this amino acid should undergo profound changes in affinity in this pH range. The observation of Klotz (1949) that binding of anions to albumin vanishes reversibly above pH 12, where the basic groups of the albumin molecule are un-ionized, is an example of the importance of the pH of the solution.

D. Competition Effects

One of the most important and practical concerns of protein binding research deals with the competition between drugs for similar sites. Drugs of similar or markedly dissimilar structure may compete for the same position (Goldbaum and Smith, 1954; Davison and Smith, 1961; Klotz et al., 1948; Anton, 1961; Solomon et al., 1968). Estimates of the expected degree of competition, which agree well with observed effects, may be made based on the relative association coefficients.

The modern clinician recognizes that multi-drug therapy may lead to alterations in plasma concentrations and rate of excretion of drugs not only because of induction of metabolic enzymes, but also because of competition for binding sites. Anton (1961) showed that plasma levels of sulfaethylthiadiazole in the rat were reduced about two-thirds by co-administration of sulfinpyrazone, an extensively bound compound bearing no apparent similarity in structure other than a negative charge. Simultaneously, tissue levels of sulfaethylthiadiazole increased. Clearances of the sulfonamide were also affected in the dog with co-administered sulfinpyrazone.

The known effect of drugs on bilirubin distribution, notably deposition in the brain of the newborn, was discussed in Chapter 3. Another extensively investigated example of clinically important competition effects is in the area of anticoagulant and analgesic therapy. Solomon et al. (1968) found antagonism of warfarin or phenylbutazone binding in vitro by substances as varied as tolbutamide, indomethacin, sulfamethoxypyridazine, chlorophenoxyisobutyric acid and fatty acids. A number of such competing compounds have been tested in vivo in mouse and man and shown to enhance the anticoagulant response to hydroxycoumarin (Schrogie and Solomon, 1967). Aggeler et al. (1967) reported that phenylbutazone and warfarin competed for the same binding sites on plasma albumin since the apparent warfarin-albumin association constant was reduced in the presence of phenylbutazone. The potentiation of the anticoagulant response was postulated to be due to an increase in the concentration of free warfarin which had been displaced by phenylbutazone. The increase in concentration of unbound drug also resulted in its more extensive metabolism.

An unusual example of interaction in binding was the observation of Dollery et al. (1961) that chlorothiazide could increase fourfold the binding of the ganglionic blocking agent pempidine. Since these two drugs are commonly given together this finding may be significant. It seems likely that the anionic chlorothiazide is acting as an intermediary between the albumin and the cationic pempidine.

E. Nuclear Magnetic Resonance Measurements

Exciting advances in determining the exact position of the binding receptor within the protein are being accomplished with high resolution nuclear magnetic resonance (Meadows *et al.*, 1967). One can assign certain NMR peaks to specific protons of given amino acids and observe changes in such peaks if the drug interaction occurs at this position. For example, the entire structure of ribonuclease is known and the position of its four histidine moieties has been ascertained and correlated with four known peaks on the NMR scan. The investigators were able to select the precise binding site of cytidine phosphate and cytosine on these histidine residues. Unfortunately, the amino acid sequence of more complex proteins has not been fully elucidated nor is their NMR spectrum so nicely defined. The structural interaction of penicillin and of sulfonamides with the albumin molecule has also been elucidated by such techniques (Jardetzky and Wade-Jardetzky, 1965).

F. Ultraviolet Absorption Spectral Measurements

As mentioned in Section III, the drug-protein complex can show an altered ultraviolet spectrum which can be used not only to measure the degree of binding but can also provide clues as to the nature of the site of interaction. The binding of anionic detergents to bovine serum albumin is accompanied by spectral shifts which are believed to be due to an interaction of the detergents with the tryptophan moieties of the protein (Polet and Steinhardt, 1968).

G. Thermodynamic Functions of Binding, ΔF, ΔH, ΔS

These values have been calculated in a few cases (Klotz, 1948; Clausen, 1966) by carrying out binding experiments at more than one temperature. Binding energies (ΔF) ranging from -3.7 kcal/M for the chloride ion to -11 kcal/M for dodecyl sulfate indicate the magnitude of the hydrophobic forces as opposed to the ion-ion attraction. Small heats of reaction (ΔH) are observed, but entropy changes, ΔS, have always been found to be positive. It would be anticipated that a negative entropy change should have been found since complexing would increase the order of the system—the positive entropy changes suggest that water molecules adhering to the protein are being liberated.

In conclusion: the study of plasma protein binding provides information whereby not only the number of sites and binding affinities can be measured, but the chemical nature of the site and interaction may be evaluated. The competition between molecules is a very important clinical aspect of such experiments. Unfortunately, comparable studies on tissue binding, which are of manifest importance in determining over-all drug distribution, are not yet possible.

REFERENCES

Anton, A. H.: A drug-induced change in the distribution and renal excretion of sulfonamides. J. Pharmacol. Exp. Ther. *134:* 291–303, 1961.

Aggeler, P. M., O'Reilly, R. A., Leong, L., and Kowitz, P. E.: Potentiation of anticoagulant effect of warfarin by phenylbutazone. New Eng. J. Med. *276:* 496–501, 1967.

Bickel, M. H. and Bovet, D.: Relationships between structure and albumin-binding of amines tested with crossing-paper electrophoresis. J. Chromat. *8:* 466–474, 1962.

Borgå, O., Azarnoff, D. L. and Sjöeqvist, F.: Species differences in the plasma protein binding of desipramine. J. Pharm. Pharmacol. *20:* 571–72, 1968.

Clausen, J. Binding of sulfonamides to

serum proteins: physicochemical and immunochemical studies. J. Pharmacol. Exp. Ther. *153:* 167–175, 1966.

Davison, C. and Smith, P. K.: The binding of salicylic acid and related substances to purified proteins. J. Pharmacol. Exp. Ther. *133:* 161–170, 1961.

Dollery, C. T., Emslie-Smith, D. and Muggleton, D. F.: Action of chlorothiazide on the distribution, excretion and hypotensive effect of pempidine in man. Br. J. Pharmac. Chemother. *17:* 488–506, 1961.

Fletcher, J. E. and Spector, A. A.: A procedure for computer analysis of data from macromolecule-ligand binding studies. Computers and Biomedical Research. *2:* 164–175, 1968.

Froese, A., Sehon, A. H. and Eigen, M.: Kinetic studies of protein-dye and antibody-hapten interactions with the temperature-jump method. Canad. J. Chem. *40:* 1786–1797, 1962.

Ganshorn, A. and Kurz, H.: Unterschiede zwischen der Proteinbindung Neugeborener und Erwachsener und ihre Bedeutung für die pharmakologische Wirkung. Arch. Pharmakol. Exp. Pathol. *260:* 117–118, 1968.

Goldbaum, L. R. and Smith, P. K.: Interaction of barbiturates with serum albumin and its possible relation to their disposition and pharmacological actions. J. Pharmacol. Exp. Ther. *111:* 197–209, 1954.

Goldstein, A.: The interactions of drugs and plasma proteins. Pharm. Rev. *1:* 102–165, 1949.

Goodman, D. S.: The interaction of human serum albumin with long chain fatty acid anions. J. Am. Chem. Soc. *80:* 3892–3898, 1958.

Hummel, J. P. and Dreyer, W. J.: Measurement of protein-binding phenomena by gel filtration. Biochim. Biophys. Acta *63:* 530–532, 1962.

Jardetzky, O. and Wade-Jardetzky, N. G.: On the mechanism of binding of sulfonamides to bovine serum albumin. Mol. Pharmacol. *1:* 214–230, 1965.

Klotz, I. M.: The nature of some ion-protein complexes. Cold Spr. Harb. Symp. *14:* 97–112, 1949.

Klotz, I. M., Triwush, H. and Walker, F. M.: The binding of organic ions by proteins. Competition phenomena and denaturation effects. J. Am. Chem. Soc. *70:* 2935–2941, 1948.

Klotz, I. M., Walker, F. M. and Pivan, R. B.: Binding of organic ions by proteins. J. Amer. Chem. Soc. *68:* 1486–1490, 1946.

McMenamy, R. H. and Oncley, J. L.: The specific binding of L-tryptophan to serum albumin. J. Biol. Chem. *233:* 1436–1447, 1958.

Meadows, D. H., Markley, J. L., Cohen, J. S. and Jardetzky, O.: Nuclear magnetic resonance studies of the structure and binding sites of enzymes. I. Histidine residues. Proc. Natn. Acad. Sci. *58:* 1307–1312, 1967.

Nozaki, Y., Gurd, F. R. N., Chen, R. F. and Edsall, J. T.: The association of 4-methylimidazole with the ions of cupric copper and zinc; with some observations on 2,4-dimethylimidazole. J. Am. Chem. Soc. *79:* 2123–2129, 1957.

O'Reilly, R. A.: Mechanism for pharmacodynamics of Warfarin in man. Clin. Res. *16:* 311, 1968.

Polet, H. and Steinhardt, J.: Binding induced alterations in ultraviolet absorption of native serum albumin. Biochemistry *7:* 1348–1356, 1968.

Potter, G. D. and Guy, J. L.: A micro method for analysis of plasma salicylate. Proc. Soc. Exp. Biol. Med. *116:* 658–660, 1964.

Rehberg, P. B.: A centrifugation method of ultrafiltration using cellophane tubes. Acta Physiol. Scand. *5:* 305–310, 1943.

Reynolds, J., Herbert, S. and Steinhardt, J.: The binding of some long-chain fatty acid anions and alcohols by bovine serum albumin. Biochemistry *7:* 1357–1361, 1968.

Scatchard, G.: The attractions of proteins for small molecules and ions. N. Y. Acad. Sci. *51:* 660–692, 1949.

Scatchard, G., Scheinberg, I. H. and Armstrong, S. H.: Physical chemistry of protein solutions. IV. The combination of human serum albumin with chloride ion. J. Am. Chem. Soc. *72:* 535–540, 1950.

Schrogie, J. J. and Solomon, H. M.: The anticoagulant response to bishydroxycoumarin. II. The effect of D-thyroxine, clofibrate and norethandrolone. Clin. Pharm. Ther. *8:* 70–77, 1967.

Solomon, H. M., Schrogie, J. J. and Williams, D.: The displacement of phenylbutazone-^{14}C and warfarin-^{14}C from human albumin by various drugs and fatty acids. Biochem. Pharmac. *17:* 143–151, 1968.

Starr, P., Nicoloff, J. T. and Pilleggi, V. J.: Elevation of the protein bound iodine (PBI) and thyroxine-binding globulin (TBG) in preadolescent negro children. Clin. Res. *15:* 127, 1967.

Sturman, J. A. and Smith, M. G. H.: The binding of salicylate to plasma proteins in different species. J. Pharm. Pharmacol. *19:* 621–623, 1967.

Tata, J. R., Windnell, C. C. and Gratzer, W. B.: A systematic study of factors affecting the binding of thyroxine and related substances to serum proteins. Clin. Chem. Acta. *6:* 597–612, 1961.

Teresi, J. D. and Luck, J. M.: The combination of organic anions with serum albumin. J. Biol. Chem. *194:* 823–834, 1952.

5

Drug Entry into Brain and Cerebrospinal Fluid

DAVID P. RALL

I. INTRODUCTION

The blood brain barrier and the blood cerebrospinal fluid barrier are complex systems of passive barriers and active transport systems which appear to subserve a number of important functions (Rall, 1964). Through the formation and accumulation of cerebrospinal fluid (CSF), a hydraulic cushion is provided to float and protect the delicate brain against mechanical injury. The barriers and transport systems maintained very tight control on a concentration of certain ions within the CSF and the extracellular fluid of the brain (Bradbury, 1965; Cserr, 1965; Oppelt et al., 1963a; Oppelt et al., 1963b). These ions, calcium, magnesium and potassium, profoundly influence neuronal excitability. Therefore, if the brain is to function properly, their concentration must be controlled very finely. These barriers and transport systems exclude lipid insoluble compounds, including organic acids, bases and other compounds such as proteins. Lastly, the systems provide a path for clearance from deep within the brain of either chemical debris, such as plasma protein which has leaked in from micro-insults or the lipid insoluble products of neuronal or glial metabolism (Rall, 1967).

The brain and its fluids comprise what is basically a three compartment system (fig. 5.1). It is impossible, except under special highly artificial circumstances, to describe the exchange by two compartment analyses. The three compartments are, of course, blood or the plasma, cerebrospinal fluid, and the brain. Each can exchange, within the limitations of the system, with each other. Drugs present in the plasma, in general, enter brain and cerebropsinal fluid at about the same rate. Exchange is possible by diffusion between CSF and the extracellular fluid (ECF) of the brain. The composition of CSF is given in Table 5.1; brain ECF seems to be of similar composition. The extracellular fluid of the brain and the cerebrospinal fluid act, in a pharmacologic sense, as if they are intracellular fluids (Rall et al., 1959). In general terms if a compound is able to pass cell membranes freely and enter typical somatic cells such as muscle cells, it can pass freely into the brain and cerebrospinal fluid. Conversely, compounds which are restricted to the extracellular fluid space of the muscle, or other peripheral tissues, are not able to enter the brain and cerebrospinal fluid in any significant amount. It should be pointed out that these systems, like all biological systems, are not perfect. Any compound present in the blood will enter the brain and cerebrospinal fluid to a certain, if very limited, extent.

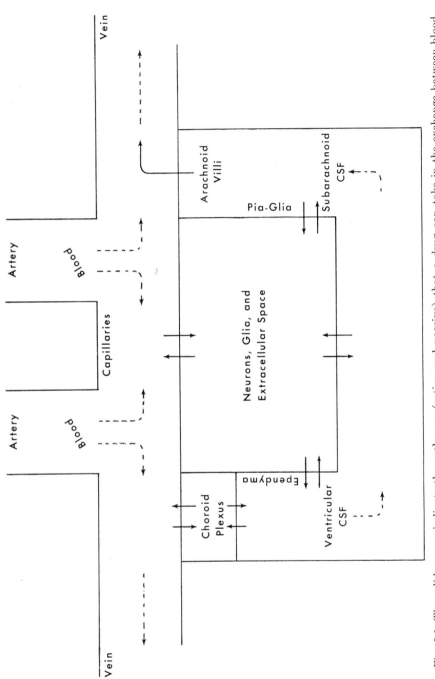

Fig. 5.1. The solid arrows indicate the pathways (active and passive) that a drug can take in the exchange between blood, brain and cerebrospinal fluid. Dashed arrows indicate blood and CSF flow.

TABLE 5.1
Composition of typical mammalian cerebrospinal fluid

	Conc CSF/Conc Pl
Na^+	0.98
Cl^-	1.10
K^+	0.615
Ca^{++}	0.49
Mg^{++}	1.39
HCO_3^-	0.87
Br^-	0.37
Protein	0.003

After Davson (1967), concentrations are in CSF and plasma water and corrected for protein binding.

II. ANATOMICAL BASIS OF BLOOD, BRAIN, AND CSF BARRIERS

In the capillary endothelial junctions in muscle, slits 50–100Å wide are present (Reese and Karnovsky, 1967). The capillaries of the brain are unlike the capillaries in muscle tissue and most other tissues. The capillary endothelial cells in brain capillaries are joined one to another by continuous tight intercellular junctions. These junctions appear to represent complete apposition of the neighboring cell membranes This suggests that materials must pass through the cells rather than between them to move from blood to brain or vice versa, as illustrated in Figure 5.2. In the choroid plexus the capillaries have open junctions leading to the interstitial space within the choroid plexus. However, the choroidal cells themselves are joined one to another with continuous tight junctions similar to those in the brain capillary. Thus, for a compound to move from blood into cerebrospinal fluid, it must pass through the choroidal epithelial cells, shown in Figure 5.3.

There are within the brain certain areas such as the area postremia and the subfornical body in which the capillaries appear to be like typical muscle capil-

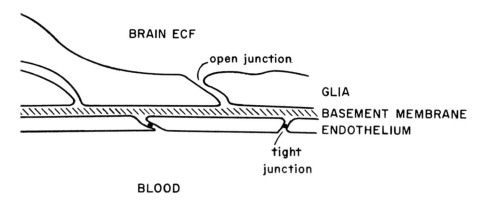

Fig. 5.2. The blood brain barrier. For a drug to diffuse from blood to brain extracellular fluid (ECF), it must move through the capillary endothelium, since the continuous band of tight junctions between the endothelium cells block intercellular passage. The basement membrane does not seem to be a barrier. (After Cserr, Fenstermacher and Rall, 1970.)

laries. Materials can pass between the capillary endothelial cells and diffuse into the substance of the brain. These areas, without a blood brain barrier, are of considerable interest; but their function at the present is unknown. They may, however, provide for the entry of small amounts of compounds which would not ordinarily enter the brain and CSF (Hoffman and Olszewski, 1961).

In many animal species, the blood brain is undeveloped at birth and becomes intact at some time during the postnatal period. This is highly species dependent (Davson, 1967). The rat appears to be quite immature at birth whereas the preliminary evidence suggests the dog, for instance, is quite mature at birth.

III. BLOOD-CSF RELATIONSHIPS

The cerebrospinal fluid is formed largely by the choroid plexuses of the lateral, third, and fourth ventricles (Davson, 1967). In man CSF production is approximately 0.5 ml/min with a total CSF volume of about 120 ml. CSF flows through the ventricular system into the subarachnoid space surrounding not only the brain, but the spinal cord as seen in Figure 5.4. Fluid formed by the choroid plexus of each lateral ventricle flows through the foramen of Monro to the third ventricle. Fluid is added by the choroid plexus at the third ventricle and moves through the aqueduct of Sylvius to the fourth ventricle, located above the medulla. Fourth ventricular choroid plexus also adds fluid and CSF moves out the foramina of Luschka and Magendie to the subarachnoid space in the cisterna magna, located at the base of the skull at the junction of brain and spinal cord. Fluid can then flow either down the subarachnoid space surrounding the spinal cord, or up through the basal cisterns, and over the convexities of the brain.

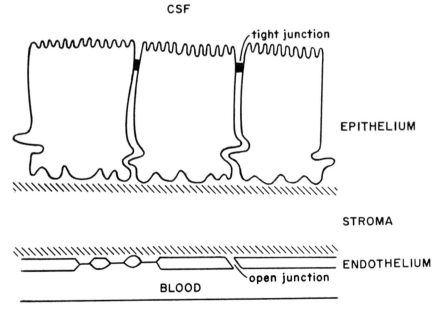

Fig. 5.3. The blood-cerebrospinal fluid barrier. For a drug to enter CSF from blood, it can pass through the open junctions, between capillary endothelial cells, through the basement membranes and stroma but is blocked from going between the epithelial cells by the continuous tight junctions. The drug must pass through the choroidal epithelial cells. (After Cserr, Fenstermacher and Rall, 1970.)

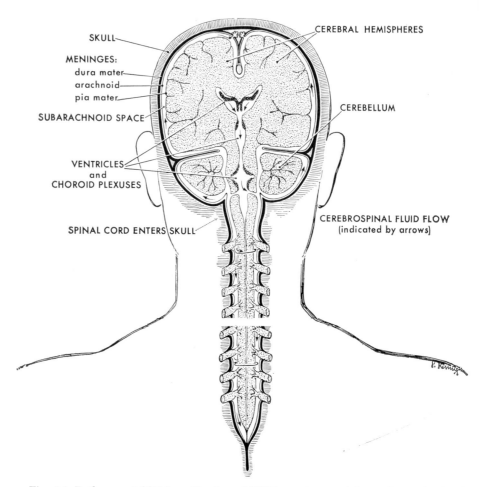

Fig. 5.4. Pathways of CSF flow. The flow of CSF from the ventricles to the cerebral and spinal subarachnoid space is shown.

The normal volume in man of the ventricular spaces is 20 ml (see Millen and Woollam, *The Anatomy of the Cerebrospinal Fluid*, 1962). CSF returns to the general circulation via a number of pathways. One, the most important, is the arachnoid granulations (Welch and Friedman, 1960). These have been shown to act as if they were one way pressure sensitive flap valves. If the hydrostatic pressure in the subarachnoid space is higher than that of the venous sinus, these valves open and CSF in bulk moves into the blood stream. If the cerebrospinal venous sinus pressure, on the other hand, exceeds that of the subarachnoid system, then these valves are forced shut and blood does not regurgitate to the CSF.

There exists, in normal situations, both an electrical potential gradient and a hydrogen ion gradient between CSF and blood. Both factors can influence drug distribution. In mammals the steady state DC potential between blood and cerebrospinal fluid averages 3–4 millivolts with the CSF positive (Held *et al.*, 1964). The magnitude and direction of this gradient is a function of pH of the blood. As the blood becomes more alkaline, the gradient becomes negative with respect to CSF so that when the blood pH is 7.5 the CSF has a negative gradient of a few millivolts. There is normally a small pH gradient between plasma and CSF with the CSF slightly more acid (Rall *et al.*, 1959). This would favor the slight concentration in CSF of weak organic bases and exclusion from CSF of organic acids. In metabolic acidosis, however, this gradient can become reversed, i.e., CSF is alkaline to blood, and often is quite pronounced. As the blood becomes increasingly acid, the CSF maintains an essentially unchanged pH because of the impermeability of the barrier to bicarbonate and the diffusability of CO_2. The opposite happens in metabolic alkalosis. Thus, in the instance of metabolic acidosis or alkalosis, rather large pH gradients can be generated between blood and CSF. These gradients can affect distribution of weak organic acids or bases. It might be mentioned that in respiratory acidosis or alkalosis, the gradient is obliterated and the blood and CSF pH move up or down together.

IV. CSF-BRAIN RELATIONSHIPS

The ependyma is that barrier which separates ventricular fluid from brain and is similar to the pia-glia which separates the subarachnoid fluid from the brain or spinal cord (Brightman, 1965). In these barriers, tight intercellular junctions do not exist and materials of large molecular size, such as ferritin, can move freely between the cells into the extracellular fluid of the brain. In spite of considerable controversy over the past decade, it seems now clear that there exists an extracellular fluid space in the brain approximately similar to that of muscle and other body tissues, i.e., 15–20% (Rall, 1967; Rall *et al.*, 1962). It can be demonstrated that materials can diffuse relatively freely in either direction between cerebrospinal fluid and extracellular fluid deep into brain tissue.

V. DRUG ENTRY INTO CSF AND BRAIN FROM BLOOD

It might be instructive to describe the problems a typical drug might have in entering the brain and cerebrospinal fluid from plasma. First, if the drug is plasma protein bound, that fraction which is bound cannot enter the CSF and brain. Therefore, it is only the free fraction which can be expected to equilibrate with CSF or brain ECF across either the choroid plexus or the brain capillary. Its ability to pass through the choroidal cells or capillary endothelial cells will be a function of its lipid solubility at body pH. If it is lipid soluble, it will diffuse rapidly and if it is partially ionized and moderately lipid soluble it will move in, but at a much slower rate. Such relationships for certain drugs are listed in Tables 5.2 and 5.3 for CSF entry, and graphically for three typical drugs in Figure 5.5. If it is lipid insoluble, or a very large molecule, or totally ionized, it will not be able to cross these cell membranes unless it belongs to a very small group of compounds which are actively transported into the brain and CSF, such as certain sugars and amino acids (Fishman, 1964).

If it is able to diffuse through the choroidal endothelial cells, its rate of equilibration within the CSF on one hand or the extracellular fluid of the brain on the other would be a function of the permeability of the respective barriers to that compound. A higher concentration may exist in one fluid than the other and therefore the possibility exists for diffusion across the ependyma either from CSF in the brain or vice versa. In the CSF the compound will move by bulk flow out of the ventricular system into the subarachnoid space, over the convexity of the brain and be removed from the CSF by return to the blood stream through the

TABLE 5.2

Partition coefficients and permeability coefficients for drugs mainly unionized at body pH with respect to entry into CSF

	% Un-ionized	Chloroform: Water Partition Coeff.	Heptane:Water Partition Coeff.	Blood-CSF Permeability Coeff. (min⁻¹)
Thiopental	61.3	102	0.95	0.50–0.69
Aniline	99.8	17	0.55	0.40–0.69
Aminopyrine	99.6	73	0.15	0.25–0.69
4-Aminoantipyrine	99.9	15	.03	0.69
Pentobarbital	83.4		<.05	0.17
Antipyrine	>99.9	28	0.04	.12–0.21
Acetanilide	>99.9	3	.01	.039
Barbital	55.7–71.5	2	.005	.026–.029
N-Acetyl-4-aminoantipyrine	>99.9	1.5	.004	.0051–0.012
Sulfaguanidine	>99.8		<0.001	.003

* This table compiled from Mayer *et al.*, J. Pharmacol. Exp. Ther. *127:* 205–211, 1959; and Brodie *et al.*, J. Pharmacol. Exp. Ther. *130:* 20–25, 1960.

TABLE 5.3

Physical characteristics and permeability coefficients for drugs mainly ionized at pH 7.4 with respect to entry into CSF

	pKa	% Un-ionized at pH 7.4	Blood-CSF Perm. Coeff. (min⁻¹)
5-Sulfosalicylic Acid	Strong	0	<0.0001
N-Methyl Nicotinamide	Strong	0	0.0005
5-Nitrosalicylic Acid	2.3	0.001	0.001
Salicylic Acid	3.0	0.004–.01	0.0026–.006
Sulfanilic Acid	3.2	0.01	0.005
Mecamylamine	11.2	0.016	0.021
Quinine	8.4	9.09	0.078

* This table compiled from Rall *et al.*, J. Pharmacol. Exp. Ther. *125:* 185–193, 1959; Mayer *et al.*, J. Pharmacol. Exp. Ther. *127:* 205–211, 1959; and Brodie *et al.*, J. Pharmacol. Exp. Ther. *130:* 20–25, 1960.

arachnoid granulation. If a compound enters the CSF only very slowly, it will never achieve a very high concentration because of its bulk flow and removal of CSF. Albumin is present in the plasma at a concentration of about 30 mg/ml. In CSF, depending on location and sampling site, the albumin concentration is about 0.15 mg/ml. Thus, for years normal mammals maintain a CSF/plasma ratio of this large molecule of 0.005. This low ratio which can be demonstrated also by the use of isotopically labelled albumin, is largely due to the brisk flow and bulk removal of CSF. If the compound is a weak organic acid or base, there is a possibility that it might be removed by an active process (analogous to that in the proximal renal tubule) at the choroid plexus (Rall and Sheldon, 1961). It can be pumped from CSF to blood by the choroidal cells.

The two other potential entry sites for compounds into the brain and CSF are first those areas within the brain which are without a blood brain barrier, which might allow small amounts of materials to enter and second there exists the possibility that the vessels within the subarachnoid space may allow certain

DRUG ENTRY INTO RABBIT BRAIN

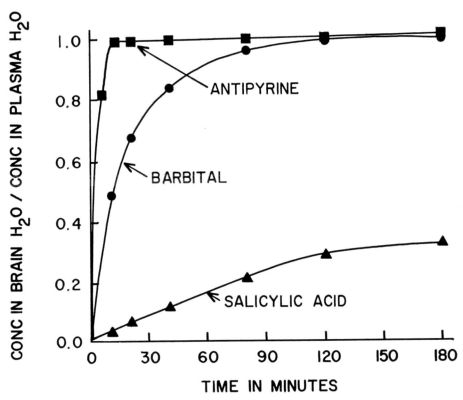

Fig. 5.5. Entry of antipyrine, barbital and salicylic acid (see Tables 5.2 and 5.3 for ionization and lipid solubility) into rabbit brain during a period of constant plasma concentration. Data from Mayer et al., 1959.

compounds to diffuse into the subarachnoid cerebrospinal fluid. If a compound enters brain at some site which is devoid of the barrier aspect of the typical brain capillary intercellular junctions, such as the area postrema in the medulla, it can diffuse through the extracellular space of the brain, either to the ventricular or subarachnoid space and be washed away by the CSF. Hoffman and Olszewski (1961) demonstrated such a pattern with fluorescein. It is clear, through all this process, that there are differing rates of equilibration, not only in different parts of the cerebrospinal fluid, but in different parts of the brain as a compound approaches a steady state. Roth and Barlow (1961) utilizing autoradiographic technics have demonstrated the patterns of equilibration of a number of drugs as they enter the brain from plasma.

VI. METHODS FOR STUDYING DRUG ENTRY AND EXIT

There are three general methods for studying the exchange of drugs between blood, brain and CSF: 1) utilizing intravenous drug administration; 2) utilizing ventricular perfusion; and 3) utilizing in vitro choroid plexus incubation. The entry of drugs from the blood into the cerebrospinal fluid after intravenous administration is straight forward and appropriate analogies can be made with renal studies (Rall *et al.*, 1959). The plasma concentration must be maintained constant during the experiment and the cerebrospinal fluid can be sampled serially from the ventricle, the cisterna magna or in certain species the lumbar sac to obtain meaningful data for kinetic analysis. If only a single dose of the drug has been given and the plasma concentration is falling, the kinetics of entry in the face of the falling concentration is so complex as to make simple analysis impossible. In general, drugs will enter the ventricles more rapidly than the cisterna magna and the lumbar sac. It is possible to sample the brain at different sites at the end of such experiments. It is also feasible, with radio-labelled compounds, to perform radioautography of the whole brain. This can yield very useful information. It is important in such studies to relate the concentrations in CSF and brain to the drug concentration in plasma which is not bound to plasma protein. It is also important, if the compounds are partially ionized, to consider the effects of the pH gradient and the DC potential difference.

The various techniques of ventricular perfusion are less useful for the simple study of the entry of compounds in the brain and CSF, but are more useful for the analysis of mechanisms of entry and special problems (Cserr *et al.*, 1970; Rall, 1967; Rall *et al.*, 1962). If the ventricular system is perfused with an inert compound such as inulin (of which very little will diffuse into the brain), the dilution of the inulin in the effluent is an index that can be used to measure the rate of newly formed cerebrospinal fluid (Davson, 1967). This is a useful method of measuring the effect of agents which affect CSF production.

The movement of compounds from CSF into brain can be studied using the ventricular perfusion technic. After the perfusion, serial samples of brain tissue can be taken on an axis perpendicular to the ependyma and assayed for the tracer. With inert extracellular markers such as sucrose it is possible to demonstrate a diffusion gradient from the ventricular surface deep into the brain. This technique has been useful in estimating extracellular space of the normal brain and could be useful for similar studies in diseased and pathological situations. If such an experiment is done with a compound which is highly diffusible with respect to capillaries of the brain, very little will be found in the brain tissue. The material will diffuse into the first few capillaries beneath the ependyma and be removed. No compound can be detected beyond the first millimeter or two of brain tissue. Pentothal and tritiated water are examples. More interesting are intermediate situations in which the compound will slowly move into cells, neurons or glia and at the same time slowly diffuse out of the brain capillary. Intermediate gradient profiles are then obtained which cannot be strictly accounted for by diffusion. Further, if the compound is metabolized or bound by cells within the brain, characteristic profiles will be observed (Cserr *et al.*, 1970). These relationships are shown in Figure 5.6.

Ventricular perfusion may be used to study the extraction of compounds by the active transport processes at the choroid plexus (Davson, 1967). In a typical experiment, if phenol red and inulin are perfused through the ventriculocisternal system, it can be demonstrated that the removal of phenol red is much greater than that of inulin and the difference between the two would represent the active removal of this organic acid by the choroid plexus.

The perfusion of the ventriculocisternal system by synthetic CSF, at the same

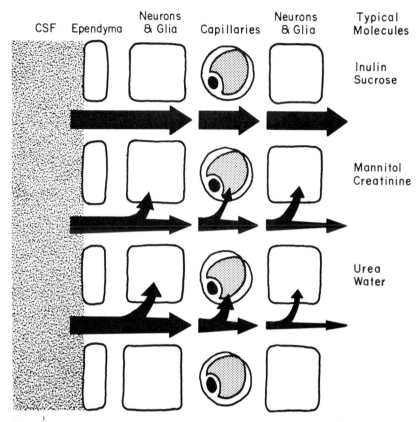

Fig. 5.6. The cerebrospinal fluid-brain barrier. Potential pathways for diffusion of typical substances from CSF into brain extracellular fluid, the cells of the brain, and into cerebral capillaries. The width of the arrow indicates the concentration of the substance.

time drug is infused intravenously into the animal, can allow for qualitative study of the entry of the compound into CSF. It must be recognized, however, that this is not purely entry into CSF, but a mixture of entry directly into CSF and entry by diffusion through brain capillaries and extracellular space of the brain across the ependyma and into the CSF. Whether future techniques will allow the resolution of these two mechanisms of entry by ventricular perfusion is yet uncertain.

The final technique is to incubate the isolated choroid plexus in artificial cerebrospinal fluid solutions and to assay it for the uptake of organic acids and bases (Rall and Sheldon, 1961). Many organic bases, such as choline, are concentrated by the choroid plexus. The effects of competition with analogs, temperature and metabolic poison can be demonstrated.

VII. PATHOLOGICAL SITUATIONS

Disease and altered physiological states can alter the blood brain and CSF barriers. Hypercarbia induced by breathing high concentrations of CO_2 can increase the concentration ratios for a number of compounds in brain and CSF (Goldberg *et al.*, 1961), possibly by capillary dilatation induced by increased blood pCO_2. Bacterial infection (meningitis) accompanied by leucocyte infiltration can increase the permeability of the blood CSF barrier (Petersdorf and Harter, 1961). Infiltration of leukemic cells in the meninges and in the CSF, however, fails to increase the permeability of the blood CSF barrier to normally poorly permeable antileukemic agents (Rieselbach *et al.*, 1963). Recent studies have shown that experimental brain tumors increase the permeability of the central portion of the tumor such that no significant barrier exists to such ionized and lipid-insoluble drugs as p-aminohippurate and inulin. The area of mixed tumor and normal brain located at the growing edge of the tumor is only slightly more permeable to these drugs than is normal brain. Shapiro and Ausman (1969), therefore, have suggested that a functional barrier at the growing edge of the tumor, the area in which tumor cells are actively proliferating and most sensitive to antineoplastic agents, may help explain the general failure of chemotherapeutic agents in the treatment of brain tumors. It is clear that as precise technics are developed for the study of drug exchange in normal brain, these technics must be applied to situations involving pathology of the brain.

REFERENCES

Bradbury, M. W. B. and Davson, H.: The transport of potassium between blood, cerebrospinal fluid and brain. J. Physiol. (London) *181:* 151–174, 1965.

Brightman, M. W.: The distribution within the brain of ferritin injected into cerebrospinal fluid compartments. II. Parenchymal distribution. Amer. J. Anat. *117:* 193–220, 1965.

Cserr, H.: Potassium exchange between cerebrospinal fluid, plasma and brain. Amer. J. Physiol. *209:* 1219–1226, 1965.

Cserr, H. F., Fenstermacher, J. D. and Rall, D. P.: Permeabilities of the choroid plexus and blood-brain barrier to urea. *Proc. Int. Colloquim on Urea and the Kidney*, Sarasota, Florida. Excerpta Medica, Amsterdam, pp. 127–137, 1970.

Davson, H.: *Physiology of Cerebrospinal Fluid*, Little Brown Co., Boston, Mass., 1967.

Fishman, R. A.: Carrier transport of glucose between blood and cerebrospinal fluid. Amer. J. Physiol. *206:* 836–844, 1964.

Goldberg, M. A., Barlow, C. F., and Roth, L. J.: The effects of carbon dioxide on the entry and accumulation of drugs in the central nervous system. J. Pharmacol. Exp. Ther. *131:* 308–318, 1961.

Held, D., Fencl, V. and Pappenheimer, J. R.: Electric potential of cerebrospinal fluid. J. Neurophysiol. *27:* 942–959, 1964.

Hoffman, H. J. and Olszewski, J.: Spread of sodium fluorescein in normal brain tissue. Neurology, Minneap. *11:* 1081–1085, 1961.

Mayer, S., Maickel, R. P. and Brodie, B. B.: Kinetics of penetration of drugs and other foreign compounds into cerebrospinal fluid and brain. J. Pharmacol. Exp. Ther. *127:* 205–211, 1959.

Oppelt, W. W., MacIntyre, I. and Rall,

D. P.: Magnesium exchange between blood and cerebrospinal fluid. Amer. J. Physiol. *205:* 959–962, 1963a.

Oppelt, W. W., Owens, E. S. and Rall, D. P.: Calcium exchange between blood and cerebrospinal fluid. Life Sci. *8:* 599–605, 1963b.

Petersdorf, R. G. and Harter, D. H.: The fall in cerebrospinal fluid sugar in meningitis. Some experimental observations. Arch. Neurol. *4:* 21–28, 1961.

Rall, D. P.: The structure and function of the cerebrospinal fluid. In *The Cellular Functions of Membrane Transport*, ed. by J. F. Hoffman, p. 269, Prentice-Hall, Englewood Cliffs, N. J., 1964.

Rall, D. P.: Transport through the ependymal linings. In *Progress in Brain Research*, ed. by A. Lajtha and D. H. Ford, p. 159, Elsevier Publishing Company, Amsterdam, 1967.

Rall, D. P.: Comparative pharmacology and cerebrospinal fluid. Proc. Int. Symposium on Comparative Pharmacology, Washington, D. C. Fed. Proc. *26:* 1020–1023, 1967.

Rall, D. P., Oppelt, W. W. and Patlak, C. S.: Extracellular space of brain as determined by diffusion of inulin from the ventricular system. Life Sci. *2:* 43–48, 1962.

Rall, D. P. and Sheldon, W.: Transport of organic acid dyes by the isolated choroid plexus of the spiny dogfish, *S. acanthias*. Biochem. Pharmacol. *11:* 169–170, 1961.

Rall, D. P., Stabenau, J. R., and Zubrod, C. G.: Distribution of drugs between blood and cerebrospinal fluid: general methodology and effect of pH gradients. J. Pharmacol. Exp. Ther. *125:* 185—193, 1959.

Reese, T. S. and Karnovsky, M. J.: Fine structural localization of a blood-brain barrier to exogenous peroxidase. J. Cell Biol. *34:* 207–217, 1967.

Rieselbach, R. E., Morse, E. E., Rall, D. P., Frei, E., III, and Freireich, E. J.: Intrathecal aminopterin therapy of meningeal leukemia. Arch. Internal Med., *111:* 620–630, 1963.

Roth, L. J. and Barlow, C. F.: Drugs in the brain. Science *134:* 22–31, 1961.

Shapiro, W. R. and Ausman, J. I.: Chemotherapy of brain tumors: A clinical and experimental review. In *Recent Advances in Neurology*, ed. by F. Plum, pp 149–235, F. A. Davis Co., 1969.

Welch, K. and Friedman, V.: The cerebrospinal fluid valves. Brain *83:* 454–469, 1910.

6

Placental Transfer of Drugs

JOSEPH ASLING
E. LEONG WAY

I. INTRODUCTION

Among all the membrane systems of the body, the placenta is unique. It separates two distinct individuals with differing genetic compositions, physiologic responses and sensitivities to drugs. Through the placenta the fetus obtains nutrients and eliminates metabolic waste products without depending on its own immature organs. This dependence, however, places the fetus at the mercy of the placenta when foreign substances appear in the mother's blood.

Pregnant women in the United States take an average of four prescription drugs, plus proprietary compounds, and have an undetermined exposure to potentially toxic substances in food, cosmetics, and household chemicals, as well as in the general environment (Barnes, 1968). The effects of these substances in pregnancy are poorly known. The ultimate concern when studying placental transfer of foreign substances is the effect on the fetus. In many cases, this effect is undesirable; however, with advances in intrauterine diagnosis, treatment of fetal diseases by medicines administered to the mother may be practical in the future.

Drug effects on the fetus are of two major types. Early in pregnancy during formation of the organ systems, the primary concern is morphologic abnormalities (i.e., congenital anomalies). The most dramatic example of such an effect is thalidomide which, when given to women between the fifth and seventh weeks of pregnancy, produces a high incidence of phocomelia in the fetus (Lenz, 1963). Later in pregnancy, functional considerations are of greater significance, and during delivery such factors as respiratory depression of the neonate and inability of the neonate to metabolize or eliminate a drug should be considered.

II. MECHANISMS OF PLACENTAL TRANSFER

The basic mechanisms by which substances may cross the placenta are the same as those of other biological membranes; they have been reviewed in detail by several authors. See Chapters 1 and 3. (Page, 1957; Moya and Thorndike, 1962).

A. Diffusion

Simple diffusion is the commonest mode of transport, and is presumably the mechanism of transfer for virtually all drugs and foreign substances that have been studied. Diffusion involves no metabolic energy and must, of course, result in net transfer of a substance in the direction of its concentration gradient. Depending on the physical characteristics of the transferred substance, up to several hundred milligrams per minute may cross the placenta by passive diffusion.

B. Facilitated Diffusion

Facilitated diffusion involves a carrier substance within the placenta, which acts to increase the rate of transfer beyond that which would be expected for a given substance. Glucose is apparently transferred in this manner (Folkart et al. 1960). Again, no metabolic energy may be required, and transfer is in the direction of the concentration gradient.

C. Active Transport

Some biological materials apparently cross the placenta by active transport. Demonstrating this phenomenon requires evidence (1) that the material is transferred in the direction opposite to a concentration gradient (or demonstrating the presence of a concentration gradient at equilibrium in the absence of complicating factors), (2) that the transport system may be saturated, (3) that it may be inhibited by metabolic poisons, and (4) that competition for transfer exists between structurally similar materials (Seeds, 1968). Essential amino acids are transferred to the fetus against a concentration gradient and, in the case of histidine, the natural L-isomer has been shown to cross several times as fast as the D-isomer (Page et al., 1957).

D. Pinocytosis

Pinocytosis involves active transport of specific materials across a membrane by vacuolization. Large molecules, such as immunoproteins, may be transferred by this process; such transport has been demonstrated in intestinal epithelium (Clark, 1959). If pinocytosis does occur in the placenta, it appears too slow and unimportant for the transfer of most drugs.

E. Membrane Discontinuities

The presence of small breaks in the placental membranes has been demonstrated (Page, 1957). This is apparently the mechanism by which erythrocytes cross the placenta, but the role of such pores in the transport of drugs is unknown. Since the umbilical circulation operates at a hydrostatic pressure 20–25 mm Hg above the intervillous space pressure (Page, 1959), any transfer of drugs by this method would probably be from fetus to mother.

III. PLACENTAL STRUCTURE

A. Morphology of the Placenta

The morphology of the placenta varies considerably from species to species. Six major types of placenta have been described, based on the number of membranes between maternal and fetal circulations and on the type of implantation (Martin, 1968). Considerable variation in both structure and function occurs, however, and placental morphologic characteristics may change even within a single species as gestation progresses. It is not always valid, therefore, to make inferences in one species based on quantitative data obtained in another. As a consequence it has been necessary to develop a "functional profile" for the pla-

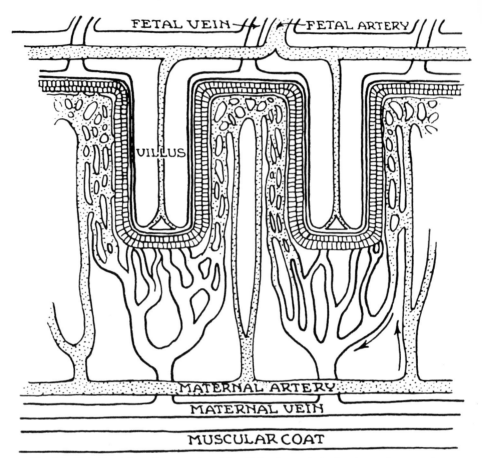

Fig. 6.1. Relationships of maternal and fetal blood vessels in the sheep placenta, demonstrating countercurrent blood flow. (From Bancroft and Barron, Anat. Rec. 1946.)

centa of each species, based on multiple physiologic criteria (Page, 1957; Greene et al., 1965).

The human placenta is of the hemochorial type. Maternal blood from the uterine arteries enters a pool called the intervillous space. Here it is exposed directly to fetal membranes, and materials need only cross the fetal trophoblast basement membrane and endothelium to enter the fetal circulation. The blood flow to the fetal side of the placenta comes from the umbilical arteries, and the fetal placental veins converge into the umbilical vein, which returns blood to the fetus. Maternal blood from the intervillous space drains into the uterine and ovarian veins and thence to the maternal systemic circulation (Fig. 6.1).

B. Fetal and Maternal Blood Supply

In recent years considerable debate has occurred concerning the relative direction of maternal and fetal blood flow. Assuming that maternal and fetal placental capillaries run parallel to each other, blood might flow in the same direction (concurrent) or in the opposite direction (countercurrent). The countercurrent system would provide for more efficient transfer of materials, for as fetal blood flowed from umbilical artery to umbilical vein, it would be exposed increasingly to arterial maternal blood, containing more of all the substances to be transferred from mother to fetus. Transfer of metabolic waste from fetus to mother would be similarly enhanced (Shapiro et al., 1967). In the human placenta, however, it would appear that direction of blood flow is neither entirely concurrent nor countercurrent, but rather a random mixture (Bartels et al., 1962).

In theory the placenta is not the only area available for maternal-fetal transfer. Fetal membranes line the entire uterine cavity, and transfer should be able to occur throughout this system. It has been held that this extraplacental transfer is significant in the transfer of some biological substances, notably large proteins (Hemmings and Brambell, 1961), but the larger surface area and blood flow of the vascular, convoluted placenta make it the only important area of diffusion for relatively small molecules such as most drugs.

Page, in his 1957 review of placental transfer mechanisms, noted that rate of transfer of materials is dependent not only on the maternal and fetal blood volumes, but on several fluid compartments within each organism. He defined six compartments (maternal and fetal extracellular and intracellular compartments, placenta, and amniotic fluid), which involve a total of fourteen unidirectional fluxes, all of which affect the rate at which a given substance disappears from maternal and fetal plasma. Plentl (1968) and Sternberg (1962) have given detailed mathematical treatments of the use of tracer techniques for placental transfer analysis.

IV. FACTORS INFLUENCING DIFFUSION ACROSS PLACENTAL MEMBRANES

A. Diffusion Equation

Simple diffusion of materials across the placenta follows the general principles of Fick's diffusion equation (Seeds, 1968):

$$(1) \qquad \frac{dQ}{dt} = \frac{KA(C_2 - C_1)}{d}$$

where: dQ/dt = rate of transfer of a substance
K = diffusion constant of the substance being transferred
A = surface area of membrane
d = thickness of membrane
C_1 and C_2 = concentrations of the substance on each side of the membrane
so that $C_2 - C_1$ represents the concentration gradient across the membrane.

According to Battaglia (1963), there are six concentration gradients involving the placenta, which may be divided into two groups of three gradients each (Fig. 6.2).

Group A: reflect gradients across the various fetal membranes, and depend on placental permeability, changes in uterine and umbilical blood flow, and changes in the metabolism of the substance in maternal and fetal tissues.

1. Maternal pool—fetal pool (chorionic gradient)
2. Fetal pool—amniotic fluid pool (amnionic gradient)
3. Maternal pool—amniotic pool (chorioamnionic gradient)

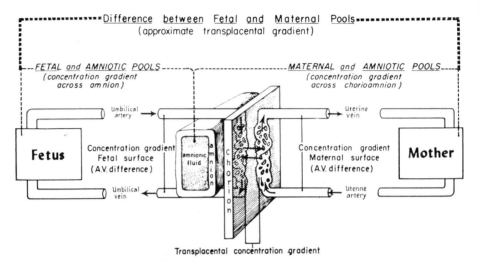

Fig. 6.2. Schematic representation of concentration gradients across the primate placenta. The three concentration differences of Group A are labelled in the upper part of the drawing with broken lead lines; the three concentration differences of Group B are labelled with solid lead lines. (From Battaglia, 1963.)

Group B: reflect specific placental transfer gradients. These are the gradients usually measured in placental transfer studies.
1. Maternal arteriovenous difference
2. Fetal arteriovenous difference
3. Transplacental concentration gradient

B. Placental Characteristics Limiting Diffusion

The placenta is not an absolute barrier; the relative rates of diffusion between different substances vary greatly. The permeability of the placenta is a function of several characteristics of both the membranes and the substance transferred. The cross-sectional area of the placenta corresponds to the functional region over which maternal and fetal blood are closely approximated. It can be enlarged by increasing either the size or the vascularity of the placenta. Fetal needs increase as gestation progresses, and these requirements are met primarily by an increase in vascularity of the placenta (Wilkin and Bursztein, 1958). Functional placental area is obviously difficult to determine directly, and consequently is usually calculated from equation 1. Direct planimetric measurements indicate that the exchange area at term is about twelve square meters. Placental accidents (infarcts, placental abruption) may suddenly decrease the effective area available for transfer, and some disorders (notably toxemia of pregnancy) are frequently associated with small placentas. Either of these conditions can compromise fetal status by decreasing placental transmission of nutrients.

The thickness of the placenta, or the distance between maternal and fetal capillary systems, depends on the number and thickness of the individual membrane layers. The diffusion rate of a given substance varies inversely with placental thickness. Since placental thickness is also difficult to estimate, it is sometimes combined with the placental area and the diffusion constant to give a "membrane resistivity" factor (d/KA):

$$(2) \qquad \frac{d}{KA} = \frac{C_2 - C_1}{dQ/dt}$$

This indicates the concentration difference necessary for a given quantity of a substance to diffuse across the placenta in a given time.

C. Drug Characteristics Limiting Diffusion

The rate of diffusion of a substance also depends on its physical characteristics. Diffusability decreases with increasing molecular weight. Substances with a molecular weight of less than 500 generally cross the placenta easily; those with a molecular weight around 1000 or higher, with difficulty. The carbohydrates raffinose (m.w. 594) and stachyose (m.w. 666) cross the chorion readily, but inulin (m.w. 6000) does not (Moore et al., 1966). Since most drugs have a molecular weight of less than 500, this is rarely a factor in limiting the rate of diffusion.

Among substances of similar molecular weight, compounds which have high lipid/water solubility ratios cross the placenta more quickly than those which are poorly lipid-soluble. Thus, placental transmission of barbital is much slower than that of the more lipid-soluble thiopental (Flowers, 1959). Some investigators have compared the placenta with the blood-brain barrier in this respect (Moya and Thorndike, 1962). Whether or not the comparison is appropriate, the similarity of these two "barriers" to each in terms of transmission of lipid-soluble materials has complicated the search for a potent anesthetic agent which does not reach the fetus in depressant quantities.

Related to lipid solubility is the ionization constant. Most ionizable compounds cross membranes in their non-ionized, more lipid-soluble form, as opposed to their more water-soluble salt. Bases with an extremely high pK_a and acids with an extremely low pK_a cross the placenta poorly. The muscle relaxants D-tubocurarine and succinylcholine are quaternary bases with high pK_a's, and their negligible placental transfer has been well utilized in Cesarean section (Cohen et al., 1953). In contrast, organic bases which are not completely dissociated at the pH of blood, cross the placenta readily. This has been demonstrated, for example, with certain local anesthetics (Shnider and Way, 1968) as well as for meperidine (Way et al., 1949).

D. Uterine and Umbilical Blood Flow

The diffusion equation discussed above (Eq. 1) does not take into account the uterine and umbilical blood flow rates, but these can be of great importance. Diffusion of molecules whose net transfer rate across the placenta is small compared with their blood concentrations (e.g., urea, sodium, chloride) is primarily limited by placental permeability, but diffusion of some substances (e.g., oxygen, water) is influenced by placental perfusion rates (Faber and Hart, 1967). If maternal placental blood flow decreases, the rate at which substances in the maternal blood are presented to the fetus decreases. Transfer rates of substances which diffuse across the placenta very slowly, will be little affected by this. The transfer rates of most drugs and nutrients which cross the placenta rapidly and in large quantities, however, will decrease, because the transplacental concentration gradient ($C_2 - C_1$) will decrease for those substances. A decrease in umbilical flow rate, by decreasing the rate at which fetal blood can clear substances which have crossed the placenta, will similarly decrease the rate of transplacental diffusion. Clinically, these changes are most commonly seen with maternal hypotension, which decreases uterine blood flow (Lucas, 1965) and umbilical cord compression, which decreases umbilical blood flow (Dawes, 1968). Either condition may be disastrous for the fetus because of decreased transfer of respiratory gases across the placenta.

Total flow may be adequate on both sides of the placenta, but distribution may still be uneven. If areas of greater maternal placental flow are opposite areas of lesser placental flow, the efficiency of transfer will decrease. This problem, which is roughly equivalent to the ventilation/perfusion defect in the lung (Comroe, 1965), has been little studied in the placenta; one would expect that such functional shunts (and anatomic shunts) may greatly affect the transfer of highly diffusable substances.

E. Protein Binding

To avoid making erroneous conclusions concerning the placental concentration gradient of a drug, several other factors need to be considered. Some substances are bound to a different extent by fetal plasma protein than by maternal plasma protein. When transplacental equilibrium exists for the unbound form of such a substance, the concentration of the bound form is higher on the side on which more protein binding has occurred. The classical example is that of oxygen and hemoglobin. Fetal hemoglobin has more affinity for oxygen than maternal hemoglobin under similar conditions of pH and temperature (Metcalfe et al., 1964). If incompletely oxygen-saturated fetal and maternal blood are allowed to equilibrate across a membrane, the partial pressure of oxygen (P_{O_2}) will be identical on both sides of the membrane, but the oxygen *content* of the fetal blood will be higher than that of the maternal blood.

F. Effect of pH

A difference in pH between maternal and fetal blood can also influence the fetal/maternal concentration gradient. Consider an organic base with pK_a approximating the pH of maternal arterial blood (7.40). Since the pH of maternal arterial blood is normally 0.10 to 0.15 pH units higher than that of umbilical vessel blood, the concentration of undissociated base will tend to be higher in the maternal blood than the fetal blood. Since the undissociated base crosses the placenta much more rapidly than the salt (see Section IV,C above) there will be a net transfer of drug from mother to fetus, and the total drug concentration will be higher in the fetus than the mother at equilibrium. This influence is not often significant, but it must be considered when dealing with ionizable compounds having pK_a's near the pH of blood.

G. Trans-placental Electro-chemical Gradient

The electro-chemical gradient across the placenta, which equals 20 millivolts (Widdas, 1961), may affect the maternal/fetal concentration gradient of ionizable compounds. Cations are attracted to the negatively charged fetal side of the placenta, introducing a potential concentration gradient.

H. Solvent Drag

The transfer of relatively large amounts of water across the placenta, in response to hydrostatic or osmotic gradients, may result in "solvent drag," increasing the transfer rate of solute beyond that which would be expected with simple diffusion (Seeds, 1968). The importance of this in drug transfer has not been defined.

I. Uptake of Drugs by Placenta and Transfer of Metabolites of Drugs

The uptake and metabolism of drugs by the placenta and the transfer of their metabolic products have rarely been studied. An apparent placental barrier exists to fluoride, not because it is impermeable, but because some is trapped by calcium-containing crystals in the placenta (Ericsson and Ullberg, 1958). Meperidine and its metabolites normeperidine and meperidinic acid traverse the placenta with ease (Tsurumi, Wilkinson and Way, unpublished). Both procaine and its biotransformation product, para-aminobenzoic acid, cross the placenta readily (Usubiaga et al., 1968). Trichloroethanol and trichloroacetic acid have been found in the fetus following maternal administration of chloral hydrate (Bernstine et al., 1954). O-toluidine, a metabolite of propitocaine, can cause fetal as well as maternal methemoglobinemia (Poppers, 1966). Ketophenylbutazone and benzopyrazone do not cross the placenta readily, but metabolites of both compounds have been found in fetal tissues (Uher et al., 1966). A drug administered to the mother might thus have a totally unexpected effect on the fetus.

V. TECHNIQUES OF INVESTIGATION OF PLACENTAL TRANSFER OF DRUGS

A. In Vivo

Investigation of placental transfer of drugs in the intact animal including humans provides information that is generally more relevant clinically than that obtained with an *in vitro* preparation. The difficulty in performing experiments on the fetus is considerable, however, and methods of obtaining human fetal blood specimens have only recently been developed.

1. **Qualitative studies of fetal pharmacologic effects.** The simplest method of determining whether a drug crosses the placenta is to administer it to the mother and look for its effect on the fetus or neonate. This technique is of value when the doses of drug involved are so small that chemical analysis is impractical, and when the fetal effect is readily observed. The placental transmission of atropine was demonstrated by administering 0.6 mg intravenously to the mother and observing an increase in the fetal heart rate (John, 1965). Infants born to opiate-addict mothers have exhibited withdrawal symptoms (Kunstadter et al., 1958). Infants of mothers who received dicumarol orally (for thrombophlebitis) have demonstrated a bleeding diathesis and a prolonged prothrombin time (Kraus et al., 1949). Such techniques need not involve biochemical analysis, and they demonstrate not only placental transfer but also fetal effect. The data obtained are only qualitative, however, and a lack of fetal changes may represent either lack of placental transfer or lack of fetal susceptibility to the drug. Moreover, such parameters as fetal heart rate are influenced by a number of factors including fetal distress, uterine contractions, and changes

in uterine blood flow. A "fetal drug effect" might, therefore, be coincidental or related to drug-induced physiologic changes in the mother. Histamine, for example, increases placental permeability to other substances, presumably by vasodilation (Dancis et al., 1962), and oxytocin decreases the rate of placental transmission of ascorbic acid (Hensleigh and Krantz, 1966).

2. Quantitative studies in animals. Early physiologic disposition studies in animals usually involved administration of the drug to the mother, followed by Cesarean section and sacrifice of the fetus. Determination of the concentration of the drug in maternal blood, fetal blood, and fetal tissue could then be carried out providing quantitative indication of the maternal/fetal concentration gradient at a specific time following injection. Only one determination per animal is possible, and to obtain a curve of fetal concentration with respect to time requires a relatively large number of animals. If animals with multiple fetuses are used, one fetus may be sacrificed at a time, but this may affect perfusion of the remaining fetuses. The demonstration of placental transmission of D-tubocurarine was made by injecting approximately ten times the paralyzing dose directly into the uterine artery of laparotomized dogs, observing the flaccidity of the fetal pups in utero, then sacrificing the pups and obtaining maternal and fetal plasma levels of D-tubocurarine (Pittinger and Morris, 1953).

Within the last ten years a more sophisticated animal preparation for study of the fetus in utero has been developed. The animal (usually a sheep, but goats and monkeys have also been used) is anesthetized with inhalation or low spinal anesthesia and the fetus or a fetal leg is delivered via a uterotomy. Umbilical and fetal vessels are then cannulated, and the fetus is either replaced in the uterus or submerged in a warm bath. The experimental conditions are then induced, and the effect on fetal blood pressure and heart rate may be monitored continuously. Samples of fetal arterial and venous blood may be withdrawn as desired through the catheters. Umbilical and uterine blood flow are measured with electromagnetic flowmeters, or by determining arterio-venous concentration differences of a continuously infused substance such as 4-aminoantipyrine (Rudolph and Heymann, 1967b). Dawes (1968) has published detailed instructions and advice regarding this sheep preparation. So far, studies using it have involved determination of regional blood flow in the fetus (Rudolph and Heymann, 1967a) and investigation of the effects of maternal hypotension on the fetus (Lucas et al., 1965), but it might easily be adapted to the study of placental transmission of drugs. Studying placental clearance of drugs by administering them to the fetus is also possible with this preparation. The experiment may be done on the day of surgery, or the incision may be closed and the experiment performed at a later date after recovery of the animals from the surgery and anesthesia. The advantages of the latter preparation are that the animal is more stable physiologically and that it may be used for several experiments. It requires, however, great care in preventing infection and other surgical complications.

3. Quantitative studies in humans. The investigation of placental transmission of drugs in humans is even more difficult than in laboratory animals since preparations such as that described above are obviously unacceptable. Most studies of drug transmission involve administering the drug to the mother just prior to vaginal delivery and obtaining fetal blood at birth by isolating a section of umbilical cord ten to fifteen inches long with two clamps. Blood is easily removed from the umbilical arteries and vein with a syringe and needle—this is superior to squeezing the contents of the cord into a test tube. Maternal blood drawn at the moment of birth makes possible the determination of fetal/maternal concentration ratios. Only one fetal sample per delivery is obtainable by this technique, and the changes in uterine and umbilical perfusion which occur as a result of labor and separation of the placenta introduce a potentially major source of error. Morishima *et al.* (1966) measured maternal and umbilical mepivacaine concentrations in patients who had mepivacaine epidural blocks for analgesia during labor; they found a fetal/maternal concentration ratio of 0.71 at equilibrium, and observed an increased incidence of neonatal depression when the concentration of mepivacaine in umbilical blood was greater than 3 μg/ml.

Alternatively, a drug may be given to the mother during elective Cesarean section. The umbilical cord is double-clamped at birth, and a maternal blood sample is obtained simultaneously. The physiologic changes occurring during vaginal delivery are replaced by the (presumably milder) changes of anesthesia and surgery. Even so, only one determination is possible per patient. Shnider and Way (1968) have analyzed the placental transfer of lidocaine by administering 3 mg/kg intravenously to women during elective Cesarean section as well as vaginal delivery and obtaining simultaneous maternal arterial, umbilical arterial, and umbilical venous blood samples. They demonstrated that the maternal decay curve of lidocaine has at least two components, with half-lives of thirty seconds and thirty minutes, respectively (Fig. 6.3) and that a significant fetal/maternal gradient exists for at least 40 minutes after injection.

The most recently developed method for determining drug concentrations of human fetal blood *in utero* was modified from the fetal scalp sampling technique introduced by Saling (1964). During labor, the fetal head is exposed transvaginally, using a modified speculum or metal cone. The scalp is sprayed with ethyl chloride, to induce reactive hyperemia. A small nick is made in the scalp with a guarded knife tip, and the arterialized capillary blood produced is drawn into a long capillary tube. The technique is used by Saling and by others to determine carbon dioxide tension and pH in cases of fetal distress. Using this technique, several samples of fetal blood may be obtained during labor in addition to the sample which may be drawn from the umbilical cord at birth. The primary disadvantage is that sample size is small (about 0.2 ml) and extremely sensitive analytic techniques must therefore be used. Scalp hematomata and infections can occur, but with proper technique and nursery care, their incidence is extremely low. Only one drug has yet been studied using this technique. Maternal and fetal blood mepivacaine concentrations have been determined following paracervical block, demonstrating that the fetal bradycardia which occasionally follows paracervical block is associated with a high fetal blood mepivacaine concentration (Fig. 6.4) (Asling *et al.*, 1970; Gordon, 1968).

B. In Vitro

In vitro methods for determining placental transfer involve either perfusion of the placenta or mounting placental membrane between two chambers. Neither method has been used extensively for the study of drug transport.

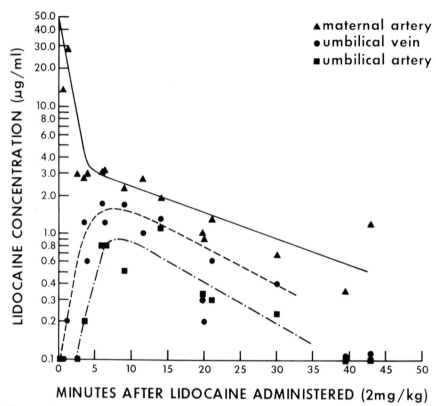

Fig. 6.3. Concentrations of lidocaine in plasma from maternal vein, umbilical vein, and umbilical artery blood following maternal intravenous injection of 2 mg/kg lidocaine. (From Shnider and Way, 1968.)

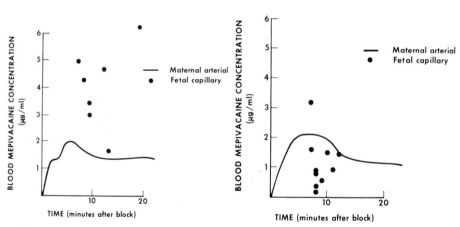

Fig. 6.4. Mepivacaine concentrations in maternal and fetal blood following paracervical injection of 200 mg mepivacaine in 17 patients. Solid lines indicate mean maternal arterial blood level curves, and points indicate fetal scalp blood samples (one point for each fetus). Fetuses which developed bradycardia following the block (*left*) had higher mepivacaine blood levels than fetuses who did not develop bradycardia (*right*). (From Asling *et al.*, 1970.)

Placental perfusion studies. Placental perfusion preparations have been described by several authors. Faber and Hart (1967) have performed Cesarean sections on rabbits, removed one fetus, and perfused the fetal side of the placenta with fresh rabbit blood using a pump which duplicated the fetal heartbeat. The maternal side of the placental circulation was left intact. Using radioactive tracers, they were able to measure the effect of umbilical perfusion rate on the flux of water, electrolytes, and acetylene. The maternal side of the placenta can be perfused either by clamping the aorta and perfusing distally to the clamp, or by removing the uterus and perfusing both uterine arteries.

The fetal side of the human placenta has been perfused following delivery (Panigel, 1962; Hensleigh and Krantz, 1966), but since the placenta has been removed from the uterus, the maternal circulation cannot be supplied and drug transport cannot be studied. Perfusion of the fetal side of the human placenta at Cesarean section, leaving the placenta in the uterus, has not been reported to the author's knowledge.

Separation of the layers of the placenta is technically difficult. This has, however, been done with both animal and human tissue, and the permeability of the various layers to water, carbohydrates and urea has been investigated (Barton and Baker, 1957; Battaglia, 1964; Moore et al., 1966). Studies of drug transport in such preparations have not been done.

Placental slices and tissue culture are not designed to measure placental transmission. They can be used, however, to investigate placental metabolism of drugs, and the effect of drugs on placental metabolism of physiological materials. Uher and co-workers (1966) have made trophoblast tissue cultures, and demonstrated that ketophenylbutazone interferes with carbohydrate metabolism of trophoblast. Sulfamethoxypyrimidine also decreases glucose utilization by trophoblast, and substantial amounts of this drug are acetylated by this tissue.

VI. TRANSMISSION OF SPECIFIC DRUGS

The placental transmission of numerous drugs has been demonstrated; those drugs frequently administered during pregnancy and labor have been studied most. A few examples are given in Table 6.1. Detailed data on these and many other drugs are available in numerous published reviews (Baker, 1960; Hagermann and Villee, 1960; Moya and Thorndike, 1962; Nyhan and Lampert, 1965; Moya and Smith, 1965; Shnider, 1966). With few exceptions, these compounds cross the placenta readily, presumably by passive diffusion.

Detailed mathematical analysis of transfer characteristics of individual drugs has rarely been done. The time required for a drug to appear in the fetus following maternal administration and the time required to reach fetal/maternal equilibrium give some indication of comparative rates of placental transfer, but they are influenced by numerous variables other than placental permeability and drug characteristics. First, the route of maternal administration in these studies may be intravenous, submucosal, intramuscular, epidural or oral, with varying rates of uptake into the maternal circulation. Second, the time required between the administration of a drug to the mother and its earliest detection in fetal blood is as much a function of the sensitivity of the analysis as the rate of placental transmission. Third, the circulatory changes which accompany expulsion

TABLE 6.1

Placental transmission data for some commonly used drugs

Compound	Time to Appear in Fetus	Time to Fetal/Maternal Concentration Equilibrium	Fetal/Maternal Concentration Ratio	Fetal or Neonatal Effect	References
Inhalation Anesthetics					
Nitrous Oxide	6 min.		0.6	None observed	Cohen et al (1953)
Cyclopropane	1.5 min.		0.8	Neonatal depression	Apgar et al (1957)
Diethyl ether		8 min.	0.96	Neonatal depression	Smith and Barker (1942)
Halothane	2 min.			Neonatal depression	Sheridan and Robson (1959)
Trichlorethylene	2 min.	6 min.	1.0		Helliwell and Hutton (1950)
Local Anesthetics					
Lidocaine	1.5 min.	6 min.	0.6	Neonatal depression	Shnider and Way (1968)
Mepivacaine	2 min.	12 min.	0.7	Neonatal depression	Morishima et al (1966) Asling et al (1970)
Procaine	0.5 min.	1.5 min.	0.6	Neonatal depression	Usubiaga et al (1968)
Prilocaine			1.0	Methemoglobinemia, cardiac arrhythmias	Poppers (1966) Epstein and Coakley (1967) Marx (1967)
Sedative-Hypnotics					
Barbital	2 min.	5 min.		None observed	Flowers (1959)
Secobarbital	0.5 min.	3 min.	0.7	Neonatal depression	Root et al (1961) Flowers (1959)
Pentobarbital	1 min.	3 min.	0.75	Neonatal depression	Fealy (1958) Flowers (1959)
Thiopental	0.75 min.	2 min.	1.0	Neonatal depression	McKechnie and Converse (1955) Flowers (1959)
Thioamylal	1 min.	1.5 min.		None observed	Flowers (1959)
Chloral Hydrate		15 min.	0.95	None observed	Bernstine et al (1954)
Ethanol			0.8	Neonatal depression	Belinkoff and Hall (1950) Chapman and Williams (1951)
Paraldehyde			0.94	Neonatal depression	Gardner et al (1940)
Tranquilizers					
Promethazine	1.5 min.	6 min.	0.7	Neonatal depression	Potts and Ullery (1961) Moya and Thorndike (1962)

TABLE 6.1—*Continued*

Compound	Time to Appear in Fetus	Time to Fetal/ Maternal Concentration Equilibrium	Fetal/ Maternal Concentration Ratio	Fetal or Neonatal Effect	References
Imipramine	3 min.	10 min.	2.0	None observed	Douglas and Hume (1967)
Narcotics					
Morphine	2–3 min.			Respiratory depression; Withdrawal signs	Shute and Davis (1933)
Meperidine	1.5 min.	6 min.	0.7	Respiratory depression; Withdrawal signs	Shnider and Way (1966) Way et al (1949)
Skeletal Muscle Relaxants					
D-tubocurarine	No transfer with clinical doses				Cohen et al (1953) Pittinger and Morris (1953)
Gallamine	3 min.	Traces only in fetus	None observed		Crawford (1956)
Succinylcholine	No transfer with clinical doses				Krisselgaard and Moya (1961)
Chemotherapeutic Compounds					
Sulfanamides	15 min.			Kernicterus	Moya and Thorndike (1962)
Penicillin		60 min.	0.2–0.7	None observed	Charles (1954) Moya and Thorndike (1962)
Oxacillin	2 hrs.		1.0	None observed	Prigot et al (1962)
Ampicillin	15 min.	45 min.	0.8	None observed	MacAulay et al (1962)
Streptomycin	1.7 hrs.		0.5	Deafness (?)	Charles (1954)
Tetracycline	2 hrs.		0.7	Bone and tooth defects	Cohen et al (1961) Gibbons and Reichelderfer (1969)
Chloramphenicol	71 min.		0.8	"Gray baby" syndrome	Scott and Warner (1960)
Cephaloridine	30 min.	5 hrs.		None observed	Bass and Graham (1967)
Isonicotinic a. hydrazide	12 min.	30 min.	0.9	None observed	Bromberg et al (1955)
Miscellaneous					
Atropine	6 min.			Tachycardia	John (1965)
Epinephrine				Tachycardia Hyperglycemia	Zuspan et al (1960)
Reserpine				Lethargy; nasal and bronchial congestion	Desmond et al (1957)

TABLE 6.1—*Continued*

Compound	Time to Appear in Fetus	Time to Fetal/Maternal Concentration Equilibrium	Fetal/Maternal Concentration Ratio	Fetal or Neonatal Effect	References
Antipyrine	1 min.	5 min.	0.98	None observed	McGaughey et al (1958)
Salicylates			0.6	None with clinical doses	Jackson (1948)
Bishydroxycoumarin				Severe hemorrhage	Kraus et al (1949)
Heparin	No apparent transfer to fetus			None observed	Flessa et al (1965)
Insulin	10 min.	60 min.	0.25	None with clinical doses	Gitlin et al (1965)
Thiouracil	10 min.	40 min.	1.0	Goiter and Pituitary hyperplasia	Hayashi and Gilling (1967) Peterson and Young (1952)
Thyroxin				Thyroid and Pituitary atrophy	Peterson and Young (1952)
Dextran (10 & 40)	No transfer to fetus				Falk et al (1967)
Chlorothiazide	60 min.		1.1	Thrombocytopenia	Garnet (1963) Nyhan and Lampert (1965)

impede drug transmission to the fetus, and therefore affect the accuracy of umbilical cord blood samples.

VII. SUMMARY

Within the past ten years, numerous studies on the basic mechanisms involved in placental transfer of drugs have been initiated. Most foreign substances cross the placenta by simple diffusion, the rate of transfer being determined primarily by the molecular weight, configuration, charge and lipid solubility of each compound, as well as the size, vascularity, and blood flow of the placenta. Even for many commonly used drugs, only qualitative or semiquantitative data on transfer characteristics are available. Information on drugs with respect to their distribution within, effect on, and excretion from the fetus and neonate, is even less available. Correlations between fetal plasma levels and drug effects are known for very few compounds. Until details of these effects are known and appreciated, the fetus will continue to be "treated" with its mother in an empiric manner, often inappropriately and sometimes with tragic results.

REFERENCES

Apgar, V., Holaday, D. A., James, L. S., Prince, C. E., Weisbrot, I. M. and Weiss, I.: Comparison of regional and general anesthesia in obstetrics, with special reference to the transmission of cyclopropane across the placenta. J.A.M.A. *165:* 2155–2161, 1957.

Asling, J. H., Shnider, S. M., Margolis, A. J.,

Wilkinson, G. L. and Way, E. L.: Paracervical block anesthesia in obstetrics. Am. J. Obstet. Gynec. *107:* 626–634, 1970.

Baker, J. B. E.: The effects of drugs on the fetus. Pharmacol. Rev. *12:* 37–90, 1960.

Barnes, A. C.: The fetal environment: Drugs and chemicals. In: *Intrauterine Development*, ed. by Barnes, Lea and Febiger, pp. 366–367, Philadelphia, 1968.

Barr, W. and Graham, R. M.: Placental transmission of cephaloridine. J. Obstet. Gynaec. Brit. Cwlth. *74:* 739–745, 1967.

Bartels, H., Moll, W. and Metcalfe, J.: Physiology of gas exchange in the human placenta. Am. J. Obstet. Gynec. *84:* 1714–1730, 1962.

Barton, T. C. and Baker, C.: Permeability of human amnion and chorion membrane. Am. J. Obstet. Gynec. *98:* 562–567, 1967.

Battaglia, F. C.: Some theoretical aspects of placental metabolism. J. Pediat. *62:* 926–932, 1963.

Battaglia, F. C.: Comparison of permeability of different layers of the primate placenta to D-arabinose and urea. Am. J. Physiol. *207:* 500–502, 1964.

Belinkoff, S. and Hall, O. W.: Intravenous alcohol during labor. Am. J. Obstet. Gynec. *59:* 429–432, 1950.

Bernstine, J. B., Meyer, A. E. and Hayman, H. B.: Maternal and foetal blood estimation following the administration of chloral hydrate during labor. J. Obstet. Gynaec. Brit. Emp. *61:* 683–685, 1954.

Bromberg, Y. M., Salzberger, M. and Bruderman, I.: Placental transmission of isonicotinic acid hydrazide. Gynaecologia *140:* 141–144, 1955.

Chapman, E. R. and Williams, P. T.: Intravenous alcohol as obstetrical analgesia. Am. J. Obstet. Gynec. *61:* 676–679, 1951.

Charles, D.: Placental transfer of antibiotics. J. Obstet. Gynaec. Brit. Emp. *61:* 750–757, 1954.

Clark, S. L.: The ingestion of proteins and colloid materials by columnar absorptive cells of the small intestine in suckling rats and mice. J. Biophys. Biochem. Cytol. *5:* 41–50, 1959.

Cohen, E. N., Paulson, W. J., Wall, J. and Elert, B.: Thiopental, curare, and nitrous oxide anesthesia for cesarean section with studies on placental transmission. Surg. Gynec. and Obstet. *97:* 456–462, 1953.

Cohlan, S. Q., Bevelander, G. and Bross, S.: Effect of tetracycline on bone growth in the premature infant. *Antimicrob. Agents and Chemotherapy:* 1961 Ed. pp. 340–347. Braun-Brumfield, Ann Arbor, Michigan.

Comroe, J. H.: *Physiology of Respiration,* pp. 147–159. Year Book, Chicago, 1965.

Crawford, J. S.: Some aspects of obstetric anesthesia. Brit. J. Anes. *28:* 146–158, 1956.

Dancis, J., Brenner, M. A. and Money, W. L.: Some factors affecting the permeability of guinea pig placenta. Am. J. Obstet. Gynec. *84:* 570–576, 1962.

Dawes, G. S.: *Fetal and Neonatal Physiology.* pp. 143–146 and 231–237. Year Book, Chicago, 1968.

Desmond, M. M., Rogers, S. F., Lindley, J. E. and Moyer, J. H.: Management of

toxemia of pregnancy with reserpine. Obstet. and Gynec. *10:* 140–145, 1957.

Douglas, B. H. and Hume, A. S.: Placental transfer of imipramine, a basic, lipid-soluble drug. Am. J. Obstet. Gynec. *99:* 573–575, 1967.

Epstein, B. and Coakley, C. S.: Passage of lidocaine and prilocaine across the placenta. Anesthesiology *28:* 246–247, 1967.

Ericsson, Y. and Ullberg, S.: Autoradiographic investigations of the distribution of F^{18} in mice and rats. Acta Odont. Scand. *16:* 363–382, 1958.

Faber, J. J. and Hart, F. M.: Transfer of charged and uncharged particles in the placenta of the rabbit. Am. J. Physiol. *213:* 890–894, 1967.

Falk, V., Forkman, B. and Arfors, K.: Permeability of the placenta to dextrans. Acta Obstet. Gynec. Scand. *46:* 414–418, 1967.

Fealy, J.: Placental transmission of pentobarbital. Obstet. and Gynec. *11:* 342–349, 1958.

Flessa, H. C., Kapstrom, A. B., Glueck, H. I. and Will, J. J.: Placental transport of heparin. Am. J. Obstet. Gynec. *93:* 570–573, 1965.

Flowers, C. E.: Placental transmission of barbiturates and thiobarbiturates and their pharmacological action on the mother and the infant. Am. J. Obstet. Gynec. *78:* 730–742, 1959.

Folkart, G. R., Dancis, J. and Money, W. L.: Transfer of carbohydrates across guinea pig placenta. Am. J. Obstet. Gynec. *80:* 221–223, 1960.

Gardner, H. L., Levine, H. and Bodansky, M.: Concentration of paraldehyde in the blood following its administration during labor. Am. J. Obstet. Gynec. *40:* 435–439, 1940.

Garnet, J. D.: Placental transfer of chlorthiazide. Obstet. and Gynec. *21:* 123–125, 1963.

Gibbons, R. J. and Reichelderfer, T. E.: Transplacental transmission of dimethylchlortetracycline and toxicity studies in premature and full term, newly born infants. Antibiot. Med. Clin. Ther. *7:* 618–622, 1960.

Gitlin, D., Kumate, J. and Morales, L.: On the transport of insulin across the human placenta. Pediat. *35:* 65–69, 1965.

Gordon, H. R.: Fetal bradycardia after paracervical block. New Eng. J. Med. *279:* 910–914, 1968.

Greene, J. H., Duhring, J. L. and Smith, K.: Placental function tests. Am. J. Obstet. Gynec. *92:* 1030–1058, 1965.

Hagemann, D. D. and Villee, C. A.: Transport functions of the placenta. Physiol. Rev. *40:* 313–330, 1960.

Hayashi, T. T. and Gilling, B.: Placental

transfer of thiouracil. Obstet. and Gynec. *30:* 736–740, 1967.

Helliwell, P. J. and Hutton, A. M.: Trichlorethylene anaesthesia: 1. Distribution in the fetal and maternal circulation of pregnant sheep and goats. Anaes. *5:* 4–13, 1950.

Hemmings, W. A. and Brambell, F. W. R.: Protein transfer across the foetal membranes. Brit. Med. Bull. *17:* 96–101, 1961.

Hensleigh, P. A. and Krantz, K. E.: Extracorporeal perfusion of the human placenta; 1. Placental transfer of ascorbic acid. Am. J. Obstet. Gynec. *96:* 5–13, 1966.

Jackson, A. V.: Toxic effects of salicylate on the fetus and mother. J. Path. and Bact. *60:* 587–593, 1948.

John, A. H.: Placental transfer of atropine and the effect on foetal heart rate. Brit. J. Anes. *37:* 57–60, 1965.

Kraus, A. P., Perlow, S. and Singer, K.: Danger of dicumarol treatment in pregnancy. J.A.M.A. *139:* 758–762, 1949.

Krisselgaard, N. and Moya, F.: Investigation of placental thresholds to succinylcholine. Anesthesiology *22:* 7–10, 1961.

Kunstadter, R. H., Klein, R. I., Lundeen, E. G., Witz, W. and Morrison, M.: Narcotic withdrawal symptoms in newborn infants. J.A.M.A. *168:* 1008–1010, 1958.

Lenz, M. W.: Chemicals and malformations in man, pp. 263–268. In: *Congenital Malformations, 2nd International Conference,* New York City, 1963. Pub.: Internat. Med. Congress: New York.

Lucas, W., Kirschbaum, T. and Assali, N. S.: Spinal shock and fetal oxygenation. Am. J. Obstet. Gynec. *93:* 583–587, 1965.

Macaulay, M. A., Abou-Sabe, M. and Charles, D.: Placental transfer of ampicillin. Am. J. Obstet. Gynec. *96:* 943–950, 1966.

Martin, C. A.: The anatomy and circulation of the placenta. pp. 35–67. In: *Intrauterine Development,* Ed. Barnes, Lea and Febiger, Philadelphia, 1968.

Marx, G. F.: Fetal arrhythmia during caudal block with prilocaine. Anesthesiology *28:* 222–226, 1967.

McGaughey, H. S., Jones, H. C., Talbert, L. and Anslow, W. P.: Placental transfer in normal and toxic gestation. Am. J. Obstet. Gynec. *75:* 482–495, 1958.

McKechnie, F. B. and Converse, J. G.: Placental transmission of thiopental. Am. J. Obstet. Gynec. *70:* 639–644, 1955.

Metcalfe, J., Moll, W. and Bartels, H.: Gas exchange across the placenta. Fed. Proc. *23:* 774–780, 1964.

Moore, W. M. O., Hellegers, A. E. and Battaglia, F. C.: In vitro permeability of different layers of human placenta to carbohydrates and urea. Am. J. Obstet. Gynec. *96:* 951–955, 1966.

Morishima, H. O., Daniel, S. S., Finster, M., Poppers, P. J. and James, L. S.: Transmission of mepivacaine across the human placenta. Anesthesiology *27:* 147–154, 1966.

Moya, F. and Thorndike, V.: Passage of drugs across the placenta. Am. J. Obstet. Gynec. *84:* 1778–1798, 1962.

Moya, F. and Smith, B. E.: Uptake, distribution and placental transport of drugs and anesthetics. Anesthesiology *26:* 465–476, 1965.

Nyhan, W. L. and Lampert, F.: Response of the fetus and newborn to drugs. Anesthesiology *27:* 487–500, 1965.

Page, E. W.: Transfer of materials across the human placenta. Am. J. Obstet. Gynec. *74:* 705–718, 1957.

Page, E. W., Glendening, M. B., Margolis, A. J. and Harper, H. A.: Transfer of D- and L-histidine across the human placenta. Am. J. Obstet. Gynec. *73:* 589–597, 1957.

Page, E. W.: Functions of the human placenta. Kaiser Found. Med. Bull. *7:* 112–121, 1959.

Panigel, M.: Placental perfusion experiments. Am. J. Obstet. Gynec. *84:* 1664–1683, 1962.

Peterson, R. R. and Young, W. C.: Placental permeability for thyrotrophin, propylthiouracil and thyroxine in guinea pig. Endocrin. *50:* 218–225, 1952.

Pittinger, C. B. and Morris, L. E.: Placental transmission of D-tubocurarine chloride from maternal to fetal circulation in dogs. Anesthesiology *14:* 238–244, 1953.

Plentl, A. V.: Placental transfer: pp. 203–249. In: *Biology of Gestation,* Vol. 1, Ed. Assali, Acad. Press, N.Y. 1968.

Poppers, P. J.: Practical and theoretical considerations on the use of prilocaine in obstetrics. Acta Anes. Scand. Supp. 25, pp. 385–388, 1966.

Potts, C. R. and Ullery, J. C.: Maternal and fetal effects of obstetric analgesia: Intravenous use of promethazine and meperidine. Am. J. Obstet. Gynec. *81:* 1253–1259, 1961.

Prigot, A., Froix, C. J. and Rubin, E.: Absorption, diffusion, and excretion of a new penicillin, oxacillin. *Antimicrob. Agents and Chemother.,* 1962 ed. pp. 402–410. Braun-Brumfield, Ann Arbor, Michigan.

Root, B., Eichner, E. and Sunshine, I.: Blood secobarbital levels and their clinical correlation in mothers and newborn infants. Am. J. Obstet. Gynec. *81:* 948–956, 1961.

Rudolph, A. M. and Heymann, M. A.: The circulation of the fetus in utero: methods for studying distribution of blood flow, cardiac output, and organ blood flow. Circ. Res. *21:* 163–184, 1967a.

Rudolph, A. M. and Heymann, M. A.: Validation of the antipyrine method for measuring fetal umbilical blood flow. Circ. Res. *21:* 185–190, 1967b.

Saling, E.: Mikroblutuntersuchungen am Feten. Ztschr. f. Geburtsch. u Gynäk. *162:* 56–75, 1964.

Scott, W. C. and Warner, R. F.: Placental transfer of chloramphenicol. J.A.M.A. *142:* 1331–1332, 1950.

Seeds, A. E.: Placental transfer, pp. 103–128. In: *Intrauterine Development,* Ed. Barnes, Lea and Febiger, Philadelphia, 1968.

Shapiro, N. Z., Kirschbaum, T. and Assali, N. S.: Mental exercises in placental transfer. Am. J. Obstet. Gynec. *97:* 130–137.

Sheridan, C. A. and Robson, J. G.: Fluothane in obstetrical anaesthesia. Canad. Anaesth. Soc. J. *6:* 365–374, 1959.

Shnider, S. M., Way, E. L. and Lord, M. J.: Rate of appearance and disappearance of meperidine in fetal blood after administration of narcotic to the mother. Anesthesiology *27:* 227–228, 1966.

Shnider, S. M.: Fetal and neonatal effects of drugs in obstetrics. Anesth. and Analg. *45:* 372–378, 1966.

Shnider, S. M. and Way, E. L.: The kinetics of transfer of lidocaine across the human placenta. Anesthesiology *29:* 944–950, 1968.

Shute, E. and Davis, E.: Effect on the infant of morphine administered in labor. Surg. Gynec. and Obst. *57:* 727–736, 1933.

Smith, C. A. and Barker, R. H.: Ether in the blood of the newborn infant. Am. J. Obstet. Gynec. *43:* 763–774, 1942.

Sternberg, J.: Placental transfers: Modern methods of study. Am. J. Obstet. Gynec. *84:* 1731–1748, 1962.

Uher, J., Dvorak, K., Queissnerova, M., Konickova, L. and Turinova, J.: Movement and metabolism of some drugs in the fetoplacental unit. Am. J. Obstet. Gynec. *95:* 1005–1008, 1966.

Usubiaga, J. E., Laiuppa, M., Moya, F., Wikinski, J. A. and Velazco, R.: Passage of procaine hydrochloride and para-aminobenzoic acid across the human placenta. Am. J. Obstet. Gynec. *100:* 918–923, 1968.

Way, E. L., Gimble, A. I., McKelway, W. P., Ross, H., Sung, C. and Ellsworth, H.: The absorption, distribution, and excretion of isonipecaine (Demerol). J. Pharmacol. Exp. Ther. *96:* 477–484, 1949.

Widdas, W. F.: Transport mechanisms in the fetus. Brit. Med. Bull. *17:* 107–111, 1961.

Wilkin, P. and Bursztein, M.: La permeabilite placentaire, pp. 224–228. In: *Le Placenta Human,* Ed. Snoeck, Masson et Cie, Paris, 1958.

Zuspan, F. P., Whaley, W. H., Nelson, G. H. and Ahlquist, R. P.: Placental transfer of epinephrine: 1. Maternal-fetal metabolic alterations of glucose and nonesterified fatty acids. Am. J. Obstet. Gynec. *95:* 284–289, 1966.

7

Pulmonary Disposition of Drugs

EDWIN S. MUNSON
EDMOND I. EGER, II

I. INTRODUCTION

The introduction of a foreign gas or vapor into the lungs results in a rise in the alveolar concentration (partial pressure) of that gas. Because anesthetic gases possess many of the extreme properties of foreign gases, the commonly used inhalation anesthetic drugs will be used to illustrate the relationship between the alveolar and inspired concentrations. In addition, the effect on alveolar concentration of alterations of certain physiologic systems also will be discussed.

II. VENTILATORY INPUT

If unimpeded, ventilation would cause the alveolar concentration to rapidly reach the inspired concentration. With a "normal" alveolar ventilation of four liters per min, and a functional residual capacity of three liters, the alveolar concentration would approach the inspired within a few minutes. However, the effect of ventilatory input is opposed by gas uptake. Just as ventilation increases alveolar concentration by bringing gas into the lungs, gas uptake decreases the alveolar concentration by removing gas through distribution to peripheral tissues. Ignoring for the moment the effect of concentration (Section III, E), the alveolar concentration is determined principally by the balance between ventilatory input and gas loss through uptake by pulmonary blood.

III. GAS UPTAKE

A. Solubility

The higher the solubility in blood and body tissues, the greater is gas uptake. Solubility is expressed as a ratio of the gas concentrations in two phases, as the gas distributes following equilibrium between the two phases. This is a partition coefficient which numerically is equal to the Ostwald solubility coefficient (Eger and Larson, 1964). By convention, the gas phase is always expressed as the denominator. Solubility coefficients collected from various sources are shown in Table 7.1. The numerator may be any liquid, tissue or other substance. For example, if at equilibrium alveolar nitrous oxide concentration were 80 volumes %, and if this concentration were in equilibrium with 37.6 volumes % in the pulmonary blood, the nitrous oxide blood/gas partition coefficient would be 0.47 (37.6/80). In other words, for every 100 molecules per ml of nitrous oxide in the alveolar gas there are 47 molecules of nitrous oxide per ml of blood. Nitrous

TABLE 7.1

Ostwald solubility coefficients (37°C)

Agent	$\dfrac{\text{Water}}{\text{Gas}}$	$\dfrac{\text{Blood}}{\text{Gas}}$	$\dfrac{\text{Oil}}{\text{Gas}}$
Helium	0.0097	0.0098	0.016
Nitrogen	0.014	0.014	0.075
Ethylene	0.08	0.14	1.26
Xenon	0.10	0.20	1.9
Cyclopropane	0.20	0.42	11.9
Nitrous oxide	0.44	0.46	1.4
Teflurane	0.32	0.60	29
Fluroxene	0.84	1.4	48
Forane	0.7	1.4	98
Ēthrane	0.82	1.9	98
Halothane	0.74	2.3	224
Divinyl ether	1.40	2.8	58
Trichloroethylene	1.55	9.2	960
Chloroform	3.8	10.3	265
Diethyl ether	13.1	12.1	65
Methoxyflurane	4.5	13	970
Acetone		333	
Ethyl Alcohol		2000	

oxide has a relatively low blood/gas partition coefficient compared, for example, to methoxyflurane which has a blood/gas partition coefficient of 13. Thus, for a given alveolar concentration, methoxyflurane is taken up in greatest quantity, halothane less so, and nitrous oxide least. The greatest difference between inspired and alveolar concentrations occurs, therefore, with methoxyflurane, a lesser but sizable difference with halothane, while only a small difference exists for nitrous oxide. When gases are administered in relatively low concentration the rate at which the alveolar concentration rises toward that inspired is inversely proportional to solubility. The effect of solubility for 5 gases is shown in Figure 7.1.

These gases are anesthetic agents. However, many nonanesthetic gases have solubility characteristics outside the limits illustrated above. For example, some of the inert gases and Freons are relatively insoluble. This property of insolubility forms the basis for the use of nitrogen and helium in pulmonary function testing. In contrast, other compounds show relatively greater solubility. The alcohols and acetone are examples of these. When these agents are inhaled they are almost completely absorbed.

B. Cardiac Output

Increase in cardiac output (pulmonary blood flow) increases gas loss from the lung, thereby delaying the rate of rise of the alveolar concentration. This is simply a function of a larger volume of blood exposed to the gas within the lung. Increase in cardiac output, as during exercise or excitement may increase the rate of gas uptake. In conditions of decreased cardiac output, as for example during shock, the reverse occurs. Resultant decreased uptake of alveolar gas effects an unusually rapid rise in alveolar gas tension, which may lead to overdosage when an anesthetic is being administered. This is particularly true of the soluble agents. Figure 7.2 shows 3 families of curves for gases of varying solu-

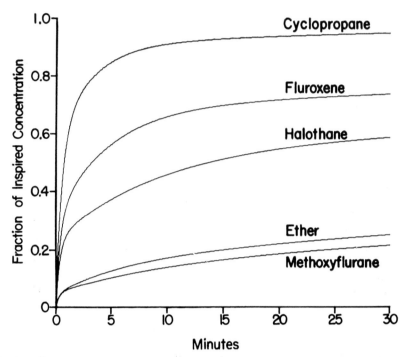

Fig. 7.1. Effect of solubility on the rate of rise of the alveolar concentration (partial pressure) toward the inspired. The greatest difference between inspired and alveolar concentrations occurs with the most soluble gases, such as ether and methoxyflurane. These and subsequent alveolar curves were obtained from a mathematical model (Munson and Bowers, 1967) that assumes the physical characteristics of normal resting man (Section III, C). Alveolar ventilation and cardiac output were 4 and 5 liters per min, respectively.

bility when cardiac output is reduced to one-half normal and increased to twice normal. Hypothetically, the cessation of pulmonary blood flow with continued ventilatory input, would result in a rapid rise of alveolar concentration. A secondary effect of alterations in cardiac output is that redistribution of flow to the viscera and lean tissues may also influence the rate of rise of alveolar concentration (Section IV, C).

C. Alveolar-venous Difference

Gas uptake increases in proportion to the magnitude of the gas partial pressure difference between alveoli and pulmonary venous blood. This difference diminishes when all body tissues achieve equilibrium with the alveolar (arterial) partial pressure. When the alveolar-venous gas partial pressure difference equals zero, gas loss (uptake) from the lung ceases. Conversely, the difference is greatest at the time of least saturation; for anesthetic gases this would be the period of anesthetic induction.

To understand what factors determine the changes in the alveolar-venous gas partial pressure difference during inhalation of a foreign gas, consider the relative distribution of blood in the body (Fig. 7.3). In the normal 70 kg man, roughly 75% of the cardiac output is directed to nearly 9% of the body tissues. These tissues consist of the brain and other tissues of the vessel rich group (VRG), in-

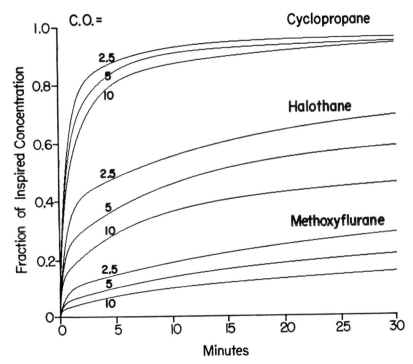

Fig. 7.2. The effect on alveolar concentration of varying cardiac output from 2.5 to 10 liters per min. The relative distribution of cardiac output remains unchanged. Changes in cardiac output have relatively little effect on an insoluble gas such as cyclopropane but show greater influence on the more soluble gases, such as methoxyflurane.

cluding the heart, kidneys, hepatoportal and digestive systems, and the endocrine glands. Because of the high blood flow/mass ratio, the VRG rapidly attains equilibrium with the gas partial pressure in arterial blood. As equilibrium is approached, the partial pressure in the venous blood leaving these tissues also rises until at equilibrium it equals the arterial (and tissue) partial pressure. If no concomitant rise in arterial concentration occurs, this process is complete within 10 to 15 minutes. Thus, after this time 75% of the blood returning to the lungs is at the same partial pressure as that in the alveoli (arterial blood). The alveolar-venous partial pressure difference is, therefore, reduced rapidly to 25% of its initial value and gas uptake is similarly reduced.

Three other tissue groups continue to remove anesthetic from arterial blood long after saturation of the VRG. Skin and muscle (MG) form 50% of the body volume and at rest receive about 18% of the cardiac output. Saturation of this group proceeds slowly and is not complete for at least 90 minutes, even when arterial partial pressure is held constant. Fat (FG) comprises roughly 20% of the body volume and has a blood flow per unit volume slightly less than the MG. The FG receives approximately 5% of the cardiac output. However, saturation of the FG proceeds more slowly than that of the MG since most gases are considerably more soluble in fat. The last tissue group, the vessel poor group (VPG), is so poorly perfused that it has little or no effect on uptake, although it makes up a significant fraction of the body mass (about 20%). Bone, cartilage,

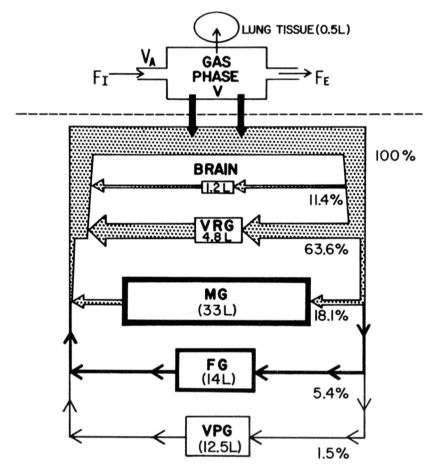

Fig. 7.3. The lung (V), alveolar ventilation (V_A), inspired (F_I) and alveolar (F_E) concentrations (partial pressures) are shown above the dashed line representing the alveolar-capillary membrane. The various body compartments are noted. Percentages refer to the normal distribution of cardiac output. (Reprinted from Munson, E. S. and Bowers, D. L.: Effects of hyperventilation on the rate of cerebral anesthetic equilibration. Anesthesiology *28:* 377–381, 1967.)

tendons, ligaments and other relatively avascular tissues are in this group. The percentages of inspired partial pressure in the alveoli and in the various tissue groups for three anesthetic agents are shown in Figure 7.4.

From the above the alveolar-venous blood difference may be seen to go through at least three stages. Initially all tissue groups are unsaturated and remove most of the gas from the blood perfusing them. The partial pressure in venous blood leaving all tissues is relatively low. Initially the VRG rapidly becomes saturated and the venous partial pressure rises thereafter to about 75% of arterial partial pressure. The remaining 25% of the alveolar-venous difference is slowly reduced over a period of hours as equilibrium is reached in the MG. During this entire period and beyond, the FG remains unsaturated and thus with the relatively soluble gases, venous and arterial (alveolar) partial pressures may not reach equality for many hours.

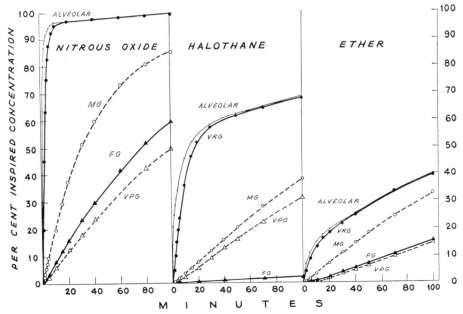

Fig. 7.4. Percent inspired partial pressures in alveoli and various tissue groups for nitrous oxide 70%, halothane 1%, and ether 10%. The relative height to which each curve rises is inversely related to solubility. The vessel rich group (VRG) closely follows the alveolar curves. Equilibration of muscle (MG) and fat (FG) with alveolar anesthetic partial pressure occurs most rapidly with nitrous oxide, slightly less so with ether and relatively more slowly with halothane. (Reprinted from Eger, E. I., II: Applications of a mathematical model of gas uptake. In: *Uptake and Distribution of Anesthetic Agents.* Papper and Kitz, Eds. New York, McGraw-Hill, 1963, Ch. 8.)

D. Metabolism

One further factor, metabolism, may influence the partial pressure of gas in the returning venous blood. Many substances are partially or even completely removed by the liver. Even the anesthetics, which were once thought to be excreted unchanged, are now known to be biodegradable (Van Dyke and Chenoweth, 1965). The importance of metabolism lies in the fact that 25% of the cardiac output flows through the liver. If extraction is complete this means that the alveolar to venous partial pressure difference will always be at least 25%. In contrast to the effect of time on tissue uptake, metabolism is greater as time passes. This is because metabolism is a function of partial pressure (unless the metabolizing enzymes become saturated) and partial pressure rises with time. In a manner similar to metabolism the percutaneous loss of gases also tends to oppose the progressive diminution of the alveolar-venous partial pressure difference (Stoelting and Eger, 1969b).

E. Concentration

1. Primary gas effect. The inspired concentration of a gas may exert profound influence on the rate at which the alveolar concentration rises (Eger, 1963). It is intuitively obvious that the higher the inspired concentration (partial pressure) the higher will be the alveolar concentration. Increasing the inspired

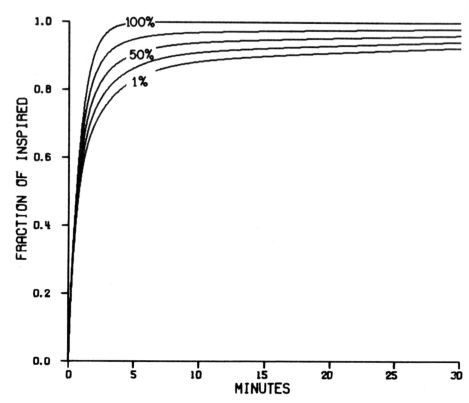

Fig. 7.5. The effect on alveolar concentration on varying inspired concentration of nitrous oxide from 1 to 100%. The higher the inspired concentration the more rapid the approach of the alveolar to inspired concentration. The magnitude of the concentration effect increases with increasing solubility and at 100% concentration the alveolar approach to the inspired is identical for all gases, irrespective of solubility.

concentration results in a more than proportional rise in the alveolar concentration. Figure 7.5 shows the relatively more rapid rise in alveolar nitrous oxide concentration when the inspired concentration is increased from 1 to 100%. At 100% concentration the rise of alveolar concentration is determined solely by the relation between the volume of the lung and the rate of ventilatory input; that is to say, the effect of ventilation (Section II) overrides the effect of solubility (Section III, A). As a result, if any gas were administered in 100% concentration the alveolar concentration would rise toward that inspired equally rapidly irrespective of differences in solubility. In other words, the effect of solubility predominates at *low* concentration; the effect of ventilation predominates at *high* concentration. A soluble gas such as methoxyflurane (Fig. 7.1) would demonstrate a relatively greater increase in alveolar concentration if it were possible to administer the gas in (high) concentrations similar to nitrous oxide.

The concentration effect results, in part, from the absolute large uptake of gas which produces an increase in the total volume of gas inspired. This additional ventilatory input is proportional to the amount of gas removed from the lungs and occurs when either the inspired concentration, or the blood solubility results in a relatively large volume of gas uptake. The effect of concentration opposing gas uptake in determining alveolar concentration has also been described as an "uptake-ventilation" effect (Mapleson, 1964).

2. Second gas effect. It has been shown that the increased inspiratory volume carries with it any other gas given concomitantly and hence will accelerate the rise of the alveolar concentration of the second gas (Epstein *et al.*, 1964). For example, uptake of large volumes of gas may occur during induction of anesthesia with high concentrations of nitrous oxide or diethyl ether (first gas). The rate of rise of the alveolar concentration of a second gas also will be accelerated when administered simultaneously with the primary gas. The respiratory gases are also subject to the second gas effect if the first gas is administered in sufficient concentration.

Recently, an additional explanation, termed the "concentrating" effect, was proposed to give further explanation for the second gas effect (Stoelting and Eger, 1969a). Administration of 70% nitrous oxide, after equilibrium of the second gas, caused the alveolar concentration of the second gas to rise above the inspired concentration (Fig. 7.6). This observation precludes the possibility that the second gas effect is due solely to an increased volume of inspired gas. The concentrating effect is greatest with the less soluble (second) gases and is inversely proportional to the magnitude of pulmonary ventilation.

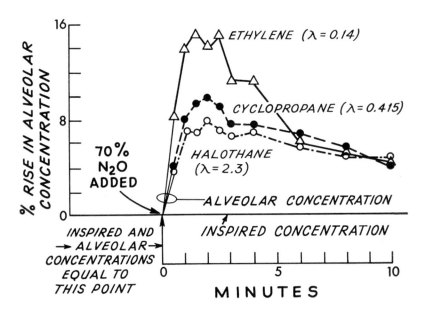

Fig. 7.6. Effect of solubility on the magnitude of the second gas effect. The average% rise in the alveolar concentration of the second gas above that inspired, after equilibrium and following the addition of 70% nitrous oxide (first gas) is shown relative to time. Inspired concentrations were held constant after the introduction of nitrous oxide; P_ACO_2 equalled 80 mm Hg. (Reprinted from Stoelting, R. K. and Eger, E. I., II: An additional explanation for the second gas effect: A concentrating effect. Anesthesiology *30*: 273–277, 1969.)

IV. INFLUENCING FACTORS

A. Ventilation and Circulation

Each of the above factors, i.e., ventilation, solubility, cardiac output and the alveolar-blood difference may interact with the other. For example, an increase in ventilation reduces the difference between inspired and alveolar concentrations by bringing more gase into the lung per unit time. However, the relative effect of an increase in ventilation varies for gases of different solubilities. Figure 7.7 shows families of curves for three anesthetics of varying solubility in blood. Changes in ventilation have a small effect on the alveolar concentration of the least soluble agents, such as nitrous oxide and cyclopropane, but have a profound effect on the very soluble gases such as methoxyflurane and ether. A doubling of ventilation during induction of anesthesia may result in a near doubling of alveolar concentration with the soluble agents, whereas essentially no change will occur with a relatively insoluble gas. Conversely, an increase in cardiac output results in an increased inspired to alveolar difference. This change is small for the less soluble agents and large for the very soluble agents (Fig. 7.2 and Section III, B).

These relationships may be viewed in another light. If a gas is relatively insoluble then the alveolar concentration essentially equals that inspired and

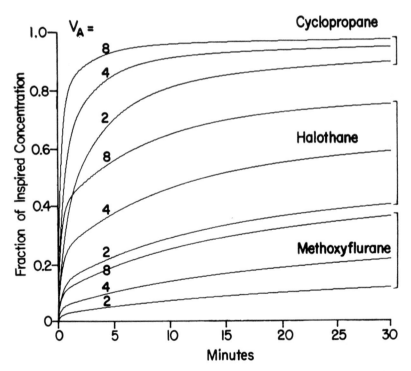

Fig. 7.7. The effect on alveolar concentrations of varying alveolar ventilation from 2 to 8 liters per min. Since uptake has little effect in determining alveolar concentration with insoluble gases, ventilation has a lesser effect on the relative alveolar concentration of nitrous oxide as compared with the more soluble methyoxyflurane. Note that increase in ventilation and cardiac output (Fig. 7.2) produce opposite changes in alveolar concentration.

uptake becomes primarily a function of cardiac output and secondarily of distribution and metabolism. If the gas is extremely soluble the alveolar-inspired concentration ratio is very small. That is, most of the gas brought into the lungs is removed and uptake is primarily a function of ventilation. Most gases lie between these extremes.

B. Pulmonary Disease

Thus far, it has been assumed that ventilation-perfusion relationships throughout the lung were equal. Ventilation-perfusion inequalities, including arteriovenous shunts across the lung, result in an alveolar-arterial difference which is proportional to the degree of abnormality (Eger and Severinghaus, 1964). When alveolar-arterial partial pressure differences, with and without ventilation-perfusion abnormalities are compared, the greatest difference occurs with the gas of least solubility (Eger et al., 1966).

C. Other Considerations

The use of mathematical models for the simulation of gas uptake and distribution usually considers physiologic variables such as ventilation, cardiac output, and tissue blood flows as linear, that is, static functions (Kety, 1951). However, that is frequently not the case, particularly when considering the effects of hyperventilation and other clinical situations (Munson and Bowers, 1967). Physiologic parameters during these conditions may vary from the "normal" during induction of anesthesia and show further changes in response to continuing anesthetic partial pressure rises. For example, theoretical calculations show that circulatory changes associated with shock and excitement increase and decrease respectively, the rates of rise of the alveolar concentration (Eger, 1964). Alterations in the distribution of cardiac output, through application of both proportional and differential tissue blood flows, result in solubility dependent and quantitatively different changes in the rate of cerebral anesthetic equilibration (Munson et al., 1968). The increased rate of rise of alveolar concentration in infants and children similarly is related, in part, to distribution of cardiac output predominately to the VRG (Salanitre and Rackow, 1969). Considerations of gas kinetics during hypothermia also would predict that the rise of alveolar concentration would be slowed as a result of reduced ventilation, cardiac output and peripheral tissue perfusion (Munson and Eger, 1970).

V. GAS EXCRETION

Elimination of foreign gases occurs nearly as an inverted reproduction of gas uptake. For example, the excretion of less soluble anesthetics is high initially but rapidly declines to a lower level. The output level continues to fall thereafter at a slow and ever decreasing rate. The output of soluble gases is high initially, but gradually decreases with time. The effects of variations in ventilation and cardiac output on reducing alveolar concentration during recovery are similar to the effects that occur during gas inhalation (Section IV, A). However, perfect inversion of the alveolar concentration curves shown in Figure 7.1 only occurs if total body equilibration with the gas is achieved. This is seldom the case, particularly when considering gases of relatively high solubility.

The duration of gas inhalation is of prime importance in considerations of gas excretion (Stoelting and Eger, 1969c). Following relatively short exposures to soluble agents such as halothane and methoxyflurane, failure of equilibration of the muscle and fat groups results in a much greater decrease in alveolar anesthetic concentration as compared to the increase observed during induction. While little difference was observed for the relatively insoluble nitrous oxide, relatively greater uptake of the more soluble agents delays the rate of alveolar concentration decrease as the duration of anesthetic exposure is prolonged. Furthermore, decrease in alveolar halothane concentration is augmented most by changes in ventilation, while the maximum effect of ventilation on excretion of the more soluble gases is delayed.

During recovery from nitrous oxide anesthesia, the outpouring of gas far exceeds the uptake of inspired gas (air). This is due to the relatively increased solubility of nitrous oxide in blood (about 34 fold) as compared with nitrogen. As a result, there occurs: (1) displacement or dilution of the inspired oxygen concentration, and (2) diminution of the inspired volume required to maintain alveolar (arterial) carbon dioxide partial pressure constant. Both factors tend

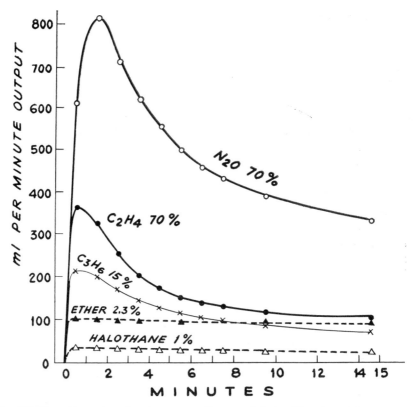

Fig. 7.8. Excretion rates of various gases after complete equilibration at the percentages noted. Ventilation is maintained constant at 4 liters per min. Note that gas output is greatest with nitrous oxide. Diffusion anoxia, which is related to the dilution of alveolar respiratory gases by nitrous oxide postanesthetically, has been reported only with this agent.

to decrease the alveolar and therefore the arterial oxygen partial pressure (Rackow *et al.*, 1961). This effect may result with any gas when the absolute volume of gas excretion by pulmonary blood is high. The bulk outpouring of a number of anesthetic agents, following complete equilibration at the percentages noted is shown in Figure 7.8. A clinical condition resulting from the use of nitrous oxide has been termed "diffusion anoxia" (Fink, 1955). Since this (inverted) process resembles the concentration effect, consideration of this phenomenon as a "dilution effect" provides a more accurate descriptive term.

VI. SUMMARY

Inhalation of a foreign gas causes the alveolar concentration of that gas to rise. The relationship between inspired and alveolar concentrations is dependent on three factors: ventilation, uptake, and inspired concentration. Ventilation causes the concentration to rise whereas gas loss through uptake opposes that rise. Gas uptake is determined by solubility in blood and tissues, cardiac output and its distribution, and metabolic degradation of gas. The inspired concentration modifies the effect of uptake. As the inspired concentration increases, uptake has less influence on the rate of rise of alveolar and therefore arterial blood and tissue partial pressure.

Acknowledgment

The authors are indebted to Mr. Donald L. Bowers, of the University of Virginia Medical Center, Charlottesville, Virginia, for his assistance in the preparation of Figures 7.1, 7.2, 7.5 and 7.7.

REFERENCES

Eger, E. I., II: The effect of inspired anesthetic concentration on the rate of rise of alveolar concentration. Anesthesiology *24:* 153–157, 1963.

Eger, E. I., II: Respiratory and circulatory factors in uptake and distribution of volatile anaesthetic agents. Brit. J. Anaesth. *36:* 155–171, 1964.

Eger, E. I., II, and Larson, C. P.: Anaesthetic solubility in blood and tissues: values and significance. Brit. J. Anaesth. *36:* 140–149, 1964.

Eger, E. I., II, and Severinghaus, J. W.: Effect of uneven pulmonary distribution of blood and gas on induction with inhalation anesthetics. Anesthesiology *25:* 620–226, 1964.

Eger, E. I., II, Babad, A. A., Regan, M. J., Larson, C. P., Shargel, R., and Severinghaus, J. W.: Delayed approach of arterial to alveolar nitrous oxide partial pressures in dog and in man. Anesthesiology *27:* 288–297, 1966.

Epstein, R. M., Rackow, H., Salanitre, E., and Wolf, G. L.: Influence of the concentration effect on the uptake of anesthetic mixtures: the second gas effect. Anesthesiology *25:* 364–371, 1964.

Fink, B. R.: Diffusion anoxia. Anesthesiology *16:* 511–519, 1955.

Kety, S. S.: The theory and applications of the exchange of inert gas at the lungs and tissues. Pharmacol. Rev. *3:* 1–41, 1951.

Mapleson, W. W.: Mathematical aspects of the uptake, distribution and elimination of inhaled gases and vapours. Brit. J. Anaesth. *36:* 129–139, 1964.

Munson, E. S. and Bowers, D. L.: Effects of hyperventilation on the rate of cerebral anesthetic equilibration. Calculations using a mathematical model. Anesthesiology *28:* 377–381, 1967.

Munson, E. S. and Eger, E. I., II: The effects of hyperthermia and hypothermia on the rate of induction of anesthesia. Calculations using a mathematical model. Anesthesiology *33:* 515–519, 1970.

Munson, E. S., Eger, E. I., II, and Bowers, D. L.: Effects of changes in cardiac output and distribution on the rate of cerebral anesthetic equilibration. Calculations using a mathematical model. Anesthesiology *29:* 533–537, 1968.

Rackow, H., Salanitre, E., and Frumin, M. J.: Dilution of alveolar gases during nitrous oxide excretion in man. J. Appl. Physiol. *16:* 723–728, 1961.

Salanitre, E. and Rackow, H.: The pulmonary exchange of nitrous oxide and halothane in infants and children. Anesthesiology *30:* 388–394, 1969.

Stoelting, R. K., and Eger, E. I., II: An additional explanation for the second gas effect: A concentrating effect. Anesthesiology *30:* 273–277, 1969a.

Stoelting, R. K. and Eger, E. I., II: Percutaneous loss of nitrous oxide, cyclopropane, ether and halothane in man. Anesthesiology *30:* 278–283, 1969b.

Stoelting, R. K., and Eger, E. I., II: The effects of ventilation and anesthetic solubility on recovery from anesthesia: An *in vivo* and analog analysis before and after equilibration. Anesthesiology *30:* 290–296, 1969c.

Van Dyke, R. A. and Chenoweth, M. B.: Metabolism of volatile anesthetics. Anesthesiology *26:* 348–357, 1965.

8

Renal Excretion of Drugs

EDWARD J. CAFRUNY

I. INTRODUCTION

There are times when investigators in the field of drug metabolism need to know something about urinary excretion of a drug and its biotransformed products. Often, all they require is information about rate of excretion. But there are also occasions when it is necessary to know how the kidney is handling a chemical substance, or why it is being excreted rapidly or slowly. This article is addressed to those who have not performed such studies but expect to do so. In it, I consider conceptual as well as practical matters pertaining to studies of renal excretion of drugs. Since this article is a written lecture rather than a review of literature, all cited references except those in the tables should be read. The papers contain valuable information (methods, discussion, instructions) which I cannot present in detail here. These particular references were chosen because they were considered to be especially informative and relevant. For those who want to probe the subject in depth, the selected review articles listed at the end of the chapter provide additional references and discussion.

II. GENERAL PLAN OF A NEPHRON UNIT

The ability of an organ to perform a task is intimately related to the structure of the organ. This is so evident in the case of the mammalian kidney that one merely needs to look at the general plan of a nephron unit in order to appreciate what the kidney can and cannot do to eliminate drugs from the body.

The most important feature of the mammalian renal system is its highly developed anatomical arrangement in which renal cells are interposed between blood and urinary passages. This arrangement is illustrated in Figure 8.1, a diagram of one of the million or more nephron units in a single human kidney. As shown in the figure, arterial blood enters a glomerular capillary network through an afferent arteriole. Since the intra-capillary pressure is higher than the pressure in the tubular lumen, fluid containing most of the solutes found in plasma is filtered across the thin walls of the capillaries and through pores of the adjacent epithelial layer of cells into the lumen of the tubule. Arterial blood flows out of the glomerulus through an efferent arteriole. The efferent vessel then divides to form a capillary network adjacent to and surrounding the tubular portion of the nephron. Glomerular filtration of solutes is limited by the size and shape of each solute present in plasma. Elongated molecules of high molecular weight are not freely filtered. The pores are too small to admit them. Conse-

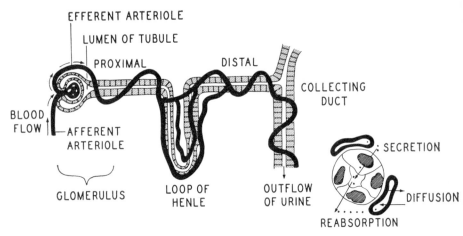

Fig. 8.1. Diagram showing a nephron unit. The small insert is a cross section of the proximal tubule and two adjacent capillaries.

quently, in normal kidneys, the glomerular filtrate is essentially free of proteins that have molecular weights of 60–70 thousand or more. Filtered fluid passes progressively through lumens of the proximal tubule, loop of Henle, and distal tubule before entering the collecting duct and eventually exiting through the renal pelvis and ureter and on into the bladder. During their passage through the tubule, filtered molecules can diffuse or be actively transported from lumen to blood (reabsorption). Molecules present in capillary blood around the tubules can also move passively into cells, or be transported into the lumen (secretion). Rate of diffusion is dependent on electrochemical or concentration gradients as well as on solubility in membranal lipoprotein.

From an evolutionary standpoint, the accession to a glomerular kidney was a major step forward for those vertebrates, especially warm-blooded land animals, that developed it. Operationally, the glomerular kidney behaves in large measure as an extension of the cardiovascular system in the performance of its excretory function. The advantages of this cardiovascular-renal system for animals subjected to the vagaries of a life on land, with its attendant chemical instability, are many. In the first place, the heart, a powerful muscular organ, supplies all the energy needed to propel fluid through the urinary passages of the kidney. This relieves the kidney of the burden of performing a task for which it is not structurally designed. Secondly, the kidney cannot toss away water and electrolytes wastefully when the circulatory system fails; when blood pressure falls glomerular filtration slows or stops. The fluid conserved thereby helps to correct disturbances of the circulation. Finally, animals with glomerular kidneys are not confronted with the problem of developing numerous specialized systems for excreting the large variety of unwanted molecules to which they are exposed. By way of contrast, the kidneys of certain aglomerular vertebrates that live in an unchanging oceanic environment must rely on special transporting mechanisms. For example, aglomerular fish actively secrete certain molecules and allow others to diffuse into urine. Fortunately, secretory systems in glomerular kidneys are merely accessory systems, albeit relatively important in some instances. Glomerular kidneys tend to excrete all filtered solutes; the most highly developed mechanisms and those that require the expenditure of large amounts of energy are the reabsorptive systems. The price of the specific advantages glomerular kidneys possess is high, for circulatory disorder usually interfere with renal function, even when the kidneys are healthy, and uremia is always just around the corner.

III. GLOMERULAR FILTRATION OF DRUGS

As mentioned above, glomerular filtration of solutes is a non-selective process in that glomerular membranes do not restrict the passage of most molecules. In general, medicinal compounds are far too small to be kept out of the urinary passages. However, their rate of filtration is frequently limited because they react with and bind to plasma proteins. It is virtually impossible to determine the extent to which protein binding impedes the glomerular filtration of a drug. The reason for this is that measurements of protein binding cannot be made under conditions even roughly equivalent to those that prevail within glomerular capillaries. Most workers use the method of Toribara *et al.* (1957) to prepare ultrafiltrates of plasma obtained from animals treated with the drug under study. Only ultrafilterable drug is considered to be "free" to enter renal tubular lumens by means of glomerular filtration. The method provides at best an approximation of the retarding effect of plasma proteins and at worst introduces a serious error. Nevertheless, it is the best procedure available and the data obtained when it is used must be accepted until better methods are devised.

If a drug is not bound to plasma protein, it is presumed to be filtered freely in amounts equal to

$$Pd \times GFR$$

where Pd = plasma concentration of drug and GFR is the rate of glomerular filtration. Approximately one-fifth to one-fourth of the volume of the renal plasma flow (RPF) is filtered into tubular lumens. Thus the filtration fraction (FF) is calculated as follows:

$$FF = GFR/RPF = 0.20 \text{ to } 0.25$$

An exception is the kidney of the dog in which FF may be as high as 0.35. Given a drug X, the total amount filtered is the product of GFR and the concentration of the free drug in arterial plasma. The renal clearance of inulin (C_{IN}) where

$$C_{IN} = \frac{\text{Urinary concentration of inulin} \times \text{urine flow rate}}{\text{Arterial plasma concentration of inulin}} = \frac{U_{IN}V}{P_{IN}}$$

provides an estimate of GFR when P_{IN} is relatively constant. In practice, inulin is injected intravenously and then infused continuously. The concentration in plasma stabilizes in about an hour. If one administers a test drug in the same way, the total amount filtered/unit time can be calculated. Complete directions for measuring inulin clearance are given by Smith (1956). The only reliable method for estimating the rate of filtration of a drug involves the separate simultaneous measurement of the GFR. The formula

$$t_{\frac{1}{2}} = (0.7 \text{ Vd})/C$$

where $t_{\frac{1}{2}}$ = the half-life in plasma, Vd = volume of distribution, and C = renal clearance, cannot be used to calculate the renal clearance of a drug. The term C does not truly represent renal clearance since drugs may be "cleared" from the body through extra-renal channels.

It is also necessary to know what the rate of glomerular filtration is because a given drug may alter it. Any pharmacologically active substance that lowers blood pressure or constricts renal arterioles will reduce the GFR. Even so, renal excretion of the substance may not be affected to the degree expected if it is secreted by the renal tubules (see below).

IV. TUBULAR TRANSPORT OF DRUGS

Although the production of glomerular filtrate is an essential step in the formation of urine, the final chemical composition of urine is largely dependent on the ease with which solutes are transported across the renal tubules. Inulin is one of the few substances that cannot enter renal cells from either direction. Most other molecules can penetrate the cellular membranes of tubules and some are carried across the cells by special processes.

As a general rule movement of solutes is from lumen to blood rather than from blood to lumen (see Figure 8.1). There is a simple explanation for this polarity. In at least three distinct portions of the nephron (proximal tubule, ascending limb of Henle's loop, distal tubule) sodium is pumped out and reenters the renal circulation. Together the pumps remove 99% or more of the sodium present in the original glomerular filtrate. Thus, in man, approximately 17 mEq of sodium are filtered each minute (plasma sodium = 140 mEq/liter; GFR = 125 ml/min) and 0.2 mEq or less is excreted. The osmotic force generated by this movement of the positively charged sodium ion and its accompanying anions from tubular lumens to blood forces water to move out as well. The solutes that remain are progressively concentrated as they flow down the length of the nephron. In this fashion a concentration gradient that favors outward movement (reabsorption) develops.

Operation of this process is depicted in panel A of Figure 8.2. A cluster of drug molecules present in the lumen of a renal tubule creates a simple diffusion gradient so that molecules move into the adjacent cell. As the concentration of the drug in the cell builds up, molecules begin to diffuse across the peritubular membrane into the surrounding interstitial space and finally into a blood vessel. Although egress by simple diffusion is theoretically possible for all drugs, it is most significant when a drug or one of its metabolites is highly lipid soluble. An excellent example of the ease with which lipid soluble drugs move out of tubular urine may be found in the work of Weiner et al. (1960). They showed that the rate of excretion of N-substituted analogues of probenecid varied inversely with the lipid solubility of each one. The pK_a of all compounds tested was 3.3–3.4. Reabsorption of probenecid was markedly dependent on the concentration of the unionized free acid, the lipid soluble form, in the tubular urine. Excretion was most rapid at high rates of flow of persistently alkaline urine, a condition in which relatively large amounts of probenecid exist in the ionized (poorly lipid soluble) form and the diffusion gradient was smaller than usual because the drug was less concentrated.

This study emphasizes the importance of urinary pH for the excretion of weak acids that are highly lipid soluble in their uncharged form. Assuming that the

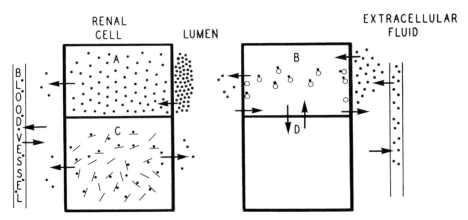

Fig. 8.2. Diagram showing different ways drugs can move into and out of renal cells. Each rectangle represents a renal tubular cell. Dots are drug molecules; circles are carrier protein molecules; short lines in cell C are macromolecules with which drugs can react. Different modes of transport are illustrated: Panel A: Simple diffusion. Molecules of drug are filtered into the tubular lumen, diffuse into and across the cell, and then pass from extracellular fluid into an adjacent capillary; Panel B: Carrier-mediated transport. Molecules diffuse from a capillary into extracellular fluid. On entering the peritubular membrane of the cell, they are picked up by a carrier, transported across the cell, and released into the lumen. As the arrows show, this process may be bidirectional; Panel C: Macromolecular facilitation. Molecules of drug diffuse into the cell and interact with a macromolecular constituent. Since the cellular concentration of free drug builds up slowly, total drug in the cell may exceed considerably the concentration in the lumen and extracellular fluid. Subsequent dissociation of drug molecules permits the cell to unload.

Arrows between B and D indicate that two adjoining cells may exchange solutes. See text for further discussion.

ionized form of the acid cannot penetrate renal cells, the distribution between plasma and tubular urine *at equilibrium* may be calculated from the equation

$$R = \frac{1 + 10(pH_u - pK_a)}{1 + 10(pH_p - pK_a)}$$

where R is the ratio of the urinary concentration and the plasma concentration of the acid, pH_u is the pH of urine, pH_p is the pH of plasma, and pK_a is the dissociation constant of the acid. When the pK_a of the acid is in the proper range (about 3 to 7), raising the pH of the urine will increase the ionization and larger amounts will be retained and excreted in urine. For bases

$$R = \frac{1 + 10(pK_a - pH_u)}{1 + 10(pK_a - pH_p)}$$

Theoretically, a significant increase in the acidity of urine will increase measurably the excretion of bases with pK_a values of 7–11.

It is obviously mandatory, if we are to describe accurately the distribution and excretion of weak acidic or basic drugs that are lipid-soluble, to conduct our experiments in such a way that the pH and the rate of formation of urine varies over a wide range. An excellent discussion of the many factors involved in pH dependent excretion of acids and bases is presented in the paper of Milne

TABLE 8.1
Common drugs with variable renal clearances

Drugs	Reference
BASES (Clearance greater in acidic urine)	
Amphetamine	Asatoor et al. (1965)
Chloroquine	Jailer et al. (1947)
Imipramine	Asatoor and Milne (1965)
Levorphanol	Braun et al. (1963)
Mecamylamine	Baer et al. (1956)
Quinine	Haag et al. (1943)
ACIDS (Clearance greater in alkaline urine)	
Acetazolamide	Maren (1956)
Nitrofurantoin	Woodruff et al. (1961)
Phenobarbital	Waddell and Butler (1957)
Probenecid	Weiner et al. (1960)
Salicylic acid	Weiner et al. (1959)
Sulfathiazole	Dalgaard-Mikkelsen and Poulsen (1956)

(Modified from table of M. D. Milne in *Renal Disease*, ed. by D. A. K. Black. F. A. Davis Co., Philadelphia, 1967.)

et al. (1958). Some of the important drugs the clearances of which are influenced by urinary pH are listed in Table 8.1.

In addition to simple passive diffusion, active transport of drugs may also occur. The term active transport denotes movement of molecules against an existing electrochemical gradient (i.e., uphill) into or out of cells. Such a process clearly requires the expenditure of energy derived from metabolic reactions of the cells. In view of the fact that active transport mechanisms can also transport molecules in the direction of a concentration gradient (i.e., downhill), the term is inexact and should either be abandoned or not be applied so rigorously. I prefer the substitutive term "carrier-mediated transport." The essentials of this process are shown in Figure 8.2B. Molecules diffuse from a neighboring blood vessel into extracellular fluid and from there into a cellular membrane. Either in the membrane itself or within the confines of the cell, the molecule is picked up by a transporting carrier that eventually releases it into the lumen of the tubule. Whether the carrier follows a predetermined path or moves randomly has not been ascertained. It is possible that two, or even a chain of carriers, participate in the transfer of a single organic substrate. The most important characteristics of carrier-mediated transport are: (1) high velocity of passage, (2) susceptibility to interference by metabolic or competitive inhibitors, and (3) a maximal capacity of the transporting mechanism. Because they are amenable to experimental analysis, points 2 and 3 are used as the major criteria for deciding whether a substance is handled by a carrier-mediated process. Workers in the field generally try to show that transport of a drug can be blocked. They

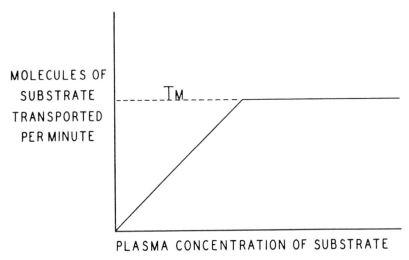

Fig. 8.3. Diagram showing saturation of a transporting carrier by the transported substrate. T_M = tubular maximal capacity of the carrier.

then try to find out whether the capacity of the tubules to transport the drug is limited. This is done in the case of a drug that is secreted by increasing its plasma concentration stepwise. A tubular maximal capacity (T_M) is demonstrable if the total amount transported (amount excreted minus the amount filtered) reaches a peak that does not increase further with additional increments in the plasma concentration of substrate (see Figure 8.3). The procedure for obtaining reabsorptive T_M values is similar except that reabsorbed drug (filtered minus excreted drug) is plotted along the ordinate. The existence of a T_M is perhaps the best indication that a carrier-mediated process subject to saturation with a substrate is involved in the renal transport of a drug. Unfortunately, it is not always possible to obtain a T_M. Some drugs are too toxic to be administered in the amounts required; others may be transported simultaneously in opposite directions (see below).

The list of organic substances whose passage through renal cells is carrier-mediated is long. Included are various sugars and amino acids, weak organic acids, and many organic bases. Examples of drugs handled in this fashion are listed in Table 8.2. Although the carriers have not been identified, at least one associated with secretion of organic bases appears to be a protein (Magour et al., 1969). The segment of the nephron that transports organic compounds is the proximal tubule, but in one instance (ascorbic acid) there is evidence for distal tubular secretion (Kleit et al., 1965).

There are now several examples of substrates that are transported by carrier-mediated processes bidirectionally across the mammalian proximal tubule. Notably, all are organic acids: p-aminohippuric acid (Cho and Cafruny, 1967); uric acid (Zins and Weiner, 1968a); taurocholic acid (Zins and Weiner, 1968b); and m-hydroxybenzoic acid (May and Weiner, 1969). How bidirectional transport takes place is one of the unsolved problems of the field of renal physiology. Perhaps the carriers in some cells or in individual tubules are oriented in different directions, or two carriers in a single cell, one reabsorptive and one secretory,

TABLE 8.2

Common drugs secreted in the proximal tubule of mammalian kidney

Drugs	Reference	
BASES		
dihydromorphine	Hug et al.	(1965)
dopamine	Rennick	(1968)
merpiperphenidol	Beyer et al.	(1953)
N-methylnicotinamide	Beyer et al.	(1950)
neostigmine	Roberts et al.	(1965)
quinine	Torretti et al.	(1962)
tetraethylammonium	Farah and Rennick	(1956)
ACIDS		
acetazolamide	Weiner et al.	(1959)
ethacrynic acid	Beyer et al.	(1965)
furosemide	Gayer	(1965)
mersalyl	Cafruny et al.	(1966)
penicillin	Beyer et al.	(1944)
phenylbutazone	Gutman et al.	(1960)
salicylate	Weiner et al.	(1959)

compete for the same substrate. Movement from one cell to another as between B and D of Figure 8.2 may take place. A confusing fact also is the observation that certain neutral molecules appear to be secreted by the organic acid transport system (O'Connell *et al.*, 1962).

It is decidedly incorrect ever to claim that a drug is transported by a carrier-mediated process unless there are supporting data showing that the process can be inhibited. Consider the following case which is illustrated in panel C of Figure 8.2: a drug has a high affinity for a cellular macromolecule. When given by injection, large amounts enter renal cells and bind to the macromolecule. In a short time blood and urinary levels fall precipitously, the drug-protein complex dissociates, and free drug leaves the cells to enter blood (large compartment) and urine (small compartment). When this happens, the renal clearance of the compound turns out to be greater than the GFR. The neutral compound, chlormerodrin, probably behaves in this fashion (Cafruny *et al.*, 1966). Large amounts react with protein-bound sulfhydryl groups of the proximal tubule. When the drug is injected in a single dose, its stop-flow curve resembles those of secreted organic acids. Yet, probenecid, an inhibitor of organic acid transport, does not alter the shape of the stop-flow curve. It is perfectly proper to consider this particular phenomenon as a form of transport, but it is certainly not a rapid, carrier-mediated process dependent on metabolic energy.

V. METHODS FOR STUDYING RENAL TRANSPORT OF DRUGS

Many questions about the renal transport of any organic compound can be answered rather quickly and expeditiously, and without resorting to the use of difficult or complicated methods. It is usually best to begin with a simple renal clearance determination. A priming dose of the drug in question is given intravenously along with a priming dose of inulin. Both substances are then infused at a constant rate for the duration of the experiment. When the plasma levels stabilize, several successive clearance determinations (UV/P) are made. It is essential that the plasma concentration of the drug used in the clearance formula does not include a non-filterable fraction bound to plasma protein. If the ratio (UV/P) drug/(UV/P) inulin is greater than 1.0, the drug is probably excreted in part by means of a carrier-mediated process; if the ratio is less than 1.0, the drug must be reabsorbed either in response to a concentration gradient or with the assistance of a carrier. These conclusions are valid only when the plasma concentration of the drug is not rising or falling rapidly. It is important to keep in mind that ratios greater than 1.0 do not rule out the simultaneous occurrence of reabsorption; nor do ratios less than 1.0 mean that secretion does not take place. As mentioned in an earlier section (see above), a weak organic acid may be secreted in the proximal tubule only to be reabsorbed passively from the more acid urine of distal segments. If the non-ionic form of the weak acid is highly lipid-soluble, passive reabsorption is almost certain to occur. In such an instance, the clearance of the drug will vary directly with the rate of urine flow and with a rise in the pH of urine.

The importance of the inulin clearance cannot be over emphasized. Without it, there can be no evaluation of the role of tubules in the transport of the drug. Moreover, a change in the inulin clearance may provide the first clue that the drug influences renal blood flow. Many workers routinely use the clearance of p-aminohippuric acid (PAH) as an estimate of renal plasma flow. I cannot recommend this practice for three reasons: 1) the renal extraction of PAH is quite variable even when plasma concentration is low, 2) PAH is reabsorbed, 3) PAH may suppress the renal transport of the test drug if it is a weak organic acid.

Once the participation of tubules in the transport of a drug has been established, it may be useful or necessary to identify the tubular segments involved. For this purpose the stop-flow method of Malvin et al. (1958) is ideal. Ureteral catheters are inserted and pushed upward until the tips reach the renal pelves. A brisk osmotic diuresis is initiated by infusing large amounts of mannitol along with the drug to be tested. When the rate of urine flow is in the range of 20–25% of the GFR (about 7–9 ml/min from one kidney of a dog weighing 15 kg), one or both catheters are occluded. During the period of occlusion, renal blood flow is not markedly affected. Solutes can diffuse or be carried across renal cells from blood to urine or from urine to blood. After a suitable period of time, the catheters are reopened and the urine is collected serially in volumes of 0.5–1.0 ml. Although a considerable amount of mixing takes place, the first collected samples in large part represent urine derived from the distal segments of nephrons; samples collected later represent urine from proximal segments. An idealized stop-flow pattern is shown in Figure 8.4. The curve marked A is that expected in the case of a drug secreted in the proximal tubule; B is one for a substance reabsorbed in distal tubules and possibly in collecting ducts. The osmotic pressure of mannitol in tubular urine slows the rate of reabsorption of water, but a certain amount of reabsorption of fluid still occurs. To correct for this, all values for concentrations of drugs in urine samples are factored by the concentration of inulin in the same samples. As shown in Figure 8.4, when (U/P) drug/(U/P) inulin is

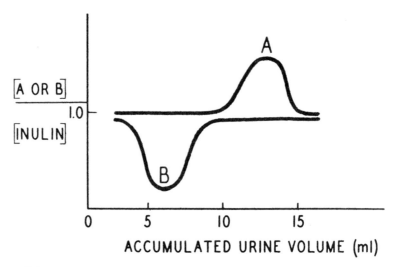

Fig. 8.4. Schematic representation of stop-flow curves for a substance secreted in the proximal tubule (curve A) and one reabsorbed in distal segments (curve B). [A or B] = concentration of drug A or B in urine samples divided by the concentration of free A or B in plasma; [Inulin] = concentration of inulin in urine samples divided by concentration of inulin in plasma. Values on the abscissa represent 1.0 ml samples collected serially following reopening of the urinary catheter. The last samples, 10–15 ml, are derived principally from the proximal tubule.

greater than 1 (curve A from samples 11–14), a secretory process may be invoked; with a value less than 1.0 (curve B from samples 4–8), a reabsorptive process may be postulated. Stop-flow analysis has been most fruitful in providing evidence for the participation of tubules in the transport of drugs and in revealing grossly the site of transport (i.e., proximal or distal segment of the nephron). In certain special cases, modified stop-flow procedures are required, and have been used successfully to demonstrate both secretion and reabsorption of organic molecules (Gussin and Cafruny, 1966; Zins and Weiner, 1968a and 1968b). Most of the stop-flow literature deals with the procedure in dogs but there are also data for other species commonly used in investigative work (Williamson et al., 1961; Vander and Cafruny, 1962).

Although the stop-flow procedure and ordinary clearance studies suffice to answer many questions regarding renal transport and excretion of drugs, in some instances certain special methods may offer distinct advantages. Thus in vitro slice techniques (Cross and Taggart, 1950) are valuable for studying highly toxic compounds and for looking at the individual components of the transporting systems. The renal portal system of the chicken is especially useful for studying secretory transport. Quebbemann and Rennick (1969) used this technique most effectively to study transport of catecholamines. Reabsorptive transport as a carrier-mediated process on the other hand, can best be examined by the technique of retrograde intraluminal injection (Cafruny et al., 1966; Cho and Cafruny, 1969). Micropuncture and microperfusion techniques have not been applied, except in a limited way, to the analysis of transport of drugs simply because they are difficult to perform and require extremely sensitive analytical techniques.

Thus far, our discussion has centered on the separate mechanisms by which the kidney recognizes and ultimately excretes or returns drugs to the circulation. Implicitly, we assign no vitalistic function to renal cells. Recognition primarily involves physico-chemical processes. Small nonpolar compounds are filtered, but as a general rule are excreted slowly because they cross tubular cells with ease. Small polar compounds, the usual products of metabolizing enzymes, are excreted rapidly because they are quite soluble in an aqueous medium. In addition, tubular secretory systems augment the excretion of many charged molecules. The involvement of secretory systems, apparently designed to promote the excretion of endogenous metabolites, in the excretion of drugs appears to be a fortuitous event, for polar drugs are apt to bind to plasma protein and thus to escape being filtered. How fortunate that the secretory systems can handle a variety of substrates—that they do not possess the specificity of most enzymes! By putting all the separate mechanisms together, we gain a better appreciation of the role of the kidney as the major organ that terminates the action of drugs and their metabolites.

REFERENCES

Asatoor, A. M., Galman, B. R., Johnson, J. R., and Milne, M. D.: The excretion of dexamphetamine and its derivatives. Brit. J. Pharmacol. *24:* 293–300, 1965.

Asatoor, A. M. and Milne, M. D.: Unpublished observations, 1965.

Baer, J. E., Paulson, S. F., Russo, H. F., and Beyer, K. H.: Renal elimination of 3-methyl-aminoisocamphane hydrochloride (mecamylamine). Am. J. Physiol. *186:* 180–186, 1956.

Beyer, K. H., Woodward, R., Peters, L., Verwey, W. F., and Mattis, P. A.: The prolongation of penicillin retention in the body by means of para-aminohippuric acid. Science *100:* 107–108, 1944.

Beyer, K. H., Russo, H. F., Gass, S. R., Wilhoyte, K. M., and Pitt, A. A.: Renal tubular elimination of N^1-methylnicotinamide. Am. J. Physiol. *160:* 311–320 1950.

Beyer, K. H., Tillson, E. K., Russo, H. F., and Paulson S. F.: Physiological economy of Darstine, 5-methyl-4-phenyl-1-(1-piperidyl)-3-hexanol methobromide, visceral anticholinergic agent. Am. J. Physiol. *175:* 39–44, 1953.

Beyer, K. H., Baer, J. E., Michaelson, J. K. and Russo, H. F.: Renotropic characteristics of ethacrynic acid: a phenoxyacetic saluretic diuretic agent. J. Pharmacol. Exp. Ther. *147:* 1–22, 1965.

Braun, W., Hesse, I., and Malorny, G.: Zur Bedeutung pH-abhängiger Diffusionvorgänge für die Nierenfunktion. Arch. Exp. Path. Pharmakol. *245:* 457–470, 1963.

Cafruny, E. J., Cho, K. C., and Gussin, R. Z.: The pharmacology of mercurial diuretics. Ann. N. Y. Acad. Sci. *139:* 362–374, 1966.

Cho, K. C., and Cafruny, E. J.: Renal reabsorption of p-aminohippuric acid (PAH) disclosed by means of the technique of retrograde intraluminal infusion. Pharmacologist *9:* 208, 1967.

Cross, R. J. and Taggart, J. V.: Renal tubular transport: accumulation of p-aminohippurate by rabbit kidney slices. Am. J. Physiol. *161:* 181–190, 1950.

Dalgaard-Mikkelsen, S. and Poulsen, E.: Renal excretion of sulfathiazole and sulphadimidine in pigs. Acta Pharmacol. (Kbh) *12:* 233–239, 1956.

Farah, A. and Rennick, B.: Studies on the renal tubular transport of tetraethylammonium ion in renal slices of the dog. J. Pharmacol. Exp. Ther. *117:* 478–487, 1956.

Gayer, J.: Die renal Exkretion des neuen Diureticum Furosemid. Klin. Wschr. *43:* 898–902, 1965.

Gussin, R. Z. and Cafruny, E. J.: Renal sites of action of ethacrynic acid. J. Pharmacol. Exp. Ther. *153:* 148–158, 1966.

Gutman, A. B., Dayton, P. G., Yu, T. F., Berger, L., Chen, W., Sicam, L. E., and Burns, J. J.: A study of the inverse relationship between pKa and rate of renal excretion of phenylbutazone analogs in man and dog. Am. J. Med. *29:* 1017–1033, 1960.

Haag, H. B., Larson, P. S., and Schwartz, J. J.: The effect of urinary pH on the elimination of quinine in man. J. Pharmacol. Exp. Ther. *79:* 136–139, 1943.

Hug, C. C., Jr., Mellett, L. B., and Cafruny, E. J.: Stop flow analysis of the renal excretion of tritium-labeled dihydromorphine. J. Pharmacol. Exp. Ther. *150:* 259–269, 1965.

Jailer, J. W., Rosenfeld, J., and Shannon, J. A.: The influence of orally administered alkali and acid on the renal excretion of quinacrine, chloroquine and santoquine. J. Clin. Invest. *26:* 1168–1172, 1947.

Kleit, S., Levin, D., Perenich, T., and Cade, R.: Renal excretion of ascorbic acid by dogs. Am. J. Physiol. *209:* 195–198, 1965.

Magour, S., Farah, A., and Sroka, A.: The partial purification of a carrier-like protein for organic bases from the kidney. J. Pharmacol. Exp. Ther. *167:* 243–252, 1969.

Malvin, R. L., Wilde, W. S., and Sullivan, L. P.: Localization of nephron transport by stop-flow analysis. Am. J. Physiol. *194:* 135–142, 1958.

Maren, T. H.: Carbonic anhydrase inhibitors. The effects of metabolic acidosis on the response to Diamox. Bull. Johns Hopkins Hosp. *98:* 159–183, 1956.

May, D. G. and Weiner, I. M.: m-Hydroxybenzoate (M-HB): Bidirectional active transport in proximal renal tubule of the dog. Fed. Proc. *28:* 523, 1969.

Milne, M. D., Scribner, B. H., and Crawford, M. A.: Non-ionic diffusion and the excretion of weak acids and bases. Am. J. Med. *24:* 709–729, 1958.

O'Connell, J. M. B., Romeo, J. A., and Mudge, G. H.: Renal tubular secretion of creatinine in the dog. Am. J. Physiol. *203:* 985–990, 1962.

Quebbemann, A. J. and Rennick, B. R.: Effects of structural modifications of catecholamines on renal tubular transport in the chicken. J. Pharmacol. Exp. Ther. *166:* 52–62, 1969.

Rennick, B. R.: Dopamine: Renal tubular transport in dog and plasma binding studies. Am. J. Physiol. *215:* 532–534, 1968.

Roberts, J. B., Thomas, B. H., and Wilson, A.: Distribution and excretion of (^{14}C)-neostigmine in the rat and hen. Brit. J. Pharmacol. Chemotherap. *25:* 234–242, 1965.

Smith, H. W.: *Principles of Renal Physiology.* New York, Oxford University Press, 1956.

Toribara, T. Y., Terepka, A. R., and Dewey, P. A.: The ultrafilterable calcium of human serum. I. Ultrafiltration methods and normal values. J. Clin. Invest. *36:* 738–748, 1957.

Torretti, J., Weiner, I. M., and Mudge, G. H.: Renal tubular secretion and reabsorption of organic bases in the dog. J. Clin. Invest. *41:* 793–804, 1962.

Vander, A. J. and Cafruny, E. J.: Stop-flow analysis of renal function in the monkey. Am. J. Physiol. *202:* 1105–1108, 1962.

Waddell, W. and Butler, T. C.: The distribution and excretion of phenobarbital. J. Clin. Invest. *36:* 1217–1226, 1957.

Weiner, I. M., Washington, J. A., II, and Mudge, G. H.: Studies on the renal excretion of salicylate in the dog. Bull. Johns Hopkins Hosp. *105:* 284–297, 1959.

Weiner, I. M., Washington, J. A., II, and Mudge, G. H.: On the mechanism of action of probenecid on renal tubular secretion. Bull. Johns Hopkins Hosp. *106:* 333–346, 1960.

Williamson, H. E., Skulan, T. W., and Shideman, F. E.: Effects of adrenalectomy and desoxycorticosterone on stop-flow patterns of sodium and potassium in the rat. J. Pharmacol. Exp. Ther. *131:* 49–55, 1961.

Woodruff, M. W., Malvin, R. L. and Thompson, I. M.: The renal transport of nitrofurantoin. Effect of acid-base balance on its excretion. J.A.M.A. *175:* 1132–1135, 1961.

Zins, G. R. and Weiner, I. M.: Bidirectional transport of uric acid, exclusively a proximal tubular function in the mongrel dog. Am. J. Physiol. *215:* 411–422, 1968a.

Zins, G. R. and Weiner, I. M.: Bidirectional transport of taurocholate by the proximal tubule of the dog. Am. J. Physiol. *215:* 840–845, 1968b.

Recommended Review Articles

Cafruny, E. J.: Renal Pharmacology. Ann. Rev. Pharmacol. *8:* 131–150, 1968.

Forster, R. P.: Renal transport mechanisms. Fed. Proc. *26:* 1008–1019, 1967.

Mudge, G. H.: Renal Pharmacology. Ann. Rev. Pharmacol. *7:* 163–179, 1967.

Peters, L.: Renal tubular excretion of organic bases. Pharmacol. Rev. *12:* 1–35, 1960.

Weiner, I. M. and Mudge, G. H.: Renal tubular mechanisms for excretion of organic acids and bases. Am. J. Med. *36:* 743–762, 1964.

Weiner, I. M.: Mechanisr s of drug absorption and excretion. Ann Rev. Pharmacol. *7:* 39–56, 1967.

Willbrandt, W. and Rosenberg, T.: The concept of carrier transport and its corollaries in pharmacology. Pharmacol. Rev. *13:* 109–183, 1961.

9

Biliary and Other Routes of Excretion of Drugs

GABRIEL L. PLAA

I. BILIARY EXCRETION

The excretion of drugs into the bile is now receiving a considerable amount of attention. This subject has been reviewed by a number of authors (Sperber, 1959; Brauer, 1959; Schanker, 1962; Smith, 1966; Stowe and Plaa, 1968); the review by Smith (1966) is by far the most comprehensive and detailed survey of our current knowledge.

A. Types of Substances Secreted into the Bile

Bile is a composite secretion of widely varying composition. Brauer (1959) has divided these constituents into three classes on the basis of their bile/plasma concentration ratios. Class A substances, whose ratio is nearly 1, include sodium, potassium and chloride ions, and glucose. Class B substances, whose bile plasma ratios usually range from 10 to 1000, include bile salts, bilirubin glucuronide, sulfobromophthalein (BSP) conjugates, fluorescein, rose bengal, and creatinine. Class C compounds consist of those in which the ratio is less than 1, and are inclusive of sucrose, inulin, phosphates, phospholipids, and mucoproteins.

B. Biliary Transfer Systems

Quite an interest is now developing in elucidating the mechanisms involved in bile secretion. The state of knowledge has recently been reviewed by Wheeler (1969). From earlier work (Brauer, 1959) it is quite clear that bile is not a product of filtration analogous to the glomerular filtrate of the kidney; bile secretion can continue up to a limiting pressure which is greater than the blood pressure. Therefore, three theoretical mechanisms exist for translating metabolic energy into bile flow: active transport of water, active transport of solute leading to osmotic flow, and secretory vacuole formation (Wheeler, 1969). Of these, active transport of water seems least likely, whereas several models have been proposed for the active transport of solute; little is known about the possibility of secretory vacuole formation in the region of the bile canaliculi or the Golgi complex. One of the major determinants of bile production is the rate of bile salt secretion. Light *et al.* (1959) demonstrated that when the cholic acid concentration in bile was reduced by interruption of the enterohepatic circulation, the rats also exhibited a parallel decrease in bile volume.

While most of the formation of bile appears to take place in the canaliculi, the bile ducts themselves may not be without effect. Secretin has been found to exert a choleretic effect in a number of species; secretin apparently increases bile flow by increasing inorganic electrolytes, but has no effect on bile salts or bile pigments. Wheeler (1969) feels that secretin acts on the bile ducts, rather than on the canaliculi, to stimulate fluid output. Brauer (1959) demonstrated that electrolyte exchange can occur between bile and plasma as the bile passes through the biliary tree; he was tempted to propose that this exchange process occurs in the bile ducts rather than in the canaliculi.

Present concepts indicate that bile flow is the result of secretory activity of the hepatic cells aligning the bile canaliculi. As this bile passes through the biliary tree, it can be modified by exchanges occurring with the blood; these exchanges presumably occur in the bile ductular region.

Much of the work that has been carried out in studying the excretion of drugs into the bile has dealt primarily with class B compounds. It appears that the transport of these substances across the biliary epithelium into bile requires an active secretory process. These substances compete for transport. The transport mechanism can be saturated by an excess of compound. Metabolic inhibitors have been shown to inhibit the secretion of some of these substances, and hypothermia has been shown to decrease their excretory rates (Brauer, 1959; Roberts et al., 1967).

The effect of hypothermia is illustrated in Table 9.1. Roberts et al. (1967) found that in rats the BSP biliary excretion maximum decreased about 7 % per °C (about 0.1 mg/kg/min) while the bilirubin excretion rate decreased about 5 % per °C (about 0.04 mg/kg/min). In mice the bilirubin excretion rate was found to decrease about 4 % per °C (about 0.01 mg/kg/min). In both species the major effect of temperature seemed to be on the rate of flow of bile although an effect on the concentrative capacity was also evident.

Hanzon (1952) has visualized the transfer of fluorescein from blood to bile in vivo. However, little is known about the actual transfer system. There appears to be at least three such systems—one for organic acids, one for bases, and one for nonionic substances. A number of carboxylic and sulfonic acids have been shown to compete for a common transport process. These substances include BSP, phenol red, fluorescein, p-acetylaminohippuric acid (PAAH), and penicillin. Recently, chlorothiazide, an acid which is neither sulfonic or carboxylic, has

TABLE 9.1

Effect of temperature on the biliary excretion of BSP and bilirubin during infusions in rats[a]

Temperature (°C)	Maximum Biliary Excretion Rate mg/kg/min		Bile Flow Rate (µl/kg/min)	
	BSP	Bilirubin	BSP	Bilirubin
31	0.58	0.55	32	35
33	0.70	0.63	47	45
35	0.88	0.70	65	53
37	1.03	0.78	80	61
39	1.20	0.88	95	71

[a] Data obtained from Roberts et al. (1967).

been shown (Hart and Schanker, 1966) to be actively secreted into bile by the same system that secretes the other organic acids. In rats with ligated renal pedicles, it was shown that 20% of the administered dose (20 mg/kg) of chlorothiazide was excreted into the bile within 20 min; the bile/plasma ratio of the nonprotein bound drug was about 80. Probenecid, a substance which inhibits the transport of a number of carboxylic and sulfonic acids, was shown to inhibit the hepatic transport of chlorothiazide. A 100 mg/kg dose of probenecid reduced the amount of chlorothiazide excreted to 8% and reduced the bile/plasma ratio to 16. It was also shown that chlorothiazide can inhibit the excretion into bile of PAAH; control rats excreted 38% of the PAAH in 90 min, whereas chlorothiazide-treated rats excreted only 6%. Recently, Guarino and Schanker (1968) have shown that 29% of a dose (50 mg/kg) of probenecid was excreted into bile within 90 min in rats with ligated renal pedicles. The proportion of the total excreted as conjugates was about 50%; the bile/plasma concentration ratio was 21.9. The biliary excretion of probenecid could be reduced by coadministering phenolphthalein.

Schanker and Solomon (1963) have also demonstrated that a number of bases can be excreted into the bile in high concentrations. The quaternary ammonium ion, procaine amide ethobromide (PAEB), rapidly appears in the bile of rats in high concentrations. After administering PAEB (5 mg/kg), 4.2% of the dose was excreted within 30 min into the bile of rats with ligated renal pedicles. The composition of the PAEB in the bile was equally distributed between the free and conjugated forms. The bile/plasma ratios for each form were between 70 and 90. Schanker and Solomon (1963) report that the following quaternary compounds are excreted into the bile of rats within 4 hours: carbidium ethanesulfonate, 10%; benzomethamine 31%; oxyphenonium, 11%; mepiperphenidol, 11%; and glycopyrrolate, 10%. Mepiperphenidol, benzomethamine, oxyphenonium and glycopyrrolate were shown to cause a 49–80% depression of the biliary excretion of free PAEB. On the other hand, quaternary ammonium compounds (tetraethyl ammonium, cetyltrimethylammonium and SQ-3576), which are not excreted into bile in large proportions failed to depress PAEB excretion. Therefore, it appears that the excretable derivatives compete for a common transport system. After studying a number of quaternary ammonium compounds, Schanker (1965) concluded that, in order to be excreted into the bile, these substances would have to contain a highly polar quaternary amine group at one end of the molecule and one or more nonpolar ring structures at the opposite end. Those bases which were poorly excreted lacked the nonpolar ring. The transport system appears to be different from the one responsible for the secretion of organic acids since BSP and glycocholate had no effect on the biliary excretion of PAEB (Schanker and Solomon, 1963).

The presence of a nonionic transport system has recently been demonstrated in rats by Kupferberg and Schanker (1968). They found that ouabain was rapidly excreted into the bile in high concentrations; bile/plasma ratios ranged from 147 to 557. Large doses of organic ions (probenecid, PAAH, PAEB, and benzomethamine) failed to depress the rate of excretion of ouabain. A number of other cardiac glycosides (digitoxin, digoxin, lanatoside C, and scillaren A) were found to inhibit the hepatic uptake of ouabain by liver slices. Cox and Wright (1959) have shown the importance of the biliary excretory route for lanatoside A and C, digoxin, and digitoxin (Table 9.2).

TABLE 9.2

Biliary excretion of glycosides in rats after 5 hrs[a]

Glycoside	% Dose Excreted		
	Parent Compound	Metabolites	Total
Lanatoside A	75	0	75
Lanatoside C	70	0	70
Digoxin	11	29	40
Digitoxin	6	4	10
Digitoxigenin	—	—	15
Digoxigenin	—	—	14

[a] Data obtained from Cox and Wright (1959). All glycosides were given at a dose of 1 mg/kg.

TABLE 9.3

Comparison of biliary excretion parameters of various substances in rats

Compound	Biliary Concentration (mg/ml)	Bile/Plasma Ratio
BSP	15	90
Chlorothiazide	0.7	80
PAEB	0.2	80
Bilirubin	12	30
Ouabain	0.05	500
Indocyanine green	0.9	30

Thus, it appears clear that there are at least three different transport systems involved in the transfer of class B substances into bile. Table 9.3 contains data obtained in the rat for a number of these substances. It can be seen that the bile/plasma ratios are quite high for all these substances, but it can also be seen that the actual biliary concentration is not necessarily very high for all of these substances.

C. Structure and Molecular Weight Considerations

A number of generalizations have been made regarding the chemical characteristics necessary for high biliary excretion. Williams *et al.* (1965) studied aniline and substituted benzoic acid derivatives. They proposed that substances of low molecular weight (less than 300) would be excreted into the bile in less than 5% of the dose. With various iodinated derivatives of p-aminobenzoic acid, they concluded that the increase in molecular weight associated with iodination resulted in increased biliary secretion. Cox and Wright (1959) proposed that the presence of very polar groups was necessary for the excretion of cardiac glycosides. Therefore, it appears that a molecular weight greater than 300 and the presence of polar groups facilitate biliary excretion.

Conjugation is also regarded as important in the biliary excretion of substances, and of particular interest is the conjugation of a compound or its metabolites with glucuronic acid. Many substances with diverse structures are known (Smith and Williams, 1966) to be excreted into the bile; these include the glucuronides of menthol, bilirubin, thyroxine, morphine, stilbestrol, glutethimide, phenolphthalein, iodopanoic acid, and some polycyclic hydrocarbons. Smith and Williams (1966) have attempted to explain how glucuronidation can enhance biliary excretion: conjugation can result in the production of an anionic polar molecule; glucuronidation can produce a molecule having a molecular weight in excess of 400; it is possible that a substance requires a balance of hydrophilic and lipophilic properties, and that glucuronidation facilitates this balance. Recently, the biliary excretion of three structurally related aryl sulphate esters has been studied (Hearse *et al.*, 1969). It was found that the parent esters with molecular weights of less than 300 were not excreted in the bile; however, those esters which were conjugated *in vivo* with glucuronic acid (m.w. greater than 400) were eliminated in the bile to a large extent. The balance between lipophilic and hydrophilic properties seemed minimal in this study. The authors felt that the limiting factor in the biliary elimination of these aryl sulphate esters was the ability of the compounds to form glucuronic acid conjugates at appropriate sites in the liver.

There are a number of exceptions to these generalizations. With BSP, conjugation has been presumed to be necessary for biliary excretion. However, a dibrominated analogue of BSP (phenol-3, 6-dibromphthalein disulfonate, DBSP) has been found to be excreted into the bile in an unchanged form (Javitt, 1964; Klaassen and Plaa, 1968a). A comparative study of BSP and DBSP excretion in three species was carried out and the nonconjugated derivative, DBSP, was found to be excreted in a manner similar to that of BSP conjugate (Table 9.4). With other phthalein derivatives, it has been found that the tri- and tetra-halogenated fluoresceins and the tetrachloro-tetrabromo-derivative are excreted to a major extent in rat bile in forms which are indistinguishable from the parent compound (Webb *et al.*, 1962). Indocyanine green and some azo dyes are also excreted into the bile in an unchanged form (Wheeler *et al.*, 1958; Ryan and Wright, 1961).

There are also some exceptions to the correlation between polarity and excretion. Haddock *et al.* (1965) studied the relative excretion rates of a series of chelated iron complexes. They found that those chelates possessing a net neutral charge and lipid solubility were excreted more extensively than those possessing a charged anionic site. They felt that the preference for biliary excretion of these substances over urinary excretion was due to the relative nonpolar nature of the derivatives. Meyer-Brunot and Keberle (1968) studied the excretion of a series of sideramine ferrioxamine derivatives which possessed different lipid-to-water partition coefficients. These substances were all neutral compounds. The studies were carried out in perfused rat livers and verified in intact animals. They found that in this series of compounds, the greater the lipid affinity of the derivatives, the more pronounced their biliary excretion and the higher their bile/plasma ratio. The most lipophilic derivative was present in an approximately 100-fold concentration in the bile, whereas the least lipophilic substance did not accumulate in the bile. A summary of these data is shown in Table 9.5.

TABLE 9.4

Hepatic disposition of BSP and DBSP in rat, rabbit, and dog[a]

Parameter	Compound	Rat	Rabbit	Dog
% conjugates in bile	BSP	69	75	70
	DBSP	0	2	2
Hepatic Storage (μmoles/μmoles %/ kg)	BSP	0.51	0.57	2.45
	DBSP	0.61	0.39	1.97
Biliary Excretion Rate (μmoles/kg/ min)	BSP	1.14	1.35	0.20
	DBSP	1.22	1.43	0.28
Biliary Concentration (μmoles/ml)	BSP	19.1	19.1	13.1
	DBSP	16.2	16.2	19.2

[a] Data obtained from Klaassen and Plaa (1968a).

TABLE 9.5
Biliary excretion of ferrioxamine derivatives by perfused rat liver[a]

Compound	Water:Butanol Partition Coefficient	% Excreted in Bile in 2 hr	Excretion Rate (nmoles/g/min)	Bile/Plasma ratio
Ferrioxamine (FO)	98:2	5	0.8	1.4
Carbamido-FO	80:20	18	5.3	7.6
Formyl-FO	77:23	42	7.2	9.1
Acetyl-FO	76:24	35	9.4	8.9
Valeryl-FO	22:78	82	34	70
Benzoyl-FO	17:83	85	42	63
p-Ethoxyphenylacetyl-FO	10:90	83	32	115

[a] Data obtained from Meyer-Brunot and Keberle (1968).

D. Importance of Biliary Excretion and the Enterohepatic Circulation

The relative importance of the biliary excretion route depends entirely upon the species and the substance concerned. The quantitative relationships for a number of substances has been reviewed by Stowe and Plaa (1968) (see Table 9.6 for a summary of these data). For those substances where the biliary route is an important route of excretion, it is evident that quantitative alterations in this pathway could have marked effects on the duration of action or even the depth of action of the pharmacological agent. Gibson and Becker (1967) have shown that the lethality of ouabain is markedly increased in mice whose bile ducts have been occluded. Keberle *et al.* (1962) demonstrated that, in the rat, the presence of the enterohepatic circulation can have a marked effect on the persistence of glutethimide in the body. The half-life for glutethimide in normal rats was about 24 hours, while in animals with a biliary fistula, the half-life was only about 6 hours. Biliary excretion can influence toxicity in those situations in which biotransformation reactions yielding toxic products occur in the lower portions of the intestinal tract. With chloramphenicol, the glucuronide has been shown to be excreted in the bile of rats, converted to arylamines and reabsorbed in this form. These arylamines can exert a toxic action on the thyroid (Thompson *et al.*, 1954). Williams *et al.* (1965) point out the possibility that the intestinal carcinogenic activity of aromatic amines in rats may be due to the biliary excretion as glucuronides of o-hydroxyamines formed in the liver and that these conjugates are then broken down in the intestine to free o-hydroxyamines which are carcinogenic. Unfortunately, no generalizations can be made about the relative importance of the enterohepatic circulation since it depends not only upon the compounds concerned but also the species being tested. However, it has become evident that research in this area would be extremely worthwhile.

Increased biliary flow has also been shown to affect the excretion of a number of substances. The choleresis which follows the administration of bile salts has been shown to increase BSP excretion (O'Maille *et al.*, 1966; Ritt and Combes, 1967). The biliary excretion of bilirubin, BSP and DBSP have been shown to be increased in rats treated with phenobarbital (Roberts and Plaa, 1967; Klaassen and Plaa, 1968b) (Table 9.7); the increase in bile flow associated with phenobarbital treatment seems to be implicated in the increased excretion of these substances.

TABLE 9.6

Excretion of various drugs into bile[a]

Compound	Species	Dose mg/kg	Time hr	Total	Parent	Metabolite
Sulfonamides						
Sulfanilamide	Rat	50	24	4	3	1
Sulfacetamide	Rat	50	24	0.5	0.5	—
Sulfapyridine	Rat	50	24	11	—	11
Sulfadiazine	Rat	50	24	2	2	—
Sulfathiazole	Rat	50	24	2	2	—
Sulfamethoxypyridazine	Rat	50	24	8	—	8
Sulfadimethoxine	Rat	50	24	11	—	11
Sulfadimethoxine glucuronide	Rat	100	24	78	78	—
Hormones						
Thyroxine	Rat	0.028	24	24	1	23
Thyroxine	Man	0.3[b]	96	10	—	—
Triiodothyronine	Dog	0.001	24	27	3	24
Progesterone	Rabbit	0.020	5	40	—	40
Hydrocortisone	Rat	0.25	3	83	—	83
Estrone	Man	0.37[b]	48	50	—	50
Estradiol	Man	0.37[b]	48	50	—	50
Testosterone	Man	1	24	13	—	13
Norethynodrel	Rabbit	5	7	33	0.3	32.7
Norethynodrel	Man	5[b]	24	30	—	—
Stilbestrol	Rat	10	24	94	3	91
Corticosterone	Cat	0.04	240	86	—	86
Antibiotics						
Methicillin	Rat	300	24	4	—	—
Methicillin	Dog	50	24	22	—	—
Ampicillin	Rat	100	18	15	—	—
Penicillin-V	Rat	100	6	5	—	—
Penicillin-T	Rat	100	2.5	20	—	—
Penicillin-G	Dog	50	24	9	—	—
Nafcillin	Dog	50	24	97	—	—
Cloxacillin	Rat	100	3	21	—	—
Metacycline	Dog	10	24	3	—	—
Oxytetracycline	Dog	10	22	2	—	—
Demethylchlortetracycline	Dog	10	24	2	—	—
Erythromycin	Rat	66	2	15	7	8
Erythromycin	Man	250[b]	20	13	—	—
Oleandomycin	Rat	100	4	10	—	—
Carbomycin	Rat	100	4	0.3	—	—
Chloramphenicol	Rat	100	4	30	—	—
Chloramphenicol	Man	1000[b]	20	3	—	—
Autonomic Agents						
Epinephrine	Rat	0.032	7	10	—	10
Norepinephrine	Rat	0.0005	8	14	—	14
Isoproterenol	Rat	0.0005	8	38	—	38
Atropine	Rat	1	4	50	—	50
Neostigmine	Rat	0.2	6	2.6	0.1	2.5

TABLE 9.6—*Continued*

Compound	Species	Dose mg/kg	Time hr	Percent of Dose Excreted		
				Total	Parent	Metabolite
Analgetics						
Morphine	Dog	30	12	40	0.2	39.8
Morphine	Monkey	30	4	12	0.1	11.9
Methadone	Rat	3	1	20	—	—
Methadone	Dog	10	5	4	1.6	2.4
Codeine	Rat	40	3	10	—	10
Diuretics						
Chlorothiazide	Dog	20	4	41	—	—
Hydrochlorothiazide	Dog	2	1	4	—	—
CNS Agents						
Thioridazine	Rat	100	72	80	0.1	79.9
Thiethylperazine	Rat	20	48	87	—	—
Prochlorperazine	Rat	25	24	37	—	—
Prochlorperazine	Dog	10	10	63	—	—
Chlorpromazine	Dog	20	10	22	—	—
Trifluoperazine	Dog	2.5	10	72	—	—
Amitriptyline	Rat	0.8	6	50	—	50
Phenyramidol	Dog	25	7	2	—	2
Methohexital	Rat	10	8	75	—	—
Methohexital	Dog	10	8	20	—	—
Glutethimide	Rat	40	15	60	3	57

[a] Data obtained from Stowe and Plaa (1968), where individual references can be found.
[b] Total dose.

TABLE 9.7

Effect of phenobarbital on biliary excretion of BSP and bilirubin in rats[a]

Parameter	BSP		DBSP		Bilirubin	
	Control	Pheno-barbital	Control	Pheno-barbital	Control	Pheno-barbital
% conjugates in bile	86	87	0	0	—	—
Enzyme conjugating activity (mg of BSP/g/5 min)	15	18[b]	—	—	—	—
Hepatic storage (mg/mg%/kg)	0.60	0.48	0.87	1.09	—	—
Biliary excretion rate (mg/kg/min)	1.30	1.60[b]	0.94	1.16[b]	0.57	0.75[b]
Bile flow (μl/kg/min)	67	83[b]	57	78[b]	49	79[b]
Biliary concentration (mg/ml)	16	15	15	13[b]	12	10

[a] BSP and DBSP data from Klaassen and Plaa (1968b); bilirubin data from Roberts and Plaa (1967).
[b] Significantly different from control ($p < 0.05$).

E. Species Variation in Biliary Excretion

Some of the data in Table 9.8 indicate that species vary in their ability to excrete drugs into the bile. The data in Table 9.4 show that the dog has a much lower maximum biliary excretion rate for BSP and DBSP than do the rat and rabbit. The maximum excretion rate for bilirubin is slower in the mouse (0.32 mg/kg/min) than in the rat (0.78 mg/kg/min) (Roberts et al., 1967). With indocyanine green, it has been shown that the rat has a higher maximum biliary excretion rate (0.065 mg/kg/min) than does the rabbit (0.05 mg/kg/min) or the dog (0.027 mg/kg/min) (Klaassen and Plaa, 1969). Abou-El-Makarem et al. (1967) compared the biliary excretory capabilities of various species. They measured the total amount of drug excreted in 3 hours (Table 9.8). For substances which had high molecular weights, good biliary excretion was demonstrated in the rat, dog, and hen, whereas poor excretion was present in the rabbit, guinea-pig and monkey; cats and sheep exhibited intermediate capacity. From these data, it is evident that one must distinguish between rate and amount when one speaks about excretion and that rankings of species depend upon the compounds themselves.

F. Techniques Employed for Determining Biliary Excretion

1. Cannulation techniques. One can get an indirect idea regarding the importance of the biliary route of excretion by following the content of a given drug and metabolite in the feces. Naturally, this technique is usually only applicable if the agent has been administered parenterally. Therefore, this approach has limitations. Investigators who have been interested in the quantitative aspects of biliary excretion have found it necessary to employ preparations in which bile is collected directly and analyzed. In the rat, the common approach has been to insert a catheter into the common bile duct. In acute preparations involving only a short time span, this type of experiment is usually carried out in anesthetized animals. However, in the rat it is possible to carry out such determinations in the unanesthetized state, provided the investigator has a means of restraining the animal. In larger species this same approach has been employed. In addition, in dogs it is possible to insert a Thomas fistula into the duodenum, through which one can catheterize the bile duct directly through the sphincter of Oddi when bile samples are desired. Such preparations have the advantage of permitting studies in the chronic state.

TABLE 9.8

Biliary excretion of various compounds in different species[a]

Compound	MW	% of Dose Excreted in 3 hrs							
		Rat	Guinea-Pig	Rabbit	Dog	Cat	Hen	Monkey	Sheep
Benzoic acid	122	1.2	1.7	0.7	0.8	1.2	0.5	—	—
Aniline	93	5.7	5.6	2.6	2.7	0.3	1.6	—	—
4-amino-hippuric acid	194	3.3	6.7	3.0	3.4	0.7	0.5	—	—
4 - acetoamido - hippuric acid	236	1.3	0.4	1.5	3.5	0.9	0.4	1.2	3.8
Succinyl-sulphathiazole	355	29	0.9	1.1	20	7	25	0.3	16
Stilbestrol glucuronide	445	95	20	32	65	77	93	—	—
Sulphadimethoxine N[1]-glucuronide	487	43	12	10	43	—	—	—	—
Phenolphthalein glucuronide	495	54	—	13	81	34	71	13	32

[a] Data obtained from Abou-El-Makarem et al. (1967).

a) *Effect of temperature.* Since the rat is the animal which is usually employed in metabolism studies, it appears appropriate to point out several technical aspects regarding these animals. First of all, body temperature can have a very marked influence on the flow of bile in rats. Roberts *et al.* (1967) carried out a study in which they compared bilirubin and BSP excretion in rats during anesthesia-induced alteration of rectal temperature. Table 9.1 shows the maximal excretory rate for these two substances and also the effect of temperature on bile flow. A linear relationship was found to exist between temperature and the excretion rate; the same relationship was found to exist in the flow of bile. Their results indicated that the decrease in rectal temperature which occurs in the period of time usually involved in such experiments is sufficient to cause a decrease in the apparent excretory maximum for both of these substances. In light of these results, one might envision the possibility that a loss of thermoregulation, in response to certain experimental treatments, could result in an alteration in the biliary excretion rate, but that this effect could be erroneously attributed to an effect of the treatment on the hepatic parenchyma. Roberts and Plaa (1966) studied the effect of environment on temperature in rats placed in restraining cages or housed in individual, open cages. Some of the rats were also subjected to a surgical laparotomy prior to the experiment. Those rats who were subjected to a surgical procedure, placed in an individual restrainer, and exposed to circulating room air had a profound loss in rectal temperature; at 24 hours, the average rectal temperature was 28°C. This same phenomena was also exhibited in rats who had had no surgery but were placed in individual restrainers and subjected to a cold draft; at 24 hours the average rectal temperature was 31.5°C. With this in mind and considering the data in Table 9.1, one can see that the biliary excretion rate for an animal whose rectal temperature was 28° could be as low as 50% of the actual control value. The complicating effect of body temperature has been demonstrated in a study in which the effects of norethandrolone on bilirubin excretion were measured in rats whose body temperatures were found to vary (Roberts *et al.*, 1968). In one set of experiments, the body temperature of the animals was maintained at 36.5° throughout the experiment. In the second set of experiments, the rectal temperature was not controlled; control animals had a rectal temperature of 33.8° and norethandrolone-treated animals had a temperature of 31.7°. In those experiments in which body temperature was maintained, norethandrolone was found to increase the bilirubin excretory rate (control, 1.04; norethandrolone, 1.50 mg/kg/min), whereas in those experiments in which body temperature was not maintained, norethandrolone was found to decrease the excretory rate (control, 0.96; norethandrolone, 0.65 mg/kg/min). These effects could be accounted for by the changes in bile flow induced by the changes in body temperature. The experimental conditions can complicate interpretation of such data.

2. Hepatic slice techniques. Other techniques have been employed to measure indirectly biliary excretion capacity. Schanker and his co-workers have employed the uptake of substrate by isolated rat liver slices (Kupferberg and Schanker, 1968; Solomon and Schanker, 1963). This has been particularly useful for those substances in which the toxicity precludes the determination of such characteristics as a transport maximum or competition with other substances. However, it should be pointed out that this procedure is an indirect method and has certain limitations in interpretation.

3. Isolated liver perfusion. Another *in vitro* technique which lends itself well to the study of biliary excretion is perfusion of the isolated liver. The development of viable and reproducible rat liver preparations is largely due to the pioneering work of Brauer *et al.* (1951) and Miller *et al.* (1951); the effects of temperature, perfusate composition, perfusion pressure and perfusate flow have all been studied (Brauer *et al.*, 1953, 1954; Brauer, 1959). Tuttle *et al.* (1962) demonstrated that choleresis could be induced in perfused rat livers by administering dehydrocholate. This preparation has been employed for a great variety of studies. It has often served as a bridge between other *in vitro* techniques and the intact animal. A few examples relating directly to biliary excretion would be the following: effect of CCl_4 on BSP excretion (Plaa and Hine, 1960); excretion of ferrioxamines of varying liposolubility (Meyer-Brunot and Keberle, 1968); excretion of related aryl sulphate esters (Hearse *et al.*, 1969); and the effect of temperature on the excretion of sulfanilamide, atropine, procaine and pentobarbital (Kalser *et al.*, 1965, 1968a, b, 1969).

4. General interpretation. Mention should also be made regarding the difference between capacity and affinity and how these relate to the biliary excretion of drugs. Usually when one intends to determine whether a substance can be excreted by the liver, the experiments are designed in a manner which eliminates other excretory pathways. A common procedure has been to carry out such experiments in animals whose renal pedicles have been ligated, thus eliminating the renal route of excretion. These types of preparations denote capacity to excrete. Also those experiments in which drugs are given by constant infusion to elicit maximum excretion rates denote capacity. However, in the intact animal, it is important to determine not only whether the liver can excrete a given substance, but whether it usually excretes it under normal conditions. Therefore, it seems important that investigations regarding the biliary excretion of drugs should be carried out under both types of conditions, i.e., those in which the liver only can excrete the substances and finally under those conditions in which the liver is competing with other routes of excretion for the material.

II. MAMMARY SECRETION, SWEAT AND SALIVARY SECRETION

A. Salivary Secretion

Although biliary excretion is probably the major route by which substances in the blood can enter into the gastrointestinal tract, it should be remembered that other types of secretions occur in this system. It has been shown that the pKa of a substance has a marked influence on whether it is secreted into the stomach or not (Shore *et al.*, 1957). Bases with pKa values greater than five have been found to be secreted into the gastric contents of dogs in high concentrations; on the other hand, weak acids have been found to be minimally secreted. Nonionic diffusion explains these differences. In addition, it has been demonstrated that drugs can enter the gut by salivary secretion. Again nonionic diffusion seems to afford the best explanation for the entrance of these substances into these secretions. On the other hand, there is evidence that perhaps active secretory processes are involved. Borzelleca and Cherrick (1965) were able to demonstrate that probenecid substantially reduces penicillin excretion into the saliva.

B. Mammary Secretion

Considerable interest has been generated recently concerning the excretion of drugs into milk. This has been particularly important because of the pesticide residue problem and also because of the use of antibiotics in cows. The mammary excretion of drugs has been extensively reviewed by Rasmussen (1966). Recently, a brief review (Stowe and Plaa, 1968) has also appeared. Generally speaking, it appears that nonionic diffusion also applies to the secretion of drugs into milk. The techniques which have been employed to study this phenomenon are usually similar to the steady-state approaches employed in studying drug passage into the gastrointestinal tract. A wide variety of substances have been found to be secreted into milk in a quantitative manner which is in close agreement with the theoretically derived values one would get from equations based on nonionic diffusion. However, one notable exception seems to be the tetracyclines. Table 9.9 summarizes some of these data obtained from the work of Sisodia and Stowe (1964).

C. Sweat

The excretion of drugs into sweat has been known for some time. Prior to 1911, iodine, bromine, benzoic acid, salicylic acid, lead, arsenic, boron, mercury, iron, alcohol and antipyrine were reputed to appear in human sweat (Stowe and Plaa, 1968). Since that time, a large number of drugs have been detected in sweat. The mechanism by which drugs appear in sweat is not well understood. However, it appears again that nonionic diffusion plays an important role. Thaysen and Schwartz (1953) studied the excretion of various compounds in methacholine-induced sweating in man and found that a relationship existed between the concentration in the sweat and the degree of ionization at pH 7.4. Compounds

TABLE 9.9

Distribution of various compounds in bovine milk[a]

Compound	pKa	Milk/Plasma Ratio	
		Experimental	Theoretical
Organic Acids			
Sulfanilamide	10.4	1.00	1.00
Sulfapyridine	8.4	0.86	0.94
Sulfamethazine	7.37	0.51	0.58
Sulfathiazole	7.14	0.43	0.46
Sulfamerazine	7.06	0.52	0.56
Sulfadiazine	6.5	0.21	0.20
Sulfadimethoxine	6.0	0.20	0.19
Sulfacetamide	5.4	0.08	0.13
Penicillin	2.7	0.25	0.16
Organic Bases			
Tetracycline	3.3, 7.7, 9.7	1.60	0.71
Quinine	8.4	4.8	4.7
Erythromycin	8.8	8.7	6.1
Penethamate	8.5	6.1	5.7
Antipyrine	1.4	1.0	1.0

[a] Data obtained from Sisodia and Stowe (1964).

TABLE 9.10
Excretion of various compounds during sweating in man[a]

Compound	Sweat/Plasma Ratio	pKa
Urea	1.84	13.8
Sulfanilamide	0.69	10.4
Sulfapyridine	0.58	8.4
Sulfathiazole	0.13	7.1
Sulfadiazine	0.11	6.5
p-Aminohippuric acid	0.02	3.8
Inulin	0.00	—

[a] Data obtained from Thaysen and Schwartz (1953).

which were mainly nonionized were excreted with high sweat/plasma ratios, a relationship shown in Table 9.10. They further showed that the sweat/plasma ratios were independent of the plasma concentration and the rate of sweating. All these data are consistent with the concept of passive nonionic diffusion.

D. Other Routes of Excretion

An extremely important route of excretion not discussed in this chapter is the expired air. The reader is referred to Chapter 7 for details concerning the role of the lungs in the elimination of drugs. To a minor extent, drugs can also be excreted into the lachrymal and reproductive tract secretions; these topics have been reviewed by Stowe and Plaa (1968).

REFERENCES

Abou-El-Makarem, M. M., Millburn, P., Smith, R. L., and Williams, R. T.: Biliary excretion of foreign compounds. Species differences in biliary excretion. Biochem. J. *105:* 1289–1293, 1967.

Borzelleca, J. F. and Cherrick, H. M.: The excretion of drugs in saliva, antibiotics. J. Oral Ther. Pharmacol. *2:* 180–187, 1965.

Brauer, R. W.: Mechanism of bile secretion. J.A.M.A. *169:* 1462–1466, 1959.

Brauer, R. W., Pessotti, R. L., and Pizzolato, P.: Isolated rat liver preparation. Bile production and other basic properties. Proc. Soc. Exp. Biol. Med. *78:* 174–181, 1951.

Brauer, R. W., Leong, G. F., and Pessotti, R. L.: Vasomotor activity in the isolated perfused rat liver. Amer. J. Physiol. *174:* 304–312, 1953.

Brauer, R. W., Leong, G. F., and Holloway, R. J.: Mechanics of bile secretion. Effect of perfusion pressure and temperature on bile flow and bile secretion pressure. Amer. J. Physiol. *177:* 103–112, 1954.

Cox, E. and Wright, S. E.: The hepatic excretion of digitalis glycosides and their genins in the rat. J. Pharmacol. Exp. Ther. *126:* 117–122, 1959.

Gibson, J. E. and Becker, B. A.: Demonstration of enhanced lethality of drugs in hypoexcretory animals. J. Pharm. Sci. *56:* 1503–1505, 1967.

Guarino, A. M. and Schanker, L. S.: Biliary excretion of probenecid and its glucuronide. J. Pharmacol. Exp. Ther. *164:* 387–395, 1968.

Haddock, E. P., Zapolski, E. J., Rubin, M., and Princiotto, J. V.: Biliary excretion of chelated iron. Proc. Soc. Exp. Biol. Med. *120:* 663–668, 1965.

Hanzon, V.: Liver cell secretion under normal and pathologic conditions studied by fluorescence microscopy on living rats. Acta Physiol. Scand. *28:* Suppl. 101, 1–267, 1952.

Hart, L. G. and Schanker, L. S.: Active transport of chlorothiazide into bile. Am. J. Physiol. *211:* 643–646, 1966.

Hearse, D. J., Powell, G. M., Olavesen, A. H., and Dodgson, K. S.: The influence of some physico-chemical factors on the biliary excretion of a series of structurally related aryl sulphate esters. Biochem. Pharmacol. *18:* 181–195, 1969.

Javitt, N. B.: Phenol 3,6 dibromphthalein disulfonate, a new compound for the study of liver disease. Proc. Soc. Exp. Biol. Med. *117:* 254–257, 1964.

Kalser, S. C., Kelvington, E. J., Randolph, M. M., and Santomenna, D. M.: Drug metabolism in hypothermia. II. C^{14}-atropine uptake, metabolism and excretion by the isolated, perfused rat liver. J. Pharmacol. Exp. Ther. *147:* 260–269, 1965

Kalser, S. C., Kelvington, E. J., Kunig, R., and Randolph, M. M.: Drug metabolism in hypothermia. Uptake, metabolism and excretion of C^{14}-procaine by the isolated, perfused rat liver. J. Pharmacol. Exp. Ther. *164:* 396–404, 1968a.

Kalser, S. C., Kelvington, E. J., and Randolph, M. M.: Drug metabolism in hypothermia. Uptake, metabolism and excretion of S^{35}-sulfanilamide by the isolated, perfused rat liver. J. Pharmacol. Exp. Ther. *159:* 389–398, 1968b.

Kalser, S. C., Kelly, M. P., Forbes, E. B., and Randolph, M. M.: Drug metabolism in hypothermia. Uptake, metabolism and biliary excretion of pentobarbital-2-C^{14} by the isolated, perfused rat liver in hypothermia and euthermia. J. Pharmacol. Exp. Ther. *170:* 145–152, 1969.

Keberle, H., Hoffmann, K., and Bernhard, K.: The metabolism of glutethimide (Doriden). Experientia *18:* 105–111, 1962.

Klaassen, C. D. and Plaa, G. L.: Hepatic disposition of phenoldibromphthalein disulfonate and sulfobromophthalein. Am. J. Physiol. *215:* 971–976, 1968a.

Klaassen, C. D. and Plaa, G. L.: Studies on the mechanism of phenobarbital-enhanced sulfobromophthalein disappearance. J. Pharmacol. Exp. Ther. *161:* 361–366, 1968b.

Klaassen, C. D. and Plaa, G. L.: Plasma disappearance and biliary excretion of indocyanine green in rats, rabbits and dogs. Toxicol. Appl. Pharmacol. *15:* 374–384, 1969.

Kupferberg, H. J. and Schanker, L. S.: Biliary secretion of ouabain-^{3}H and its uptake by liver slices in the rat. Am. J. Physiol. *214:* 1048–1053, 1968.

Light, H. G., Witmer, C., and Vars, H. M.: Interruption of the enterohepatic circulation and its effect on rat bile. Am. J. Physiol. *197:* 1330–1332, 1959.

Meyer-Brunot, H. G. and Keberle, H.: Biliary excretion of ferrioxamines of varying liposolubility in perfused rat liver. Am. J. Physiol. *214:* 1193–1200, 1968.

Miller, L. L., Bly, C. G., Watson, M. L., and Bale, W. F.: The dominant role of the liver in plasma protein synthesis. J. Exp. Med. *94:* 431–453, 1951.

O'Maille, E. R. L., Richards, T. G., and Short, A. H.: Factor determining the maximal rate of organic anion secretion by the liver and further evidence on the hepatic site of action of the hormone secretin. J. Physiol. (London) *186:* 424–438, 1966.

Plaa, G. L. and Hine, C. H.: The effect of

carbon tetrachloride on isolated perfused rat liver function. Arch. Indust. Hlth. *21:* 114–123, 1960.

Rasmussen, F.: *Studies on the Mammary Excretion and Absorption of Drugs*, Carl F. Mortensen, Copenhagen, 1966.

Ritt, D. J. and Combes, B.: Enhancement of apparent excretory maximum of sulfobromophthalein sodium (BSP) by taurocholate and dehydrocholate. J. Clin. Invest. *46:* 1108–1109, 1967.

Roberts, R. J., Klaassen, C. D., and Plaa, G. L.: Maximum biliary excretion of bilirubin and sulfobromophthalein during anesthesia-induced alteration of rectal temperature. Proc. Soc. Exp. Biol. Med. *125:* 313–316, 1967.

Roberts, R. J. and Plaa, G. L.: The effect of bile duct ligation, bile duct cannulation, and hypothermia on α-naphthylisothiocyanate-induced hyperbilirubinemia and cholestasis in rats. Gastroenterology *50:* 768–774, 1966.

Roberts, R. J. and Plaa, G. L.: Effect of phenobarbital on the excretion of an exogenous bilirubin load. Biochem. Pharmacol. *16:* 827–835, 1967.

Roberts, R. J., Shriver, S. L., and Plaa, G. L.: Effect of norethandrolone on the biliary excretion of bilirubin in the mouse and rat. Biochem. Pharmacol. *17:* 1261–1268, 1968.

Ryan, A. J. and Wright, S. E.: The excretion of some azo dyes in rat bile. J. Pharm. Pharmacol. *13:* 492–495, 1961.

Schanker, L, S.: Passage of drugs across body membranes. Pharmacol. Rev. *14:* 501–530, 1962.

Schanker, L. S.: Hepatic transport of organic cations. In: *The Biliary System*, Taylor, W., Ed., Blackwell, Oxford, 469–480, 1965.

Schanker, L. S. and Solomon, H. M.: Active transport of quaternary ammonium compounds into bile. Am. J. Physiol. *204:* 829–832, 1963.

Sisodia, C. S. and Stowe, C. M.: The mechanism of drug secretion into bovine milk. Ann. N.Y. Acad. Sci. *111:* 650–661, 1964.

Shore, P. A., Brodie, B. B., and Hogben, C. A. M.: The gastric secretion of drugs: a pH partition hypothesis. J. Pharmacol. Exp. Ther. *119:* 361–369, 1957.

Smith, R. L.: The biliary excretion and enterohepatic circulation of drugs and other organic compounds. Proc. Drug. Res. *9:* 299–360, 1966.

Smith, R. L. and Williams, R. T.: Implication of the conjugation of drugs and other exogenous compounds. In: *Glucuronic Acid Free and Combined*, Dutton, G. J., Ed., Academic Press, New York, 457–491, 1966.

Solomon, H. M. and Schanker, L. S.:

Hepatic transport of organic cations: active uptake of a quaternary ammonium compound procaine amide ethobromide by rat liver slices. Biochem. Pharmacol. *12:* 621–626, 1963.

Sperber, I.: Secretion of organic anions in the formation of urine and bile. Pharmacol. Rev. *11:* 109–134, 1959.

Stowe, C. M. and Plaa, G. L.: Extrarenal excretion of drugs and chemicals. Ann. Rev. Pharmacol. *8:* 337–356, 1968.

Thaysen, J. H. and Schwartz, I. L.: The permeability of human sweat glands to a series of sulfonamide compounds. J. Exp. Med. *98:* 261–268, 1953.

Thompson, R. Q., Sturtevant, M., Bird, O. D., and Glazko, A. J.: The effect of metabolites of chloramphenicol "chloromycetin" on the thyroid of the rat. Endocrinology *55:* 665–681, 1954.

Tuttle, W. W., Eisenbrandt, L. L., and Scott, P. M.: Hydrocholeresis in the isolated perfused rat liver. J. Pharm. Sci. *51:* 161–164, 1962.

Webb, J. N., Fonda, M., and Brouwer, E. A.: Metabolism and excretion patterns of fluorescein and certain halogenated fluorescein dyes in rats. J. Pharmacol. Exp. Ther. *137:* 141–147, 1962.

Wheeler, H. O.: Secretion of bile. In: *Diseases of the Liver,* Schiff, L., Ed., 3rd Ed., J. B. Lippincott Company, Philadelphia, 84–102, 1969.

Wheeler, H. O., Cranston, W. I., and Meltzer, J. I.: Hepatic uptake and biliary excretion of indocyanine green in the dog. Proc. Soc. Exp. Biol. Med. *99:* 11–14, 1958.

Williams, R. T., Millburn, P., and Smith, R. L.: The influence of enterohepatic circulation on toxicity of drugs. Ann. N.Y. Acad. Sci. *123:* 110–124, 1965.

DRUG BIOTRANSFORMATION AND FACTORS WHICH MODIFY DRUG METABOLISM

10

Pathways of Drug Biotransformation: Biochemical Conjugations

H. GEORGE MANDEL

I. BIOTRANSFORMATION AND ITS GENERAL FUNCTIONS

It has been known since early history that chemical substances can alter normal physiological functions of animals and man, but it was recognized only relatively recently that contact with biological material could also affect the structure of a chemical compound. Considerable study of this latter process, especially during the past 25 years, has provided a great wealth of information and has led to the introduction of drug metabolism as a subdiscipline of pharmacology. Strictly speaking, drug metabolism refers exclusively to the chemical alterations of a drug produced by the biological environment, and thus represents one aspect of the physiological disposition, or fate, of the agent.

Drug metabolism first became an organized scientific endeavor through the work of Williams (1947), who published the first text on the subject. The more recent and greatly enlarged second edition of this book (Williams, 1959) now serves as the most authoritative source on the routes of metabolism for drugs and other chemicals. Its title, *Drug Detoxication*, is indicative of one of the major natural functions of drug metabolism, i.e., the formation of more polar and water-soluble derivatives which results in reduction of the pharmacological activity of a drug and its rapid excretion. Brodie (1964) has stated that if there were no such process as drug metabolism, it would take the body about a hundred years to terminate the action of pentobarbital, which is lipid-soluble and thus cannot be readily excreted without being metabolized.

Detailed examination of biological and physico-chemical properties of drugs or other chemicals and their metabolites indicates that the effects of drug metabolism are complex. Usually drug metabolites are more water-soluble than the original drug because the derivatives normally contain more hydrophilic functional groups, or are conjugated with relatively lipophilic moieties. Table 10.1 lists relative solubilities in water for a number of compounds and their metabolic products. Although water solubility is frequently increased by drug biotransformation, there are many exceptions. It should be kept in mind, however, that the metabolites are rarely concentrated to the limit of their water-solubility in biological systems but are usually excreted before that time.

Furthermore, metabolites tend to be more ionized at physiological pH values than the parent compounds, and hence would more likely be in the form of water-soluble salts (Table 10.2). Again, such compounds being more polar

TABLE 10.1

Solubilities of compounds and their metabolites

Compound	Solubility in Water mg/100 ml	Metabolite	Solubility in Water mg/100 ml
Benzoic acid	184	Hippuric acid (mammals)	463
Phenylacetic acid	915	Phenaceturic acid (dogs)	1145
		Phenacetylglutamine urea (man, chimpanzee)	117
o-Chlorophenylacetic acid	311	o-Chlorophenaceturic acid	457
p-Chlorophenylacetic acid	222	p-Chlorophenaceturic acid	117
m-Aminobenzoic acid	730	m-Acetamidobenzoic acid	100
Sulfanilamide	1480	N^4-Acetylsulfanilamide	534

From Williams, 1959.

TABLE 10.2

pK_a *Values of compounds and their metabolites*

Compound	pK_a	Metabolite	pK_a
Phenol	10.0	Phenylglucuronide	3.4
2,4-Dimethylpentan-3-ol	ca. 18	2,4-Dimethylpentyl-3-glucuronide	3.9
Veratric acid	4.4	Veratroylglucuronide	3.5
Diethylacetic acid	4.7	Diethylacetylglucuronide	3.4
Benzoic acid	4.2	Hippuric acid	3.7
o-Chlorobenzoic acid	2.9	o-Chlorohippuric acid	3.8
Salicylic acid	3.2	Salicyluric acid	3.6
p-Aminobenzoic acid	4.9	p-Aminohippuric acid	4.0
	4.9	p-Acetamidobenzoic acid	4.3
Phenylacetic acid	4.25	Phenaceturic acid	3.7
Benzene	—	Phenylmercapturic acid	3.6

From Williams, 1959.

would be expected to exhibit reduced lipid solubility. o-Chlorobenzoic and salicylic acids are more unusual than most compounds examined in that they are converted to metabolites of slightly higher pK_a. The acidic metabolites are frequently secreted by the renal tubules, and thus are rapidly removed from the body. For these reasons drug metabolism usually leads to an accelerated termination of pharmacological activity.

Although most drug metabolites are less biologically active than their parent compounds, in quite a few instances a more toxic metabolite is actually produced. In Table 10.3, sulfadiazine, sulfamerazine, and pyridine, for example, are transformed to more toxic products. Thus, drug metabolism does not necessarily imply detoxication or loss of pharmacological activity. Indeed, there are a number of cases where compounds are produced by metabolism which exhibit increased therapeutic or toxic effects. For example, in the case of the sulfonamides, several of the drugs and their acetyl metabolites are very water-insoluble, and kidney damage results from intratubular crystallization of the compounds (Table 10.4). In the case of sulfathiazole, particularly, this drug of limited water solubility is converted to a product of greater water insolubility. Whether a

TABLE 10.3

Toxicity of compounds and their metabolites

Compound	Toxicity[a]	Metabolite	Toxicity
Benzoic acid	2.0	Hippuric acid	4.15
p-Aminobenzoic acid	2.85	p-Aminohippuric acid	4.93
		p-Acetamidohippuric acid	5.25
Sulfadiazine	1.6	N^4-Acetylsulfadiazine	0.6
Sulfamerazine	1.4	N^4-Acetylsulfamerazine	0.7
Sulfamethazine	0.9	N^4-Acetylsulfamethazine	1.3
Aminopyrine	0.24	4-Aminoantipyrine	1.2
Hydrogen cyanide	0.003–0.005	Sodium thiocyanate	0.4–0.6
Pyridine	1.2	N-Methylpyridinium chloride	0.22

[a] Toxicity usually expressed as LD_{50} in g/kg for mice. For details see compilation by Williams, 1959.

TABLE 10.4

Water solubility of sulfonamides and renal damage

Compound	Solubility mg/100 ml at 37°		Occurrence of Kidney Blockage by Crystalline Deposits
	Free Drug	Acetyl Metabolite	
Sulfanilamide	1500	530	not encountered
Sulfacetamide	1100	215	not encountered
Sulfamethazine	75	115	rare
Sulfadiazine	13	20	frequent
Sulfamerazine	37	79	frequent
Sulfapyrazine	5	5	very frequent
Sulfathiazole	98	7	very frequent

From Williams, 1959.

metabolite is more or less pharmacologically active than its parent drug depends on the specific compound being studied, the biological properties measured, and the sensitivity of individual tissues or organs.

Numerous other examples have now been recognized where the administered drug is really only a "pro-drug" which is biotransformed into a pharmacologically active or more active metabolite. By this transformation process, first referred to as "lethal synthesis" by Peters (1952), the formation of fluorocitrate apparently accounts for the toxic effects observed following fluoroacetate administration. Structural analogs of purines, pyrimidines and their sugar derivatives are converted to ribomononucleotides which have potent carcinostatic activity (Mandel, 1959). The classical examples of organic pentavalent arsenicals, or of prontosil, which had chemotherapeutic activity *in vivo* but not *in vitro*, also involve pharmacological activation reactions, and the metabolically derived trivalent arsenicals and sulfanilamide are active *in vivo* as well as *in vitro*. The demethylation of imipramine to desmethylimipramine; the desulfuration of parathion to paraoxon; the oxidation of diethylene glycol to oxalate; and the conversion of α-methyldopa to α-methylnorepinephrine, all are other instances where drug metabolism has produced compounds of enhanced pharmacological potency.

II. MAJOR PATHWAYS OF DRUG BIOTRANSFORMATION

Most drugs are metabolized in the liver, and metabolizing enzymes can occur in the soluble, mitochondrial, or microsomal fractions. The most common routes of drug metabolism involve oxidation, reduction, hydrolysis, and conjugation. Very often a drug is subjected to several competing pathways *simultaneously*, and the extent of formation of the various metabolites depends on the relative rates of the various interactions. In addition, very commonly metabolic reactions proceed *sequentially*, and oxidation, reduction, or hydrolysis reactions are followed by conjugation of these derivatives. For example, the alkyl side chain of a drug may be oxidized to an alcohol which then forms a conjugate with glucuronic acid; an ester may be hydrolyzed to a carboxylic acid which then is coupled with glycine; or an aromatic azo compound is reduced to an amine derivative which is subsequently acetylated. It has not been possible to predict precisely the pathways of metabolism in a given species. Enough information is available at this time, however, that by analogy the major routes of metabolism for most drugs can be anticipated.

It is rare that a drug forms a double conjugate, since one such adduct already increases the likelihood for excretion. A few doubly conjugated drugs have been isolated, however.

This chapter will deal primarily with conjugation of drugs. For purposes of completeness, however, Table 10.5 lists the characteristic oxidation, reduction and hydrolysis reactions to which drugs are subject. Most of the oxidation reactions are catalyzed by microsomal enzymes and require oxygen and NADPH. Chapters 12 and 14 describe these reactions and their mechanisms in greater detail.

The terms anabolism and catabolism have been used to describe specific directions in drug alterations. Anabolism has been used to refer to the biosynthesis of more complex molecules, usually requiring energy, whereas catabolism implies degradation to simpler structures. On the other hand, with metabolite analogs, anabolism is used to describe the process of pharmacological activation whereby a substrate analog, for instance, forms a conjugate with greater biological activity than the parent compound, and catabolism relates to those processes involving deactivation and drug destruction. Because of the lack of a strict relationship between molecular size and drug activity (e.g., the biosynthesis of a pharmacologically inactive drug glucuronide derivative) it becomes necessary to define anabolism and catabolism carefully, or otherwise to avoid these terms. In the present chapter we have taken the latter alternative to prevent confusion.

The purpose of this chapter is to provide a general review of the subject of conjugation of drugs rather than to make available extensive details on particular reactions. Additional references and more specific information will be found in the various reviews and papers cited.

The author is most indebted to Professor R. T. Williams, who has written several excellent reviews of drug conjugations (Williams, 1959; 1963, 1967). In particular, the chapter by Williams (1967) in Bernfeld's *Biogenesis of Natural Compounds* provides several tables which represent the best overall summary of conjugation reactions undergone by specific classes of chemical agents. Those have been reproduced in this chapter almost without change. For other major source books on conjugation reactions the reader is referred to Volume 6 of the

TABLE 10.5

Major pathways of drug biotransformation other than conjugation

Microsomal oxidation

1. Side chain oxidation

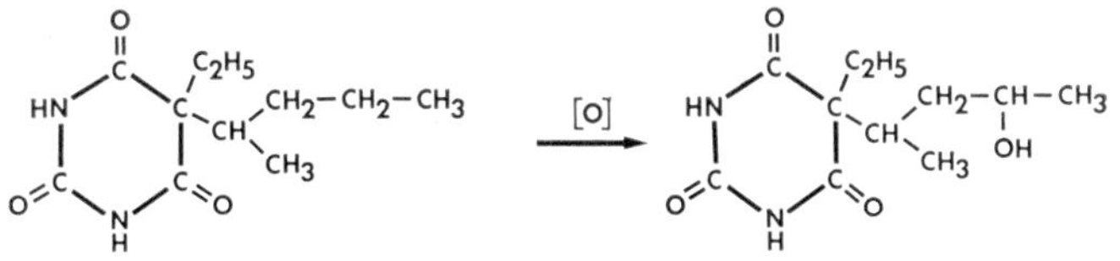

pentobarbital   "pentobarbital alcohol"

2. Hydroxylation

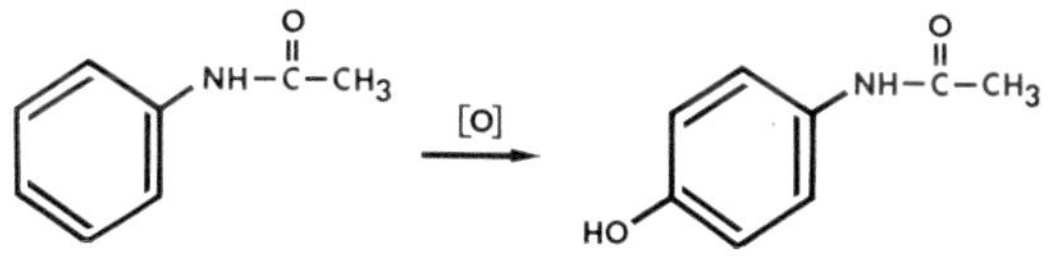

acetanilid   *p*-hydroxyacetanilid

3. N-oxidation

$$(CH_3)_3N \xrightarrow{[O]} (CH_3)_3N=O$$

trimethylamine   trimethylamine oxide

4. Sulfoxidation

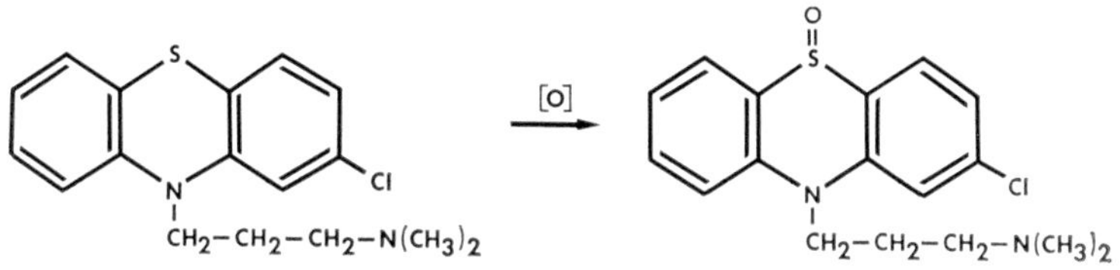

chlorpromazine   chlorpromazine sulfoxide

5. N-dealkylation

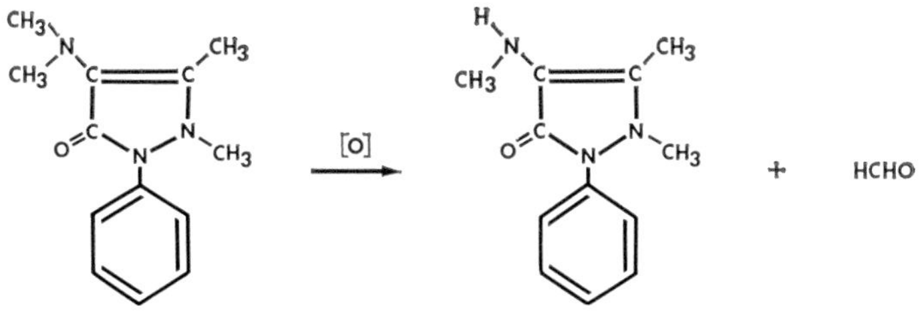

aminopyrine   4-methylaminoantipyrine   +   HCHO

6. O-dealkylation

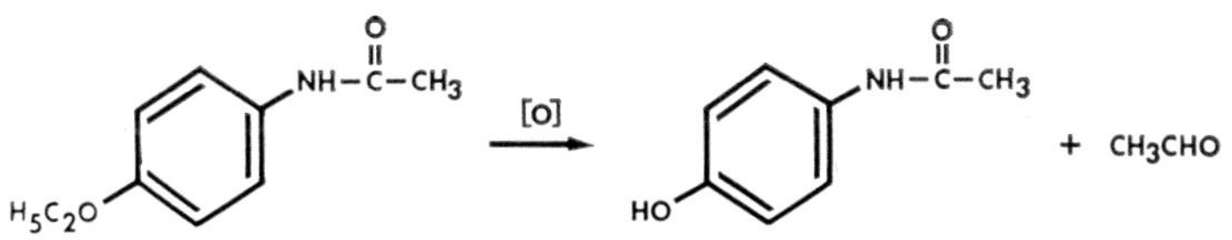

acetophenetidin   *p*-hydroxyacetanilid   + CH_3CHO

TABLE 10.5 (*continued*)

7. S-dealkylation

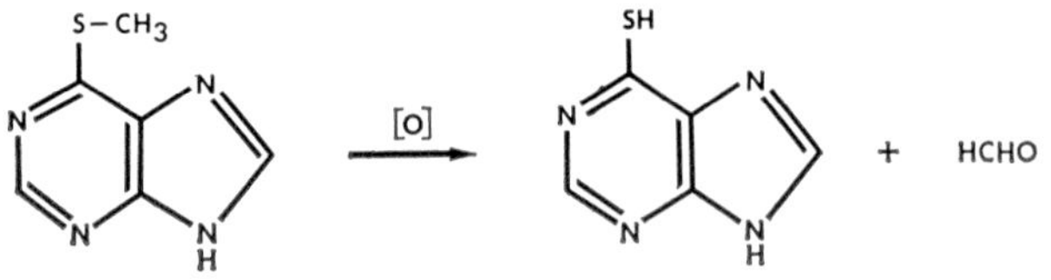

$S-CH_3$ (6-methyl thiopurine) $\xrightarrow{[O]}$ SH (6-mercaptopurine) $+$ HCHO

6-methyl thiopurine　　　　　6-mercaptopurine

8. Deamination

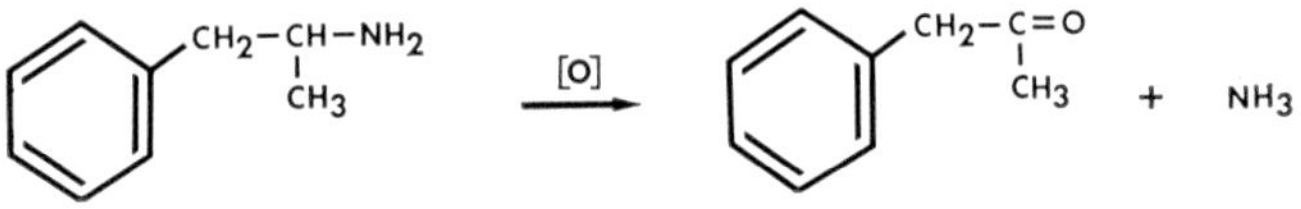

$CH_2-CH-NH_2$ / CH_3 (amphetamine) $\xrightarrow{[O]}$ $CH_2-C=O$ / CH_3 (phenylacetone) $+$ NH_3

amphetamine　　　　　phenylacetone

9. Desulfuration

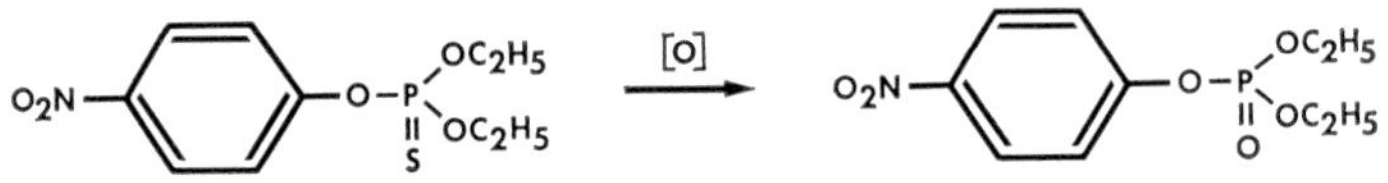

O_2N-⟨benzene⟩$-O-P(\overset{S}{\underset{OC_2H_5}{\parallel}})OC_2H_5$ (parathion) $\xrightarrow{[O]}$ O_2N-⟨benzene⟩$-O-P(\overset{O}{\underset{OC_2H_5}{\parallel}})OC_2H_5$ (paraoxon)

parathion　　　　　paraoxon

Nonmicrosomal Oxidation
1. Alcohol oxidation

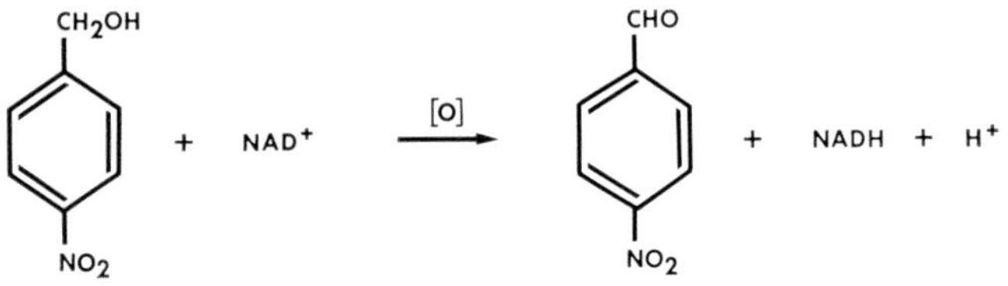

CH_2OH / NO_2 (p-nitrobenzyl alcohol) $+$ NAD^+ $\xrightarrow{[O]}$ CHO / NO_2 (p-nitrobenzaldehyde) $+$ $NADH$ $+$ H^+

p-nitrobenzyl alcohol　　　　　*p*-nitrobenzaldehyde

2. Aromatization

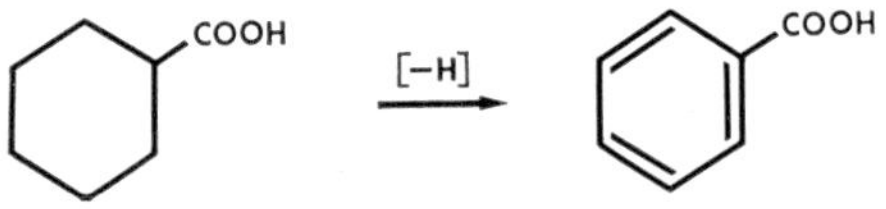

cyclohexane carboxylic acid (COOH) $\xrightarrow{[-H]}$ benzoic acid (COOH)

cyclohexane
carboxylic acid　　　　　benzoic acid

Reductions
1. Nitroreductase

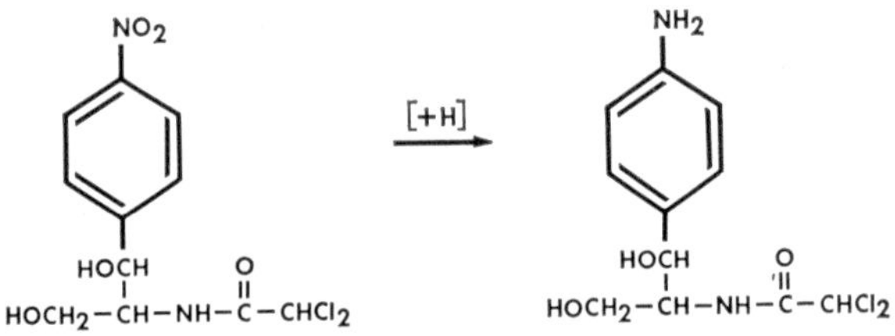

NO_2 / chloramphenicol $\xrightarrow{[+H]}$ NH_2 / "arylamine"

$\underset{HOCH_2-CH-NH-\overset{O}{\overset{\parallel}{C}}-CHCl_2}{HOCH}$

chloramphenicol　　　　　"arylamine"

TABLE 10.5 (*continued*)

2. Azoreductase

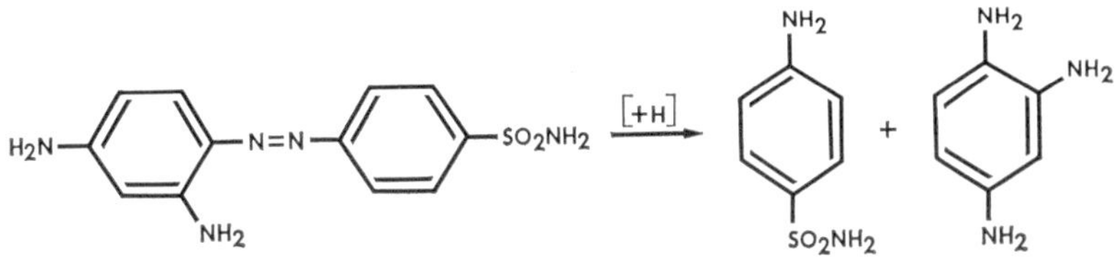

prontosil   sulfanilamide

3. Alcohol dehydrogenase

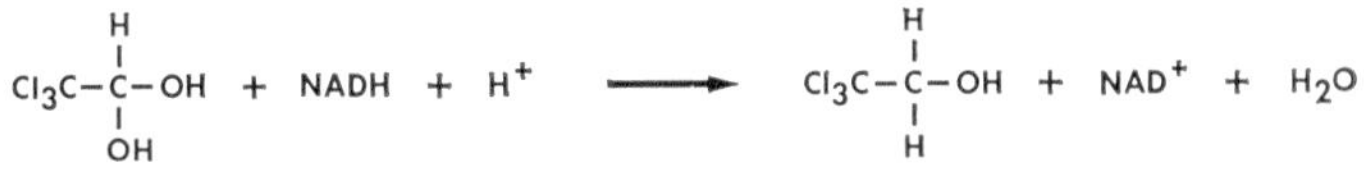

chloral hydrate   trichloroethanol

Hydrolysis

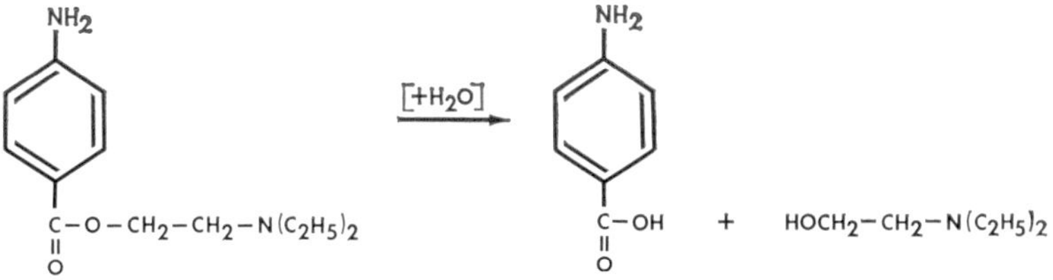

procaine   *p*-amino-   diethylaminoethanol
                                             benzoic acid

Proceedings of the First International Pharmacology Meetings (Brodie and Erdös, 1962); the monograph by Parke (1968); and the detailed text on glucuronic acid by Dutton (1966a). Additional but briefer reviews on the subject have been prepared by Gillette (1963), Smith (1964), and Goldstein *et al.* (1968).

III. DRUG CONJUGATION PATHWAYS

A. Glucuronic Acid Conjugation

1. Mechanism of the reaction. Because of the general availability of glucose in biological systems, glucuronide formation is one of the more common routes of drug metabolism for many drugs, and quantitatively may account for a major share of the metabolites. The reaction involves the condensation of the drug or its biotransformation product with D-glucuronic acid. This route of metabolism has been the subject of a detailed monograph (Dutton, 1966a). The reaction does not take place directly, but requires the activation of glucuronic acid by the synthesis of uridine diphosphate glucuronic acid (UDPGA). The normal route of synthesis requires a series of reactions from UDP-glucose, as shown below. The C^1 atom of glucuronic acid is present in the α configuration in UDPGA but forms a β configuration complex with drugs. It should be noticed that all glucuronide derivatives have a free carboxyl group.

glucose-1-phosphate + UTP $\xrightarrow{\text{pyrophosphorylase}}$

$$\text{UDP-glucose} + \text{pyrophosphate}$$

UDP glucose + 2 NAD$^+$ + H$_2$O $\xrightarrow[\text{dehydrogenase}]{\text{UDPG-}}$

$$\text{UDP-glucuronic acid} + 2\text{ NADH} + 2\text{H}^+$$

UDP-glucuronic acid + RZH $\xrightarrow[\text{transferase}]{\text{glucuronyl}}$ RZ-glucuronic acid + UDP

where **Z** is

$$\text{O, } \overset{\overset{\text{O}}{\|}}{\text{CO}}\text{, NH or S.}$$

phenol   UDPGA   phenyl glucuronide

The formation of UDPGA from UDP glucose is mediated by a dehydrogenase present in the supernatant fraction of liver. The interaction of UDPGA with the acceptor drug is catalyzed by glucuronyl transferase, a microsomal enzyme which has been solubilized (Isselbacher *et al.*, 1962) and which occurs mainly in the liver but also in other organs and tissues such as kidney, GI tract and skin. Numerous such transferases are known to exist, but the exact substrate specificity is unclear. Competition can be shown between substrates for the same transferase enzyme. A critical evaluation of the evidence for the multiplicity of mammalian glucuronyl-transferases has been provided by Dutton (1966b).

2. Substrates for the reaction. Several types of drugs tend to form glucuronides (see Table 10.6). Alcohols and phenols, which form "ether type" glucuronides, are the most common examples. Aromatic but also some aliphatic carboxylic acids form "ester type" glucuronides. Various amines, especially aromatic compounds, form N-glucuronides (Axelrod *et al.*, 1958), some of which may even form spontaneously, i.e., without the catalytic action of a glucuronyl transferase. Certain thiol compounds form S-glucuronides. In addition, normally occurring substrates, such as steroids, thyroxine and bilirubin, also conjugate with glucuronic acid.

3. Consequences of the reaction. Conjugation of drugs with glucuronic acid produces several changes characteristic of drug metabolism in general (*see* Section I), and the implications of this biotransformation have been examined most carefully with glucuronides. The products become more water-soluble than the parent drugs because of the large hydrophilic carbohydrate moiety, and

TABLE 10.6
Types of compounds conjugating with glucuronic acid

Type	Example	Formula
(a) Hydroxyl Primary alcoholic	Trichloroethanol	Cl_3C-CH_2OH
Secondary alcoholic	Butan-2-ol	$C_2H_5(CH_3)CHOH$
Tertiary alcoholic	*Tert*-butyl alcohol	$(CH_3)_3COH$
Phenolic	Phenol	⬡—OH
Enolic	4-Hydroxy-coumarin	C(OH)=CH ... O—CO
Hydroxylamine	N-Hydroxy-2-acetylaminofluorene	—NOH, COCH₃
(b) Carboxyl Aromatic Carbocyclic	Benzoic acid	⬡COOH
Heterocyclic	Nicotinic acid	pyridine-COOH
Aliphatic Alkyl	2-Ethylhexoic acid	$C_4H_9CH(C_2H_5)COOH$
Aryl-alkyl	Phenylacetic acid	⬡CH_2COOH
(c) Amino Aromatic	Aniline	⬡NH_2
Carboxyamide	2-Methyl-2-propyl 1,3-propanediol dicarbamate (meprobamate)	CH_3 C(CH₂OCONH₂)₂ $CH_2CH_2CH_3$
Sulfonamide	Sulfadimethoxine	$NH_2C_6H_4SO_2NH$ pyrimidine OCH₃, OCH₃
Heterocyclic	Sulfisoxazole	$NH_2C_6H_4SO_2NH$ isoxazole H₃C, CH₃

Arrow points to H atom replaced by glucuronide or to point of attachment of glucuronic acid. From Williams, 1967.

TABLE 10.6 (*continued*)

Type	Example	Formula
(d) *Sulfhydryl* Sulfhydryl	2-Mercaptobenzo- thiazole	
Carbodithioic	*N*,*N*-Diethyldi- thiocarbamic acid	$(C_2H_5)_2N \cdot CS \cdot SH$

thereby the partition ratio between a lipid and an aqueous solvent is considerably reduced. At the same time, the glucuronides usually are stronger acids than the parent drugs (Table 10.2), and thus are more ionized at physiological pH values. Such compounds are less likely to penetrate membranes than the parent drugs, are poorly reabsorbed by the kidney tubules, and are more readily excreted (see Smith and Williams, 1966).

In general, glucuronide formation abolishes the biological properties of a drug. In those few instances where biological activity is encountered following the administration of a drug-glucuronide, it is likely that some degree of reconversion to the aglycone derivative, probably via β-glucuronidase, has occurred (Smith and Williams, 1966). This enzyme, usually localized in lysosomes, degrades glucuronides, although its exact function still is not clear. The enzyme differs entirely from the glucuronyl transferases (see Dutton, 1966b); for example, β-glucuronidase is inhibited by glucurolactone, whereas the glucuronyl transferases are not affected. A drug-glucuronide conjugate may be hydrolyzed by β-glucuronidase in specific tissues to restore the aglycone in sufficiently high concentration to produce toxicity. Occasionally β-glucuronidase may also alter the pattern of glucuronide formation by catalyzing the transfer of glucuronyl moieties from ether glucuronides to aliphatic alcohols (see Parke, 1968).

4. General methodology. Although it is possible to isolate glucuronides by precipitation from solutions followed by crystallization (Fishman, 1961), it is more customary to identify such derivatives by the use of β-glucuronidase preparations. The recovery of aglycones by this treatment serves as a measure of the specifically hydrolyzed glucuronide derivative, and can be used as a quantitative assay. The enzyme is usually prepared from liver, snails or bacteria. Details on the methodology used in identification and estimation of glucuronides are found in the chapter by Marsh (1966), and have received additional emphasis in Chapter 18. Table 10.7 shows stability characteristic of various glucuronides. It should be noted that there are numerous individual variations among these categorical properties.

5. Excretion of glucuronides. Glucuronides are frequently excreted by the kidney by tubular secretion, using the characteristic but not very specific excretory route for organic acids. Not all glucuronides are excreted by tubular secretion, however. Conjugates of higher molecular weight, such as the glucuronides of androsterone and pregnanediol, are eliminated by glomerular filtration alone, whereas those of menthol, phenol and resorcinol, which are of lower molecular

TABLE 10.7

Stability of glucuronides

Treatment	Glucuronide			
	O-ester	O-ether	N-ether	S-ether
β-glucuroni-dase[a]	hydro-lyzed	hydrolyzed	slowly hydrolyzed[d]	hydrolyzed
0.2 N HCl[b]	stable	slowly hydrolyzed	hydrolyzed	hydrolyzed
0.2 N NaOH[c]	hydro-lyzed	stable	slowly hydrolyzed	slowly hydrolyzed

[a] 700 enzyme units, pH 7.4, 15 min at 37°. [b] 5 min at 25°. [c] 20 hr at 37°. [d] non enzymatic? Adapted from Axelrod *et al.*, 1958.

weight, are secreted by the tubules in addition to glomerular filtration (Smith and Williams, 1966).

Glucuronides may also be eliminated via the bile, which in some cases may be the predominant route of excretion. This pathway is relatively more common for the rat, dog, hen and cat than other species. For the rat, for example, glucuronide conjugates with a molecular weight greater than 400 (i.e., aglycone about 200) are usually actively secreted into the bile, whereas lower molecular weight derivatives are less likely to be transferred by this route. Thus, the glucuronides of bilirubin, thyroxine, pregnanediol, diethylstilbestrol, morphine, glutethimide and chloramphenicol are mostly excreted into the bile. Following the passage of these conjugates into the gut, they may be subjected to hydrolysis by intestinal β-glucuronidase. If the conjugates are readily hydrolyzed, the aglycone (e.g., diethylstilbestrol, morphine, glutethimide and chloramphenicol) then can undergo reabsorption, transport to the liver, reconjugation and re-excretion (enterohepatic circulation). Conjugates more stable to hydrolysis, such as the glucuronide of sulfadimethoxine, will be excreted in the feces without extensive recirculation (Smith and Williams, 1966).

6. Glucuronide formation in various species. Glucuronide conjugation of drugs takes place in most mammalian species with the exception of the cat, which forms such conjugates with few if any drugs. In this animal, phenols, for example, are conjugated as sulfates rather than glucuronides. It should be noted that in the cat, however, various endogenous compounds, such as bilirubin, thyroxine and steroids, are conjugated as glucuronides. It has been demonstrated that the cat can synthesize UDPGA, but apparently lacks those glucuronyl transferases used in drug conjugation (see Dutton, 1966b). In fish, a deficiency of UDPGA seems to be responsible for the observed lack of glucuronide excretion.

The Gunn strain of Wistar rats is characteristic in its diminished ability of conjugating certain compounds with glucuronic acid. In this strain, even though UDPGA levels are normal, O-glucuronyl transferases have decreased levels of activity. Although aniline and *p*-nitrophenol are excreted as glucuronides, bilirubin, *o*-aminophenol and *o*-aminobenzoic acid do not form glucuronide derivatives (Arias, 1961). Because of this abnormality the animals develop acholuric jaundice. A similar situation appears to obtain in infants with congenital nonhemolytic jaundice, such as Crigler-Najjar syndrome (Dutton, 1966b). In these individuals there is insufficient conjugation of bilirubin with glucuronic acid leading to high serum bilirubin levels, kernicterus, and cerebral damage. The capacity to form glucuronide conjugates with salicylic acid, menthol and hydrocortisone is also diminished under these conditions, indicating that several transferase systems are reduced in activity. Drugs which are normally conjugated with glucuronic acid may aggravate kernicterus in these individuals by further impeding the conjugation of bilirubin. Related information for the human without this congenital condition is provided in the next section.

7. Factors affecting glucuronide formation. Various factors influence the extent of glucuronide conjugation. In the rat, for example, male animals produce more of the conjugate than do females; testosterone enhances glucuronide formation in the female rat while estradiol reduces that in the male. The sex difference does not hold for the human, however.

The activity of glucuronyl transferase is increased by the administration of benzpyrene or other microsomal drug metabolism inducers. Thyroxine administration may also lead to such an increase.

Glucuronide conjugation may be impaired in patients with liver damage. A number of drugs and hormones are known to inhibit glucuronyl transferase activity. The microsomal enzyme inhibitor, SKF 525A, inhibits the enzyme *in vivo*. Novobiocin limits glucuronide formation of drugs and normal substrates. Phenylbutazone inhibits glucuronide formation *in vitro*. Cortisone and estradiol, under certain situations, also decrease hepatic microsomal glucuronide synthesis, but the pharmacological significance of these effects is still unrecognized (Smith and Williams, 1966). The diminished conjugation with glucuronic acid during pregnancy may be due to the elevated levels of progesterone and pregnanediol, which inhibit transferase activity (Parke, 1968). The various effects of drugs on glucuronide formation, described in detail by Dutton (1966b), depend on the species, sex, stage of development and organ location of the enzymes, and occasionally may relate to competition for glucuronide formation.

Recognition is indisputably given to the fact that in the newborn certain drug metabolizing enzymes take a few weeks to develop (Brown *et al.*, 1958). The levels of glucuronyl transferase in newborn of most species, with the exception of the rat, are remarkably low (see Dutton, 1966b). The failure to metabolize chloramphenicol to the nontoxic glucuronide is related to the low enzyme level in the human neonate. The incomplete development of renal excretory function of the newborn further complicates the situation in that under these conditions chloramphenicol can accumulate to toxic levels to produce the characteristic "Gray Baby" syndrome, involving cyanosis, cardiovascular toxicity and death (Weiss *et al.*, 1960). Similarly, the inability to conjugate bilirubin to its less toxic glucuronide derivative is responsible for the development of kernicterus in the newborn. This situation is aggravated when novobiocin is administered because this drug further reduces glucuronide formation (Hargreaves and Holton, 1962). Investigators are currently attempting to prevent or treat kernicterus by inducing the enzyme in the newborn with repeated drug treatment. The administration of phenobarbital to either the mother before delivery or to the newborn leads to the enhanced rate of formation of glucuronyl transferase which then may reduce the level of bilirubin by conjugation (Yaffe *et al.*, 1966).

B. Sulfate Conjugation

1. Mechanism of the reaction. To form a sulfate derivative of a drug, sulfate must first be activated by a series of reactions involving ATP. Sulfate is converted first to adenosine-5'-phosphosulfate (APS) and then to 3'-phospho-adenosine-5'-phosphosulfate (PAPS). PAPS has been identified as the active sulfate which transfers the sulfate to the drug acceptor. These reactions, which take place in the soluble fraction of cells, are shown below.

$$SO_4^= + ATP \xrightarrow{\text{ATP-sulfurylase}}$$

adenosine-5'-phosphosulfate (APS) + pyrophosphate

$$APS + ATP \xrightarrow[\text{kinase}]{\text{APS phospho-}}$$

3'-phosphoadenosine-5'-phosphosulfate (PAPS) + ADP

$$PAPS + RZH \xrightarrow{\text{sulfokinase}}$$

R-Z-SO$_3$H + 3-phosphoadenosine-5'-phosphate (PAP)

where Z is O or NH

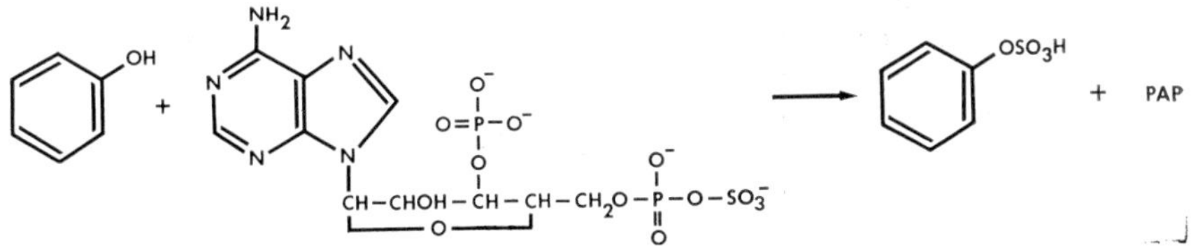

phenol   PAPS   phenyl sulfate

Several distinct sulfokinases (or sulfotransferases) have been described, and these enzymes exhibit considerable specificity (Nose and Lipmann, 1958). The enzyme which transfers sulfate to phenol, for example, is found in the soluble fraction of liver, kidney and intestine; enzymes functioning in sulfate conjugation of certain steroids act in the liver only.

2. Substrates of the reaction. Drugs such as phenols, certain aliphatic alcohols and aromatic amines may form sulfate derivatives (see Table 10.8) In the case of alcohols or phenols, these conjugates are called ethereal sulfates. Ethanol, propanol, butanol and chloramphenicol may form ethereal sulfates. The N-sulfates, or sulfamates, have been reported mainly for the rat, rabbit and guinea pig; conjugation takes place in the soluble fraction of liver (Roy, 1960a). Traces of the N^4-sulfate have been recovered as a metabolic product of sulfanilamide, and aniline and related amines are also known to form N-sulfates. The formation of S-sulfates (thiosulfates) has not been definitely established.

In addition, various normal body constituents exist as sulfates and are formed by reactions identical to those of drug sulfates, except for the individuality of the sulfokinases (Borstrum, 1965). For example, the sulfokinases which catalyze the reaction with phenols are sufficiently specific that they do not mediate those with steroids, and vice versa. These endogenous conjugates include heparin,

TABLE 10.8

Types of compounds conjugating with sulfate

Hydroxy Compounds	Example	Ethereal Sulfate
Phenols		
(i) Carbo-cyclic	Phenol	$O-SO_3H$
(ii) Hetero-cyclic	3-Hydroxy-coumarin	$O-SO_3H$
(iii) Steroidal	Estrone	HO_3S-O
Alcohols		
(i) Primary aliphatic	Ethanol	$C_2H_5O-SO_3H$
(ii) Secondary steroidal	Dehydro-epiandro-sterone	HO_3S-O
Amino compounds Aromatic amine	Aniline	$NH-SO_3H$

From Williams, 1967.

chondroitin sulfate, various sulfolipids, tyrosine sulfate, the sulfates of epinephrine, norepinephrine, and those of numerous steroids, such as progesterone, estrone, pregnenolone, androsterone, and bile acids.

3. Factors affecting sulfate conjugation. The total pool of sulfate is usually quite limited and can be readily exhausted; thus, with increasing doses of a drug, conjugation with sulfate becomes a less preponderant pathway, and may become a zero order reaction (Bray *et al.*, 1952). (See also Section V.) For this reason conjugation with glucuronic acid usually predominates over that of sulfate. Competition for the sulfate pool probably is responsible for the diminished synthesis of endogenous sulfates of such compounds as hormones.

Most species, including man, appear to be able to make sulfate derivatives, although they are not readily synthesized in the pig and, apparently, fish. At birth relatively little sulfokinase activity is present in many animals, analogously to the situation with glucuronyl transferase. In man, however, fetal liver apparently can function in sulfate conjugation with *p*-nitrophenol. In the mouse during the early postnatal development, liver sulfokinase activity is equal to or greater than the adult levels, but varies depending on the substrate used (Percy and Yaffe, 1964). In the rat a few days are required for development of sulfo-transferases to adult levels.

An entirely different group of enzymes, the sulfatases, are present in most species which can cleave the sulfate group from such derivatives (Roy, 1960b).

4. General methodology. As a rule ethereal sulfates are remarkably stable. As with glucuronide derivatives, precipitating agents may be used to isolate sulfate derivatives, or such conjugates may be assayed by difference after subjecting the metabolic products to hydrolysis, as, for example, with sulfatase enzymes from bacteria or snails. It is also possible to separate inorganic sulfates from ethereal sulfates by treatment with barium salts (Wengle, 1964). Radioactive sulfate may be helpful in locating and identifying sulfate derivatives. The sulfokinase enzymes have been described by Gregory (1962).

C. Amide Synthesis

There are several metabolic routes which involve the interaction of an acid with an amine to form an amide. Since the mechanism of this reaction is similar in all cases, it is reasonable to consider together (1) the condensation of a carboxylic acid-containing drug with an amine (actually an amino acid) such as glycine (e.g., hippuric acid formation), and (2) the reaction of an amine drug with a carboxylic acid, such as acetic acid (acetylation). In both cases the acid must be converted to an active form, and this process involves Coenzyme A. The activation system is the same one which also activates many endogenous fatty acids.

This overall series of reactions leading to amide formation is as follows, where either R COOH or R'NH$_2$ can be the drug to be conjugated.

$$\text{R COOH} + \text{ATP} \xrightarrow{\text{acyl synthetase or thiokinase}}$$

$$\text{R CO-AMP} + \text{pyrophosphate}$$

$$\text{R CO-AMP} + \text{CoA-SH} \xrightarrow{\text{acyl thiokinase}} \text{R CO-S-CoA} + \text{AMP}$$

$$\text{R CO-S-CoA} + \text{R'NH}_2 \xrightarrow{\text{transacylase}} \text{R CO NHR'} + \text{CoA-SH}$$

benzoic acid   hippuric acid

sulfanilamide   acetyl CoA   N^4-acetylsulfanilamide

These reactions normally take place in the mitochondrial fraction of liver and kidney cells of most species. The dog and chicken may differ in that only the kidney is active in these conversions.

1. Conjugation with endogenous amines

a. *Glycine.* The formation of hippuric acid from administered benzoic acid with endogenous glycine is probably the earliest demonstrated reaction in drug metabolism. Keller (1842) was the first person to isolate and identify this metabolic product after self-administration of benzoic acid. Since originally it had been isolated from the horse, the name "hippuric" acid (from hippos, Greek for horse) was chosen for the product. For other acids the ending "uric" is still applied to the metabolite, even though it has no relation to uric acid; salicyluric acid thus is the glycine conjugate of salicylic acid.

Amide formation with glycine takes place with aromatic and heterocyclic carboxylic acid drugs, as well as certain aliphatic acids, especially those with aromatic substituents (Table 10.9). Most other aliphatic acids apparently are too readily oxidized in the body so that conjugation cannot occur. Certain normal metabolites, such as bile acids, also form derivatives with glycine, but the reaction takes place in the microsomal rather than mitochondrial fraction. Glycine is the most common of the endogenous amines to conjugate organic acids. Although the body pool of glycine may be limited so that hippuric acid formation may follow zero order kinetics, this route of metabolism can be important quantitatively.

In man conjugation with glycine may be impaired in certain cases of liver disease, and hippuric acid formation following benzoic acid ingestion has been used as a test for liver function. In the newborn and in the elderly, glycine availability may be more limited, thereby reducing hippuric acid formation (Williams, 1963).

b. *Other Amino Acids.* The nature of the amine used for conjugation depends on the species. In addition to glycine, man and certain monkeys (chimpanzee, baboon, red monkey and specific species of African monkeys) can use glutamine for conjugation with organic acids, especially with phenylacetic and closely related acids (Williams, 1963). In these species, apparently a special acylating enzyme is present in liver or kidney to mediate glutamine conjugation (Moldave and Meister, 1957).

In arachnids, glycine may be replaced by arginine. In reptiles and certain birds, such as the hen, goose, duck, or turkey, ornithine is used for conjugation rather than glycine, whereas in the pigeon, glycine conjugation does take place. In the hen, for example, ornithine is conjugated to benzoic, phenylacetic, and heterocyclic aromatic acids, including furoic and nicotinic acids. Occasionally two acids may conjugate with the two amino groups of ornithine. The enzyme system for ornithurate formation has been localized in the particulate fraction of the chicken kidney, but is absent in the liver of this species. The acylating enzyme catalyzing the conjugation with ornithine is distinct from that for glycine.

In exceptional cases serine and glycyltaurine conjugates of aromatic acids have been recovered.

2. Conjugation with endogenous acids. Acetylation is the most common

TABLE 10.9
Types of acids forming glycine conjugates

(a) *Aromatic*	*Example*	
Carbocyclic	Benzoic acid	⟨benzene⟩—COOH
Heterocyclic	Nicotinic acid	⟨pyridine⟩—COOH
(b) *Substituted acetic acid*		
Monosubstituted (arylacetic acids)	Phenylacetic acid	⟨benzene⟩—CH₂—COOH
Disubstituted	Hydratropic acid	⟨benzene⟩—CH(CH₃)—COOH
(c) *β-Substituted propionic acid*	β-o-Tolylpropionic acid	⟨benzene(CH₃)⟩—CH₂—CH₂—COOH
(d) *Substituted acrylic acids*		
β-Monosubstituted carbocyclic	Cinnamic acid	⟨benzene⟩—CH=CH—COOH
Heterocyclic	Furylacrylic acid	⟨furan⟩—CH=CH—COOH
β-Disubstituted	β-Methylcinnamic acid	⟨benzene⟩—C(CH₃)=CH—COOH
α,β-Disubstituted	Phellandric acid (4-Isopropylcyclohex-1-ene-carboxylic acid)	HC=C—COOH ... CH(CH₃)₂
(e) *Steroid acids*	Cholic acid Deoxycholic acid	

Arrow points to carboxyl group conjugated with glycine. From Williams, 1967.

example of this type of reaction, which takes place in many tissues with aromatic primary amines, some endogenous primary aliphatic amines, unphysiological amino acids, hydrazines and hydrazides (Table 10.10). Sulfonamides form both N^1 and N^4 acetyl derivatives, as well as traces of the diacetyl compounds. Secondary amines are not acetylated. The reaction usually represents a minor metabolic route, in contrast to deamination, but for some compounds (e.g., isoniazid in man) it may be the major pathway. Phenols, alcohols, or thiol drugs do not form acetyl derivatives, although of course certain natural compounds with such functional groups, like choline and Coenzyme A, react in this manner. A variety of

TABLE 10.10
Types of compounds acetylated

Type	Example	Acetyl Derivative
Primary amine Natural $(R—CH_2NH_2)$	Histamine	(imidazole ring)—$CH_2CH_2NH—\underline{COCH_3}$[a]
Amino acid ω-Phenyl-sub- stituted $\underset{\underset{COOH}{|}}{\overset{\overset{NH_2}{|}}{Ar—(CH_2)_nCH—}}$	γ-Phenyl-α- aminobutyric acid	(phenyl)—$CH_2CH_2\underset{\underset{}{}}{\overset{\overset{COOH}{|}}{CH}}—NH—\underline{COCH_3}$
S-Arylcysteine $\underset{\underset{COOH}{|}}{\overset{\overset{NH_2}{|}}{Ar—S—CH_2CH—}}$	S-Phenyl- cysteine	(phenyl)—$S—CH_2\overset{\overset{COOH}{|}}{CH}—NH—\underline{COCH_3}$
Hydrazine derivatives Hydrazine (NH_2NH_2)	Hydrazine	$\underline{CH_3CO}—NH—NH—\underline{COCH_3}$
Hydrazide $(R—CONHNH_2)$	Isonicotinyl- hydrazide	(pyridine)—$CONH—NH—\underline{COCH_3}$
Sulfonamide $(Ar—SO_2NH_2)$	Sulfanilamide	H_2N(phenyl)$SO_2NH—\underline{COCH_3}$
Aromatic amine Unsubstituted $(Ar—NH_2)$	Aniline	(phenyl)$NH—\underline{COCH_3}$
Substituted $(R—Ar'—NH_2)$	Sulfanilamide	$\underline{CH_3CO}—HN$(phenyl)SO_2NH_2

[a] Acetyl group underlined. From Williams, 1967.

cysteine derivatives are acetylated, which are described under Mercapturic Acid Formation (*see* Section III, D).

Effects of acetylation of sulfonamides have been described in Tables 10.3 and 10.4. It is apparent that conjugation with acetyl groups can alter the relative solubility, and hence renal toxicity, of these drugs in either direction.

Some special comments should be made regarding acetylation. The reaction takes place in the reticuloendothelial rather than parenchymal cells of liver (Govier, 1965), and reticuloendothelial cells of lung, spleen and mucosa can also mediate the reaction. Unlike its relative inability to form glucuronides, the neonate apparently has the capacity to acetylate like the normal adult (Vest and Rossier, 1963). It is also of interest that the investigation of the acetylation of sulfonilamide led to the discovery of Coenzyme A (Lipmann, 1945).

The guinea pig cannot acetylate arylcysteines or glucosamine but can acetylate aromatic amines. The dog differs from many mammalian species in its relatively low excretion of acetylated derivatives of aromatic amines and hydrazides. It has been reported that an inhibitor of arylamine acetyl transferase is responsible for that effect (Leibman and Anaclerio, 1962). At the same time, however, the dog has the capacity to acetylate unphysiological aromatic amino acids and to form mercapturic acids. Furthermore, it can form an acetyl derivative of N^1 but not N^4-amino groups of sulfanilamide, suggesting that enzyme specificity of various transacetylases must be involved in this selectivity. The relative inability of the dog to form acetyl conjugates implies that the dog would be a poor choice of species for the preliminary prediction of the human metabolism of drugs which are aromatic amines. Acetylation of isoniazid is genetically determined in man and certain strains of monkeys, and the levels of certain of the hepatic acetyl transferases differ in certain subjects (see Chapter 15). This polymorphism related to acetylation of isoniazid in man has been demonstrated also for acetylation of hydralazine but not for that of sulfanilamide or p-aminobenzoic acid.

Because of the hydrolytic deacetylation of aromatic amine drugs in certain species, the net acetylation of a drug may depend on the relative rates of acetylation and deacetylation which usually take place in the liver and kidney, respectively. The dog, for example, rapidly deacetylates aromatic amine derivatives. In man and the rabbit, on the other hand, which lack the ability to deacetylate aromatic amine derivatives, the apparent rate of acetylation is therefore relatively great. Thus the relative lack of excretion of acetylated primary aromatic amines in the dog may be due, in part, to rapid deacetylation. Aliphatic deacetylase activity is poor in the dog and greater in the rabbit.

Besides acetylation, a few examples of formylation are known, and succinyl conjugates of drugs are also possible.

D. Mercapturic Acid Synthesis

The formation of drug mercapturates has been studied in considerable detail in animals (reviewed by Boyland and Booth, 1962). In man, however, it is a rather unlikely route of metabolism, although apparently it can occur (Williams, 1963). It is also rare in the guinea pig, probably because of a lack of a specific acetylase, but has been observed in the rabbit, dog and rat. Drugs subject to this reaction frequently contain an active halogen or a nitro group, as indicated in Table 10.11, although not all compounds with these functional groups form mercapturates. The reaction may be depicted as follows:

$$RX + \text{glutathione} \xrightarrow[\text{aryltransferase}]{\text{GSH—S—}}$$

$$
\begin{array}{c}
\text{CO—NH—CH}_2\text{COOH} \\
| \\
\text{R}\text{-}\text{—S—CH}_2\ \text{CH} \\
| \\
\text{NH—CO(CH}_2)_2\text{CH(NH}_2)\text{COOH}
\end{array}
$$

$$
\xrightarrow{\text{glutathionase}}
\begin{array}{c}
\text{CO—NH—CH}_2\text{COOH} \\
| \\
\text{R—S—CH}_2\text{—CH} \\
| \\
\text{NH}_2
\end{array}
\xrightarrow{\text{peptidase}}
$$

$$
\begin{array}{ccc}
\underset{\text{R—S—CH}_2\text{—CH}}{\overset{\overset{\displaystyle\text{COOH}}{|}}{\underset{\underset{\displaystyle\text{NH}_2}{|}}{}}} & \xrightarrow{\text{acetylase}} & \underset{\text{R—S—CH}_2\text{—CH}}{\overset{\overset{\displaystyle\text{COOH}}{|}}{\underset{\underset{\displaystyle\text{NH—CO—CH}_3}{|}}{}}}
\end{array}
$$

where RX is an aromatic ring, a halide or nitro compound

benzyl chloride   benzyl mercapturate

The drug interacts with glutathione at its reactive site. The mediating enzymes, glutathione-S-aryl (or alkyl) transferase or glutathiokinase, occur in the soluble fraction of liver, heart, and kidneys; several such enzymes are known, but for some compounds like benzyl chloride the reaction apparently may also proceed to a limited extent nonenzymatically (Booth et al., 1961). The complex first loses glutamate by transpeptidation, and then the glycine portion of the glutathione conjugate is cleaved by a peptidase. Thereafter, acetylation takes place on the free amino group of the cysteine moiety. Occasionally intramolecular rearrangements permit substitution by glutathione in different positions of an aromatic ring.

Glutathionase is most active in the kidney, and to a lesser extent in the liver, depending on the species. Peptidases are active in several tissues, mainly the kidney, liver and pancreas. Acetylation takes place in the liver and perhaps in the kidney, and the resulting mercapturic acid is then excreted in the urine. Intermediary metabolites during these conversions may appear in the bile. Newborn animals have diminished capacity to form mercapturates.

The remarkable metabolism of the normally stable, unsubstituted aromatic cyclic hydrocarbons, such as benzene, naphthalene and anthracene, does not result from replacement of a nuclear hydrogen but probably involves first an intermediary oxidation to the epoxide. This reaction requires liver microsomes, NADPH and oxygen. This product then reacts with glutathione in the presence of a special enzyme, GSH S-epoxidetransferase, to form a "premercapturate" which is excreted and which in the presence of dilute acid loses water to form the corresponding mercapturate:

phenyl premercapturate   phenyl mercapturate

TABLE 10.11
Types of compounds forming mercapturic acids in vivo

Type of Compound	Example	Formula	Group Replaced by Acetyl-cysteyl residue	Mercapturic Acid (—S—R = Acetyl-cysteyl Residue)
(a) Aromatic hydrocarbon	Benzene	(benzene ring)	H	(benzene ring)—S—R
(b) Halogenated aromatic hydrocarbon	Chlorobenzene	Cl—(benzene ring)	H	Cl—(benzene ring)—S—R
(c) Halogenated paraffin	Bromopropane	C_3H_7Br	Br	C_3H_7—S—R
(d) ω-Halogenated alkylbenzene	Benzyl chloride	(benzene ring)—CH_2Cl	Cl	(benzene ring)—CH_2—S—R
(e) Halogenated nitrobenzene	(a) p-Fluoronitrobenzene	NO_2—(benzene ring)—F	F	NO_2—(benzene ring)—S—R
	(b) Pentachloronitrobenzene	Cl Cl / Cl—(ring)—NO_2 / Cl Cl	NO_2	Cl Cl / Cl—(ring)—S—R / Cl Cl
(f) Nitroparaffin	Nitrobutane	$C_4H_9NO_2$	NO_2	C_4H_9—S—R
(g) Alkyl sulfonic ester	Ethyl methanesulfonate	CH_3—SO_3—C_2H_5	CH_3SO_3	C_2H_5—S—R
(h) Aromatic amine	Aniline	H_2N—(benzene ring)	H	H_2N—(benzene ring)—S—R
(i) Carbamic ester	Urethane	$NH_2COOC_2H_5$	NH_2	C_2H_5O—CO—S—R
(j) Sulfonamide	Benzothiazole sulfonamide	(benzothiazole)C—SO_2NH_2	SO_2NH_2	(benzothiazole)C—S—R

Mainly from Williams, 1967.

E. Methylation

Methylation usually represents a relatively minor metabolic pathway for drugs. The process differs from the other routes of conjugation reactions in that the products formed occasionally have extensive biological activity (epinephrine, 6-methylmercaptopurine). There are numerous endogenous compounds which are normally methylated, and several methylation systems are available. The reaction usually takes place via the formation of S-adenosylmethionine. The activated methyl group then reacts with various acceptors in the presence of a methyl transferase, and S-adenosylhomocysteine is the other reaction product.

$$\text{ATP} + \text{methionine} \xrightarrow[\text{transferase}]{\substack{\text{methionine} \\ \text{adenosine}}} \text{S-adenosylmethionine} + \text{pyrophosphate} + \text{phosphate}$$

$$\text{S-adenosylmethionine} + \text{RZH} \xrightarrow[\text{transferase}]{\text{methyl}}$$

$$\text{RZ CH}_3 + \text{S-adenosylhomocysteine}$$

where Z is O, NH or S

histamine   S-adenosylmethionine   methylhistamine

Epinephrine   Metanephrine

Table 10.12 shows the type of compounds which undergo methylation. There are very few examples of aliphatic amine drugs being methylated (N-methylation) but several endogenous aliphatic amines, such as norepinephrine and dimethylaminoethanol are substrates. Aromatic amines rarely undergo the reaction. Heterocyclic tertiary nitrogen atoms may be methylated and may be converted to quaternary bases. Methylation of phenols (O-methylation) and of thiol groups (S-methylation) may also take place. It is unusual for monohydric phenols to be methylated but estradiol, N-acetylserotonin and a few other endogenous compounds may undergo the reaction. For polyhydric phenols, such as catechols, orientation of methylation *in vivo* is usually quite specific and is normally confined to only one of the hydroxyl groups (Williams, 1967).

The methyl transferases differ from each other in terms of cofactor requirements and demonstrate substrate and species specificity, variations in tissue distribution and sensitivity to different inhibitory drugs. These enzymes are summarized in Table 10.13.

In addition to methylation, demethylation may also occur. Liver, for instance, contains a demethylase enzyme which cleaves the methyl group to form the desmethyl derivatives. The sequential methylation, demethylation and remethylation of a compound may be misinterpreted as a migration of the methyl group from one position to another. The more rapid demethylation of *p*-methoxy than *m*-methoxy catechols probably accounts for the greater excretion of the *meta* derivatives, since the catechol O-methyl transferases can methylate in either of the two positions *in vitro* (Williams, 1967).

TABLE 10.12
Types of compounds methylated

Type of Compound	Example	Methylated Metabolite
N-METHYLATION *Amines* (*Aliphatic*) (a) Primary	Norepinephrine	HO— HO—C_6H_3—CHOH—CH$_2$NH—CH$_3^a$
(b) Secondary	Guanidoacetic acid	HN CH$_3$ ‖ ‖ NH$_2$—C—N—CH$_2$—COOH
(c) Tertiary	Dimethylamino-ethanol	CH$_3$ / HO—CH$_2$—CH$_2$—N$^+$—CH$_3$ \ CH$_3$
N-Heterocycles (a) Tertiary N	Pyridine	+N—CH$_3$
(b) Secondary N	Histamine	N═⟍CH$_2$CH$_2$NH$_2$ N CH$_3$
O-METHYLATION *Phenols* (a) Monohydric	4-Hydroxy-3,5-di-iodobenzoic acid	I CH$_3$O—⟍COOH I
(b) Dihydric	3,4-Dihydroxy-benzoic acid	CH$_3$O— HO—⟍COOH
(c) Trihydric	3,4,5-Trihy-droxybenzoic acid	HO— CH$_3$O—⟍COOH HO—
S-METHYLATION Thiopyrimidine	Thiouracil	H O N— CH$_3$S—⟍ N

[a] Methyl group is underlined. From Williams, 1967.

F. Conjugation of Substrate Analogs

Numerous drugs are able to utilize metabolic pathways available for normal physiological constituents. Certain structural, electronic and steric requirements must be met, but it is now realized that these limitations are not so stringent. Some of the best documented examples of compounds exhibiting metabolism by these routes are the analogs of purine and pyrimidine bases (Langen, 1968). For example, the guanine analog, 8-azaguanine, serves as a substrate for guanase, and is degraded to azaxanthine in a manner analogous to the conversion of

TABLE 10.13

Tabulation of major methyl transferases

N-methyl Transferases

Type	Substrates	Features	Location	Reference
phenylethanol	norepinephrine other phenylethanol-amines	requires Mg⁺⁺ and glutathione	adrenal medulla: supernatant	Kirshner and Goodall, 1957
non-specific 1° amines	serotonin tryptamine other endogenous and drug amines	Mg⁺⁺ and glutathione not required	*lung*; others in liver and brain: supernatant	Axelrod, 1962
2° amines	N-methylserotonin nornicotine normeperidine normorphine norcodeine			
3° amines	pyridine quinoline			
imidazole	histamine	Mg⁺⁺ or glutathione not required; inhibited by chlorpromazine and antimalarial drugs	widely distributed, especially brain	Brown *et al.*, 1959 Cohn, 1965
others, specific	nicotinamide guanidoacetic acid phosphatidylamino-ethanol polynucleotide bases	requires Mg⁺⁺ requires —SH compound, but not Mg⁺⁺	liver nucleoli	Cantoni, 1951 Fleissner and Borek, 1963

O-methyl Transferases

catechol	epinephrine norepinephrine gallic acid caffeic acid dopamine dihydroxyamphetamine other catechols	Mg^{++}, Co^{++} or Mn^{++} required; glutathione not required; monohydric phenols not substrates; inhibited by pyrogallol	liver, *kidney*, skin, blood cells, glandular tissue, nerve fibers; not skeletal muscle: supernatant	Axelrod and Tomchick, 1958
catechol	N-acetyltyramine l-epinephrine	differs from soluble enzyme in distribution and pH optimum; can be stimulated	liver: microsomes	Inscoe et al., 1965
phenol	various phenols	Mg^{++} not required	liver, lung, kidney: microsomes	Axelrod and Daly, 1968
hydroxyindole	N-acetylserotonin bufotenine hydroxyindoles	controlled by lighting, diurnal variation; Mg^{++} not required; —SH required: catechols not substrates	pineal body, not kidney or liver: supernatant	Axelrod and Weissbach, 1961
iodophenol	iodophenols	thyronine and triiodothyronine not substrates; no Mg^{++} required	liver: supernatant	Tomita et al., 1964

S-methyl Transferases

	alkyl mercaptans mercaptoethanol dimercaptopropanol thiouracil	cysteine, homocysteine and glutathione not substrates; can also transfer ethyl group from S-adenosylethionine	liver, kidney and lung: microsomes	Bremer and Greenberg, 1961

Compiled mainly from Williams (1967) and Parke (1968).

guanine to xanthine. The subsequent biochemical degradation, to urate, is not applicable for azaguanine because of the lack of an oxidizable carbon atom in position 8, and thus azaxanthine is the major excretory product. Azaguanine also uses the biosynthetic pathways of guanine and is incorporated into nucleic acids (Mandel *et al.*, 1954). In the presence of phosphorylribose pyrophosphate (PRPP), azaguanine and nucleotide pyrophosphorylase, the ribomononucleotide is synthesized *in vitro* (Way and Parks, 1958).

8-azaguanine   PRPP   8-azaguanosine-5'-phosphate

In addition, numerous other conjugates which are characteristically formed by guanine are also available for the analog. Conjugates with ribose (8-azaguanosine), deoxyribose (deoxyazaguanosine), and ribose phosphates (azaguanosine mono-, di- and triphosphates) have been identified, and the drug has been incorporated into DNA and the various RNA fractions (Fig. 10.1) (Mandel, 1959; Grünberger, 1966).

Most of the enzymes catalyzing these reactions are located in the soluble fraction of cells and are preponderant in those tissues with greatest biosynthetic activity, such as intestinal epithelium, bone marrow, and hair follicles. Tumor

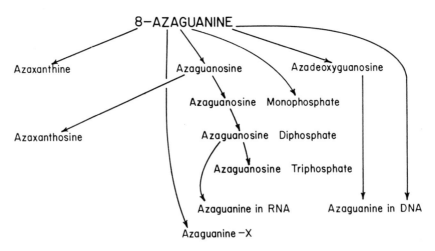

Fig. 10.1. Metabolic conversions of 8-azaguanine. (From Mandel, 1959.)

cells frequently exhibit extensive biosynthetic activity also, thus explaining in part the rational basis for the use of substrate analogs in cancer chemotherapy.

The relative affinities of substrates and substrate analogs for the enzymes catalyzing the reactions are variable, although frequently the enzyme interacts preferentially with the normal substrate. Table 10.14 represents various *in vitro* reactions indicating the enzyme affinity relationships of some normal purine derivatives and their thio analogs. The *in vivo* metabolism of the analog and its pharmacological significance is related not only to the enzyme affinity but also to the enzyme concentration, the relative pool sizes of substrate and inhibitor, and the importance of the reaction (Elion, 1967).

Another analog which has received extensive study of its metabolism in a variety of species is 5-fluorouracil (Heidelberger, 1965). This drug competes with uracil, and the drug's derivatives compete with the corresponding ones for uracil along the various biochemical pathways. A large number of analog conjugates have been isolated and identified, revealing the resemblance in the reactions of both biosynthesis and degradation (Fig. 10.2). Derivatives such as fluoroureidopropionate are formed in organs such as liver, where the reaction is localized in the soluble fraction, and are further metabolized for excretion (Chaudhuri *et al.*, 1958). In *E. coli*, fluorouridine diphospho-N-acetyl glucosamine fails to permit normal cell wall biosynthesis for which UDP-N-acetyl glucosamine normally is required, and leads to osmotic instability of newly-formed bacteria. The formation of FU-containing RNA, either by polymerization of fluorouridine triphosphate, in the presence of the natural nucleoside triphosphates, or by biosynthesis, results in abnormal polynucleotides with slight but significant alterations in biochemical and biophysical properties, both *in vitro* and *in vivo* (Mandel, 1969). For example, ribosomal RNA has different sedimentation properties when it contains fluorouracil (Fig. 10.3). It is possible to separate normal from analog-containing transfer RNA molecules by column chromatography (Fig. 10.4). The conversion of the analog to the deoxyribo-

TABLE 10.14

Inhibition by 6-mercaptopurine or its metabolites TIMP, TIDP, TITP of various biosynthetic reactions

Normal Reaction	Inhibitor	K_m	K_i
H $\rightarrow$ IMP	6-MP	1.1×10^{-5}	8.3×10^{-6}
H$_4$FA $\xrightarrow{\text{ATP}}$ FH$_4$FA	6-MP	5×10^{-4}	3.3×10^{-3}
			2.5×10^{-4}
IMP $\rightarrow$ SAMP	TIMP	3×10^{-5}	3×10^{-4}
IMP $\rightarrow$ XMP	TIMP	1.4×10^{-5}	3.6×10^{-6}
SAMP $\rightarrow$ AMP	TIMP	2.8×10^{-6}	3×10^{-4}
ADP $\rightarrow$ poly A	TIDP[a]	1.7×10^{-3}	3.3×10^{-5}
ATP + NMN $\rightarrow$ NAD	TITP	7.4×10^{-5}	5×10^{-5}

[a] Concns. for 50% inhibition.

TIMP, thioinosinate (6 MP ribonucleotide); TIDP and TITP, thioinosine diphosphate and triphosphate, respectively. ADP, adenosine diphosphate; AMP, adenylate; FH$_4$FA, formyltetrahydrofolate; H, hypoxanthine; H$_4$FA, tetrahydrofolate; IMP, inosinate; NMN, nicotinamide mononucleotide; poly A, polyadenylate; SAMP, adenylsuccinate; XMP, xanthylate; K_m and K_i in *M*. (From Elion, 1967.)

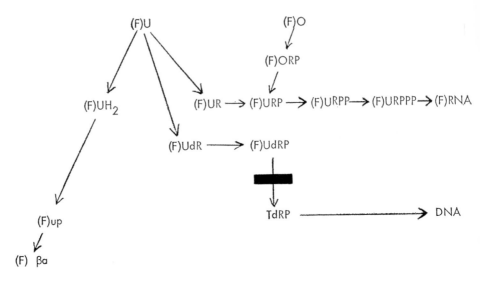

Fig. 10.2. Biochemical conversions of uracil and orotate and their 5-fluoro analogs (F) during biosynthesis (towards right) and degradation (towards left). O, orotate; U, uracil; R, ribose; P, phosphate; dR, deoxyribose; up, ureidopropionate; βa, β-alanine. ■ blocked reaction in presence of FUdRP.

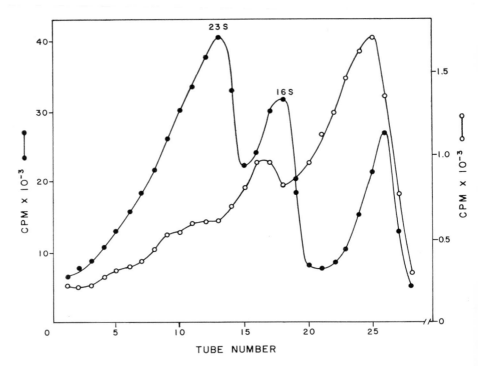

Fig. 10.3. Elution profile of RNA from *Bacillus cereus* cells grown in the absence (●) and presence (○) of FU. In normal cells (●) RNA labeled with adenine-^{14}C, elution following density gradient centrifugation of characteristic 23S and 16S rRNA, and 4S sRNA. For drug-treated culture (○) used FU-^{14}C to label RNA. Note shifted rRNA peaks, greater proportion of radioactive FU in sRNA. (From Hahn and Mandel, 1971.)

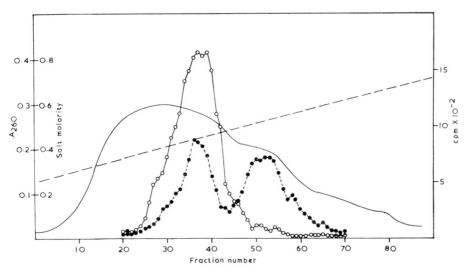

Fig. 10.4. Methylated albumin column chromatography of ³H-phenylalanine-tRNA and ¹⁴C-phenylalanine-FU-tRNA. By this procedure it was possible to resolve amino acid-charged FU-tRNA into two components, one of which behaved like the normal tRNA component formed before the addition of FU to *E. coli*, and the other was the highly FU-substituted amino acid-charged FU-tRNA. ——, absorbance at 260 mμ; (○) ³H-radio-activity; (●) ¹⁴C-radioactivity; ————, salt gradient. (From Lowrie and Bergquist, 1968.)

TABLE 10.15

Inhibition of thymidylate synthetase

Compound[a]	% Inhibition		
	10^{-8}	2×10^{-7}	3×10^{-8}
FU[b]	0		
FUR	0		
FURP	5		
FUdR	13		
FUdRP		84	40

[a] Compounds inhibiting enzyme activity at various concentrations, in *M*.   [b] FU, fluorouracil; R, ribose; P, phosphate; dR, deoxyribose. From Hartman and Heidelberger, 1961, and personal communication.

mononucleotide (FUdRP) is responsible for inhibition of thymidylate synthetase by competitively preventing methylation of the corresponding deoxyuridine (UdRP) derivative, thus preventing DNA synthesis. The activation of 5-fluoro-uracil by these conversions to a more inhibitory product is demonstrated in Table 10.15, where other drug derivatives do not show corresponding levels of potency.

It should be noted that 5-bromouracil, unlike 5-fluorouracil, does not substitute for uracil but instead replaces thymine in its conjugation reactions; thus, it forms an analog of thymidylic acid and is incorporated into DNA. The larger bromo atom resembles more closely the methyl group of thymine, whereas the fluoro atom has an atom radius more closely approximating that of hydrogen.

The chloro derivative, having a halogen of intermediate size, follows the pathways of both uracil and thymine (Dunn and Smith, 1957).

It is interesting that one of the most prevalent mechanisms by which populations of tumor cells become resistant to purine and pyrimidine analogs is causally associated with the loss of formation of ribomononucleotides of the purine or pyrimidine analogs, thus confirming the pharmacological significance of such pathways of metabolism (Brockman, 1963).

Numerous other derivatives of nucleic acid bases and ribomononucleotide derivatives have been shown to undergo metabolic alterations corresponding to those of the natural substrates, but the patterns of metabolism are not always uniform. For example, 6-azauracil, unlike 5-fluorouracil, is not usually incorporated into RNA, and 6-mercaptopurine, unlike 6-thioguanine, apparently forms insufficient nucleoside triphosphate derivatives to permit condensation into polynucleotides.

Quite similarly, structural analogs of amino acids may be metabolized along pathways available for the normal substrates (Richmond, 1962). p-Fluorophenylalanine, for example, is activated like phenylalanine, and is incorporated into polypeptides in place of phenylalanine. The antibiotic drug, puromycin, takes the place of phenylalanine-charged transfer RNA, which it resembles structurally, and, by incorporating into the nascent protein, terminates polypeptide formation and produces incomplete protein molecules.

puromycin   phe-t-RNA

where R represents the remainder of the RNA molecule.

It is well known that analogs of cofactors and vitamins may behave metabolically like the normal substances. A special case of conjugation might be the interaction of a drug molecule with its receptor. Amethopterin, for example, binds to dihydrofolate reductase like folate but differs in having greater affinity for this enzyme by a factor of 100,000 (Nichol, 1968). It has been possible to isolate this drug-enzyme complex following column chromatography.

It is apparent, as the metabolic fate of additional drugs is examined, that many compounds follow biosynthetic routes available for normal substrates, and that such pathways are not restricted to compounds with obvious structural resemblance to endogenous substrates. As in the case of puromycin and its very much larger endogenous substrate, only a portion of the molecules must be analogous for competition at the active sites.

Furthermore, such pathways of conjugation for analogs of substrates are not restricted to lipid-insoluble compounds. Puromycin is relatively lipid-soluble, as indicated by its distribution coefficient between chloroform and phosphate buffer (Mazel and Henderson, 1965).

In addition to the biosynthetic pathways described for substrate analogs, these drugs may also be metabolized by the conjugation reactions described for other drugs, as well as the microsomal oxidation reactions discussed in Chapter 12. Puromycin, for example, is demethylated by rat liver microsomes. Thus, the differences in metabolism between substrate analogs and other drugs are not absolute. The sulfanilamide derivatives represent another example. These compounds compete with p-aminobenzoic acid in the latter's conversion to folic acid. At the same time, the conjugation of sulfanilamides by acetylation, and microsomal glucuronide formation have been described earlier.

These observations are probably quite similar to the numerous examples already provided where drugs share with certain endogenous substrates the routes of conjugation, such as glucuronide and sulfate conjugation, amide synthesis and methylation. Furthermore, hydroxylation of steroids and many drugs is mediated by microsomal hydroxylases, as described in subsequent chapters. Consequently, categorical distinctions between conjugation reactions of substrate analogs and other drugs are unwarranted, as are those between drugs and normal substrates.

G. Miscellaneous Reactions

Glucoside conjugation occurs in insects and plants where it apparently replaces glucuronide conjugation. Ester and ether glucosides are formed from UDP-glucose which acts as the source of activated glucose. Mammals do not synthesize glucosides because they lack glucosyl transferases. The reaction goes as follows:

$$\text{ROH} + \text{UDP-glucose} \xrightarrow{\text{glucosyl transferase}} \text{RO-}\beta\text{-glucoside} + \text{UDP}$$

Thiocyanate formation from cyanide ion is mediated by the enzyme sulfurtransferase or rhodanese. This enzyme occurs in many organs but is found mainly in liver mitochondria of most species, and is specific for the interaction of cyanide with sulfur donors such as endogenous thiosulfate to form thiocyanate. Organic cyanides or nitriles will react only if hydrolyzed to the cyanide ion and certain oximes are metabolized to liberate cyanide. The reaction scheme is as follows:

$$\underset{\text{cyanide}}{\text{CN}^-} + \underset{\text{thiosulfate}}{\text{S}_2\text{O}_3^=} \xrightarrow{\text{rhodanese}} \underset{\text{thiocyanate}}{\text{SCN}^-} + \underset{\text{sulfite}}{\text{SO}_3^=}$$

IV. SUMMARY OF THE MAJOR PATHWAYS OF CONJUGATION

Table 10.16 represents a simplified overview of the more important routes of conjugation, together with the most common functional groups with which such reactions take place. For convenience, those animal species which differ in their general behavior with respect to a particular route are indicated.

In Table 10.17 information is provided as to the most likely routes of metabolism applicable to a particular structure or functional group. It is important to

TABLE 10.16

Types of conjugations for animals

Conjugate	Major Target Groups	Deficient Species
1. Glucuronic acid conjugation	—OH, —COOH, —NH$_2$, >NH, —SH	cat; Gunn rat
2. Sulfate conjugation	aromatic-OH, aromatic-NH$_2$, some alcohols	pig
3. Glycine conjugation	aromatic-COOH, aromatic-alkyl-COOH	certain birds and reptiles
Ornithine conjugation[a]	aromatic COOH	most
Glutamine conjugation[b]	aromatic CH$_2$COOH	most
4. Acetylation	aromatic-NH$_2$, some aliphatic-NH$_2$, hydrazides, —SO$_2$NH$_2$	dog
5. Mercapturic acid synthesis	aromatic hydrocarbons, —Cl, —Br, —F, —NO$_2$	guinea pig, man
6. Methylation	aromatic-OH, NH$_2$, >NH, —>N, —SH	

[a] Certain birds and reptiles only.   [b] Man and certain monkeys only.

TABLE 10.17

Metabolic fate of drugs with functional groups

1. Aromatic rings: hydroxylation; (mercapturic acid synthesis).
2. Hydroxyl:
     (a) aliphatic: chain oxidation; glucuronic acid conjugation; sulfate conjugation.
     (b) aromatic: ring hydroxylation; glucuronic acid conjugation; sulfate conjugation; methylation.
3. Carboxyl:
     (a) aliphatic: glucuronic acid conjugation; (amino acid conjugation).
     (b) aromatic: ring hydroxylation; amino acid conjugation; glucuronide conjugation.
4. Primary amines:
     (a) aliphatic: deamination; methylation.
     (b) aromatic: ring hydroxylation; acetylation; glucuronic acid conjugation; methylation; sulfate conjugation.
5. Secondary and tertiary amines: dealkylation; (methylation).
6. Sulfhydryl: glucuronic acid conjugation; methylation; oxidation.

remember that previous conclusions on metabolic conversions have by necessity been based on analytical procedures much less specific than those available today.

Numerous factors may influence the most likely metabolic pathways of an agent. These are described in detail in the subsequent chapters and are listed here only briefly.

1. Dose and frequency of administration of the drug (pools of conjugating metabolite may be readily exhaustible).

2. Species and strain of animal used (metabolic differences; pharmacogenetics).

3. Diet and nutritional status (may affect pools of conjugating groups, enzymes).

4. Age, sex and weight of animal (developmental factors, changes in body constituents).

5. Route of administration (delivery to organs with specific metabolic roles).

6. Time of administration (circadian rhythm, light, seasonal changes).

7. Interaction of other drugs and environmental contaminants (enzyme inhibitors and inducers, competition for conjugating groups, alterations in drug distribution, hormonal factors).

8. Subsequent interaction with other enzymes (β-glucuronidase, sulfatase, deacetylase, for which drug conjugates may be substrates).

9. Pregnancy and physiological abnormalities (tissue redistribution, functional alteration in organs with specific metabolic roles, e.g., liver).

V. CHARACTERISTIC EXAMPLES OF METABOLIC PATHWAYS FOLLOWED BY DRUGS

A brief account of the pattern of metabolism of a few characteristic drugs is provided here to indicate some quantitative relationships for the various pathways.

1. Phenol. The distribution of metabolites from phenol administered to the rabbit is presented in Figure 10.5. The rabbit excretes about 90% of the administered phenol as phenyl sulfate or phenyl glucuronide, with only traces of quinol or catechol; some of these hydroxylated derivatives may appear more slowly. At a dose of 50 mg/kg, the sulfate and glucuronide conjugates each make up about 45% of the total metabolites, but factors such as diet, temperature and fatigue may alter this ratio. When the dose of phenol is raised to 250 mg/kg, however, sulfate conjugation is reduced to only 15%, whereas glucuronides now account for 70% of the metabolites. This effect is due to the limited availability of endogenous sulfate for conjugation. When L-cystine or sulfite is provided to the animals, the percentage of phenol excreted as ethereal sulfate is raised to 30% (Williams, 1959).

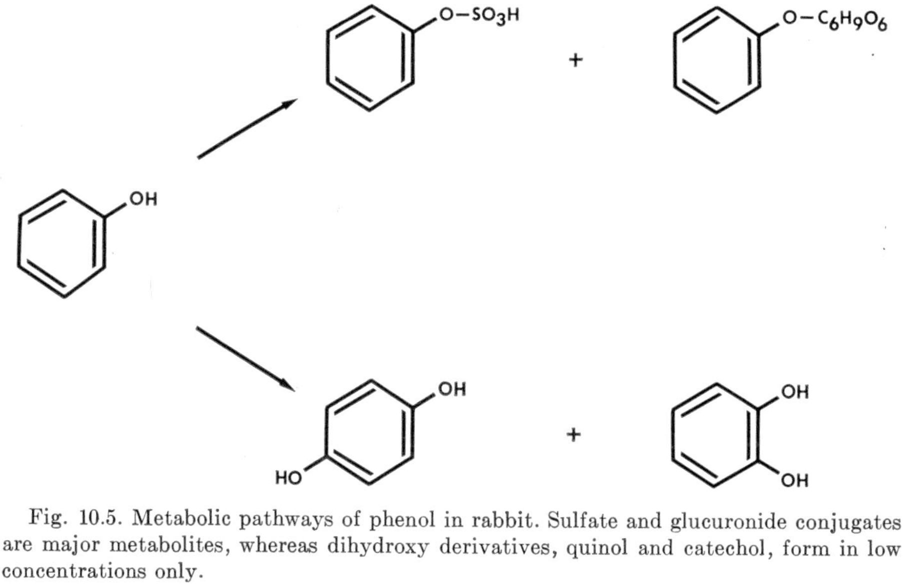

Fig. 10.5. Metabolic pathways of phenol in rabbit. Sulfate and glucuronide conjugates are major metabolites, whereas dihydroxy derivatives, quinol and catechol, form in low concentrations only.

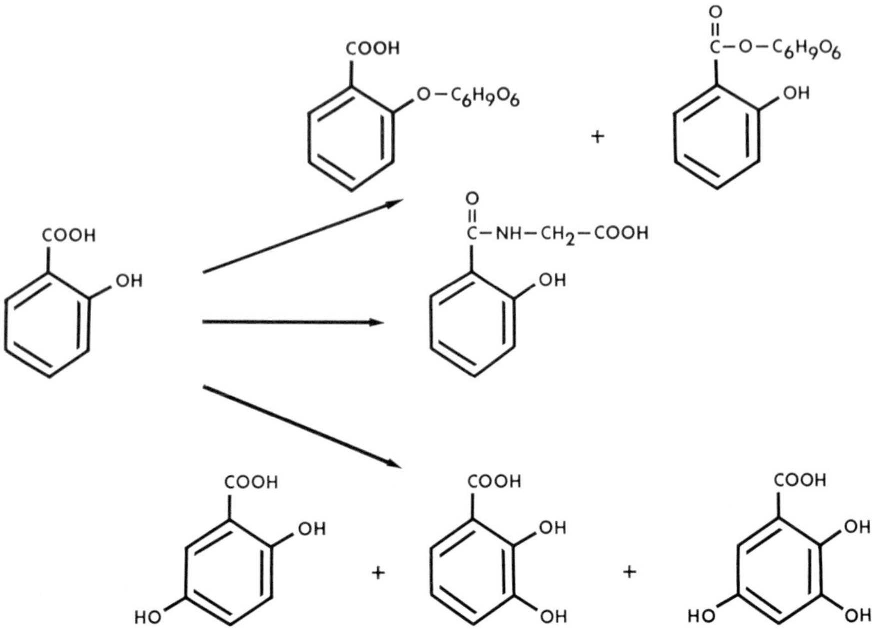

Fig. 10.6. Metabolic pathways of salicylic acid. Top line, ether and ester glucuronides; middle, salicyluric acid; bottom, hydroxylated derivatives (gentisic, 2,3-dihydroxybenzoic and 2,3,5-trihydroxybenzoic acids) are very minor metabolites.

2. Salicylic acid. The major metabolites of salicylic acid are shown in Figure 10.6. Recent studies by Hollister and Levy (1965) have revealed that in man following a 1 g oral dose of aspirin (which is rapidly converted to salicylate), 10 % of total urinary salicylate is salicylate itself, 70 % is salicylurate and 20 % appears as glucuronides. The percentage excreted as salicylic acid was only 3 % in those individuals whose urinary pH was usually between 5 and 5.6, but was up to 25 % when the pH was between 6 and 7. The variation in percentage of salicylate in the urine undoubtedly is due to the rapid excretion of salicylate at higher pH values because of diminished tubular reabsorption. The percentage excreted as salicylurate decreases with dose and becomes zero order kinetics at higher doses, but this interpretation has been disputed (Wagner, 1967). Benzoate competitively inhibits the formation of salicylurate (Levy and Amsel, 1966). Two glucuronides have been isolated in man, with the ethereal one being present in somewhat greater concentration than the ester derivative (Alpen et al., 1951). In the dog, on the other hand, no ester glucuronide has been detected; the rabbit again produces both glucuronide conjugates. Only a trace of gentisate has been isolated as a metabolite in man, the dog and the mouse. Traces of other oxidation products have also been reported. Sulfate conjugation and decarboxylation to phenolic derivatives have not been observed.

Little salicylurate is observed in blood or tissues except for the kidney, while the glucuronides occur in liver, but little in blood. It has been estimated that only 7 % of the total salicylate in blood is in the form of derivatives, and less than 1 % may be in the form of glucuronides.

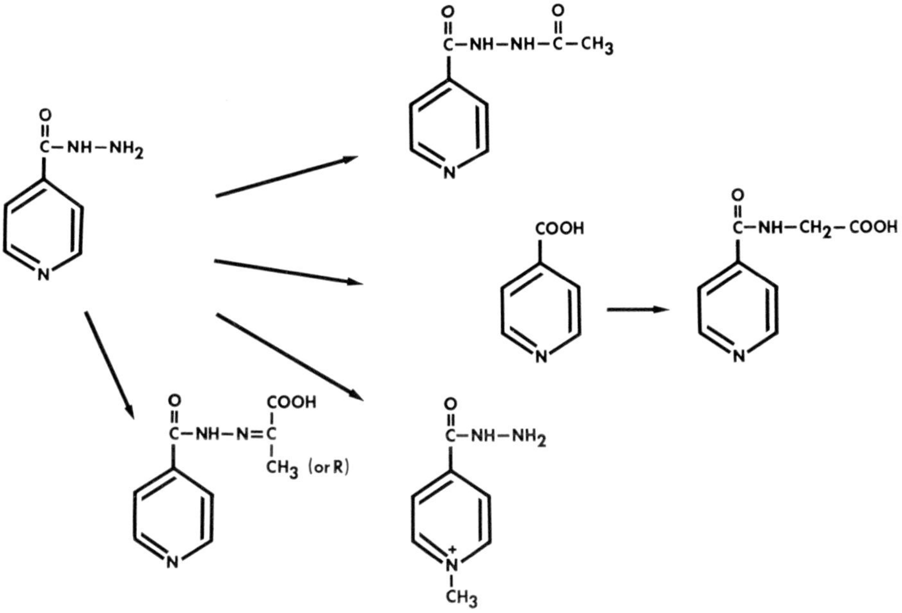

Fig. 10.7. Metabolic pathways of isoniazid. Compounds are acetyl isoniazid (top line) which is a major metabolite in man but not the dog; isonicotinic and isonicotinuric acids, present in appreciable amounts in man and especially the dog; N-methyl isoniazid, found in trace amounts in the dog; and the isonicotinylhydrazones of pyruvic and other keto acids, also present in small quantities in urine.

3. Isoniazid. Figure 10.7 indicates that isoniazid undergoes several biotransformations. In addition to the acetyl derivative, the drug is hydrolyzed to isonicotinic acid and forms a glycine conjugate, isonicotinuric acid. Small amounts of the hydrazones of α-keto acids, and the N-methyl conjugate of isoniazid are also produced.

The genetic polymorphism for isoniazid inactivation in human populations has already been mentioned and is related to the inherent capacity of individuals to acetylate the drug. It appears to be unrelated to age or sex but instead is associated with race. "Slow" inactivators of the drug usually demonstrate greater toxicity and therapeutic effectiveness after isoniazid than do the "fast" inactivators, undoubtedly because the acetylated compound is less active than isoniazid.

Analysis of urine following isoniazid administration to humans reveals a large number of urinary metabolites, although considerable variation has been reported by different investigators. For so-called rapid inactivators of the drug, an average of 4% of unchanged isoniazid was recovered, together with 4% of α-ketoglutaric and pyruvic acid isonicotinyl hydrazones, 44% as acetyl isoniazid, and 48% as isonicotinic acid and isonicotinuric acid (Peters et al., 1965); for the slow inactivators, these values were 13, 21, 34 and 32%, respectively.

In the dog very little of the isoniazid is acetylated, characteristic of the lack of excretion of acetyl derivatives of amines in this species. Traces of N-methyl isoniazid have been reported for the dog.

Acknowledgments

This chapter was supported in part by USPHS research grant GM 13749 and training grant GM 26 from the National Institute of General Medical Sciences, NIH, Bethesda, Md.

REFERENCES

Alpen, E. L., Mandel, H. G., Rodwell, V. W., and Smith, P. K.: The metabolism of C^{14} carboxyl salicylic acid in the dog and in man. J. Pharmacol. Exp. Ther. *102:* 150–155, 1951.

Arias, I. M.: Ethereal and N-linked glucuronide formation by normal and Gunn rats *in vitro* and *in vivo*. Biochem. Biophys. Res. Comm. *6:* 81–84, 1961.

Axelrod, J.: The enzymatic N-methylation of serotonin and other amines. J. Pharmacol. Exp. Ther. *138:* 28–33, 1962.

Axelrod, J. and Daly, J.: Phenol-O-methyltransferase. Biochim. Biophys. Acta *150:* 472–478, 1968.

Axelrod, J., Inscoe, J. K., and Tomkins, G. M.: Enzymatic synthesis of N-glucosyluronic acid conjugates. J. Biol. Chem. *232:* 835–841, 1958.

Axelrod, J. and Tomchick, R.: Enzymatic O-methylation of epinephrine and other catechols. J. Biol. Chem. *233:* 702–705, 1958.

Axelrod, J. and Weissbach, H.: Purification and properties of hydroxyindole-O-methyl transferase. J. Biol. Chem. *236:* 211–213, 1961.

Booth, J., Boyland, E., and Sims, P.: An enzyme from rat liver catalysing conjugation with glutathione. Biochem. J. *79:* 516–524, 1961.

Borstrum, H.: Sulfate conjugation and conjugated sulfates. (Review). Scand. J. Clin. Lab. Invest. *86:* Suppl. 17: 33–52, 1965.

Boyland, E. and Booth, J.: The metabolic fate and excretion of drugs. Annual Rev. Pharmacol. *2:* 129–142, 1962.

Bray, H. G., Humphris, B. G., Thorpe, W. V., White, K., and Wood, P. B.: Kinetic studies of the metabolism of foreign organic compounds. 4. The conjugation of phenols with sulphuric acid. Biochem. J. *52:* 419–423, 1952.

Bremer, J. and Greenberg, D. M.: Enzymic methylation of foreign sulfhydryl compounds. Biochim. Biophys. Acta *46:* 217–224, 1961.

Brockman, R. W.: Mechanism of resistance to anticancer agents. Advances in Cancer Res. *7:* 129–234, 1963.

Brodie, B. B.: Distribution and fate of drugs; therapeutic implications. In *Absorption and Distribution of Drugs*, ed. by T. B. Binns, pp. 199–255, Williams and Wilkins, Baltimore, Md., 1964.

Brodie, B. B. and Erdös, E. G., Eds., Metabolic factors controlling duration of drug action, *Proc. First International Pharmacology Meeting*, Vol. 6, Macmillan Co., N. Y., 1962.

Brown, D. D., Axelrod, J., and Tomchick, R.: Enzymatic N-methylation of histamine. Nature *183:* 680, 1959.

Brown, A. K., Zuelzer, W. W., and Burnett, H. H.: Studies with neonatal development of the glucuronide conjugating system. J. Clin. Invest. *37:* 332–340, 1958.

Cantoni, G. L.: Methylation of nicotinamide with a soluble enzyme system from rat liver. J. Biol. Chem. *189:* 203–216, 1951.

Chaudhuri, N. K., Mukherjee, K. L., and Heidelberger, C.: Studies on fluorinated pyrimidines, VII. The degradative pathway. Biochem. Pharmacol. *1:* 328–341, 1958.

Cohn, V. H.: Inhibition of histamine methylation by antimalarial drugs. Biochem. Pharmacol. *14:* 1686–1688, 1965.

Dunn, D. B. and Smith, J. D.: Effects of 5-halogenated uracils on the growth of *Escherichia coli* and their incorporation into deoxyribonucleic acids. Biochem. J. *67:* 494–506, 1957.

Dutton, G. J.: *Glucuronic Acid, Free and Combined. Chemistry, Biochemistry, Pharmacology and Medicine*, Academic Press, N. Y., 1966a.

Dutton, G. J.: The biosynthesis of glucuronides. In *Glucuronic Acid, Free and Combined. Chemistry, Biochemistry, Pharmacology and Medicine*, ed. by G. J. Dutton, pp. 185–299, Academic Press, N. Y., 1966b.

Elion, G. B.: Biochemistry and pharmacology of purine analogues. Federation Proc. *26:* 898–903, 1967.

Fishman, W. H.: *Chemistry of Drug Metabolism*, Charles C Thomas, Springfield, Ill., 1961.

Fleissner, E. and Borek, E.: Studies on the enzymatic methylation of soluble RNA. I. Methylation of the s-RNA polymer. Biochemistry *2:* 1093–1100, 1963.

Gillette, J. R.: Metabolism of drugs and other foreign compounds by enzymatic mechanisms. Prog. in Drug Res. *6:* 11–73, 1963.

Goldstein, A., Aronow, L., and Kalman,

S. M.: Principles of drug action. *The Basis of Pharmacology*, Hoeber Medical Division, Harper & Row, N. Y., 1968.

Govier, W. C.: Reticuloendothelial cells as the site of sulfanilamide acetylation in the rabbit. J. Pharmacol. Exp. Ther. *150:* 305–308, 1965.

Gregory, J. D.: Sulfate transferring enzymes. Methods in Enzymology *5:* 977–983, 1962.

Grünberger, D.: Function of ribonucleic acids containing 8-azaguanine in protein synthesis. In *Ribonucleic Acid—Structure and Function*, pp. 91–105, Pergamon Press, N. Y., 1966.

Hahn, G. A. and Mandel, H. G.: The effects of fluorouracil on RNA synthesis in *Bacillus cereus*. Biochem. Pharmacol., in press.

Hargreaves, T. and Holton, J. B.: Jaundice of the newborn due to novobiocin. Lancet *1:* 839, 1962.

Hartmann, K-U. and Heidelberger, C.: Studies on fluorinated pyrimidines, XIII. Inhibition of thymidylate synthetase. J. Biol. Chem. *236:* 3006–3013, 1961.

Heidelberger, C.: Fluorinated pyrimidines. In *Progress in Nucleic Acid Research and Molecular Biology 4:* 1–50, 1965.

Hollister, L. and Levy, G.: Some aspects of salicylate distribution and metabolism in man. J. Pharm. Sci. *54:* 1126–1129, 1965.

Inscoe, J. K., Daly, J., and Axelrod, J.: Factors affecting the enzymatic formation of O-methylated dihydroxy derivatives. Biochem. Pharmacol. *14:* 1257–1263, 1965.

Isselbacher, K. J., Chrabas, M. F., and Quinn, R. C.: The solubilization and partial purification of a glucuronyl transferase from rabbit liver microsomes J. Biol. Chem. *237:* 3033–3036, 1962.

Keller, W.: Ueber Verwandlung der Benzoësaüre in Hippursaüre. Justus Liebig's Ann. Chem. *43:* 108–111, 1842.

Kirshner, N. and Goodall, McC.: The formation of adrenaline from noradrenaline. Biochim. Biophys. Acta *24:* 658–659, 1957.

Langen, P.: *Antimetabolite des Nucleinsäurestoffwechsels. Biochemische Grundlagen der Wirkung.* Akademie Verlag, Berlin, 1968.

Leibman, K. C. and Anaclerio, A. M.: Comparative studies of sulfanilamide acetylation; an inhibitor in dog liver. In *Metabolic Factors Controlling Duration of Drug Action. Proc. First International Pharmacology Meeting*, ed. by B. B. Brodie and E. G. Erdös, pp. 91–96, Macmillan Co., N. Y., 1962.

Levy, G. and Amsel, L. P.: Kinetics of competitive inhibition of salicylic acid

conjugation with glycine in man. Biochem. Pharmacol. *15:* 1033–1038, 1966.

Lipmann, F.: Acetylation of sulfanilamide by liver homogenates and extracts. J. Biol. Chem. *160:* 173–190, 1945.

Lowrie, R. J. and Bergquist, P. L.: Transfer ribonucleic acids from *Escherichia coli* treated with 5-fluorouracil. Biochemistry *7:* 1761–1770, 1968.

Mandel, H. G.: The physiological disposition of some anticancer agents. Pharmacol. Rev. *11:* 743–838, 1959.

Mandel, H. G.: The incorporation of 5-fluorouracil into RNA and its molecular consequences. In *Progress in Molecular and Subcellular Biology, 1,* 82–135, 1969.

Mandel, H. G., Carlo, P. E., and Smith, P. K.: The incorporation of 8-azaguanine into nucleic acids of tumor-bearing mice. J. Biol. Chem. *206:* 181–189, 1954.

Marsh, C. A.: Chemistry of d-glucuronic acid and its glycosides. In *Glucuronic Acid, Free and Combined*, ed. by G. J. Dutton, pp. 4–136, Academic Press, N. Y., 1966.

Mazel, P. and Henderson, J. F.: On the relation between lipid solubility and microsomal metabolism of drugs. Biochem. Pharmacol. *14:* 92–94, 1965.

Moldave, K. and Meister, A.: Synthesis of phenylacetylglutamine by human tissue. J. Biol. Chem. *229:* 463–476, 1957.

Nichol, C. A.: Studies on dihydrofolate reductase related to the drug sensitivity of microbial and neoplastic cells. In *Advances in Enzyme Regulation*, ed. by G. Weber, pp. 304–322, Pergamon Press, N. Y., 1968.

Nose, Y. and Lipmann, F.: Separation of steroid sulfokinases. J. Biol. Chem. *233:* 1348–1351, 1958.

Parke, D. V.: *The Biochemistry of Foreign Compounds.* Pergamon Press, N. Y., 1968.

Percy, A. K. and Yaffe, S. J.: Sulfate metabolism during mammalian development. Pediatrics *33:* 965–968, 1964.

Peters, R. A.: Lethal synthesis. Proc. Roy. Soc., Ser. B, *139:* 143–170, 1952.

Peters, J. H., Miller, K. S., and Brown, P.: Studies on the metabolic basis for the genetically determined capacities for isoniazid inactivation in man. J. Pharmacol. Exp. Ther. *150:* 298–304, 1965.

Richmond, M. H.: The effect of amino acid analogues on growth and protein synthesis in microorganisms. Bact. Rev. *26:* 398–420, 1962.

Roy, A. B.: Enzymic synthesis of aryl sulphamates. Biochem. J. *74:* 49–56, 1960a.

Roy, A. B.: The synthesis and hydrolysis of sulfate esters. Advances in Enzymology *22:* 205–235, 1960b.

Smith, J. N.: Comparative biochemistry of detoxification. In *Comparative Bio-*

chemistry, ed. by M. Florkin and H. S. Mason, pp. 403–457, Academic Press, N. Y., 1964.

Smith, R. L. and Williams, R. T.: Implications of the conjugation of drugs and other exogenous compounds. In *Glucuronic Acid Free and Combined*, ed. by G. J. Dutton, pp. 457–491, Academic Press, N. Y., 1966.

Tomita, K., Cha, C-J. M., and Lardy, H. A.: Enzymic O-methylation of iodinated phenols and thyroid hormones. J. Biol. Chem. *239:* 1202–1207, 1964.

Vest, M. F. and Rossier, R.: Detoxification in the newborn: the ability of the newborn infant to form conjugates with glucuronic acid, glycine, acetate and glutathione. Ann. N. Y. Acad. Sci. *111:* 183–197, 1963.

Wagner, J. G.: Fallacy in concluding there are zero order kinetics from blood level and urinary excretion data. J. Pharm. Sci. *56:* 586–594, 1967.

Way, J. L. and Parks, R. E., Jr.: Enzymatic synthesis of 5'-phosphate nucleotides of purine analogues. J. Biol. Chem. *231:* 467–480, 1958.

Weiss, C. F., Glazko, A. J., and Weston, J. K.: Chloramphenicol in the newborn infant. A physiological explanation of its toxicity when given in excessive doses. New Engl. J. Med. *262:* 787–794, 1960.

Wengle, B.: Studies on ester sulfates. 16. Use of ^{35}S-labelled inorganic sulfate for quantitative studies of sulfate conjugation in liver extracts. Acta Chem. Scand. *18:* 65–76, 1964.

Williams, R. T.: *Detoxication Mechanisms. The Metabolism of Drugs and Allied Organic Compounds.* John Wiley & Sons, N. Y., 1947.

Williams, R. T.: *Detoxication Mechanisms. The Metabolism and Detoxication of Drugs, Toxic Substances and Other Organic Compounds.* John Wiley & Sons, N. Y., 1959.

Williams, R. T.: Detoxication mechanisms in man. Clin. Pharm. Ther. *4:* 234–254, 1963.

Williams, R. T.: The biogenesis of conjugation and detoxication products. In *Biogenesis of Natural Compounds*, ed. by P. Bernfeld, pp. 589–639, Pergamon Press, N. Y., Sec. Ed., 1967.

Yaffe, S. J., Levy, G., Matsuzawa, T., and Baliah, T.: Enhancement of glucuronide-conjugating capacity in a hyperbilirubinemic infant due to apparent enzyme induction by phenobarbital. New Engl. J. Med., *275:* 1461–1466, 1966.

11

Species Variations in Drug Biotransformations

R. T. WILLIAMS

I. INTRODUCTION

The metabolism of a drug or any other environmental chemical is important in its therapeutic activity and toxicity, but we now know that there are many factors which affect this metabolism and consequently the activity of the drug. These factors include route of administration, species, sex, age, strain, diet, temperature, time of day, season, chronic administration and the previous or concurrent administration of other drugs or chemicals. Drug metabolism is thus a very complex affair, and although we are concerned here only with the factor of species, the other factors must be kept in mind and in any comparative study kept constant if this is possible. The difficulty of keeping the other factors constant arises, for example, if one is comparing a herbivorous with a carnivorous animal, for in this case the diet may have to be varied to suit the test animal. The testing of drugs and other chemicals for their safety in use is carried out largely on the lower animals and therefore it is important to know how close a test animal is to man in its reactions to the substance being examined. The metabolism of a drug may be a criterion for this comparison, but such a comparison presupposes that the fate of the drug in man will be studied as well as in the other species. The kinds of questions raised by comparative pharmacology are relatively simple, such as "are tests on dogs or rats valid for man?" and "should monkeys be used because they are nearest to man on the evolutionary scale?" The answers to these questions are difficult to give mainly because our knowledge of comparative pharmacology and comparative drug metabolism is, as yet, limited. Recent reviews on comparative drug metabolism have been published by Williams (1967a) and Smith (1968).

II. ENZYMIC BASIS OF DRUG METABOLISM

The general pattern of drug metabolism is common to all species. The basic pattern is usually biphasic, the initial phase of the process consisting of reactions classified as oxidations, reductions and hydrolyses and the second as syntheses (Williams, 1967a). These reactions are controlled by tissue enzymes and it is mainly in the nature of these enzymes that species variation in drug metabolism lies. These enzymes may vary qualitatively and quantitatively from one species to another and some striking variations have been found. Although the main causes of species variation in drug metabolism seem to be associated with the tissue enzymes, it is becoming clear that other factors may be involved in certain cases, for it has been found that the gastrointestinal flora play a role in the overall metabolism of some foreign compounds, and these organisms are known to vary with species and with dietary habits.

Species variations in the metabolism of foreign compounds are not unexpected, since such variations often occur in the metabolism of some natural metabolites of the body and are explicable in enzymic terms. Thus the inability of man to synthesize L-ascorbic acid is due to the lack of the liver (or kidney in some other species) microsomal enzyme, L-gulonolactone oxidase, which converts L-gulonolactone to 2-keto-L-gulonolactone which then isomerises to ascorbic acid. This enzyme is also absent in the monkey and, on evolutionary grounds, one might say that this is not unexpected, but this enzyme is also missing in animals as far apart as the guinea pig, a rodent, the Indian fruit bat, and the passerine bird, the red-vented bulbul. Scurvy can be induced in these species and then cured by administration of vitamin C (Chatterjee, et al., 1961).

Species variation in the metabolism of drugs may appear as: a) qualitative differences in the actual pathways of metabolism and/or; b) quantitative differences in pathways of metabolism which are common to several species. The qualitative differences probably result from the presence in a particular species of an enzyme which is not found in others, or the absence in a species of an enzyme otherwise generally distributed in the animal world. Quantitative differences could be due to variations in the amount of an enzyme or its natural inhibitor, or to the occurrence of an enzyme, possibly located in another tissue, reversing the reaction, or to an enzyme competing for the same substrate.

Detailed examination of these possibilities has not yet been made, and it offers a wide field for future investigation. Attempts have been made to explain species variation in drug metabolism through *in vitro* studies, and whilst these studies are an important guide to what happens *in vivo*, both types of study must be made together so that factors such as absorption, tissue distribution, biliary and urinary excretion, enterohepatic circulation and the role of gut bacteria can be taken into account in the overall picture of species variation. Thus the *in vitro* demethylation of ethylmorphine by liver microsomal preparations of mouse, rat, guinea pig and rabbit shows a fourfold variation in rate, the mouse preparation being the most active and the rabbit the least active (Davies, et al., 1969). This should be a guide to the species variation in the demethylation of the drug *in vivo*. These workers show that at the enzymic level, species differences parallel differences in NADPH-cytochrome P-450 reductase and may be related to the rate of reduction of the cytochrome-P-450-substrate complex in different species.

III. SPECIES VARIATION IN PHASE I REACTIONS

Reactions which can be classified as oxidations, reductions and hydrolyses are many and varied and they are carried out by enzymes which appear to be of two kinds. The first kind consist of enzymes which are involved in the metabolism of the natural substrates of the body and thus have natural and foreign substrates (para-metabolic enzymes) and the second are the so-called "drug-metabolizing" enzymes which appear to be concerned only with foreign compounds (xenometabolic enzymes) and are located mainly in the endoplasmic reticulum of the liver cell. In an earlier paper (Williams, 1967a) it was suggested that species variation in the parametabolic reactions might be less common than in xenometabolic reactions, since the basic pattern of normal metabolism may not vary widely in mammalian species. This suggestion, however, requires that much detailed experimental work be done with this type of enzyme in different species.

A. Aromatic Hydroxylation

One of the most intensely studied of phase I reactions is aromatic hydroxylation. It has been found to occur in all species examined including insects, fish, birds, reptiles and mammals including man (Williams, 1967a; Smith, 1968) and consists usually of the replacement of a hydrogen of an aromatic ring by an OH group. Although the reaction occurs in most species, there are considerable species variations in the extent to which it occurs in a given compound, in its orientation and also in the extent to which it occurs with different compounds in the same species. A simple example is the hydroxylation of aniline which can occur in the o- and p-position. In the intact dog, cat and ferret the p/o ratio is 1 or less, whereas in other species it varies from 4–6 in the mouse, rat and rabbit to about 15 in the gerbil (see Table 11.1). This suggests that there are two aniline aromatic hydroxylases, of which the ortho-hydroxylase is more active in the carnivores and the para-hydroxylase in the other species (see Williams, 1967a).

Another compound which illustrates species differences in hydroxylation is amphetamine. The metabolism of this drug also illustrates species differences in the extent of different pathways and the occurrence of a metabolite in one species which hardly occurs in the other species at all. The two main routes of metabolism of amphetamine are aromatic hydroxylation and subsequent conjugation of the new OH group, and deamination of the side chain followed by its oxidation to benzoic acid which is then conjugated (see formulae below). Amphetamine is also partly excreted unchanged. Hydroxylation is the major reaction in the rat but a minor one in the other species (Table 11.2). Deamination and subsequent oxidation is the major reaction in the guinea pig, whilst in the rabbit deamination is a major reaction giving rise to three metabolites, two of which do not occur to any appreciable extent in the other species. In man, monkey and dog nearly a third of the drug is excreted unchanged and almost another third is de-

TABLE 11.1

Species variation in the ortho- and para-hydroxylation of aniline in vivo

Species		p/o ratio in urine	Species		p/o ratio in urine
Carnivores	Dog	0.5	Rodents	Rat	6
	Cat	0.4		Mouse	3
	Ferret	1		Hamster	10
				Guinea pig	11
	Rabbit	6		Gerbil	15
	Hen	4			

aminized to benzoic acid (*see* Table 11.2) (Dring, *et al.*, 1966; Dring, 1968). Man, rhesus monkey and dog metabolize amphetamine similarly excreting 25–30% of the dose unchanged and 20–30% as total benzoic acid. Hydroxylation is a minor reaction in these species, the main metabolic reaction being deamination followed by oxidation of the side chain. The metabolism of the drug in the mouse is not very different from that in man, except that hydroxylation is rather more extensive. The metabolism of amphetamine in the rat, guinea pig and rabbit is different from that in the other 4 species and different from that in each other. In the guinea pig amphetamine is mainly deaminated and oxidized to benzoic acid (65%), hydroxylation being barely detectable. In the rat, the drug is mainly hydroxylated (60%), deamination and oxidation being at a low level (3%). Then in the rabbit the main reaction is deamination (53%), but only about a half of the deamination product (phenylacetone) is oxidized to benzoic acid, for most of the rest is conjugated with sulphate (as the enol of phenylacetone) (Dring, *et al.*, 1968) and a lesser part is reduced to benzyl methyl carbinol (see formulae below). This metabolic study of amphetamine suggests that man could be compared with the rhesus monkey or dog or possibly with the mouse, except that although the mouse is similar to man in the excretion of unchanged amphetamine and benzoic acid, the extent of hydroxylation in mouse, although not high (15%), is 5 times that in man. But it is to be noted that hydroxylation in the mouse is only a quarter of that in the rat, a related species.

Metabolism of Amphetamine

In II and V, R = $C_6H_9O_6$; in VI R = SO_3H; in IV, R = $NHCH_2CO_2H$

An interesting example of an aromatic hydroxylation missing in some species but present in most other species examined is the 7-hydroxylation of coumarin to umbelliferone. This reaction, studied *in vitro* using the 10,000 g supernatant of liver homogenates, was found to be absent in rats and mice but present in man, pigeon, cat, rabbit, guinea pig and coypu (Creaven *et al.*, 1965).

Coumarin

TABLE 11.2

Metabolites of amphetamine in various species

Species	% of dose of ^{14}C-labeled drug excreted in the urine in 24 hr as				
	Amphetamine	4-Hydroxy-amphetamine*	Benzoic acid*	Phenyl-acetone	Benzylmethyl-carbinol*
Man	30	3	20	3	0
Monkey (rhesus)	25	6	29	0	0
Dog	30	6	28	1	1
Rabbit	3	6	23	22†	8
Guinea pig	18	1	65	0	0
Mouse	30	15	31	0	0
Rat	13	60	3	0	0

* Total including conjugates.   † Suspected to be present as the enol sulphate.

Thus the rat, which can hydroxylate aniline in the 2- and 4-positions (Table 11.1) and which hydroxylates amphetamine much more extensively than any other species (Table 11.2), is unable to insert a hydroxyl group into the 7-position of coumarin. It can, however, hydroxylate coumarin in the 3-position as can also the rabbit (Kaighan & Williams, 1961).

These studies on aniline, amphetamine and coumarin suggest that there are several microsomal hydroxylases attacking aromatic compounds, and that their occurrence depends not only upon species but also upon the nature of the aromatic compound. Furthermore, as suggested by the study of amphetamine, species variation in the hydroxylation of this drug could be due to differences in the amount of the hydroxylating enzyme or to competition with the deaminizing enzyme or both. It appears that although aromatic hydroxylation is a reaction common to all species, the distribution of specific aromatic hydroxylases amongst species can be haphazard and each aromatic compound must be treated on its merits.

IV. PHASE II REACTIONS OR CONJUGATIONS

Conjugation reactions may occur when the drug contains a group, usually OH, COOH, NH_2 or SH, which is suitable for combining with a natural compound provided by the body to form readily excreted water-soluble polar metabolites. If the drug does not contain these groups, it may acquire them through a phase I reaction, i.e., by oxidation, reduction or hydrolysis. Thus phenol, which contains a hydroxyl group, can undergo conjugation directly, but benzene, which does not contain a group suitable for conjugation, acquires one by being oxidized to phenol in the body. The compounds provided by the body for conjugation (i.e., conjugating agents) are derived from materials involved in normal carbohydrate, protein and fat metabolism and include glucuronic acid, glycine, cysteine, methionine for methylation, sulphate, acetic acid, and thiosulphate for sulphur. Apart from these, some species provide glucose (insects), glutamine (man), and ornithine (birds) for conjugation.

The majority of the known conjugating agents are shown in Table 11.3. These conjugating agents, however, do not, as a rule, react directly with the drug or its phase I metabolite but do so either in an "activated form" or with an "activated form" of the drug. These "activated forms" are usually nucleotides, and

TABLE 11.3

Compounds used in conjugation

Main Source of Conjugating Agent	Distribution of Compounds or Groups Involved in Conjugation	
	General*	Special or rare
Carbohydrates	Glucuronic acid	Glucose (insects)
		N-Acetylglucosamine (rabbits)
		Ribose (rats, mice)
Amino acids	Glycine	Glutamine (man, insects)
	Glutathione (cysteine)	Ornithine (birds)
	Methionine (CH₃)	Arginine, Agmatine (ticks, spiders)
		Glycyltaurine (cats)
		Glycylglycine (cats)
		Serine (rats, rabbits)
Miscellaneous	Acetyl	Formyl (rats, dogs)
	Sulfate	Phosphate (dogs, insects)
	Thio (S group)	

* I.e., In most species with certain exceptions.

the reaction between the nucleotide and the drug or conjugating agent as the case may be is catalysed by an enzyme. Thus for glucuronide synthesis, the glucuronic acid is used in the form of the nucleotide, uridine diphosphate glucuronic acid (UDPGA) which under the influence of the enzyme, glucuronyl transferase, transfers its glucuronyl residue to the drug. In the case of glycine conjugation, which occurs usually with aromatic acids, the foreign acid forms a nucleotide derivative with coenzyme A, that is an aroyl-CoA, which then transfers its aroyl group to glycine, the conjugating agent, under the influence of the enzyme, glycine N-acylase.

Thus a conjugation requires a conjugating agent, a nucleotide containing either the conjugating agent or the foreign compound and a transferring enzyme. Species variations in conjugation reactions can thus depend on the occurrence of the conjugating agent or the ability to form the necessary nucleotide or the amount of the transferring enzyme. It is well known, for example, that the cat has a defect in glucuronide synthesis, a defect not in the animal's ability to provide glucuronic acid or to make the nucleotide, UDPGA, but in a deficiency of the enzyme, glucuronyl transferase. Man is peculiar in being able to convert phenylacetic acid (and some other arylacetic acids) into phenylacetylglutamine (arylacetylglutamines). The rat is unable to do this because, although it can make the intermediate nucleotide derivative, phenacetyl-CoA, it does not possess the necessary transferring enzyme which, however, occurs in human liver and kidney.

A. Species Variations in Glucuronic Acid Conjugations

Glucuronic acid conjugation is one of the most widespread of phase II reactions. It occurs in fish, reptiles, amphibia, birds, marsupials and mammals (but see cat above), but not in insects (Smith, 1968). Smith and Williams (1966) have listed 16 groups (6 types of OH, 4 of NH₂ or NH, 4 of COOH and 2 of SH) which are known to form glucuronic acid conjugates *in vivo*. Nevertheless some striking variations in the extent of glucuronic acid conjugation can occur.

In insects, glucuronide formation is replaced by β-glucoside conjugation. This

TABLE 11.4

Species variation in the conjugation of phenol

Dose of ^{14}C-phenol = 25 mg/kg orally (in man 1 mg/person or 17 μg/kg)

Species	No. of metabolites	% of ^{14}C excreted in 24 hrs as the				Remarks
		Glucuronide of		Sulphate of		
		Phenol	Quinol	Phenol	Quinol	
Pig*	1	100	0	0	0	no sulphate
Indian fruit bat	2	90	0	10	0	
Rhesus monkey	2	35	0	65	0	
Cat*	2	0	0	87	13	no glucuronide
Man	3	23	7	71	0	two glucuronides and one sulphate
Squirrel monkey	3	70	19	10	0	two glucuronides and one sulphate
Ring-tailed monkey	3	65	21	14	0	two glucuronides and one sulphate
Guinea pig	3	78	5	17	0	two glucuronides and one sulphate
Hamster	3	50	25	25	0	two glucuronides and one sulphate
Rat	3	25	7	68	0	two glucuronides and one sulphate
Ferret	3	41	0	32	28	one glucuronide and two sulphates
Rabbit	3	46	0	45	9	one glucuronide and two sulphates
Gerbil	3	15	0	69	15	one glucuronide and two sulphates
Hedgehog	3	15	0	75	10	one glucuronide and two sulphates
Lemming	4	38	15	35	12	
Mouse	4	33	14	43	5	
Jerboa	4	26	4	61	12	

* The sulphate conjugation of phenol in the pig and the glucuronic acid conjugation of phenol in the cat are very small (about 2%) (unpublished data).

could be due to inability to form glucuronic acid, for insects can form and utilize uridine diphosphate glucose (UDPG) but not UDPGA. According to Smith (1968), in terms of numbers of species, glucose conjugation may be more widespread than glucuronic acid conjugation, for it occurs in most insects species tested and probably in other invertebrate groups also.

Within the vertebrates, some curious species variations in glucuronic acid conjugation have been encountered and these may be due to the occurrence of different forms of the enzyme, glucuronyl transferase. The cat is defective in its glucuronic acid mechanism (although it is not known whether this applies to other members of the cat family such as lions, tigers, etc.) and does not conjugate simple phenols (*see* Table 11.4) and alcohols, such as phenol, 7-hydroxycoumarin and borneol, with glucuronic acid (Robinson and Williams 1965); nevertheless, it is able to conjugate bilirubin with glucuronic acid as well as most vertebrates (Lathe and Walker, 1958).

The main urinary metabolite of the drugs, sulphadimethoxine and sulphamethomidine in man and the monkeys is an N^1-glucuronide, the formula of which is shown below:—

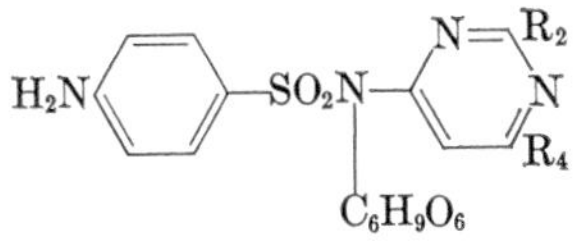

N^1-Glucuronide of sulphadimethoxine ($R_2 = R_4 = OCH_3$) and of sulphamethomidine ($R_2 = OCH_3$, $R_4 = CH_3$)

In the case of sulphadimethoxine, this glucuronide is its main urinary metabolite in the primates, man, rhesus monkey, green monkey, baboon, squirrel monkey, capuchin, giant bushbaby, slow loris and tree shrew, but not in the rat, guinea pig, rabbit and dog (Adamson *et al.*, 1966). Furthermore, the formation of this type of glucuronide in primates is limited to the two derivatives of 6-sulphanil-amidopyrimidine given above. The 2-, 4- or 5-monomethoxy, the 2,4-dimethyl, the 2,5-dimethoxy- and 4,5-dimethoxy- derivatives of 6-sulphanilamidopyrimidine do not form N^1-glucuronides in primates or other species (Bridges *et al.*, 1968; 1969a, b). This would suggest that primates possess a glucuronyl transferring enzyme which can transfer glucuronic acid from UDPGA to sulphadimethoxine and sulphamethomidine and which does not occur in other species although both the primates and the other species are able to conjugate phenols with glucuronic acid (see Table 11.4).

B. Species Variation in Sulphate Conjugation

Sulphate conjugation is mainly a reaction of phenols in which highly polar arylsulphates ($ArOSO_3H$) are formed, but it can also occur as a very minor process with aromatic amines to form arylsulphamic acids ($ArNHSO_3H$) and with aliphatic alcohols to form alkylsulphates ($ROSO_3H$). The formation of the sulphate esters of phenols is a widespread phenomenon amongst species occurring in most mammals, birds, reptiles, amphibia, insects and arachnids (Smith, 1968).

Stekol (1933) showed that the pig compared with the dog was poor in utilizing sulphur compounds for conjugation. In some recent work in the author's laboratory (French *et al.*, 1969) ^{14}C-labelled phenol was administered orally at one dose level (25 mg/kg) to 16 species of animals. The output of radioactive metabolites in the urine collected during the next 24 hours was measured by radiochromatogram scanning. At most 4 urinary metabolites were found, namely, phenylglucuronide, phenylsulphate, quinol monoglucuronide and quinol monosulphate (see formula below). The results of these experiments are summarized in Table 11.4, which shows how variable the metabolites can be in quantity and, in some cases, in nature from one species to another. Some species excrete one metabolite only, whilst others excrete two, three or four metabolites. The cat excreted two metabolites, mainly phenylsulphate and a small amount of quinol sulphate and as expected did not excrete phenylglucuronide. The pig, on the other hand, excreted only phenylglucuronide and there was no conjugated sulphate. The pig should now be examined at the enzyme level to check whether it is unable to form the ethereal sulphates of administered phenols. The metabolic fate of phenol is as follows:

R = SO₃H or C₆H₉O₆

All the species examined, except the pig, Indian fruit bat and the rhesus monkey were able to hydroxylate some of the phenol to quinol. All of the species in this study except the pig, Indian fruit bat, squirrel monkey, ring-tailed monkey, and guinea pig, tended to conjugate this dose level of phenol more with sulphate than with glucuronic acid. It is possible that dietary habit may play a role here, since there is a tendency for the herbivorous species to utilize glucuronic acid for conjugation more readily than sulphate and for the other species to use sulphate at this level of phenol dosage. This table illustrates the complexity of the quantitative detail of species variation even with a simple compound such as phenol. The general pattern of phenol metabolism, however, is similar in the majority of the species in that phenol is excreted mainly conjugated with glucuronic acid and/or sulphate and oxidized to some extent to quinol, which is also excreted conjugated.

C. Amino Acid Conjugations

Some ten amino acids or peptides are shown in Table 11.3 as being involved in the formation of conjugation products. Apart from these, one or two others have been reported to occur in plants and bacteria (see Smith, 1968). The amino acids of interest here are glycine, glutamine, ornithine, glutathione and methionine. The first three undergo a peptide synthesis with acids which are usually aromatic. The foreign acids form activated nucleotides with Coenzyme A which then react enzymically with the amino acid to give the conjugated product thus:

$$\text{Aroyl-CoA} + \text{amino acid} \xrightarrow{\text{enzyme}} \text{aroylamino acid} + \text{CoASH}$$

In hippuric acid synthesis, the reaction is:

$$\text{Benzoyl-CoA} + \text{glycine} \xrightarrow{\text{glycine N-acylase}} \text{benzoylglycine} + \text{CoASH}$$

Glutathione is involved in the synthesis of mercapturic acids which takes place in several steps all of which are controlled by enzymes and are thus subject to species variation (see Williams, 1967b, for detailed steps). One route to the mercapturic acid is as follows (all steps not shown):

$$\text{ArX} + \text{GSH} \xrightarrow{\text{glutathiokinase}} \overset{\displaystyle \text{Gly}}{\underset{\displaystyle |}{\text{Ar—Cys}}}\text{—(Glu—NH}_2) \longrightarrow \text{Ar—Cys}$$

$$\xrightarrow{\text{acetylase}} \text{ArSCH}_2\text{CH(NHAc)CO}_2\text{H}$$

(X is usually a halogen).

Methionine is involved in the methylation of various foreign compounds by transferring its methyl group via the nucleotide, S-adenosylmethionine, to the foreign compound under the influence of various methyl transferases. Species variation in methylation could arise from differences in the occurrence and amounts of these transferases.

D. Glycine and Related Conjugations

Glycine conjugation of aromatic acids has been found to occur in most species of mammals, in insects, amphibia, in the class of birds named columbiformes, which includes pigeons and doves, and in some reptiles. It is, however, replaced in some species by other amino acids. In the birds classed as anseriformes (duck, goose) and galliformes (hen, turkey), glycine is replaced by ornithine so that benzoic acid is excreted as dibenzoylornithine (ornithuric acid). It is to be noted that ornithine conjugation does not occur in all classes of birds, since pigeons and doves form hippuric acid. Although insects are able to use glycine for the

Table 11.5

The conjugation of benzoic acid on various species

Dose of ^{14}C-benzoic acid = 50 mg/kg orally (man 1 mg/kg)

Species		% of 24 hr excretion of ^{14}C as	
		Hippuric acid	Benzoyl glucuronide
Man	Primates	100	0
Rhesus monkey		100	0
Squirrel monkey		82	tr.*
Ring-tailed monkey		100	tr.
Cat	Carnivores	100	0
Dog		73	27
Ferret		70	21
Pig		89	tr.
Rabbit		100	tr.
Fruit bat		tr	80
Hedgehog		81	13
Rat	Rodents	100	tr.
Mouse		95	5
Hamster		98	1
Guinea pig		97	3
Gerbil		98	0
Lemming		100	0
Pigeon	Birds	84	1*
Hen		tr	0 (ornithuric acid 58%)

* Some free benzoic acid excreted; tr = trace.

conjugation of aromatic acids, in spiders, ticks and scorpions it is replaced by arginine.

Table 11.5 shows the results of a study carried out in the author's laboratory (Bridges *et al.*, 1970) on the fate of a single dose (50 mg/kg) of ^{14}C-labelled benzoic acid in a number of species. All the species in this table, except the Indian fruit bat and the hen, excrete almost all the benzoic acid as hippuric acid. The fruit bat forms only traces of hippuric acid. The hen, as expected, excretes mainly ornithuric acid instead of hippuric acid. The dog and ferret also call for comment, for although most other species excrete benzoic acid at this dose level almost entirely as hippuric acid, these two carnivores excrete appreciable amounts of the glucuronide. In the dog it is known that the rate of mobilization of glycine is slow and furthermore that the ability to conjugate glycine is limited to its kidney, whereas in several other species such as the rabbit, glycine conjugation occurs both in the liver and kidney (*see* Williams, 1959). The location of glycine conjugation in the ferret, however, is not known. It is therefore possible for a species variation in the extent of a conjugation to be partly dependent on a species difference in the tissue location of the conjugation. In the dog, as far as benzoic acid is concerned, only conjugation with glucuronic acid can occur in the liver.

Glycine conjugation is also a reaction of arylacetic acids (ArCH$_2$COOH), but in man the conjugation of this type of acid occurs with glutamine. Phenylacetic, indolylacetic and 3,4-dihydroxy-5-methoxyphenylacetic (a metabolite of mescaline) acids are excreted by man as the corresponding glutamine conjugates of the general formula,

$$ArCH_2CONHCHCH_2CH_2CONH_2$$

$$| \\ CO_2H$$

This type of conjugation also occurs in the chimpanzee and probably in other Old World monkeys but not in lemurs (*see* Williams, 1967a). In lower species, such as the rat and rabbit, these acids are excreted as glycine conjugates, $ArCH_2 \cdot CONHCH_2CO_2H$.

Apart from these variations in amino acid conjugations, occasional observations have been recorded of unusual conjugations of specific compounds in certain species. Thus quinoline-2-carboxylic acid (quinaldic acid) as a typical aromatic acid might be expected to form a glycine conjugate. In fact, this is what happens in the rat, but in the cat it conjugates with glycyltaurine and to a lesser extent with glycylglycine (see formula below). The meaning of such unusual mechanisms is at present obscure and much more research is needed in this area.

In rat, $R = NHCH_2CO_2H$
In cat, $R = NHCH_2CONHCH_2CH_2SO_3H$ or $NHCH_2CONHCH_2CO_2H$

E. Glutathione Conjugations

The ability to form glutathione conjugates seems to be widely distributed amongst species, and *in vitro* studies (Grover and Sims, 1964) suggest that it occurs in man, mammals, birds, reptiles, amphibia, fish and insects and other invertebrates (*see* Smith, 1968). The enzyme system, glutathiokinase, seems widely distributed, but glutathione conjugates also give rise to N-acetylcysteine conjugates or mercapturic acids (see Section IV, C). There is evidence that certain species are defective in some of the steps leading to mercapturic acid. The guinea pig, although able to conjugate suitable compounds with glutathione, is unable to produce mercapturic acids, and has a defect in the ability to acetylate arylcysteines to mercapturic acids (James and Jeffrey, 1964).

Various observations in the literature also suggest that man, the pig and the hen may be defective in mercapturic acid formation. Glutathione S-aryltransferase in the livers of these species is at a relatively low level compared with other common laboratory animals (Grover and Sims, 1964). No detectable mercapturic acid occurred in the urine of children given bromobenzene (Wainer and Lorincz, 1963). The pig, as already mentioned, utilizes sulphur compounds poorly for conjugation purposes and is not a good mercapturic acid former. In fact, Coombs and Hele (1927) reported that the pig did not form a mercapturic acid from iodobenzene, which is extensively converted to p-iodophenylmercapturic acid in the rat and rabbit. An isolated observation on the hen from this laboratory (Baldwin, 1961) failed to find a mercapturic acid in the excreta after dosing hens with bromobenzene.

Preliminary studies in this laboratory (French, 1970) on the metabolism of ^{14}C-labelled chlorobenzene in various species have shown that some 20–30% of the excreted radioactivity is present as p-chlorophenylmercapturic acid in the rat, rabbit, hamster, gerbil, mouse and ferret. The output of the mercapturic acid in man, however, was small and neither the guinea pig nor the hedgehog appeared to excrete the mercapturic acid. The main metabolite of chlorobenzene in all these species, accounting for about 70 % of the excreted radioactivity, was 4-chlorocatechol conjugated mainly with glucuronic acid and to a lesser extent with sulphate. Defects of mercapturic acid synthesis in certain species, however, require further detailed study.

F. Acetylation

Acetylation is mainly a reaction of amino groups, although acetylation of the OH and SH group occurs in special cases, e.g., choline and CoA.SH. Formylation has also been observed, but only rarely (*see* Table 11.3). The nature of the NH_2 group is important in acetylation reactions *in vivo* and from this point of view five types of amino groups have been found to undergo acetylation in the animal body. These are: 1) aromatic amino group, $ArNH_2$; 2) aliphatic amino group, RNH_2; 3) α-amino acid, $RCH(CO_2H)NH_2$; 4) hydrazino, $RNHNH_2$ or $ArNHNH_2$; and 5) sulphonamido, $ArSO_2NH_2$.

Each of these amino groups probably need different transacetylases for their acetylation and therefore species variation in acetylation could depend upon the presence or absence of any of these enzymes. Man, rat and rabbit are able to acetylate all these groups, but the dog is unable to acetylate aromatic and hydrazino NH_2 groups. The fox, like the dog, does not acetylate the aromatic amino group of sulphanilamide. Acetylation of the aromatic amino group is a reaction which is widely distributed amongst species and has been found in mammals, reptiles, fish, amphibians, plants and insects (Smith, 1968), but exceptions occur as in the case of the dog and fox, although other members of the family, Canidae, have not been studied.

The guinea pig as already mentioned does not acetylate the amino group of S-arylcysteines ($ArSCH_2CH(CO_2H)NH_2$) which are α-amino acids, but whether this inability extends to other α-amino acids is not known.

Few systematic studies of the variation in the ability of various species to carry out the acetylation of different amino groups have been carried out. Table 11.6 shows the results of a study of the ability of 13 species including man to acetylate the aromatic and sulphonamido NH_2 groups of sulphanilamide (see Williams, 1967a). This drug can give rise in the body to three acetyl derivatives, namely N^1- and N^4-monoacetylsulphanilamide and N^1,N^4-diacetylsulphanilamide.

$$H_2\overset{4}{N} \bigcirc SO_2\overset{1}{N}H_2$$

This table shows that all the species examined can convert sulphanilamide to sulphacetamide (N^1-acetylsulphanilamide), but the total N^1-acetylation (i.e., N^1-acetyl $+ N^1,N^4$-diacetyl) is less than 20 % of the dose. N^4-acetylation exceeds N^1-acetylation considerably in all the species except the dog, fox, guinea pig and cat. In the dog and fox, N^4-acetylation does not occur, whereas in the guinea pig and cat, N^4- and N^1-acetylation are approximately equal. The absence of N^4-acetylation in the dog, suggests that the N^1- and N^4-acetylation of sulphanilamide are carried out by different transacetylases.

TABLE 11.6

Acetylation of sulfanilamide in various species

Order Family	Species	% Dose Excreted in Urine in 24 hr as			
		Free drug	N^1-acetyl	N^4-acetyl	N^1, N^4-diacetyl
Galliformes	Hen	47	3	24	1
	Turkey	25	9	47	4
Columbiformes	Pigeon	60	6	23	1
Rodentia — Muridae	Mouse	49	4	13	7
	Rat	36	10	36	2
Caviidae	Guinea pig	65	9	7	7
Capromyidae	Coypu	36	4	39	5
Lagomorpha	Rabbit	22	1	39	4
Carnivora — Felidae	Cat	65	6	8	6
Canidae	Dog	82	9	0	0
	Fox	70	10	0	0
Primates	Rhesus monkey	27	1	56	4
	Man	36	7	24	2

Dose of sulfanilamide = 100 mg/kg orally, except in man where it was 10 mg/kg Williams (1967a).

V. SPECIES DIFFERENCES DEPENDENT ON THE GUT MICROFLORA

The gastrointestinal flora are able to metabolize drugs and other chemicals (Scheline, 1968). Although several of these organisms are common to many species, they have been found to vary in numbers and location in the intestine of different species and they could vary in the same species with the nature of the diet. Since many foreign compounds are taken orally, it is possible for species variation in the metabolism of some compounds to depend at least partly upon the gut flora. This is, however, a field which has hardly been explored in any detail.

A striking example of such a species variation has been found in the metabolism of *l*-quinic acid (1,3,4,5-tetrahydroxycyclohexanecarboxylic acid). It had been observed as long ago as 1863 by Lauteman that quinic acid was excreted as hippuric acid in man but not in some other species. Quinic acid is a component of chlorogenic acid which occurs in appreciable amounts in tea, coffee, fruits and vegetables (a cup of coffee contains about 300 mg) and an appreciable proportion of the hippuric acid occurring normally in human urine may be derived from chlorogenic acid thus:

Chlorogenic acid   Quinic acid   Hippuric acid

When doses (300 mg/kg) of *l*-quinic acid are given orally to various animals

TABLE 11.7

*Species variation in the aromatization of quinic acid**

Dose of *l*-quinic acid was 0.3 g/kg orally except in man where it was 0.1 g/kg

Species			% of dose aromatized and excreted in 24 hr
Primates	Man		64
	Rhesus monkey	Old World monkeys	43
	Baboon		49
	Green monkey		45
	Spider monkey	New World monkeys	10
	Squirrel monkey		0
	Capuchin		0
	Giant bushbaby	Lemurs	6
	Slow loris		1
	Tree shrew		0
	Cat	Carnivores	0
	Dog		1
	Ferret		0
	Rabbit	Lagomorph	4
	Rat	Rodents	5
	Mouse		0
	Hamster		0
	Lemming		0
	Guinea pig		0
	Hedgehog	Insectivore	0
	Indian fruit bat	Chiroptera	0
	Pigeon	Bird	2

* Data from author's laboratory; see Adamson, *et al* (1966, 1970).

(22 species), only man and the Old World monkeys show extensive (20–70 % of dose) conversion of quinic acid to benzoic acid which is excreted almost entirely by the species examined as hippuric acid (see Table 11.7). In the other species the excretion of hippuric acid from quinic acid is usually about zero and rarely up to 10 % of the dose. Earlier workers had been unable to demonstrate aromatization of quinic acid by liver preparations although cyclohexanecarboxylic acid can be aromatized to benzoic acid by such preparations (Beer *et al.*, 1951).

In the rhesus monkey, aromatization of quinic acid occurs only if it is given by mouth. If the acid is injected intraperitoneally, no aromatization occurs. If the monkey is pretreated with antibiotics to suppress gut organisms, the aromatization is also inhibited (Adamson *et al.*, 1970), but the ability of the monkey to aromatize oral quinic acid returns on withdrawal of antibiotics. All the species examined were able to excrete orally administered benzoic acid mainly as hippuric acid; hence, if benzoic acid had been formed from quinic acid, it is unlikely to have been destroyed in the gut. The aromatization of quinic acid is therefore a striking example of a species variation in the metabolism of a compound dependent upon the gut flora.

Another example of a species variation influenced by gut bacteria is to be found in the metabolism of homoprotocatechuic acid. This acid is dehydroxylated to *m*-hydroxyphenylacetic acid in the rat and rabbit, but the excretion of this metabolite is suppressed almost to zero if the animals are pretreated with antibiotics. Aromatic dehydroxylation of this compound seems therefore to depend upon the gut flora. Homoprotocatechuic acid, however, is also methylated in these animals to 4-hydroxy-3-methoxphenylacetic acid (homovanillic acid) but the output of this metabolite is unaffected by pretreatment with antibiotics. The rabbit dehydroxylates twice as much as the rat (Dacre et al., 1968) and there is now evidence that the rabbit differs from several other species in its gut flora (see Scheline, 1968). This species difference in the extent of dehydroxylation appears to depend upon the gut flora. The main metabolites and the extent of their excretion (in % of dose) are shown below:

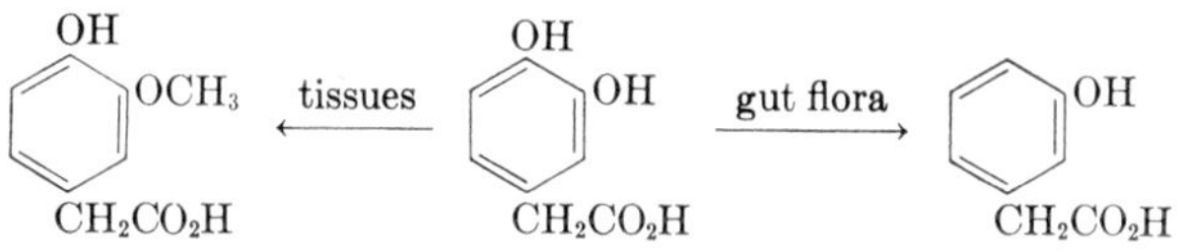

Rat	19	55	7
Rabbit	6	63	14

It is clear from these examples that more attention has to be paid to the possibility that the gut flora may, in some cases, play a role in the species variation in the metabolism of drugs. The extensive use of antibiotics may alter the activity of gut bacteria and therefore the metabolism of those drugs acted upon by these organisms.

VI. SPECIES VARIATION IN THE BILIARY EXCRETION OF FOREIGN COMPOUNDS

The main channel of excretion of foreign compounds and their metabolites is through the kidney into the urine. However, it has been known for a considerable time that some compounds are excreted partly or mainly through the liver into the bile. Those compounds excreted in the bile may then be excreted in the feces as such or after transformation by the gut flora, or they may be reabsorbed and be excreted in the urine or take part in an enterohepatic circulation. Thus any species variation in biliary excretion could give rise to differences in the overall metabolism of a drug. That species variations in the extent of the biliary excretion of certain types of foreign compounds occur has been shown by Abou-el-Makarem et al. (1967).

It is suggested by Williams et al. (1965) that the polarity and molecular weight (m.w.) of a compound were factors in determining the extent of its biliary excretion in the rat (see Millburn et al., 1967). In the rat compounds of molecular weight below about 300 were found to be poorly excreted in the bile, for less than 10% of the dose of such compounds was excreted in the bile and the rest was excreted in the urine as such or as metabolites. When the molecular weight exceeded about 325 ± 50, extensive biliary excretion of the compound occurred if it were polar or if it could be converted into a polar metabolite whose molecular weight exceeded this figure. Thus aniline (m.w. 93), benzoic acid (m.w. 122) and aminohippuric acid (m.w. 194) are poorly (<5%) excreted in the bile by the rat, but succinylsulphathiazole (m.w. 355) and phenolphthalein glucuronide (m.w. 495) are extensively (>50%) excreted in the bile.

When these compounds were examined in different species, it was found that with compounds of molecular weight less than 300 there was no species variation in the extent of their biliary excretion (see Table 11.8), even though there could

TABLE 11.8
Biliary excretion of low molecular weight compounds in various species

Species	% of dose* excreted in bile in 3 hrs after		
	Aniline	Benzoic acid	p-Aminohippuric acid
Rat	5.7	1.2	1.4
Dog	0.3	0.8	3.4
Cat	1.6	1.2	0.7
Hen	2.7	0.5	0.5
Guinea pig	5.6	1.7	6.7
Rabbit	2.6	0.7	3.0

* See text for nature of biliary metabolites.

be a species variation in the nature of the biliary metabolites. In the case of aniline, the biliary metabolites were 2- and 4-aminophenylglucuronides in all the species except the cat, which excreted 2-aminophenol only. The cat is known to be defective in glucuronide formation and, as shown in Table 11.1, hydroxylates aniline mainly in the 2-position. With benzoic acid, the main biliary metabolite in rat, cat, guinea pig and rabbit was hippuric acid; in the hen, ornithuric acid; and in the dog, benzoylglucuronide. It has already been stated that the glycine conjugation of mammals is replaced in the hen by ornithine conjugation. In the dog, hippuric acid synthesis occurs only in the kidney, so that it is reasonable to expect that the only conjugate of benzoic acid in dog bile would be the glucuronide which is synthesized mainly in the liver. The main biliary metabolite of p-aminohippuric acid in the rat, guinea pig and rabbit is p-acetamidohippuric acid, and both the free acid and its acetyl derivative are found in cat bile. In the dog, which is unable to acetylate aromatic amino groups, only p-aminohippuric acid is found. In hen bile, the free acid predominates with some acetyl derivative.

With compounds of molecular weight from 300–500 a sharp species variation in the extent of their biliary excretion is evident (*see* Table 11.9). The species in this table can be divided into three groups, namely, good biliary excretors which include the rat, dog and hen, moderate biliary excretors including the cat and sheep, and poor biliary excretors including the rabbit, guinea pig and rhesus monkey. The compounds in this table are polar anionic compounds of pKa 3–5 which are virtually fully ionized at the pH of the bile. They are excreted mainly unchanged in the bile by all the species cited in Table 11.9.

The fact that the rhesus monkey is a poor biliary excretor of compounds in this range of molecular weight might suggest that man is also a poor biliary excretor. This view is supported by observations on the biliary excretion of morphine (m.w. 285) and chloramphenicol (m.w. 323). Both these compounds are partly excreted as glucuronides of molecular weight 461 and 500, respectively. In the rat some 60% of morphine is excreted in the bile as 'bound' morphine (Way and Adler, 1962), whereas in man only 7% is excreted by this route (Elliott *et al.*, 1954). With chloramphenicol, biliary excretion is about 30–60% in the rat, whereas in man it is less than 3% (Glazko *et al.*, 1949, 1950, 1952).

There is a tendency for the extent of the biliary excretion of foreign compounds to increase with molecular weight, but this relationship is irregular and obviously

TABLE 11.9

Species variation in the biliary excretion of compounds of molecular weight 300–500

Compounds given intravenously unless otherwise indicated

Species	5,5'-Methylene disalicylic acid	Succinyl-sulphathiazole	Stilbestrol glucuronide	Phenolphthalin glucuronide
Mol. wt.	288	355	445	495
Dose in mg/kg	10	20	10	10
	% of dose excreted in 3 hr in bile			
Group I				
Rat	54	29	95	54 (i.p.)
Dog	65	20	65	81
Hen	—	25	93	71
Group II				
Cat	—	7	—	34
Sheep	—	10	—	37
Group III				
Rabbit	5	1	32	13
Guinea pig	4	0.9	20	6 (i.p.)
Rhesus monkey	—	0.3	—	9

other factors apart from molecular weight and polarity are involved (Clarke *et al.*, 1969). The minimum molecular weight for the extensive biliary excretion of polar compounds seems to be species related. For the "good" biliary excretors (rat, dog, hen) the minimum is in the region of 325 ± 50. For the "moderate" biliary excretors (cat, sheep), the minimum may be in the region of 400, whereas for the "poor" biliary excretors (guinea pig, rabbit, rhesus monkey and probably man) the minimum may be about 500. Studies on the biliary excretion of compounds of molecular weight higher than 500 in various species suggest that in all the species examined (rat, dog, mouse, guinea pig, rabbit, rhesus monkey and man) these compounds are highly excreted in the bile. This conclusion can be reached from a survey of the literature (see Millburn, 1970) on the biliary excretion of indomethacin (in bile as a glucuronide of m.w. 534), dichloromethotrexate (523), indocyanine green (752), bromsulphalein (792), rose bengal (972) and the cholecystographic agents such as pheniodol (494), iopanoic acid (571), iophenoxic acid (572), tetrabromophenolphthalein (634), iodophthalein (822) and iodipamide (1140). It would appear that species variation in the extent of biliary excretion of drugs is likely to occur with compounds of molecular weight between 300 and 500. Below 300 and above 500, species variation may not be significant.

There is a tendency for new drugs to have bigger and bigger molecules compared with those used in the past and therefore the extent of biliary excretion of drugs is becoming a matter of increased importance.

REFERENCES

Abou-El-Makarem, M. M., Millburn, P., Smith, R. L., and Williams, R. T.: Biliary excretion of foreign compounds. Biochem. J. *105:* 1289-1293, 1967.

Adamson, R. H., Bridges, J. W., Evans, M. E., and Williams, R. T.: Species differences in the aromatization of quinic acid in vivo and the role of gut bacteria. Biochem. J. *116:* 437–443, 1970.

Adamson, R. H., Bridges, J. W., and Williams, R. T.: The metabolism of quinic acid and sulphadimethoxine in primates. Biochem. J. *100:* 71P, 1966.

Baldwin, B. C.: Ph.D. Thesis, University of London (1961), p. 168.

Beer, C. T., Dicken, F., and Pearson, J.: The aromatization of hydrogenated derivatives of benzoic acid in animal tissue. Biochem. J. *48:* 222–237, 1951.

Bridges, J. W., French, M. R., Smith, R. L. and Williams, R. T. The fate of benzoic acid in various species. Biochem. J. *118:* 47–51, 1970.

Bridges, J. W., Kibby, M. R., Walker, S. R., and Williams, R. T.: Species difference in the metabolism of sulphadimethoxine. Biochem. J. *109:* 851–856, 1968.

Bridges, J. W., Kibby, M. R., Walker, S. R., and Williams, R. T.: Structure and species as factors affecting the metabolism of some methoxy-6-sulphanilamido-pyrimidines. Biochem. J. *111:* 167–172, 1969a.

Bridges, J. W., Walker, S. R., and Williams, R. T.: Species difference in the metabolism and excretion of sulphasomidine and sulphamethomidine. Biochem. J. *111:* 173–179, 1969b.

Chatterjee, I. B., Kar, N. C., Ghosh, M. C., and Guha, B. C.: Aspects of ascorbic acid biosynthesis in animals. Ann. N.Y. Acad. Sci. *92:* 36–55, 1961.

Clarke, A. G., Hirom, P. C., Millburn, P., Smith, R. L., and Williams, R. T.: Reabsorption from the biliary system as a factor influencing the biliary excretion of organic anions. Biochem. J. *115:* 62P, 1969.

Coombs, H. I. and Hele, T. S.: Studies in the sulphur metabolism of the dog. VI. The metabolism of the pig and dog compared. Biochem. J. *21:* 611–622, 1927.

Creaven, P. J., Parke, D. V., and Williams, R., T.: A spectrofluoroimetric study of the 7-hydroxylation of coumarin by liver microsomes. Biochem. J. *96:* 390–398, 1965.

Dacre, J. C., Scheline, R. R., and Williams, R. T.: The role of the tissues and gut flora in the metabolism of C^{14}-homoprotocatechuic acid in the rat and rabbit. J. Pharm. Pharmacol. *20:* 619–625, 1968.

Davies, D. S., Gigon, P. L., and Gillette, J. R.: Species and sex differences in electron transport system in liver microsomes and the relationship to ethylmorphine demethylation. Life Sci. *8:* (II): 85–91, 1969.

Dring, L. G.: Ph.D. Thesis, University of London, 1968.

Dring, L. G., Smith, R. L., and Williams, R. T.: The fate of amphetamine in man and other mammals. J. Pharm. Pharmacol. *18:* 402–404, 1966.

Dring, L. G., Smith, R. L., and Williams, R. T.: A precursor of benzyl methyl ketone in amphetamine urine. Biochem. J. *109:* 10P, 1968.

Elliott, J. W., Tolbert, B. M., Adler, T. L., and Anderson, H. H.: Excretion of carbon-14 by man after administration of morphine-N-methyl-C^{14}. Proc. Soc. Exp. Biol. Med. *85:* 77–81, 1954.

French, M. R., Ph.D. Thesis, Univ. of London, 1970.

Glazko, A. J., Dill, W. A., and Rebstock, M. C.: Biochemical studies on chloramphenicol. J. Biol. Chem. *183:* 679–691, 1950.

Glazko, A. J., Dill, W. A., and Wolf, L. M.: Observations on the metabolic disposition of chloramphenicol in rat. J. Pharmacol. Exp. Ther. *104:* 452–458, 1952.

Glazko, A. J., Wolf, L. M., Dill, W. A., and Bratton, A. C.: Biochemical studies on chloramphenicol. J. Pharmacol. Exp. Ther. *96:* 445–459, 1949.

Grover, P. L. and Sims, P.: Distribution of glutathione S-aryltransferase in vertebrate species. Biochem. J. *90:* 603–606, 1964.

James, S. P. and Jeffrey, D. J.: The biosynthesis of N-acetyl-S-hydroxyalkylcysteines. Biochem. J. *93:* 16P, 1964.

Kaighen, M. and Williams, R. T.: The metabolism of 3-^{14}C coumarin. J. Med. Pharm. Chem. *3:* 25–43, 1961.

Lathe, G. H. and Walker, M.: The synthesis of bilirubin glucuronide in animal and human liver. Biochem. J. *70:* 705–711, 1958.

Lauteman, E.: Uber die Reduktion der Chinasäure zu Benzoësäure und die Verwandlung derselben in Hippursäure im thierischen Organismus. Liebig's Ann. *125:* 9, 1863.

Millburn, P.: Factors in the biliary excretion of organic compounds. In *Metabolic. Conjugation and Metabolic Hydrolysis*, Vol 2, ed. by W. H. Fishman, Academic Press, p. 1, 1970.

Millburn, P., Smith, R. L., and Williams, R. T.: Biliary excretion of foreign compounds. Biochem. J. *105:* 1275–1281, 1967.

Robinson, D. and Williams, R. T.: Do cats form glucuronides? Biochem. J. *68:* 23P–24P, 1958.

Scheline, R. R.: Drug metabolism by intestinal microorganisms. J. Pharm. Sci. *57:* 2021–2035, 1968.

Smith, J. N.: The comparative metabolism of xenobiotics. Adv. Comp. Physiol. Biochem. *3:* 173–232, 1968.

Smith, R. L. and Williams, R. T.: Implications of the conjugation of drugs and other exogenous compounds. In *Glu-*

curonic Acid, Free and Combined, ed. by G. J. Dutton, pp. 457–491, Academic Press, N. Y., 1966.

Stekol, J. A.: Comparative studies in the sulfur metabolism of the dog and pig. J. Biol. Chem. *113:* 675–682, 1933.

Wainer, A. and Lorincz, A. E.: Studies on mercapturic acid synthesis by humans. Life Sci. *2:* 504–508, 1963.

Way, E. L. and Adler, T. K.: The biological disposition of morphine and its surrogates, pp. 19–35, W.H.O. Geneva, 1962.

Williams, R. T.: *Detoxication Mechanisms*, 2nd ed., p. 351, London, Chapman & Hall, Ltd., 1959.

Williams, R. T.: Comparative patterns of drug metabolism. Fed. Proc. *26:* 1029–1039, 1967a.

Williams, R. T.: (Chapt. 9) In *Biogenesis of Natural Compounds*, ed. by P. Bernfeld, pp. 590–639, Pergamon Press, N.Y., 2nd ed., 1967b.

Williams, R. T., Millburn, P., and Smith, R. L.: The influence of enterohepatic circulation on toxicity of drugs. Ann. N. Y. Acad. Sci. *123:* 110–124, 1965.

12

Microsomal Enzyme Systems which Catalyze Drug Metabolism

G. J. MANNERING

I. INTRODUCTION

The first description of the metabolism of a foreign compound by hepatic microsomes was given by Mueller and Miller (1949, 1953). They showed that the microsomal fraction of a liver homogenate catalyzed both the reductive splitting of the azo linkage and the oxidative N-demethylation of aminoazo dyes. The reactions required nicotinamide-adenine dinucleotide phosphate (NADP), nicotinamide adenine dinucleotide (NAD) and molecular oxygen. Brodie *et al.* (1955) showed that a similar enzyme system localized in hepatic microsomes was responsible for the metabolism of many drugs. Recombination of the various cell fractions of liver homogenates revealed the requirement for both soluble and microsomal fractions. Full activity was obtained when the soluble fraction was replaced by a NADPH generating system consisting of NADP, glucose-6-phosphate (G-6-P) and G-6-P dehydrogenase or by NADPH itself. Magnesium ion was required for full activity. The requirement of both a reducing agent and molecular oxygen places the reaction within the external mixed function oxidase classification of Mason (1957, 1965) or the monooxygenase terminology of Hayaishi (1964), which means that the enzymes catalyze the consumption of one molecule of oxygen per molecule of substrate with one atom of oxygen appearing in the product and the other undergoing two-equivalent reduction. Direct support of this view was given by Posner *et al.* (1961a), who employed $^{18}O_2$ and $H_2^{18}O$ to show that the oxygen utilized in the hydroxylation of acetanilide is derived from molecular oxygen rather than from water.

A wide variety of oxidative reactions are known to occur in microsomes: deamination, O-, N- and S-dealkylation, hydroxylation of alkyl and aryl hydrocarbons, epoxidation, formation of alkylol derivatives, N-hydroxylation, N- and S-oxidation and dehalogenation. Azo- and nitro-reductase activities are also found in hepatic microsomes. Examples of these reactions are given in Chapter 10 (Table 10.5) and they are discussed in some detail by Gillette (1966). The great versatility of the microsomal drug metabolizing system seems less remarkable when the reactions are visualized simply as different kinds of hydroxylation reactions (Brodie *et al.*, 1958; Gillette, 1963, 1966).

Aromatic hydroxylation

$$CH_3CO—NH—C_6H_5 \xrightarrow{[OH]} CH_3—CO—NH—C_6H_4—OH$$

Aliphatic hydroxylation

$$R-CH_3 \xrightarrow{[OH]} R-CH_2-OH$$

N-Dealkylation

$$R-NH-CH_3 \xrightarrow{[OH]} [R-NH-CH_2OH] \rightarrow RNH_2 + CH_2O$$

O-Dealkylation

$$R-O-CH_3 \xrightarrow{[OH]} [R-O-CH_2OH] \rightarrow ROH + CH_2O$$

Deamination

$$R-CH(NH_2)-CH_3 \xrightarrow{[OH]} [R-C(OH)(NH_2)-CH_3] \rightarrow R-CO-CH_3 + NH_3$$

Sulfoxidation

$$R-S-R' \xrightarrow{[OH]} [R-SOH-R']^+ \rightarrow R-SO-R' + H^+$$

N-Oxidation

$$(CH_3)_3N \xrightarrow{[OH]} [(CH_3)_3NOH]^+ \rightarrow (CH_3)_3NO + H^+$$

Microsomal enzymes metabolize drugs by other than oxidative or reductive mechanisms, for example, by participating in glucuronide synthesis through the action of uridine diphosphate glucuronyl transferase. Such mechanisms are discussed elsewhere in this volume; this chapter is concerned only with those microsomal enzymes involved in oxidative and reductive processes. Gillette (1963, 1966, 1969) and Mannering (1968) have reviewed certain of the material to be presented. For detailed treatment of some of the more current advances made in the field, the reader is referred to the recently published proceedings of a symposium devoted to microsomes and drug oxidations (Gillette and co-editors, 1969).

II. DRUG METABOLIZING SYSTEMS OF THE HEPATIC ENDOPLASMIC RETICULUM

The microsomal drug metabolizing system is thought of as a mixed function oxidase mechanism whereby NADPH reduces a component in microsomes which reacts with molecular oxygen to form an "active oxygen" intermediate. The "active oxygen" is then transferred to the drug. Gillette (1963) formulated the overall reaction as follows:

1. $NADPH + A + H^+ \rightarrow AH_2 + NADP^+$

2. $AH_2 + O_2 \rightarrow$ "active oxygen"

3. $\underline{\text{"Active oxygen"} + \text{drug} \rightarrow \text{oxidized drug} + A + H_2O}$
   $NADPH + O_2 + \text{drug} = NADP^+ + H_2O + \text{oxidized drug}$

Key enzymes in the overall reaction are NADPH-cytochrome c reductase, the flavin enzyme involved in the oxidation of NADPH, cytochrome P-450, which in its reduced form is generally considered to be A, and NADPH cytochrome P-450 reductase, which functions in the reduction of oxidized cytochrome P-450.

This mechanism requires that equivalent amounts of NADPH, oxygen and substrate be utilized in the reaction. Stoichiometric relationships have been obtained for the hydroxylation of phenylalanine by hepatic microsomes (Kaufman, 1957) and the hydroxylation of 17-hydroxyprogesterone by adrenal microsomes (Cooper *et al.*, 1963). Trimethylamine has been reported to stimulate NADPH oxidation by an amount equivalent to the amount of trimethylamine oxide formed (Baker and Chaykin, 1962) and hexobarbital was found to increase NADPH oxidation in accordance with stoichiometric expectations (Trivus and Spirtes, 1965). However, Gillette (Gillette *et al.*, 1957; Gillette, 1966, 1969) found that some drugs had no effect on NADPH oxidation whereas others had more of an effect than could be accounted for by the metabolism of the drug. Microsomes contain enzymes which oxidize NADPH and utilize molecular oxygen in the absence of drugs, greatly complicating the analysis. Whether or not a drug stimulates or depresses NADPH oxidation would seem to depend upon whether or not it stimulates or depresses cytochrome P-450 reductase activity; this in turn would seem to depend upon whether the drug combines with cytochrome P-450 as a type I or as a type II compound (Gillette and Gram, 1969; Gillette, 1969). This will be discussed in more detail later. Ernster and Orrenius (1965) demonstrated a 1:1:1 stoichiometry of oxygen utilization, NADPH disappearance and formaldehyde formation from the oxidative demethylation of aminopyrine. However, Estabrook and Cohen (1969) found that stoichiometry did not support the basic assumption of a mixed function oxidase reaction, that a mole of NADPH be oxidized for each mole of formaldehyde formed; two moles of NADP were formed per mole of formaldehyde, suggesting the reaction is more complex than anticipated. Sasame (1964) did not find a stoichiometric relationship between NADPH and hexobarbital oxidation; the amount of NADPH oxidized was about 50% greater than the amount of hexobarbital metabolized.

Figure 12.1 shows the electron transfer system involving cytochrome P-450

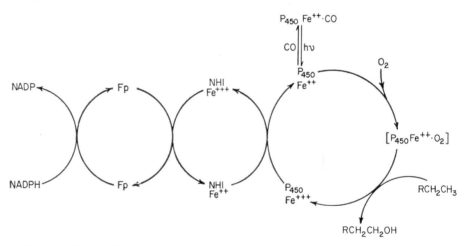

Fig. 12.1. Proposed electron transfer system employed in the microsomal metabolism of drugs (Omura *et al.*, 1965a, 1966). F_p = flavoprotein (in the liver, cytochrome c reductase; in the adrenal, adrenodoxin reductase); NHI = non-heme iron protein (in the adrenal, adrenodoxin).

as conceived by Omura *et al.* (1965a, 1966). Working in Estabrook's laboratory, these investigators fractionated sonicated mitochondria from beef adrenal cortex into a particulate fraction which contained cytochrome P-450 free of other hemoproteins, and a soluble fraction that retained the activity of the NADPH-cytochrome P-450 reductase system. This soluble fraction contained non-heme iron protein and an FAD-flavoprotein (cytochrome c reductase), both of which were necessary for the reconstitution of NADPH-cytochrome P-450 reductase activity. Direct evidence has not been presented to show that the electron transfer system of the adrenal cortex is the same as that found in the liver, but Maclennan *et al.* (1967) point out that the spectral and oxidation-reduction properties of the P-450 complex prepared from beef liver microsomes are remarkably like those described by Estabrook and associates (Cooper *et al.*, 1963, 1965) for the cytochrome P-450 complex obtained from beef adrenal cortex.

The first description of the microsomal system responsible for drug metabolism (Mueller and Miller, 1949, 1953) included a role of NADH as well as NADPH. From time to time since then NADH has been implicated in reactions involving drug metabolism (Conney *et al.*, 1957; Nilsson and Johnson, 1963; Ullrich, 1969). Using the mechanism of peroxidase action as a model, Estabrook and Cohen (1969) suggested a way in which NADH might contribute to the reaction (Fig. 12.2). NADPH may serve as an electron donor via a respiratory chain direct to cytochrome P-450 with an associated branched pathway to cytochrome b_5, the only cytochrome other than cytochrome P-450 found in microsomes. In this way cytochrome b_5 might serve as a second electron donor to cytochrome P-450 and thus satisfy the requirement of two electrons for the overall reaction.

Sih and coworkers (Sih *et al.*, 1968; Sih, 1969) question the function of NADPH as solely one of providing the reducing equivalents for cytochrome P-450 via the

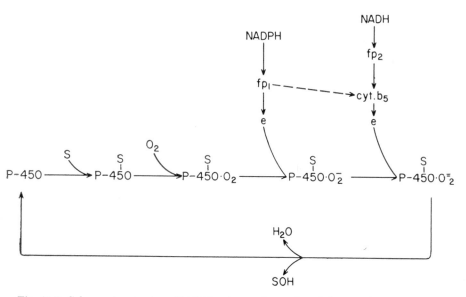

Fig. 12.2. Scheme showing how NADH and cytochrome b_5 might contribute to the electron transfer system employed in the microsomal metabolism of drugs (Estabrook and Cohen, 1969).

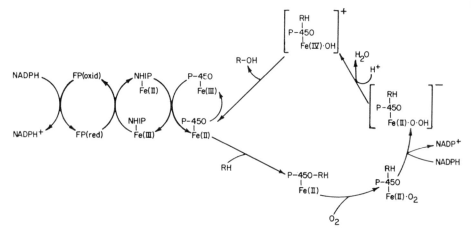

Fig. 12.3. Scheme illustrating a proposed dual role of NADPH in the oxidation of corticosteroids by mitochondria of the adrenal cortex (Sih *et al.*, 1968; Sih, 1969). FP = flavoprotein (adrenodoxin); NHIP = non-heme iron protein (adrenodoxin reductase).

electron transfer system as shown in Figure 12.1. Three lines of evidence led to the scheme given in Figure 12.3, which visualizes a dual role of NADPH in the oxidation of corticosteroids by mitochondria of the adrenal cortex.

1) With a mixture of soluble flavoprotein, soluble adrenodoxin (non-heme iron protein) and subparticles of mitochondria obtained by sonication, NADH rather than NADPH was employed to give a maximum rate of reduction of adrenodoxin. Normally, NADH is not thought to function in this reaction because of the much greater reactivity of NADPH with the flavoprotein, but if the concentration of flavoprotein is increased greatly, as was the case here, a rate of reduction can be obtained with NADH equivalent to that seen with NADPH. Under these adjusted conditions, no significant quantity of steroid hydroxylation occurred.

2) In accordance with the scheme given in Figure 12.3, NADPH and steroid combine with different enzymes. A double reciprocal plot of the velocity of steroid oxidation vs. NADPH concentration at fixed concentration of steroid should yield a series of parallel lines (Cleland, 1963). However, a series of intersecting lines was obtained indicating that NADPH and steroid either combine with the same enzyme or with a different enzyme form, but connected with reversible steps. In addition, these kinetic studies indicated that NADPH also combined with a different enzyme, in all probability flavoprotein.

3) Studies employing $NADPT_A$ and $NADPT_B$ led to the conclusion that $NADPH_B$ serves in an accessory capacity, keeping cytochrome P-450 in the ferrous level of oxidation, whereas $NADPH_A$ is involved directly in steroid hydroxylation by generating the highly reactive hydroperoxo complex, P-450-Fe^{2+}-O-OH. The proposed mechanism avoids the previous objection that a ferrous ion-oxygen complex should not be reactive enough to enter directly into oxidations such as those of unactivated carbon-hydrogen bonds, e.g., the penultimate hydroxylation of aliphatic chains so frequently encountered in drug biotransformations. Conclusions were based on the assumption that the flavoprotein, adrenodoxin and cytochrome P-450 exist in a well-defined complex which behaves as a single enzyme. In this scheme, the NADPH that keeps cytochrome P-450 in the ferrous state of oxidation does not enter into the stoichiometry of

the hydroxylation reactions, whereas the NADPH that is involved in the formation of the "active oxygen," $(Fe^{++}\text{-}O\text{-}OH)^-$, is substrate dependent. Thus the observation of Das et al. (1968) that $NADPH_A$ rather than $NADPH_B$ is involved predominantly in the microsomal oxidation of drugs is not in disagreement with the concept of Sih and associates. The existence of the transient $(Fe^{++}\text{-}O\text{-}OH)^-$ species remains to be demonstrated.

Much of the speculation regarding the components of the microsomal drug metabolizing system exists because attempts to solubilize cytochrome P-450 in active form had failed and it was necessary to employ crude microsomal preparations. Recent studies (Lu and Coon, 1968; Coon and Lu, 1969; Lu et al., 1969, 1969a) may have done much toward solving this problem. Solubilization of hepatic microsomes from the rabbit with a mixture of glycerol, dithiothreitol and sodium deoxycholate in a potassium citrate buffer produced an extract which was resolved into a fraction containing cytochrome P-450, a fraction containing an NADPH reductase and a fat soluble, heat stable fraction. All three fractions were necessary for the maximal oxidation of drugs (benzphetamine, aminopyrine, ethylmorphine, hexobarbital, norcodeine, p-nitroanisole) or for the ω-hydroxylation of laurate. The criteria for the solubilization of cytochrome P-450 was that it remained in the supernatant fraction of the preparation after centrifugation at $105,000 \times g$ for 2 hours. These fractions may provide the opportunity for purification and identification of the components of the system.

Microsomal drug metabolism is not restricted to oxidative reactions. A wide variety of azo dyes are cleaved reductively to primary aromatic amines; nitro compounds such as chloramphenicol, p-nitrobenzoic acid and nitrobenzene are reduced to primary amines. In Gillette's laboratory (Gillette, 1966; Hernandez et al., 1967, 1967a) steapsin was employed to solubilize microsomal azoreductase. The absorption spectrum of the purified enzyme was typical of a flavoprotein and at no stage of the purification was it possible to separate azoreductase and NADPH-cytochrome c reductase activities. However, microsomal azoreductase activity decreased upon solubilization, whereas NADPH-cytochrome c reductase activity increased. The second azoreductase pathway suggested by these studies was shown to involve cytochrome P-450. It was concluded that azo dyes are reduced by two mechanisms, a) a carbon monoxide and solubilization sensitive pathway requiring cytochrome P-450, and b) a carbon monoxide insensitive pathway involving NADPH-cytochrome c reductase, which is not destroyed by solubilization. A third pathway, insensitive to carbon monoxide, but sensitive to solubilization, was observed in microsomes from animals which had received 3-methylcholanthrene.

Both NADH and NADPH can act as the electron donor in the reduction of nitro compounds. The reaction is presumed to proceed to the primary amine through the formation of nitroso and hydroxylamine derivatives. Nitroreductase is only active under anaerobic conditions. Sensitivity to oxygen may be due in part to the autooxidation of the hydroxylamine intermediate (Gillette et al., 1968). In studies which employed p-nitrobenzoate as a substrate, Gillette et al. (1968) concluded that the reduction was mediated by cytochrome P-450. These investigators proposed an electron transport system which would explain both the oxidative and the reductive function of the microsomal drug-metabolizing system (Fig. 12.4).

A microsomal NADPH- and oxygen-dependent, mixed function oxidase which

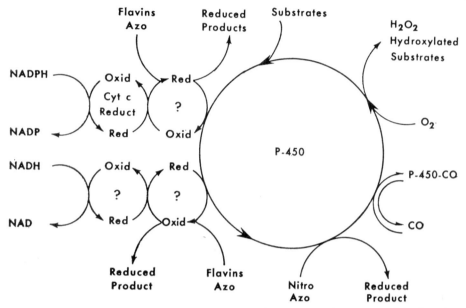

Fig. 12.4. Scheme showing how the microsomal electron transfer system might function in both the oxidation and reduction of drugs (Gillette *et al.*, 1968).

functions independently of cytochrome P-450 in the N-oxidation of a variety of N-alkyl-substituted amines has been demonstrated repeatedly (Baker and Chaykin, 1962; Coccia and Westerfeld, 1967; Ziegler and Pettit, 1966; Ziegler *et al.*, 1969). The purified enzyme, which has been concentrated about 1000-fold from pork liver, catalyzed a number of secondary and tertiary amines, including tranquilizers, antihistamines, narcotics, tropine alkaloids, and ephedrine and ephedrine-like compounds. Tertiary amines are oxidized to the amine oxide only; secondary amines are oxidatively N-dealkylated, at least partially. The purified oxidase is a flavoprotein. It contains (in mμmoles/mg of protein) FAD, 12.8, non-heme iron <2.0, cytochrome b_5, 0.55; an undetermined amount of phospholipid, and no detectable cytochrome P-450 (Ziegler *et al.*, 1969). Kinetic studies, as well as evidence based on the selective actions of inhibitors on the oxidative N-dealkylation of dialkylamines (Ziegler and Pettit, 1966; Machinist *et al.*, 1966) indicate that the amine oxides can be intermediates in the dealkylation of these amines.

III. COMPONENTS OF THE MICROSOMAL DRUG METABOLIZING SYSTEM

A. Cytochrome P-450

1. General. Cytochrome P-450, earlier referred to as the CO-binding pigment, was first described by Klingenberg (1958), Garfinkel (1958) and Omura and Sato (1962, 1964, 1964a). It is found in abundance not only in hepatic microsomes, but also in the microsomes and mitochondria from the adrenal cortex, where it functions in the hydroxylation of steroids (Estabrook *et al.*, 1963; Omura *et al.*, 1965a) although not in the oxidation of most drugs. Lesser amounts are found in the kidney and intestinal mucosa (Takesue *et al.*, 1965). The presence of cytochrome P-450 has also been reported in mitochondria from the corpus luteum (Yohro and Horie, 1967).

The hemoprotein is found in liver microsomes from a variety of vertebrates, including several mammals, a bird, a snake, a frog and a fish (Omura and Sato, 1965), in bacteria (Katagiri et al., 1968), in bacteroids (Appleby, 1967, 1968, 1969, 1969a) and in yeast (Ishidate et al., 1969, 1969a). Cytochrome P-450 should not be assumed to be identical in every tissue or species; the substrate specificities of the enzyme systems involving adrenal and hepatic cytochrome P-450 differ greatly, and differences are also seen in the substrate specificities of the drug metabolizing systems of hepatic microsomes from different species. These differences are very likely due to differences in the way in which cytochrome P-450 is associated with the microsomal membrane or in qualitative or quantitative differences in other components of the enzyme system, but it is also possible that cytochrome P-450 may exist in a variety of forms.

The following observations provide evidence for the involvement of cytochrome P-450 in drug metabolism:

1) Light reverses the inhibitory effect of carbon monoxide on the metabolism of codeine, monomethylaminopyrine and acetanilide; the active spectrum of the reversal of the inhibition of drug metabolism by light corresponds with the spectrum of the carbon monoxide complex of cytochrome P-450, with the wavelength at 450 mμ producing the maximum effect (Cooper et al., 1965).

2) Cyanide does not combine with cytochrome P-450 (Omura and Sato, 1964), nor does it inhibit drug metabolism (Cooper and Brodie, 1955; LaDu et al., 1955; Gillette et al., 1957).

3) Carbon monoxide combines with cytochrome P-450 and it inhibits drug metabolism (Conney et al., 1957; Orrenius and Ernster, 1964; Cooper et al., 1965).

4) Substances which destroy the drug metabolizing activity of microsomes, such as deoxycholate, steapsin and snake venom (Gillette et al., 1957; Posner et al., 1961) convert cytochrome P-450 to the inactive form of the hemoprotein, cytochrome P-420 (Omura and Sato, 1964, 1964a). Moreover, detergents such as isooctylphenoxypolyethoxyethanol and Triton N-101, which can be employed to partially solubilize microsomes, lower the rate of drug metabolism in direct proportion to the conversion of cytochrome P-450 to cytochrome P-420 (Gillette, 1966; Silverman and Talalay, 1967).

5) Agents that cause an increase or decrease in the cytochrome P-450 levels of microsomes frequently cause a parallel increase or decrease in the rates at which the same microsomes metabolize drugs (Orrenius and Ernster, 1964; Remmer and Merker, 1965; Mannering, 1968; Sladek and Mannering, 1969).

6) Drugs bind to cytochrome P-450 giving characteristic difference spectra; with certain drugs there is a similarity of the kinetics of this binding and the kinetics of the metabolism of the same drugs (Remmer et al., 1966; Imai and Sato, 1966, 1967; Schenkman et al., 1967).

7) The liver and the adrenal cortex oxidize steroids (Estabrook et al., 1963; Kuntzman et al., 1964, 1965); microsomes from both organs are rich in cytochrome P-450.

2. Spectral characteristics. Cytochrome P-450 is measured by the difference spectrum seen when it is reduced, usually with dithionite, and combined with carbon monoxide. NADH and NADPH reduce cytochrome P-450 only in the absence of molecular oxygen, the pigment being very autooxidizable. About 50% inhibition of hydroxylation reactions are obtained when the CO/O_2 ratio is about 1 (Omura et al., 1965a). This can be compared with the ratio of about 1/200 for the half conversion of oxyhemoglobin to carbon monoxyhemoglobin and about 10 observed by Keilin and Hartree (1939) and Warburg (1949) for 50% inhibition of cytochrome oxidase. The difference spectrum of reduced cytochrome P-450 in the presence of CO is unusual for a cytochrome and provides no clue as to the nature of the pigment (Sato et al., 1965). That the CO-binding pigment is indeed a cytochrome was shown by the spectrum of its derivative, cytochrome P-420, and by techniques which permitted the recording of the absolute spectrum of cytochrome P-450 contained in microsomal particles.

Except for traces of catalase, the only cytochromes thought to be present in microsomes are cytochrome P-450 and cytochrome b_5. Cytochrome b_5 can be selectively removed by digesting the microsomes anaerobically with 0.14% steapsin (crude pancreatic lipase) under suitable conditions (0.1 M phosphate buffer, pH 7.5, 37°C, 1 hr), leaving the CO-binding pigment attached to the undigested particles and partly in the form of cytochrome P-420. When these particles are treated anaerobically with snake venom (0.1% heated or unheated venom from Trimeresurus flavoviridis, Tris buffer, pH 8.5, 0°C, 16 hr) or with sodium deoxycholate (0.5%), all of the CO-binding pigment is solubilized and converted to cytochrome P-420. Processing of the extract yielded purified cytochrome P-420 which showed an absorption spectrum characteristic of a cytochrome of the b type; i.e., the α-, β, and Soret bands of the reduced form lie at 559, 530 and 427 mμ, respectively (Omura and Sato, 1963, 1964, 1964a; Sato et al., 1965). The Soret band of the oxidized form occurs at 414 mμ. On combination with CO the Soret peak of reduced cytochrome P-420 shifts to 422 mμ and is intensified considerably. These spectra are very similar to those of bacterial cytochrome b_1 (Fujita et al., 1963) but the bacterial cytochrome differs from cytochrome P-420 in that it does not bind CO.

Determination of the absolute spectrum of cytochrome P-450 is complicated by the presence of cytochrome b_5 and cytochrome P-420. The problem has been solved to a large degree by removing cytochrome b_5 from the microsomes and by stabilizing cytochrome P-450 with glycerol. In Sato's laboratory (Nishibayashi and Sato, 1968; Nishibayashi et al., 1968; Sato et al., 1969) the absolute spectrum of cytochrome P-450 was observed in microsomal particles that had been freed of cytochrome b_5 as a result of being treated anaerobically with Nargase, a proteinase from Bacillus subtilis, and in which the small amount of cytochrome P-420 that had been formed in the presence of glycerol was almost completely removed with H_2O_2. Maclennan and coworkers (1967) obtained a spectrum using microsomal membranes that had been reduced in size as a result of treatment with tert.-amyl alcohol, but the particles contained a cytochrome b_5-like hemoprotein and a flavin enzyme in addition to cytochrome P-450. In Mason's laboratory hepatic microsomes were treated with the nonionic detergent, Lubrol WX, to produce subparticles which gave an absolute spectrum for cytochrome P-450 with no apparent interference from cytochrome b_5 and very little interference from cytochrome P-420 (Miyake et al., 1968). The absolute spectra of cytochrome P-450 from adrenal mitochondria (Kinoshita and Horie, 1967) and from Rhizo-

bium japonicum bacteroids (Appleby, 1967, 1968) are very similar to that from hepatic microsomes.

A clever method was proposed by Kinoshita and Horie (1967) for determining the absolute spectrum in microsomes which had not been treated to remove cytochrome b_5. The method is based on the knowledge that cytochrome b_5 is the only microsomal cytochrome other than cytochrome P-450 and that the administration of inducing agents such as phenobarbital cause a large increase in the concentration of cytochrome P-450 in microsomes without affecting appreciably the cytochrome b_5 level. Suspensions of microsomes from untreated rabbits and rabbits treated with phenobarbital were diluted so that each contained an equal amount of cytochrome b_5.

With respect to the hemoprotein content, the only apparent difference between these two preparations was their cytochrome P-450 content. Using the microsomes from the untreated animals in the reference cuvette, the difference spectrum obtained with the two preparations was very similar to the absolute spectrum for cytochrome P-450 obtained by other methods. The procedure has been used extensively in Estabrook's laboratory for the recording of the absolute spectra of CO-binding pigments from animals induced with phenobarbital or 3-methylcholanthrene (Hildebrandt *et al.*, 1968; Hildebrandt and Estabrook, 1969). When the hemoprotein is placed in both cuvettes with a higher concentration in the sample cuvette, as is the case when the method of Kinoshita and Horie is employed, the resulting spectrum has the qualitative features of the absolute spectrum of the hemoprotein, but it is reduced in magnitude throughout its entirety by exactly the minus contribution of the inverted spectrum produced by the hemoprotein in the reference cuvette. Unless corrected, the resulting spectrum is therefore not a quantitative representation of the apparent absolute spectrum. Furthermore, qualitative aspects of the apparent absolute spectrum can only be meaningful if the microsomes from untreated and phenobarbital treated animals contain spectrally identical cytochrome P-450's.

That the cytochrome P-450 in microsomes from phenobarbital treated rabbits is spectrally the same as that found in the microsomes of untreated animals is evident when the apparent absolute spectrum obtained by Hildebrandt and Estabrook (1969) by the method of Kinoshita and Horie is compared with the absolute spectrum published by Sato and associates (1969). The latter spectrum was obtained by a direct spectrophotometric procedure using microsomes freed of cytochrome b_5. The observed quantitative difference in the two spectra is very close to that which can be calculated from theoretical considerations. When the cytochrome P-450's are not identical in different microsomes, as is the case when the hemoproteins from untreated animals and animals treated with 3-methylcholanthrene are compared, the "absolute" spectrum obtained by the method of Kinoshita and Horie cannot be correct qualitatively or quantitatively. This will be discussed in more detail later in this chapter under the heading of *Cytochrome P_1-450*.

In our laboratory a purified, soluble ("soluble" means that cytochrome P-450 was not sedimented from 0.1 M phosphate buffer (pH 7.4) containing 10 % glycerol and 0.5 % Triton N-101 after centrifugation for 90 min at 98,000 × g) cytochrome P-450 has been obtained by treating hepatic microsomes with the non-ionic detergent, Triton N-101, and fractionating the supernatant on a DEAE

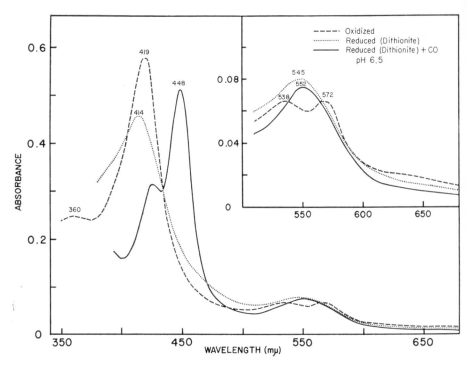

Fig. 12.5. Absolute spectra of solubilized microsomal P-450 hemoprotein (cytochrome P_1-450) from livers of rats treated with 3-methylcholanthrene (Fujita and Mannering, unpublished results). The hemoprotein was solubilized by treating microsomes with Triton N-101 and fractionating the supernatant on a DEAE cellulose column. The preparation was free of cytochrome b_5, but contained a small amount of P-420 hemoprotein. Table 12.3 summarizes the spectral properties of solubilized cytochromes P-450 and P_1-450.

cellulose column (Fujita and Mannering, unpublished observations). The preparation was free of cytochrome b_5, but it contained a small amount of cytochrome P-420. Its spectrum (Fig. 12.5) compares well with that reported for particulate cytochrome P-450. Using sodium cholate, Mitani and Horie (1969) obtained soluble cytochrome P-450 from adrenal mitochondria which gave an absolute spectrum similar to that seen with insoluble microsomal cytochrome P-450 from liver.

3. Conversion to cytochrome P-420. Cytochrome P-450 is converted to cytochrome P-420 by a wide variety of agents: snake venom containing phospholipase A (Omura and Sato, 1963, 1964, 1964a), detergents such as sodium deoxycholate (Omura and Sato, 1964, 1964a) and lysolecithin (Imai and Sato, 1967a), the metal-binding reagents, bathocuproine sulfonate and bathophenanthroline sulfonate (Mason et al., 1965, 1965a), trypsin (Mason et al., 1965; Orrenius et al., 1969), urea (Mason et al., 1965) and other ureas (Ichikawa et al., 1968), guanidine (Imai and Sato, 1967a), neutral salts (Imai and Sato, 1967a), the mercurial —SH-binding agents, p-chloromercuribenzoate (Omura et al., 1965; Mason et al., 1965), p-chloromercuriphenyl sulfate (Mason et al., 1965) and $HgCl_2$ (Mason et al., 1965; Ichikawa and Yamano, 1967), iodine (Imai and Sato, 1967a; Ullrich, 1969), aniline (Imai and Sato, 1967a), alcohols (Mason et al., 1965; Imai and Sato, 1967a; Ichikawa et al., 1968), and a variety of amides and phenols (Ichikawa *et al.*, 1968). Cytochrome P-420 is frequently solubilized as it is formed, but this need not be the case; for example, cytochrome P-420 that forms when microsomes are incubated with purified phospholipase C remains bound to the microsomes (Chaplin and Mannering, 1969).

In a critical analysis of the manner in which these diverse agents may convert cytochrome P-450 to cytochrome P-420, Imai and Sato (1967a) concluded that the ultimate effect of each agent was to disrupt the association between hemoprotein and microsomal lipid. Depending upon the agent, this may occur either by its action on the lipid or by an effect on protein associated with the lipid. Since with few exceptions it is those drugs possessing high lipid solubility which react with the drug metabolizing system, the active area of cytochrome P-450 has been assumed to be in contact with or "imbedded" in a highly hydrophobic part of cytochrome P-450 protein or in lipids of the microsomal membrane. According to Imai and Sato (1967a), "the specific structural relationship of the heme to the hydrophobic region seems to be maintained by the special ternary conformation of the P-450 protein or by the high lipid content in the membrane."

The unusual spectral properties of cytochrome P-450 are ascribed to a hydrophobic interaction of the heme with nearby components. Depending upon the agent employed, the conversion of cytochrome P-450 to cytochrome P-420 would result from the disturbance of the hydrophobic environment around the heme either by primary action of the agent or by secondary effects caused by conformational changes in the hemoprotein. These authors provide several arguments to support their view. The observation that cytochrome P-450 can be solubilized by detergents, but not by proteases which solubilize about half of the microsomal protein (Omura and Sato, 1964a), favors the concept of a strong interaction of lipid and protein. Detergents disrupt hydrophobic bonds in general and they denature proteins. The action of phospholipase A on microsomes produces lysolecithin, itself a powerful detergent. Chelating agents like bathocuproine sulfonate are soluble in both aqueous and lipid solvents and could therefore act as detergents. Proteases cause modifications in the conformation of the hemoprotein which lead to a breakdown of the hydrophobic interaction of the heme. Hydrophobic bonds could also be disrupted by the protein denaturates, urea and guanidine.

Aniline and other substrates of the drug metabolizing system produce characteristic spectral changes when they combine with cytochrome P-450, which probably reflect certain alterations in the conformation of the proteins. Alcohols in fairly high concentrations also produce these spectral changes. The effectiveness of neutral salts in causing the conversion of cytochrome P-450 to cytochrome P-420 obeys the order known as Hofmeister's lyotropic series of ions ($SCN^- > I^- > Br^- > Cl^- > SO_4^-$, CH_3COO^- for anions, and $Li^+ > K^+$, Na^+ for cations), which was originally determined for the capability of salts to precipitate proteins from aqueous solution (Hofmeister, 1888). Since, with minor exceptions, the same order of activity of ions can be applied for the destabilization of macromolecules such as ribonuclease (von Hippel and Wong, 1964, 1965), collagen (von Hippel and Wong, 1962), myosin (Tonomura *et al.*, 1962) and DNA (Hamaguchi and Geiduschek, 1962), it is suggested that the conversion of cytochrome P-450 to cytochrome P-420 by salts also involves the destabilization of macromolecules.

Electron spin resonance studies show that cytochrome P-420 can exist in four states (Mason *et al.*, 1965; Ichikawa and Yamano, 1967; Ichikawa *et al.*, 1968), designated β, γ, δ and ω by Mason's group, which show the same spectra, but which differ from one another in their spin states. Detergents, organic solvents and proteases act on cytochrome P-450 (the α state of the hemoprotein) to produce the β and γ states. Purified cytochrome P-420 prepared by the action of snake venom on microsomes is a low spin hemoprotein (δ state). The ω (high spin) state of the ferrihemoprotein can be obtained by the action of mercurials on the hemoprotein while it is in the α or γ state. This suggests that with mercurials, and perhaps with iodine, the conversion mechanism differs from that operating with other reagents. However, mercurials and iodine cause modifications of proteins, especially by reacting with sulfhydryl groups. Mason *et al.* (1965) have proposed that sulfide serves as a ligand in cytochrome P-450, in which case, these reagents could attack the ligand itself to cause the conversion to cytochrome P-420.

Ichikawa and coworkers (Ichikawa and Yamano, 1967; Ichikawa *et al.*, 1968) also visualize a stepwise conversion of cytochrome P-450 to cytochrome P-420 whereby hydrophobic binding is first disrupted by detergents, anilines, ketones, and alcohols and this is followed by the loss of ligands responsible for ESR signals.

Cytochrome P-420 formed as a result of treatment of microsomes with the detergent, sodium cholate, or the sulfhydryl reagent, p-chloromercuribenzoate, was converted back to cytochrome P-450 by polyols (glycerol, polyethylene glycol, propylene glycol, ethylene glycol monobutyl ether, diethylene glycol monoethyl ether) and reduced glutathione (Ichikawa and Yamano, 1967). Dialysis also produced partial reversal. Only the high spin form of cytochrome P-420 (ω state) was convertible to cytochrome P-450.

4. Concentration in hepatic microsomes. The molar extinction co-efficient of cytochrome P-450 has been estimated indirectly from studies employing solubilized and purified cytochrome P-420 (Omura and Sato, 1963, 1964a). Cytochrome P-450 was converted to soluble cytochrome P-420 through the combined actions of heated snake venom and deoxycholate and purified by ammonium sulfate fractionation, gel filtration through Sephadex and hydroxyl-apatite column chromatography. The final preparation represented a 4- to 6-fold purification over microsomes and contained 6–7 mμmoles of protoheme/mg of protein. From the absorption spectra it was possible to calculate the extinction coefficient on the basis of protoheme content. The following values were obtained (mM^{-1} cm^{-1}): oxidized form at 414 mμ, 124; reduced form at 426 mμ, 149; CO compound at 422 mμ, 213; CO compound (increment between 420 and 490 mμ), 111. From the last value and the change in the CO-difference spectrum accompanying the conversion of cytochrome P-450 to cytochrome P-420, the increment of molar extinction coefficient between 450 and 490 mμ was estimated to be 91 mM^{-1} cm^{-1}. Using this value, Omura and Sato found a microsomal preparation from rabbit liver to contain 1.55 mμmoles of cytochrome P-450/mg of protein. The same preparation contained 1.12 and 2.55 mμmoles/mg of protein of cytochrome b$_5$ and protoheme, respectively. Thus all of the microsomal heme was accounted for by cytochrome b$_5$ and cytochrome P-450. It has become the common practice to estimate the cytochrome P-450 content of microsomal preparations on the basis of the molar extinction increment between 450 and 490 mμ of 91 mM^{-1} cm^{-1}.

Cytochrome P-450 levels in hepatic microsomes are increased markedly by the administration of phenobarbital, 3-methylcholanthrene and many other compounds known to increase the drug metabolizing activity of the liver (reviewed recently by Conney, 1967; Mannering, 1968; Kuntzman, 1969). The increase in cytochrome P-450 after phenobarbital administration, and the subsequent decline to the normal level after the effect of the barbiturate has run its course, parallel the gradual increase and subsequent decline in the rate of drug metabolism that occurs. However, the rate of metabolism of certain drugs does not increase with the increase in the cytochrome P-450 level (Sladek and Mannering, 1966, 1969; Mannering et al., 1969). The reason for this will be discussed under the heading Cytochrome P_1-450 later in this chapter.

Cytochrome P-450 levels increase in the livers of male, but not female, rats as they age from birth to maturity (El Defrawy, 1967). Fasting increases the cytochrome P-450 content of hepatic microsomes (Ichikawa et al., 1967). Levels are lowered in male rats by morphine (Sladek and Mannering, 1969a; Mannering et al., 1969) and by thyroxin (Mannering et al., 1969) administration.

5. Binding to drugs. Narasimhulu and coworkers (1965) observed characteristic spectral changes when 17-hydroxyprogesterone was added to the cytochrome P-450 dependent steroid C-21 hydroxylase system in adrenal cortical microsomes. This prompted studies by Remmer and associates (1966) and Imai and Sato (1966), published almost simultaneously, which showed that drugs and other foreign compounds combine with hepatic cytochrome P-450 to produce difference spectra of two general types, type I and type II. Compounds giving type I or II difference spectra with hepatic microsomes have come to be known as type I or type II compounds (or drugs). Type I compounds give a difference spectrum with a λ_{max} in the general range of 385–390 mμ and a λ_{min} in the equally broad range of 418–427 mμ; the λ_{max} and λ_{min} given by type II compounds are 425–435 and 390–405 mμ, respectively (Schenkman et al., 1967). Thus, with opposing λ_{max} and λ_{min}, type I and type II spectra are approximate mirror images of each other. Type I and II spectra given by a typical type I (hexobarbital) and a typical type II (aniline) compound are shown in Figure 12.6.

The reason for the characteristic difference spectra seen when type I or type II drugs are added to microsomes can be seen when the absolute spectra of cytochrome P-450 are recorded before and after the addition of hexobarbital (type I) or aniline (type II). Using the technique of Kinoshita and Horie (vide supra) with oxidized microsomes from untreated animals (reference cuvette) and animals treated with phenobarbital (sample cuvette), Remmer and associates (1969) recorded the absolute spectra of cytochrome P-450, cytochrome P-450 + hexobarbital, and cytochrome P-450 + aniline. Hexobarbital caused a shift of the absolute spectrum in the direction of lower wavelengths with the λ_{max} shifting from 420 mμ to 415 mμ. The addition of aniline caused a shift of the absolute spectrum in the direction of higher wavelengths with the λ_{max} shifting from 420 mμ to 426 mμ. When the difference between the absolute spectra seen with and without drugs was plotted, a curve was obtained almost identical to the difference spectrum seen experimentally when either hexobarbital or aniline was employed.

Table 12.1 lists type I and II drugs as classified by the difference spectra they produced when combined with hepatic microsomes from several sources. With but one exception, type I and type II compounds produced their characteristic

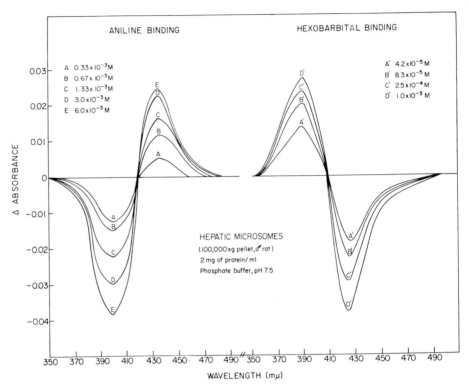

Fig. 12.6. Type I and type II binding spectra given by different concentrations of typical type I and type II compounds (hexobarbital, type I; aniline, type II).

binding spectra consistently regardless of the source of microsomes. The exception is phenobarbital, which gave a type I binding spectrum with microsomes from rats, but a type II binding spectrum with microsomes from rabbits. Assuming that type I and type II binding sites are located on a single cytochrome P-450, this would suggest a qualitative difference in the cytochrome P-450's from the two species; assuming the other possibility, that two cytochrome P-450's exist, one possessing a type I binding site and the other a type II binding site, the difference in the way phenobarbital binds with microsomes from the two species would suggest that the proportions of the two cytochromes differ markedly in rat and rabbit microsomes. It is also to be noted that in low concentrations phenobarbital produced a type I spectrum with microsomes from rabbits.

A sex difference in the binding properties of cytochrome P-450 as well as an age difference has been observed in rats. Male rats have long been known to metabolize certain drugs more rapidly than female rats, a phenomenon not seen in other laboratory animals commonly employed. This sex difference between mature male and female rats has recently been shown to relate to quantitative differences in the binding spectra produced by type I drugs (Schenkman et al., 1967a). No difference was observed between the abilities of microsomes from mature male and female rats to oxidize aniline or to combine with aniline to form the type II spectrum. However, the oxidation of aminopyrine, a type I drug, and the binding of aminopyrine and hexobarbital (type I) by microsomes from male rats were much greater than observed with microsomes from female rats. No sex

TABLE 12.1

Qualitative differences in the binding of compounds to hepatic hemoprotein as determined by difference spectra

No.	Compound	Animal Species[a]	Pretreatment of animal[b]	Type of Binding		References
				I[c]	II[d]	
1	Acetanilide	R	N		+	h
2	Acetone	Rb	N		+	f
3	Alcohols (methyl-, ethyl-, 2-propyl-, isobutyl-, isoamyl-)	Rb	P		+	f
	1-Butanol	Rb	M		+	g
4	Amines (n-propyl-, n-butyl-, n-pentyl-, n-heptyl-, n-acetyl-, n-decyl-, benzyl-, cyclohexyl-)	Rb	N		+	g
		Rb	M		+	g
		Rb	P		+	g
5	p-Aminophenol	R	N		+	h
6	Aminopyrine	R	N	+		e, h
	(Dimethylaminoantipyrine)	M	P	+		i
7	Amobarbital	R	N	+		e, h
8	Amphetamine	R	N		+	j
9	Aniline	R	N		+	e, h, j, k, l
		R	P		+	e, k, l
		R	B		+	e
		Rb	N		+	f, k
		Rb	P		+	g
		Rb	M		+	g
		G	N		+	k
		M	P		+	i
10	3,4-Benzpyrene	R	B	+		m
11	Chlorpromazine	R	N	+		h
12	Corticosterone	R	N		+	h
13	Cortisol	R	N		+	h
14	Coumarin	Rb	N	+		n
15	Cyanide	R	N		+	h
16	Cyclohexane	R	N	+		o
17	DDT	R	N	+		h
18	Desdimethylimipramine	M	P		+	i
19	Dihydrosafrole	Rb	N	+		f
20	N,N-Dimethylaniline	R	N	+		h
21	Dioxane	Rb	P		+	f
22	DPEA[p]	R	N		+	e, h, q
		M	P		+	i
23	β-Estradiol	R	N	+		h
24	Ethylbenzene	R	N	+		r
25	Ethyl isocyanide	R	N		+	h
26	Ethylmorphine	R	N	+		j, s
		R	P	+		j
		G, Rb, M	N	+		s
		M	P	+		i
27	Hexobarbital	R	N	+		e, h, l
		R	B	+		e
		R	M	+		l
		R	P	+		e, l, t
		Rb	N	+		u
		M	P	+		i

TABLE 12.1—*Continued*

No.	Compound	Animal Species[a]	Pretreatment of animal[b]	Type of Binding I[c]	Type of Binding II[d]	References
28	Imidazole	M	N		+	i
		Rb	P		+	g
29	Imipramine	R	N	+		h
30	Lilly 327-169-22B[v]	M	N	+		i, w
31	Lilly 390-378-23B[x]	M	N	+	+	i, w
32	N-Methylaniline	R	N		+	j
		Rb	P		+	g
33	3-Methyl-4-Methylaminoazobenzene	R	N		+	j
34	Methylphenidate	R	N	+		j
35	Metyrapone	R	P		+	x
		M	P		+	z
36	Monomethylaminopyrine	Rb	N		+	f, k
37	Morphine	R	N	+		j
38	Naphthalene	M	P	+		z, aa
39	Nicotinamide	R	N		+	h
		M	N		+	i
		Rb	P		+	g
40	Nicotine	R	N		+	h
41	Phenacetin	Rb	N	+		f, k
42	Phenobarbital	R	N	+		e, h, j
		Rb	N	+[bb]		g
		Rb	N		+[cc]	f, g, j, k
		Rb	M		+	g
		Rb	P		+	g
43	Phenylhydrazine	Rb	P		+	g
44	Pregnenolene	R	N	+		dd
45	Progesterone	R	N	+		dd
46	Pyridine	R	N		+	h
		Rb	N		+	f
		Rb	P		+	g
		M	N		+	i
47	Rotenone	R	N		+	h
48	SKF 525-A[ee]	R	N	+		e, h, j
		R	M	+		j
		R	P	+		j
		M	N	+		i, w
49	SKF 8742-A[ff]	R	N	+		j
		M	N	+	+	w
50	SKF 26754-A[gg]	R	N		+	j
		M	N		+	i, w
51	Testosterone	R	N	+		h

[a] G = guinea pig; M = mouse; R = rat; Rb = rabbit.

[b] N: no treatment other than vehicle for agents; B: with 3,4-benzpyrene; M: with 3-methylcholanthrene; P: with phenobarbital.

[c] Difference spectrum: λ_{max}, 385–390 mμ; λ_{min}, 418–425 mμ (Schenkman *et al.*, 1967).

[d] Difference spectra: includes both Type II (λ_{max}, 425–435 mμ; λ_{min}, 390–405 mμ) and "modified" Type II (λ_{max}, 409–445 mμ; λ_{min}, 365–410 mμ) as described by Schenkman *et al.* (1967).

[e] Remmer *et al.*, 1966.

[f] Imai and Sato, 1967.

[g] Jefcoate *et al.*, 1969.

[h] Schenkman *et al.*, 1967.

[i] Sasame and Gillette, 1969.

TABLE 12.1—*Continued*

j Shoeman and Mannering, unpublished results.

k Imai and Sato, 1966.

l Shoeman *et al.*, 1969.

m Schenkman *et al.*, 1969.

n Kratz and Staudinger, 1968.

o Ullrich, 1969.

p 2,4-dichloro-6-phenylphenoxyethyla-mine.

q Gigon *et al.*, 1969.

r McMahon and Sullivan, 1969.

s Davies *et al.*, 1969.

t Cammer *et al.*, 1966.

u Schenkman and Sato, 1968.

v 2,4-dichloro-6-phenylphenoxyethyldi-ethylamine.

w Gillette, 1969.

x Hildebrandt *et al.*, 1969.

y 2,4-dichloro-6-phenylphenoxyethyl-methylamine.

z Netter *et al.*, 1969.

aa Netter, 1969.

bb Low concentrations of phenobarbital were used.

cc High concentrations of phenobarbital were used.

dd Mitani and Horie, 1969.

ee 2-diethylaminoethyl 2,2-diphenylval-erate HCl.

ff 2-ethylaminoethyl 2,2-diphenylvaler-ate.

gg aminoethyl 2,2-diphenylvalerate HCl.

difference in the rate of metabolism of drugs is seen in immature rats, which suggests the occurrence of a qualitative change in cytochrome P-450 as male rats mature.

Microsomes are known to lose some of their ability to metabolize certain drugs when stored in the cold. This is probably due to the loss of the type I binding site. Storage of microsomes at $-5°C$ for seven days caused almost complete loss of type I binding, but had little or no effect on type II binding (Shoeman *et al.*, 1969a).

It will be noted in Table 12.1 that many of the type II compounds are amines. Comparison of tertiary, secondary and primary amines shows a shift from type I binding to type II binding with a decrease in degree of N-alkylation. Thus, the tertiary amine, SKF 525-A, is a type I compound, the secondary amine, SKF 8742-A, shows both type I and type II binding characteristics, and the primary amine, SKF 26754-A, is a type II compound. A comparable relationship is seen with the dichlorophenylphenoxyethylamines, Lilly 327-169-22B (tertiary), Lilly 390-378-23B (secondary) and DPEA (primary).

It may be of some interest that compounds which induce increased microsomal drug metabolism tend to be type I compounds. In a previous review (Mannering, 1968) Table 3.1 lists a large number of inducing agents. Although many of the compounds found in Table 12.1 are not found in Table 3.1, with but one exception, all of the compounds found in both tables are type I compounds. The one exception is nicotine, a type II compound which is reported to be an inducing agent.

Nicotinamide is a type II compound. In the past it was frequently added to incubation mixtures when drug metabolism was studied. This was to prevent the loss of NADP by inhibiting nucleotidase. However, Schenkman and coworkers (1967b) found that in concentrations used commonly, drug metabolism was inhibited by nicotinamide, probably because it combines with cytochrome P-450. As a result of this study, most investigators have learned to exclude nicotinamide from their incubation mixtures.

A number of compounds studied by Schenkman and coworkers (1967) for their binding characteristics gave type II spectra with λ_{max} and λ_{min} falling well outside the usual range. These compounds were classified as "modified type II" compounds. Representatives of this group are cortisol, corticosterone, acetanilide, ethyl isocyanide, cyanide and rotenone. Sasame and Gillette (1969) have suggested that these compounds produce their atypical spectra because they combine with the type I binding site as well as with the type II binding site. If the modified type II spectrum is simply a "typical" type II spectrum with wider ranges of λ_{max} and λ_{min}, and this greater range in the locations of the peaks and troughs is due to the ability of modified type II compounds to combine with both type I and type II sites, then the smaller range of λ_{max} and λ_{min} seen in the spectra obtained with typical type II compounds may simply reflect a lesser tendency of these compounds to combine with both sites. The possibility must therefore be considered that few if any compounds combine exclusively with either the type I or type II binding site and that compounds produce composite spectra which in varying degrees are only predominantly type I or type II. The alignments of the peaks and troughs of type I and type II compounds are such that they tend to cancel each other. However, the alignments are not perfect and this might account for the variations in λ_{min} and λ_{max} in the composite spectrum seen when type I and type II binding occurs simultaneously. A compound capable of combining equally well with both binding sites would present essentially no difference spectrum. The molar extinction of a type I compound would be reduced by whatever degree the compound also combines with the type II site and the molar extinction of a type II compound would be effected in a like manner by a type I binding component.

While there would seem to be little question that the spectral changes seen when drugs are added to microsomes result from interactions of drugs with cytochrome P-450, it might be well to pause at this point and review the evidence supporting this concept. Imai and Sato (1967) list the following lines of evidence:

1) The magnitude of the spectral change is proportional to the content of cytochrome P-450 contained in different microsomal preparations.

2) Ethyl isocyanide combines with cytochrome P-450 in aerobic microsomes to produce a difference spectrum with a peak at 434 mμ (Nishibayashi *et al.*, 1966). Aniline, a compound which gives a binding spectrum (type II) with microsomes, interferes competitively with the binding of ethyl isocyanide to cytochrome P-450.

3) Aniline gives a maximum binding spectrum with microsomes at 427 mμ. The peak seen when aniline is added to partially purified cytochrome P-420 occurs at 417 mμ and it has a much lower molar extinction than the 427 mμ peak seen with microsomes. All treatments causing a conversion of cytochrome P-450 to cytochrome P-420 caused a decrease in the aniline binding spectrum and a shift of the λ_{max} from 427 mμ toward 417 mμ. The extent of these changes in the aniline difference spectrum paralleled the extent of cytochrome P-420 formation on partial conversion of P-450. Ullrich (1969) also showed a loss of cyclohexane binding (type I) corresponding to the extent of conversion of cytochrome P-450 to cytochrome P-420.

4) Purified cytochrome b$_5$, the other hemoprotein in microsomes, produces no spectral interactions with the compounds that cause spectral changes in microsomes.

If further evidence is needed that the binding spectra result from interactions with cytochrome P-450, it can be found in the observation of Lu and Coon (Lu *et al.*, 1969, 1969a) that solubilized and partially purified cytochrome P-450 combines with type I and type II compounds to give characteristic binding spectra.

When microsomes were incubated under nitrogen at 4°C for 24 hours with 0.07 % steapsin, about 25 % of the microsomal cytochrome P-450 was converted to cytochrome P-420 and released into the medium. After removing salts with Sephadex G-25 and concentrating the clear solution to about one fourth its volume, an aggregate was formed containing a high concentration of cytochrome P-420 and no cytochrome b_5. Electron microscopy showed the aggregate to consist of microtubules with globular substructures (Shoeman *et al.*, 1969). The addition of 1.6 mM hexobarbital or 10 mM aniline to suspensions of the aggregated cytochrome P-420 resulted in typical type I and type II spectra, respectively. Soluble cytochrome P-420 did not form binding spectra with these concentrations of hexobarbital or aniline. These studies show the importance of macromolecular organization in the binding of drugs to hemoprotein. Imai and Sato (1967) demonstrated type II binding of aniline to soluble cytochrome P-420, but a high concentration of aniline (67 mM) was required and the λ_{max} was at 417 $m\mu$ rather than at 427 $m\mu$, the λ_{max} observed when aggregates of cytochrome P-420 were used.

Because cytochrome P-450 has not been obtained in highly purified form, little is known about the chemical bonds of the heme moiety or of the coordination bonds of the fifth and sixth ligands of the heme iron. Attempts to determine the nature of the binding sites of cytochrome P-450 have therefore been highly speculative. In one of the earliest publications describing drug binding, Schenkman and coworkers (1967) offered three alternative hypotheses:

1) Type I and II binding spectra result from interactions of compounds with two different molecular species of cytochrome P-450. They point out that this hypothesis is weakened because substrates causing one type of spectral change competitively inhibit the metabolism of substrates which cause the same and the other type spectral change.

2) Type I and II compounds affect different ligands of the heme with the enzyme protein thereby modifying the heme-protein ligand interaction and causing a spectral shift. An alternative of this hypothesis is that of substances causing different types of spectral change by modifying the ligand on different sides of the heme of cytochrome P-450. Spectral changes may be due to modification of the molar extinction coefficient of the hemoprotein as more or less nucleophilic substances interact near the heme iron, thus altering the heme-iron-protein interaction. Electron paramagnetic resonance (EPR) spectroscopy (Cammer *et al.*, 1966) supports the suggestion that substrate interaction modifies ligand interaction with the heme iron of cytochrome P-450.

3) Type I and II spectral changes result from an alteration of the oxidation state of cytochrome P-450. This hypothesis implies an electron transfer during interaction with the substrate. Experimental evidence provided by these authors tended to rule out this possibility. The second hypothesis was favored.

Imai and Sato (1967) offer four hypotheses:

1) The substrate substitutes a ligand for the heme iron of cytochrome P-450 thereby modifying the molecular extinction coefficient of the hemoprotein.

2) The substrate modifies the ligand state of the hemoprotein by interacting

with the porphyrin ring. They point out that this interaction is without precedent and therefore seems unlikely, if not impossible.

3) The substrate combines with a specific site located on the protein moiety of cytochrome P-450 causing a conformational change in the hemoprotein molecule to alter the ligand state. Different types of substrates may or may not combine with different sites on the protein moiety.

4) The substrate interacts indirectly with cytochrome P-450 through phospholipid surrounding the hemoprotein. This alters the hydrophobic environment of the heme group with a consequent modification of the ligand state.

Imai and Sato favor the third hypothesis for a number of reasons. Although aniline, and conceivably other type II compounds, are capable of combining with iron as a ligand, as evidenced by its ability to displace carbon monoxide (Schenkman *et al.*, 1967), most substrates of the drug hydroxylase system, as judged by their chemical structures, are unsuitable as ligands for heme iron. The established role of the heme of cytochrome P-450 as the oxygen-activating site in drug hydroxylations further excludes the possibility of direct combination of substrate with heme. Of the six ligand sites of iron, four are occupied by pyrrole nitrogens of the porphyrin ring. One of the remaining two ligands must be available for the substitution by oxygen if the hydroxylation process is to occur. Because the last ligand is situated on the opposite side of the heme molecule from that which involves the oxygen molecule, it seems unlikely, if not impossible, for the substrate bound to the sixth ligand to react with the activated oxygen. Thus while the heme iron does not seem to be suitable for substrate binding, it can be assumed that the substrate is bound closely enough to the activated oxygen molecule to react with it. The spectral changes would occur because of a secondary effect on the ligand state due to a conformational change in the protein caused by drug binding. The degree of conformational change and exact location of the peak would vary with the substrate. The concept does not exclude the possibility that certain compounds might bind to hemoprotein without producing a conformational change; thus failure of a compound to exhibit a binding spectrum would not necessarily exclude it as a substrate for the hydroxylation reaction.

The hypothesis is consistent with the observation of Imai and Sato that organic solvents caused spectral changes similar to those produced by type II drugs. The concentrations of alcohols required to produce binding spectra were of the same order of magnitude as those known to cause changes in protein conformation. Moreover, the relative intensities of spectral changes induced by a given concentration of alcohol were as follows: isoamyl > isobutyl > isopropyl > ethyl > methyl, which is the order in which alcohols are known to cause conformational changes in protein by disrupting hydrophobic bonds.

Imai and Sato do not except the possibility that the binding spectra caused by solvents may be due to a disruption of the lipid environment surrounding the hemoprotein. The finding that higher concentrations of aniline or organic solvents cause the conversion of cytochrome P-450 to cytochrome P-420 (*vide supra*) also supports the third or fourth hypothesis. Imai and Sato believe that the modifications of electron paramagnetic resonance (EPR) signals that result when drugs interact with cytochrome P-450 (Cammer *et al.*, 1966) are sufficiently small that they may be accounted for by the secondary alteration in the ligand state mediated by a conformational change in protein as well as by an alteration in heme-protein ligand interaction.

Jefcoate and coworkers (1969) have provided further evidence for the hydrophobic nature of the drug binding sites. For hydrophobic binding without steric restriction, a linear increase in binding energy with chain length has been predicted by theory (Nemethy and Scheraga, 1963) and found in practice for inhibitors of alcohol dehydrogenase (Anderson et al., 1965). Jefcoate and coworkers divided type II binding into two classes, type IIa (λ_{max} 427 mμ, λ_{min} 392 mμ) and type IIb (λ_{max} 432 mμ, λ_{min} 410 mμ). When the log of the binding constant, K, (which is proportional to binding energy) of the type IIb binding of a series of n-alkylamines was plotted against chain length, excellent linearity was obtained between C_3 and C_8. The magnitude of the binding energy produced by the addition of each methylene group was typical for hydrophobic binding of an alkyl side chain in a nonpolar cavity (Nemethy, 1967). The authors proposed that such a cavity could be provided either by the cytochrome P-450 protein or by the microsomal membrane.

Schenkman and coworkers (1967) attributed the type II spectral change to ferrihemochrome formation, a conclusion based on the characteristics of the spectrum, the fact that type II compounds were amines and the observation that aniline, a type II compound, displaced CO from cytochrome P-450. This led to the use of ferriheme solutions as a model system for binding studies (Schenkman and Sato, 1968). Spectral changes in ferriheme solutions very similar to the type I binding spectrum were produced simply by varying the pH of the solution between 5 and 8. This suggested that the type I binding spectrum results from an alteration in the electronegativity of the sixth ligand of the heme. Nonpolar substances are able to invade the hydrophobic region of the apoenzyme (possibly the active site) and displace the sixth ligand. It is suggested that two forms of cytochrome P-450 exist; one is the unreacted enzyme, the other is the substrate-bound enzyme. In the course of the metabolism of the substrate, the first form is converted to the second form and this transition is accompanied by the type I spectral change.

When microsomes are treated with iodine, cytochrome P-450 is converted to cytochrome P-420 and a spectral trough is seen at about 420 mμ corresponding to the trough produced by the type I compound, cyclohexane (Ullrich, 1969). Cyclohexane binding is lost proportionately as cytochrome P-450 is converted to cytochrome P-420 by iodine. The ΔO.D. of the trough produced by iodine, which is much larger than that seen with cyclohexane, is thought by Ullrich to be a measure of the total amount of cytochrome P-450 in microsomes, whereas the ΔO.D. of the trough produced by cyclohexane is representative of that part of the total cytochrome P-450 capable of participating in the binding interaction.

Ullrich estimates that only about 12% of the cytochrome P-450 in microsomes from untreated rats and about 32% in microsomes from phenobarbital-treated rats is capable of binding with cyclohexane. The turnover number for the hydroxylation of cyclohexane was determined using microsomes from animals that had been induced to varying degrees with phenobarbital. Microsomes from these animals contained widely different amounts of cytochrome P-450, which also varied greatly in its ability to bind with cyclohexane. The turnover number was the same regardless of source of microsomes when the amount of "bindable" cytochrome P-450 was used in the calculations, but not when the total cyto-chrome P-450 was employed as the reference.

In our laboratory, purified phospholipase C from *Clostridium welchii* was used in an attempt to evaluate the role of phospholipids in the binding and metabo-lism of drugs (Chaplin and Mannering, 1969). Phospholipase C specifically hydrolyzes phosphatidylcholines and phosphatidylethanolamines to correspond-ing phosphoryl products. Untreated and phospholipase C treated hepatic micro-somes from rats were used to study the oxidation and binding of two type I drugs, ethylmorphine and hexobarbital, and the type II compound, aniline. Phospho-lipase C virtually destroyed the type I binding site, but microsomes lost only about 40% of their ability to oxidize ethylmorphine and hexobarbital. The loss of aniline oxidation was only about 15% and the binding of aniline was increased significantly. That phospholipase C destroys type I binding, but not type II binding, provides further evidence that the two binding sites differ and supports the view that the type I binding site is closely associated with phospholipids. Phospholipids appear to be essential for the specific conformation of the type I binding site; they may even be an integral part of the sixth ligand to the heme of cytochrome P-450.

The enhanced type II binding spectrum that results after microsomes are treated with phospholipase C may be explained in at least two ways:

1) The ligand state of the hemoprotein may be affected by its association in the membrane with phospholipid. When released from this association, new dis-sociation constants for type II compounds come into effect.

2) Aniline may be reactive with both the type I site and the type II site, but more reactive with the type II site, indicated by the fact it gives a type II spec-trum. The procedure whereby difference spectra are obtained is such that any binding of aniline to the type I site would cause a corresponding reduction of the type II binding spectrum. Removal of the type I site would remove this com-petitive interference with the type II spectrum produced by aniline.

The studies employing phospholipase C show that a compound need not produce a binding spectrum to be metabolized. This does not necessarily mean that the compound does not bind to cytochrome P-450 but simply that it does not cause a conformational change in the hemoprotein. The oxidation of ethyl-morphine and hexobarbital by phospholipase C-treated microsomes was in-hibited by CO, which tends to rule out some mechanism other than one involving cytochrome P-450. While the type I binding site may not be obligatory for the oxidation of type I compounds, it would appear to be facilitative. Thus, treat-ment of microsomes with phospholipase C increased the K_m for ethylmorphine N-demethylation from 29 to 69 mM and decreased the V_{max} from 510 to 335 mμmoles of HCHO formed/mg of protein/hr.

Imai and Sato (1967) have pointed out that barbital and benzene are hy-droxylated by microsomes although they do not produce binding spectra. It is also to be noted that the ability of compounds to form binding spectra with cytochrome P-450 does not guarantee their metabolism; many n-alkylamines combine avidly with cytochrome P-450 to produce type II binding spectra, but are not metabolized (Jefcoate et al., 1969).

Phospholipase C caused about a 20% conversion of cytochrome P-450 to cytochrome P-420 while producing an almost complete loss of type I binding (Chaplin and Mannering, 1969). This would support Ullrich's contention that only a relatively small percentage of the cytochrome P-450 in microsomes is available for drug binding (Ullrich, 1969).

Of greatest interest to the observers of binding spectra was the apparent relationship between the kinetics of drug binding and the kinetics of drug metabolism. The familiar double reciprocal Lineweaver-Burk plot of the ΔO.D. of spectral change *vs* concentration of drug can be used to derive the spectral dissociation constant (K_s) in the manner that the Michaelis constant (K_m) is obtained for the oxidation of the same compound by plotting the reciprocal of the velocity of the reaction against the reciprocal of the substrate concentration. In a number of cases, the K_s and the K_m for a given compound were found to be similar and this encouraged the view that drug binding is an obligatory step in the mechanism of drug hydroxylation.

Table 12.2 summarizes the results of studies from several laboratories where comparisons were made between the K_s and K_m of compounds reacting with cytochrome P-450. To remark that the case for $K_s = K_m$ is not very convincing would be charitable. Not only does K_s fail to equal K_m in many cases, but the absolute values for K_s and K_m vary greatly from species to species and from laboratory to laboratory for a given species. Even in the same laboratory, when aniline was studied, $K_s = K_m$ one time (Remmer *et al.*, 1966), but differed by an order of magnitude another time (Schenkman *et al.*, 1967). Perhaps it is more than can be expected that the two kinetic constants will be equal under all conditions for all drugs that bind to cytochrome P-450. From the data in Table 12.2 it is obvious that conditions vary greatly from laboratory to laboratory. This may be due to differences in the age or strain of the animals employed or to variations in environmental conditions. If the K_s is to equal the K_m, a number of conditions must be met:

1) Essentially all of the hydroxylation that occurs must be associated with spectral binding. As suggested by the studies employing phospholipase C (*vide supra*), this may not be the case.

2) The compound must bind almost exclusively with either the type I binding site or the type II binding site, or if binding occurs at both sites in varying degrees, i.e., with different spectral dissociation constants for each of the sites, those spectral dissociation constants must closely match the Michaelis constants for the metabolism of the drug being mediated through each of the sites.

3) More than one molecular species of cytochrome P-450 may exist in a given source of microsomes. The relative amounts of each may differ among animal species or within a species under different conditions. If the K_s is to equal the K_m when all sources of microsomes are employed, the K_s and K_m for a given compound must be the same for each of the molecular species of cytochrome P-450, or if not, the relative amounts of each of the kinds of cytochrome P-450 must be the same in all sources of microsomes.

4) The K_m is dependent upon kinetic constants that take into account the dissociation of the enzyme-substrate complex into product and enzyme, as well as those governing the formation of the enzyme-substrate complex, whereas only the latter kinetic constants determine the K_s; the K_s can be expected to be similar to the K_m only if the constants for the dissociation of the complex to product and enzyme are minimal with respect to the constants governing the formation of the complex.

Cytochrome P-450 can be oxygenated only when in the reduced form and must

TABLE 12.2

Comparison of spectral dissociation constants (K_s) *and Michaelis constants* (K_m) *of compounds reacting with microsomal hemoprotein*

Compound	Type of Binding	Reaction Measured	Species of Animal[a]	K_s (M × 10⁴)	K_m (M × 10⁴)	Reference
Aminopyrine	I	N-demethylation	R	4	8	b
				3.3	3.6	c
Aniline	II	Hydroxylation	R	8	7	b
				3.6	0.4	c
				5–10	5–10	d
				3.3	0.4	e
				5.4[f]	1.0[f]	e
				38	0.5	g
			Rb	26	17–20	d
			G	50	60	d
Coumarin	I	Hydroxylation	Rb	9[h]	0.06	i
Cyclohexane	I	Hydroxylation	R[j]	7.4	4.3	k
Ethylmorphine	I	N-demethylation	R ♂	2.5	3.2	l
			♂	1.9	3.4	g
			♀	3.5	5.6	l
			G ♂	10.8	12.5	l
			♀	13.2	13.1	l
			M ♂	9	11	l
			♀	6	9	l
			Rb ♂	9.5	20.5	l
			♀	9.0	20.8	l
Hexobarbital	I	Hydroxylation	R	0.8	1	c
				6.8	—	g
				—	12	m
Monomethylamino-pyrine	II	N-demethylation	Rb	18	17	d
SKF 525-A[n]	I	N-deethylation	R	0.067	1.4	g

[a] G = guinea pig; M = mouse; R = rat; Rb = rabbit.

[b] Remmer *et al.*, 1966.

[c] Schenkman *et al.*, 1967.

[d] Imai and Sato, 1967.

[e] Guarino *et al.*, 1969.

[f] Microsomes were obtained from animals that had been pretreated with phenobarbital.

[g] Bidleman and Mannering, unpublished results

[h] Microsomes from both untreated and phenobarbital treated animals gave the same value.

[i] Kratz and Staudinger, 1968.

[j] Animals were treated with phenobarbital.

[k] Ullrich, 1969.

[l] Davies *et al.*, 1969.

[m] Rubin *et al.*, 1964.

[n] 2-diethylaminoethyl 2,2-diphenylvalerate.

therefore be in the reduced state when the activated oxygen reacts with the substrate. With the exception of metyrapone (Hildebrandt *et al.*, 1969), drugs do not bind to microsomes reduced by $Na_2S_2O_4$. Under anaerobic conditions aniline gives a binding spectrum with cytochrome P-450 reduced with NADPH (Imai and Sato, 1967). However, spectrophotometric studies show that in the presence of both oxygen and NADPH, cytochrome P-450 is mostly in the oxidized state. The reduction of cytochrome P-450 is believed to be the rate-limiting step in the overall process of microsomal metabolism (Davies *et al.*, 1969; Gigon *et al.*, 1969; Gillette and Gram, 1969). If the binding of drugs to oxidized cytochrome P-450 is to have any significance with respect to participation in the overall reaction, some means must be found for the drug-cytochrome P-450 (ox) complex to become the drug cytochrome P-450 (red) complex. The following scheme was proposed by Imai and Sato (1967) for aniline hydroxylation:

1. $P\text{-}450^{+++}$ + aniline → $[P\text{-}450^{+++}]$ − aniline (type II binding)

2. $[P\text{-}450^{+++}]$ − aniline $\xrightarrow{\text{specific microsomal electron}}_{\text{transfer system}}$ $[P\text{-}450^{++}]$ − aniline

3. $[P\text{-}450^{++}]$ − aniline + O_2 → $[P\text{-}450^{++}\cdot O_2]$ − aniline

4. $[P\text{-}450^{++}\cdot O_2]$ − aniline → $[P\text{-}450^{+++}]$ +p-aminophenol

where $[P\text{-}450^{+++}]$ −aniline and $[P\text{-}450^{++}\cdot O_2]$ indicate that aniline and oxygen are bound to a nonheme site and the heme iron of cytochrome P-450, respectively.

In the following scheme, Gillette (1969) presents a variety of ways in which oxidized cytochrome P-450, reduced cytochrome P-450, oxygen and drugs might interact during drug hydroxylation:

1. NADPH cytochrome c reductase + H^+ ⇌ $NADP^+$ + H_2-cytochrome c reductase

2. Cytochrome P-450 (Fe^{+3}) + substrate ⇌ cytochrome P-450 (Fe^{+3}) − ubstrate
S

3a. H_2-cytochrome c reductase + cytochrome P-450 (Fe^{+3}) $\xrightarrow{\text{carrier?}}$ cytochrome c reductase + cytochrome P-450 (Fe^{+2}) + $2H^+$ + e^-

3b. H_2-cytochrome c reductase + cytochrome P-450 (Fe^{+3}) − substrate $\xrightarrow{\text{carrier?}}$ cytochrome c reductase + cytochrome P-450 (Fe^{+2}) − substrate + $2H^+$ + e^-

4. Cytochrome P-450 (Fe^{+2}) + substrate ⇌ cytochrome P-450 (Fe^{+2}) − substrate

5a. Cytochrome P-450 (Fe^{+2}) + O_2 ⇌ cytochrome P-450 (FeO_2)

5b. Cytochrome P-450 (Fe^{+2}) − substrate + O_2 ⇌ cytochrome P-450 (FeO_2) − substrate

6. Cytochrome P-450 (FeO_2) + substrate ⇌ cytochrome P-450 (FeO_2) − substrate

7a. Cytochrome P-450 (FeO_2) + $2H^+$ + e^- → cytochrome P-450 (Fe^{+3}) + H_2O_2

7b. Cytochrome P-450 (FeO_2) − substrate + $2H^+$ + e^- → cytochrome P-450 (Fe^{+3}) + oxidized substrate + H_2O

Leibman and coworkers (1969) believe that many of the inconsistencies in the kinetics of binding and metabolism can be explained by the interconvertibility of type I and type II cytochrome P-450 complexes. This conclusion was drawn partly from kinetic studies in which either a type I or II compound (modifier) was added to a suspension of microsomes placed in both cuvettes of a dual beam spectrophotometer. Graded amounts of either a type I or type II compound (substrate) were added to the sample cuvette and the difference spectrum recorded. The sum of the absorbance changes at the wavelengths of the peak and the trough was determined. These data were then treated in the classical enzyme-substrate-inhibitor models using absorbance change in place of initial velocity. When the modifier was a type II compound and the substrate a type I compound, competitive "inhibition" was observed. When modifier and substrate were type II compounds, "inhibition" was never competitive, and in certain cases kinetics were analogous to classical non-competitive inhibition. Both competitive and non-competitive "inhibition" were seen when the modifier and substrate were type I compounds. When the modifier was a type I substance and the substrate a type II compound, "stimulation" rather than "inhibition" was seen.

They suggested that some of these results might be explained as illustrated in Figure 12.7. E represents the form of the oxidized hemoprotein whose absolute spectrum shows a peak at 395 mμ, and EX that form which may represent a complex of E with an endogenous substrate or membrane constituent. It has a peak at about 420 mμ. E can react with type II substrates to give spectral properties similar to those given by EX. The resulting increase in absorbance at 420 mμ and the decrease at 395 mμ result in a type II difference spectrum. Similarly, reaction of EX with a type I compound gives a complex similar to E, and the resulting increase in the 395 mμ peak and decrease in the 420 mμ peak gives rise to a type I difference spectrum. EI and EII are pictured as interconvertible. After maximal conversion of EX to EI, all of the hemoprotein is in a form in which it can react readily with a type II substrate. This would explain why "stimulation" was seen when the modifier was a type I compound and the substrate a type II compound. However, it does not explain why "stimulation" did not occur when the modifier was a type II compound and the substrate a type I compound. The authors suggest that other, unreactive complexes may be formed.

Netter and coworkers (1969) concluded from inhibition studies that type I and II binding sites reside on the same molecule and that the binding properties of one site are influenced by the reaction of substrate or inhibitor with the other site. In these studies, the inhibitor, metyrapone, a type II compound, was considered a counterpart of the inhibitor, SKF 525-A, a type I compound. They presented a "highly speculative schematic representation" (Fig. 12.8) of a possible molecular configuration of a microsomal hydroxylase, presumably cytochrome P-450. The converging arrows symbolize competition for binding sites. The wavy arrows denote allosteric interactions which mutually modify the properties of the binding sites.

The presence of more than one molecular species of cytochrome P-450 has been suggested from studies demonstrating the different patterns of products formed during microsomal oxidation of substrates, the wide diversity of substrates metabolized oxidatively, the preferential effect of inducing agents for causing the increased metabolism of some drugs, but not others, and the variation in the relative rates of metabolism observed with different animal species, between sexes in the rat, and in response to starvation, thyroxin and alloxan (Mannering, 1968). While there appears to be at least one other molecular species

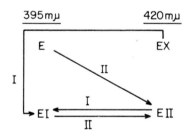

Fig. 12.7. Diagram showing proposed interaction of type I and type II cytochrome P-450-drug complexes (Leibman and coworkers, 1969). The diagram is discussed in the text.

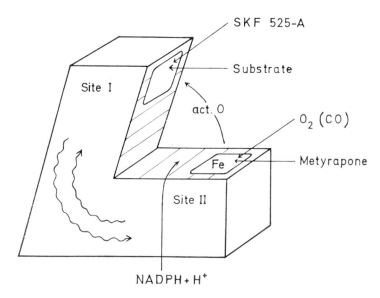

Fig. 12.8. Schematic representation of a molecular configuration of a microsomal hydroxylase illustrating possible interaction of type I and II binding sites. The converging arrows symbolize competition for binding sites. The wavy arrows denote allosteric interactions which mutually modify the properties of the binding sites. (Reprinted by permission from Netter *et al.* 1969).

of cytochrome P-450, as will be discussed under the heading *Cytochrome P_1-450*, most of these studies which purported to demonstrate the existence of more than one hydroxylase system can also be interpreted to mean that a single molecular species of cytochrome P-450 exists which reacts with different drugs in varying degrees through the type I or the type II binding site or via both sites in varying degrees. These differences between species, sexes and responses to environmental changes might simply reflect differences in the environment of the hemoprotein which in turn determine the degree of binding of drugs to type I or type II sites. Differences in the formation of an endogenous substance binding strongly to the type I site might represent one way in which the environment of the hemoprotein could be altered. The sex difference in the ability of rats to metabolize certain drugs has already been explained by an increase in the type I binding site that occurs in the male rat as it reaches maturity (Schenkman *et al.*, 1967a).

B. Cytochrome P_1-450 (P-448, P-446, High Spin P-450, Type a P-450)

The mechanism by which phenobarbital and many other drugs stimulate the synthesis of the microsomal drug metabolizing system has long been considered to be different from the mechanism whereby polycyclic hydrocarbons produce their inductive effects (reviewed by Mannering, 1968). This early assumption was based on the knowledge that drugs such as phenobarbital induce the increased metabolism of a much larger number of drugs and other foreign substances than do the polycyclic hydrocarbons such as 3-methylcholanthrene or 3,4-benzpyrene. Attempts in our laboratory to measure some of the differences between the two inductive processes led to the conclusion that polycyclic hydrocarbons cause the synthesis of a modified cytochrome P-450. For lack of a more suitable nomenclature for the microsomal hemoproteins, we named the hemoprotein *cytochrome P_1-450* (Sladek and Mannering, 1966, 1969, 1969a; Shoeman *et al.*, 1969a; Mannering *et al.*, 1969). A number of observations led to the recognition of cytochrome P_1-450:

1) In low concentrations, SKF 525-A (2-diethylaminoethyl 2,2-diphenylvalerate HCl), a potent inhibitor of drug metabolism, inhibited the N-demethylation of 3-methyl-4-methylaminoazobenzene (3-CH_3-MAB) by microsomes from untreated and phenobarbital-treated rats and the N-demethylation of ethylmorphine by microsomes from untreated and from phenobarbital- and 3-methylcholanthrene-treated rats, but much higher concentrations of SKF 525-A were required to inhibit the N-demethylation of 3-CH_3-MAB by microsomes from 3-methylcholanthrene-treated rats (Sladek and Mannering, 1969a). Because SKF 525-A is thought to inhibit drug metabolism in certain cases by acting as an alternative substrate (Anders and Mannering, 1966), this observation suggested that 3-methylcholanthrene had produced a change in the N-demethylating system such that the oxidation of SKF 525-A was retarded, but that of 3-CH_3-MAB was not.

2) Two-substrate kinetic studies employing ethylmorphine and 3-CH_3-MAB supported the view that the microsomal system responsible for 3-CH_3-MAB N-demethylation in rats treated with 3-methylcholanthrene is not the same as that found in untreated rats or in rats treated with phenobarbital (Sladek and Mannering, 1969a). These studies also suggested that a single enzyme system was responsible for the N-demethylations of both ethylmorphine and 3-CH_3-MAB when microsomes from untreated and phenobarbital-treated rats were used, but that when microsomes from 3-methylcholanthrene-treated rats were employed, two N-demethylating systems were involved, one of which reacted poorly with ethylmorphine.

3) The K_m of 3-CH_3-MAB N-demethylation of 10.1×10^{-5} M observed with microsomes from untreated rats was reduced to 2.9×10^{-5} M when microsomes from rats treated with 3-methylcholanthrene were employed (Sladek, 1966). No change in K_m was seen when ethylmorphine was the substrate.

4) In contrast to the hemoproteins from microsomes of untreated rats or rats treated with phenobarbital, which combine with both type I and type II compounds, the hemoprotein from 3-methylcholanthrene-treated rats appeared largely incapable of binding with type I compounds (Shoeman *et al.*, 1969a).

5) The parallel increases in rates of metabolism of certain drugs and cytochrome P-450 levels in the livers of animals during the administration of phenobarbital and their subsequent parallel decreases to normal values after the withdrawal of the barbiturate (Orrenius, 1965; Remmer and Merker, 1965) led to the conclusion that cytochrome P-450 may be the rate-limiting component of the microsomal drug metabolizing system. The observation that polycyclic hydrocarbons cause an increase in cytochrome P-450 (i.e., CO-binding hemoproteins) levels in the liver and an increase in the N-demethylation of 3-CH_3-MAB without increasing ethylmorphine N-demethylase activity (Sladek and Mannering, 1966, 1969, 1969a) suggested either that cytochrome P-450 is not the rate-limiting component in the overall reaction involving the N-demethylation of ethylmorphine by microsomes from untreated rats or that polycyclic hydrocarbons cause the production of a P-450 hemoprotein differing from that which existed previ-

ously in that it functions in the N-demethylation of 3-CH$_3$-MAB, but not in that of ethylmorphine.

6) Using ethyl isocyanide rather than carbon monoxide as the ligand for reduced microsomal hemoprotein, Imai and Sato (1966a) observed Soret peaks at 430 mμ and 455 mμ. The relative sizes of the two peaks were pH dependent, but the sum of the heights of the two peaks were about the same regardless of pH, which led to the conclusion that reduced cytochrome P-450 exists in two interconvertible forms. With the thought in mind that the effect of pH on this interconvertibility might differ from hemoprotein to hemoprotein, spectral measurements of the binding of ethyl isocyanide to hemoprotein were made at different pH's. In developing their concept, Imai and Sato plotted the heights of the 430 and 455 mμ peaks obtained at different pH's. The curves intercepted at pH 7.4, the pH at which the heights of the two peaks are equal. When similar curves were constructed using microsomes from untreated or phenobarbital-treated rats, the intercepts were the same as those observed by Imai and Sato, who used microsomes from untreated rabbits. However, the microsomes from 3-methylcholanthrene-treated rats gave an intercept at pH 6.9. This was taken as good evidence that a different hemoprotein was formed as the result of 3-methylcholanthrene administration. The relationships between N-demethylase activities, cytochrome P-450 levels, relative heights of peaks at 430 and 455 mμ (at pH 7.4), and the pH-dependent intercepts of the interconvertible forms of the hemoproteins in microsomes from untreated, phenobarbital-treated and 3-methylcholanthrene-treated rats are shown in Figure 12.9. More recent studies showed that the inductive potencies of different polycyclic hydrocarbons related to the amount of cytochrome P$_1$-450 formed, as determined by the lowering of the "pH intercept" and by the increase in type II binding to aniline that occurred (Parli and Mannering, 1970).

Soon after we presented evidence for the existence of cytochrome P$_1$-450, Alvares et al. (1967) and Hildebrandt et al. (1968) showed that the λ_{max} of reduced microsomal protein bound to CO obtained after the administration of polycyclic hydrocarbons differed slightly from that observed in microsomes from untreated animals. Alvares et al. observed a λ_{max} at 448 mμ; cytochrome P$_1$-450 is therefore sometimes called cytochrome P-448. They also observed that 3-methylcholanthrene caused a reduction in the K$_m$ of 3,4-benzpyrene hydroxylation from 1.4×10^{-5} M, obtained with microsomes from control rats, to 0.2×10^{-5} M. Hildebrandt and associates observed a λ_{max} at 446 mμ; thus cytochrome P$_1$-450 is referred to as cytochrome P-446 by some investigators. The shift from 450 mμ to 448 mμ is slight, but real. On the other hand, the peak at 446 mμ can only be observed when the method of Kinoshita and Horie (vide supra) is employed and does not represent the true λ_{max} of cytochrome P$_1$-450. Instead, it is the λ_{max} of the composite spectrum that results when the spectrum of cytochrome P$_1$-450 (λ_{max}, 448 mμ) is superimposed upon the inverted spectrum of cytochrome P-450 (λ_{max}, 450 mμ) obtained when microsomes from untreated animals are placed in the reference cuvette of the dual beam spectrophotometer. Thus there is no rational basis for applying the term cytochrome P-446 to cytochrome P$_1$-450.

The electron paramagnetic resonance (EPR, electron-spin resonance, ESR) examination of hepatic microsomes exhibits an anisotropic 3-line spectrum

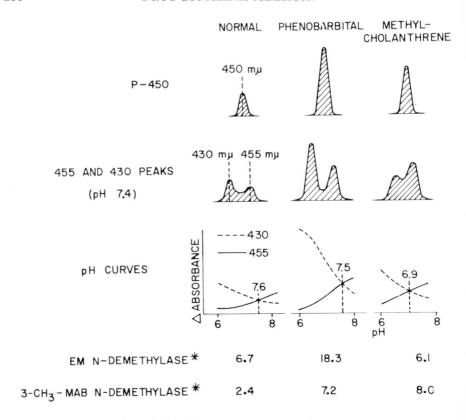

Fig. 12.9. Relationship between ethylmorphine (EM) and 3-methyl-4-methylamino-azobenzene (3-CH₃-MAB) N-demethylase activities, P-450 hemoprotein (reduced microsomes + CO), relative heights of absorption peaks at 430 and 455 mμ (reduced microsomes + ethyl isocyanide), and pH-dependent intercepts of the 430 and 455 mμ peaks from untreated, phenobarbital-treated, and 3-methylcholanthrene-treated rats (Mannering, 1968). (Reprinted by permission of Marcel Dekker, Inc., New York.)

(g = 2.41, 2.25 and 1.91) typical of ferric iron with one unpaired electron ("low-spin" iron, Mason *et al.*, 1965). The close correlation between the concentrations of low-spin iron and cytochrome P-450 in microsomes from either untreated or phenobarbital-treated animals led to the conclusion that the EPR spectrum is due to cytochrome P-450, whose iron is in a low-spin state. Oxidized cytochrome P-450 has been characterized as a low-spin hemoprotein in microsomes (Hashimoto *et al.*, 1962; Mason *et al.*, 1965; Cammer *et al.*, 1966; Ichikawa *et al.*, 1967; Whysner *et al.*, 1969; Jefcoate and Gaylor, 1969, Miyake *et al.*, 1969, Ichikawa and Yamano, 1970), in submicrosomal particles (Maclennan *et al.*, 1967; Miyake *et al.*, 1968, 1969, Ichikawa and Yamano, 1970), and in solution (Lu *et al.*, 1969a). Hildebrandt *et al.* (1968) observed an EPR spectrum produced by microsomes from animals treated with 3-methylcholanthrene indicative of a high spin form of cytochrome P-450 (5 unpaired electrons; g, about 6). The high-spin iron was identified with the new form of cytochrome P-450 that results when polycyclic hydrocarbons are given to animals. Jefcoate and Gaylor (1969) confirmed this observation and assigned a g value of 6.6 to the high-spin hemoprotein.

Primary aliphatic amines bind to oxidized cytochrome P-450 to produce two superimposed difference spectra: (a) λ_{max} 424 mμ, λ_{min} 392 mμ; (b) λ_{max} 432 mμ, λ_{min} 410 mμ (Jefcoate et al., 1969). Pretreatment of rabbits with 3-methylcholanthrene increased the amount of type a cytochrome P-450 in microsomes, whereas pretreatment with phenobarbital increased both a and b forms of the hemoprotein. Types a and b forms of cytochrome P-450 correspond to high- and low-spin cytochrome P-450, respectively.

While it is agreed that the administration of polycyclic hydrocarbons cause a change in microsomal hemoprotein, there is much controversy as to whether the change reflects the formation or revelation of a new molecular species of hemoprotein, the alternative being that the change simply represents an alteration in the relative amounts of interconvertible forms of a single hemoprotein. It is our opinion that cytochrome P-450 and cytochrome P_1-450 are similar, but separate entities, each of which can exist in two interconvertible forms. This opinion was originally based on indirect measurements as cited previously.

Recently, direct comparison of cytochrome P-450 and cytochrome P_1-450 was made possible through solubilization and partial purification of the microsomal hemoproteins from phenobarbital- and 3-methylcholanthrene-treated rats (Fujita and Mannering, unpublished observations).

The absolute spectrum of soluble purified cytochrome P_1-450 is shown in Figure 12.5; some properties of cytochromes P-450 and P_1-450, Table 12.3. The absolute spectra of the two hemoproteins are very much alike, but there are differences. The Soret peaks at 448 mμ and 450 mμ (reduced + CO) shown by cytochrome P_1-450 and cytochrome P-450, respectively, accords with what was ex-

TABLE 12.3

Absorption peaks and molar extinction coefficients of absolute spectra of soluble cytochromes P-450 and P_1-450[a]

Conditions	Cytochrome P-450[b]		Cytochrome P_1-450[c]	
	λ_{max} (mμ)	ϵ (mM^{-1}cm^{-1})	λ_{max} (mμ)	ϵ (mM^{-1}cm^{-1})
Oxidized	δ 360	49.2	360	45.7
	Soret 418	104.2	419	120.3
	β 537	12.9	537	13.5
	α 568	12.3	568	13.4
Reduced	Soret 418	86.0	414	90.1
	545	14.9	545	16.4
Reduced + CO	423	65.8	423	60.0
	Soret 450	89.1	448	108.0
	548	13.9	551	15.4

[a] The hemoproteins were solubilized by treating microsomes with Triton N-101 and fractionating the supernatant on a DEAE cellulose column (Fujita and Mannering, unpublished observations). The preparations were free of cytochrome b_5, but they contained small amounts of P-420. The absolute spectrum of cytochrome P_1-450 is shown in Figure 12.5.

[b] The preparation contained 3.24 mμmoles of P-450 hemoprotein/mg of protein, an increase of 4.3 fold over that contained in the microsomes from which the preparation was obtained. Recovery of hemoprotein was 15.5%.

[c] The preparation contained 4.42 mμmoles of P-450 hemoprotein/mg of protein, an increase of 3.5 fold over that contained in the microsomes from which the preparation was obtained. Recovery of hemoprotein was 13.9%.

pected from spectral studies employing microsomes. The Soret peak at 414 mμ rather than at 418 mμ (reduced hemoprotein) also distinguishes cytochrome P_1-450 from cytochrome P-450. Particularly to be noted is the absence of a peak at about 395 mμ. Putatively, a peak at 395 mμ characterizes the form of the P-450 hemoprotein that results when polycyclic hydrocarbons are administered (Hildebrandt *et al.*, 1968; Schenkman *et al.*, 1969). The most likely explanation for the peak at 395 mμ is that 3,4-benzpyrene, a type I compound (Schenkman *et al.*, 1969), or a metabolite binds with hemoprotein to produce a type I spectrum. The polycyclic hydrocarbon or its metabolite binds more avidly than most type I compounds and is not lost during preparation of the microsomes. However, the loss of 3-methylcholanthrene or its metabolite occurs when the hemoprotein is solubilized.

The extinction coefficient of 89 mM^{-1} cm^{-1} for cytochrome P-450 agrees with the value of 91 mM^{-1} cm^{-1} given originally by Omura and Sato (1963, 1964a), but the value of 108 mM^{-1} cm^{-1} for cytochrome P_1-450 does not agree with the value of 220 mM^{-1} cm^{-1} proposed by Hildebrandt *et al.* (1968). The latter value was derived from equations that could not be solved because they dealt with more unknown factors than the equations could accommodate.

Further evidence for the existence of two molecular species of P-450 hemoprotein was obtained by comparing the cytochrome P-420's derived from cytochromes P-450 and P_1-450 (Shoeman *et al.*, 1970). When hepatic microsomes from untreated rats were incubated under nitrogen at 4°C for 24 hours with 0.07 % steapsin, about 25 % of the P-450 hemoprotein was solubilized as P-420 hemoprotein. After desalting and concentrating the clear solution to about one-fourth its volume, an aggregate of cytochrome P-420 was formed consisting of microtubules with globular substructures (Shoeman *et al.*, 1969). Microsomes from rats that had received 3-methylcholanthrene, when treated in the same manner, also yielded aggregates, but only small numbers of the tubular structures were seen, their presence possibly being due to the existence of some residual cytochrome P-450 in the microsomes. Aggregates of cytochrome P-420 showed both type I and type II binding with drugs, but aggregates of cytochrome P_1-420 bound only with type II compounds. On the basis of heme content, the molar absorbancy of cytochrome P-420 was determined to be 110 mM^{-1} cm^{-1}, whereas that of cytochrome P_1-420 was 134 mM^{-1} cm^{-1}. Disc electrophoresis of aggregates solubilized with 8 M urea disclosed differences in the ionic mobilities of the two P-420 hemoproteins.

Estimates of the amount of cytochrome P_1-450 in microsomes from untreated animals ranged from negligible (Sladek and Mannering, 1969a) to as high as 25 % (Hildebrandt and Estabrook, 1969; Jefcoate and Gaylor, 1969). In both cases where high estimates were made, certain factors were ignored which, when taken into account, greatly alter the interpretation of data. Hildebrandt and Estabrook (1969) used the method of Kinoshita and Horie (*vide supra*) to obtain an apparent absolute spectrum from which extinction coefficients of 218 and 56 m$_M$$^{-1}$ cm^{-1} were calculated for cytochrome P-450 and cytochrome P_1-450 (P-446). The observed absorbance is equal to the sum of the products of the concentration of each species of hemoprotein and its extinction coefficient. To calculate the extinction coefficient of a different hemoprotein requires that its concentration be known. As the only other measurable quantities are absorbance of total P-450 hemoprotein, total heme and cytochrome b_5, it is obvious that there is insufficient information to determine either the extinction coefficient of the different hemoprotein or the relative amounts of each hemoprotein.

Jefcoate and Gaylor (1969) concluded from EPR studies that in microsomes from 3-methylcholanthrene-treated animals, about half of the P-450 hemoprotein was in a high-spin state and that the two types of P-450 hemoprotein were therefore present in a ratio of about 1:1. From measurements of type a and b amine binding spectra (*vide supra*), microsomes from untreated and phenobarbital-treated rabbits were calculated to contain 20–25 % of the high spin hemoprotein. It is difficult to reconcile these conclusions with the failure of these investigators to detect any high-spin signal in the EPR spectrum of microsomes from phenobarbital-treated animals. One can calculate from their data that the microsomes from phenobarbital-treated animals should have contained at least as much high-spin hemoprotein per milligram of microsomal protein as the microsomes from 3-methylcholanthrene-treated animals; thus, the high-spin signal should have been observed with the microsomes from phenobarbital-treated rabbits. That storage of the microsomes from 3-methylcholanthrene-treated animals caused a loss of the high-spin signal without an alteration in the type a binding spectrum should suggest that type a binding and the high spin state of the hemoprotein may not be related.

More doubt is cast on the validity of identifying the new hemoprotein with a high spin EPR signal by the EPR studies of Ichikawa and Yamano (1970), who found all cytochrome P-450 to be in "pure low spin form" regardless of its source, whether from microsomes from untreated, phenobarbital-treated or 3-methylcholanthrene-treated rabbits. No EPR signals between $g = 5.0$ and $g = 7.0$ were seen with microsomes, even at 100°K. Small high-spin signals observed with submicrosomal particles were attributed to traces of cytochrome P-420, which was established as a high-spin hemoprotein. The absolute spectra of P-450 hemoprotein published by Jefcoate and Gaylor (1969) show the presence of appreciable amounts of cytochrome P-420. Cytochrome P-420 is much more susceptible to degradation than cytochrome P-450 and this might account for the disappearance of the high-spin signal when their microsomes were stored. The peak in the vicinity of 650 mμ of the visible absolute spectra of microsomal hemoproteins is often equated with a high-spin state. Ichikawa and Yamano (1970) believe this is due to the presence of small amounts of cytochrome P-420.

The administration of δ-aminolevulinic acid-3,5-^{3}H to immature male rats introduces radioactivity into microsomal cytochrome P-450. The incorporated radioactivity decreases *in vivo* in two distinct phases, a rapid phase with a half-life of 7–8 hours, and a slow phase with a half-life of 46–48 hours (Levin and Kuntzman, 1969, 1969a, 1969b). The ratios of the fast to slow component are 3.8, 3.3 and 1.0 in untreated, phenobarbital-treated and 3-methylcholanthrene-treated animals, respectively. These ratios are very similar to the ratios of type a to type b binding hemoproteins reported by Jefcoate and coworkers (Jefcoate *et al.*, 1969; Jefcoate and Gaylor, 1969), which suggests that the investigators from each laboratory may be measuring the same thing by different methods.

Schenkman and associates (1969) proposed that the changes in the hemoprotein seen after the administration of polycyclic hydrocarbons result simply from the irreversible addition of the inducing agent or a metabolite to the type I binding site of native cytochrome P-450. This conclusion was based on the observations that 3,4-benzpyrene is a type I binding compound and that the "absolute" spectrum obtained by the method of Kinoshita and Horie (*vide supra*) showed a peak at about 395 mμ, which is what would be expected if type I binding had occurred. They concluded that cytochrome P-450 exists in only two forms, the native enzyme and the enzyme-substrate complex. A number of arguments weaken this hypothesis:

1. Phospholipase C treatment of microsomes eliminates the type I binding site (Chaplin and Mannering, 1969), but the reduced hemoprotein-CO spectrum remains at 450 mμ; it does not shift to 448 mμ, as might be expected. Neither does the "pH intercept" shift to a lower pH when ethyl isocyanide is employed as the ligand, as is the case with cytochrome P_1-450 (Fig. 12.2).

2. SKF 525-A binds irreversibly to the type I binding site when added to microsomes (Bidleman and Mannering, unpublished results). Microsomes treated in this manner remain unchanged with respect to the reduced hemoprotein-CO peak at 450 mμ and the "pH intercept" with ethyl isocyanide.

3. When 3-methylcholanthrene was incubated with microsomes in a medium commonly employed in drug metabolism studies, microsomes took up an amount of polycyclic hydrocarbon which was about 30 times that found in microsomes from animals treated with the compound. These microsomes showed CO, ethyl isocyanide and type I binding (hexobarbital) spectra that were no different qualitatively or quantitatively from those obtained with microsomes not incubated with 3-methylcholanthrene (Shoeman and Mannering, unpublished results). Gnosspelius *et al.* (1969/70) also observed no cytochrome P_1-450 (P-448) formation when microsomes were incubated with 3,4-benzpyrene with or without added NADPH.

4. Formation of cytochrome P_1-450 was not observable until 16 hours after 3-methylcholanthrene administration (Gnosspelius *et al.*, 1969/70). This suggests that if the polycyclic hydrocarbon is combining with native hemoprotein, it must do so while it is being formed. This view is supported by the observation that the inhibitors of protein synthesis, ethionine and actinomycin D, prevent the formation of cytochrome P_1-450 caused by 3-methylcholanthrene treatment (Alvares *et al.*, 1967, 1968; Kuntzman *et al.*, 1969).

5. The concept of direct binding of a polycyclic hydrocarbon or a metabolite to native cytochrome P-450 to produce a polycyclic hydrocarbon-hemoprotein derivative implies that the formation of this derivative is independent of the inductive effect produced by the compound. This would mean that the polycyclic hydrocarbon would induce the increased synthesis of native cytochrome P-450, much as phenobarbital and many other compounds induce increased amounts of native cytochrome P-450, and that the polycyclic hydrocarbon or a derivative would then combine with it. This being the case, it would be expected that the polycyclic hydrocarbon would combine with native cytochrome P-450 whether it was caused to be formed as a result of phenobarbital or of 3-methylcholanthrene administration. When phenobarbital and 3-methylcholanthrene were administered to rats simultaneously, each in an amount known to produce its maximum inductive effect, the amount of P-450 hemoprotein produced was additive. The amount of cytochrome P_1-450 formed, as judged from the relative heights of the 455 mμ and 430 mμ peaks seen when reduced microsomes were liganded

with ethyl isocyanide, was not consistent with the concept of equal combination of 3-methylcholanthrene with newly formed, native cytochrome P-450, resulting from induction by both phenobarbital and 3-methylcholanthrene (Sladek and Mannering, 1969a). The 455 mμ:430 mμ peak height ratio with microsomes from 3-methylcholanthrene-treated rats was 1.37, that obtained with microsomes from phenobarbital-treated rats was 0.56, and that seen with microsomes from rats treated with both compounds was 0.94. This implies that the formation of cytochrome P_1-450 is part of the inductive process, not incidental to it.

6. Microsomes from rats obtained 20 hours after the last of 4 daily doses of tritiated 3-methylcholanthrene (20 mg/kg/day) contained only 1/10 the counts required for a 1:1 molar ratio of 3-methylcholanthrene to P-450 hemoprotein (Shoeman et al., 1970). Gas chromatographic analysis of the microsomes established the radioactivity as being due to 3-methylcholanthrene rather than to a metabolite. This agrees with Jefcoate and Gaylor (1969), who used ^{14}C-labeled 3-methylcholanthrene to show that the new hemoprotein cannot arise from direct 1:1 binding of the compound with cytochrome P-450. Solubilized cytochrome P_1-450 prepared by Dr. Fujita in our laboratory (Fig. 12.5, Table 12.3) from animals injected with tritiated 3-methylcholanthrene contained only 0.04 mole of 3-methylcholanthrene per mole of P-450 hemoprotein. Aggregates of cytochrome P_1-420 obtained from the same animals showed no measurable radioactivity (Shoeman et al., 1970).

In summary, the preponderance of evidence leads to the following conclusions:

1) The administration of polycyclic hydrocarbons causes the biosynthesis of cytochrome P_1-450, a molecular species of cytochrome P-450 not normally detectable in appreciable amounts in microsomes from untreated or phenobarbital-treated animals. This does not exclude the possibility that small amounts of cytochrome P_1-450 may be found in untreated animals; in fact, this can be expected to be the case. Polycylic hydrocarbons or other substances capable of inducing the synthesis of cytochrome P_1-450 may be present in the diet or atmosphere or may be produced by the intestinal flora. The earliest recognition of an exogenous inductive effect on the metabolism of a foreign substance was made by Miller and coworkers (Brown et al., 1954; Reif et al., 1954) who observed that rancid diets contained oxidized steroids which stimulated the N-demethylation of aminoazo dyes.

2) Cytochrome P-450 and cytochrome P_1-450 both exist in their own interconvertible forms.

3) Cytochrome P_1-450 does not form as a result of the combination of native cytochrome P-450 with polycyclic hydrocarbons or their metabolites.

C. Non-Heme Iron Protein

Adrenodoxin, a non-heme iron protein, is a component of the electron transport system that functions in the hydroxylation of steroids by adrenal microsomes and mitochondria (Omura et al., 1965a, 1966; Suzuki and Kimura, 1965; Kimura and Suzuki, 1965, 1967). In this system, adrenodoxin acts as the electron carrier between flavin enzyme (adrenodoxin reductase) and cytochrome P-450 (Figs. 12.1 and 12.3). Because of the similarities of the microsomal hydroxylase systems of the adrenal and liver, it has been assumed that adrenodoxin or some other non-heme iron protein is involved in the microsomal drug metabolizing system. There is no evidence for this, but insufficient work has been done to exclude the possibility. In the presence of NADPH, a mixture of adrenodoxin and adrenodoxin reductase caused the reduction of cytochrome P-450 contained in submicrosomal liver particles, but the essentiality of adrenodoxin was not determined (Miyake *et al.*, 1968). Kimura (1968) concluded that tissues capable of producing steroid hormones (adrenals, testis, ovary) contain adrenodoxin, but liver and other tissues do not. This does not exclude the possibility that a different non-heme protein may function in the hepatic drug hydroxylase system.

Purified adrenodoxin was estimated to have a molecular weight of 15,000–20,000 (Kimura and Suzuki, 1967). Assuming a molecular weight of 15,000, there are two atoms of iron per mole of adrenodoxin. No heme iron was detectable. Absorption maxima were seen at 455, 414 and 320 mμ.

D. Reductases

1. NADPH-cytochrome c reductase. NADPH-cytochrome c reductase was first observed by Horecker (1950) in whole-liver acetone powder. Horecker recognized its particulate origin, but methods available at the time did not permit its identification with microsomes. NADPH-cytochrome c reductase activity in microsomes had been observed by Strittmatter and Velick (1956). Phillips and Langdon (1962) and Williams and Kamin (1962) documented its microsomal origin and solubilized and purified the enzyme. The prosthetic group was identified as FAD (Williams and Kamin, 1962), which was shown to be present in the amount of two moles per mole of enzyme (Masters *et al.*, 1965). Purification of the enzyme revealed NADPH-cytochrome c reductase activity to be associated with a single protein capable of catalyzing the reduction of ferric ions, ferricyanide, tetrazolium compounds, menadione, FAD and azo-compounds. An excellent review of the properties of NADPH-cytochrome c reductase has been written by Kamin and associates (1965).

Microsomal NADPH-cytochrome c reductase catalyzes the following reactions (Williams and Kamin, 1962):

1. $NADPH + H^+ + 2\ Cyt\ c^{3+} \rightarrow NADP^+ + 2\ Cyt\ c^{2+} + 2H^+$
2. $NADPH + H^+ + dye \rightarrow Reduced\ dye + NADP^+$
3. $NADPH + H^+ + O_2 \rightarrow NADP^+ + H_2O_2$ (?)

It is seen that this enzyme can reduce both one-electron and two-electron acceptors. Studies in Kamin's laboratory (Masters *et al.*, 1965, 1965a; Kamin *et al.*, 1965) showed that the oxidation states of the flavin are the same for catalysis of reduction of both one- and two-electron acceptors and demonstrated a mechanism not previously described for flavins, namely, an alternation of the flavin between the fully reduced form ($FADH_2$) and the half-reduced form ($FADH$). The oxidized form (FAD) does not appear to be involved in catalysis.

NADPH-cytochrome c reductase is currently thought to reduce cytochrome P-450 directly or indirectly through a non-heme iron protein or some other unidentified carrier. The possibility that NADPH-cytochrome c reductase might be a component of the microsomal drug metabolizing system was suggested by the finding that cytochrome c and other electron acceptors inhibited microsomal drug metabolism (Gillette *et al.*, 1957; Gillette, 1966). Because cytochrome c is not present in microsomes, and there is no other known natural substrate for the reductase in these organelles, NADPH-cytochrome c reductase was considered particularly eligible to play a role in the transfer of electrons from NADPH to cytochrome P-450.

The enhancement of NADPH-cytochrome c reductase activity seen in microsomes when microsomal drug metabolizing activity is caused to be increased as a result of phenobarbital administration (Remmer and Merker, 1963; Orrenius and Ernster, 1964) provides another indirect association of the reductase with the microsomal hydroxylating system. On the other hand, highly purified NADPH-cytochrome c reductase did not substitute for the flavin fraction in Lu and Coon's solubilized microsomal system (Lu et al., 1969a). This does not necessarily eliminate NADPH-cytochrome c reductase as the flavin enzyme involved in drug metabolism; the highly purified reductase may have been partially denatured so as to lose its activity in the hydroxylase system while retaining its reactivity with cytochrome c. This denaturation could involve the loss of a component which enables the reductase to reform an intimate association with the multi-enzyme hydroxylase complex.

Highly purified cytochrome c reductase was also unable to substitute for the adrenal cortex flavoprotein in the re-establishment of NADPH-cytochrome P-450 reduction (Omura et al., 1965a). On the other hand, as has already been mentioned, a mixture of adrenodoxin and adrenal cortex flavoprotein (adrenodoxin reductase) was able to perform in the reduction of cytochrome P-450 contained in submicrosomal liver particles (Miyake et al., 1968).

Cytochrome c reductase catalyzed the reduction of azo dyes without benefit of cytochrome P-450 (Gillette, 1966; Hernandez et al., 1967, 1967a). The microsomal amine oxidase which functions independently of cytochrome P-450 in the N-oxidation of a variety of N-alkyl-substituted amines (vide infra) is a flavoprotein with an FAD prosthetic group; its relationship to cytochrome c reductase, if any, has not been established.

2. NADPH-cytochrome P-450 reductase. The measurement of NADPH-cytochrome P-450 reductase activity is based on the knowledge that CO forms a complex with reduced, but not with oxidized, cytochrome P-450 to give a Soret peak at 450 mμ. A suspension of oxidized microsomes is saturated with oxygen-free CO and placed in a cuvette under strictly anaerobic conditions. An NADPH generating system consisting of NADP, sodium isocitrate and isocitrate dehydrogenase is introduced and mixed very rapidly and the absorbancy of the reduced cytochrome P-450-CO complex at 450 mμ is recorded on a rapidly moving chart (Gigon et al., 1969). When the logarithm of the unoxidized percentage of cytochrome P-450 was plotted against time, the rate of cytochrome P-450 reduction was observed to be biphasic. The first phase was very rapid and appeared complete within 3 or 4 seconds. The second phase came into prominence immediately afterward, at which time about half of the cytochrome P-450 had been reduced. The slower rate of reduction continued linearly over the next 50 or 60 seconds during which time the percentage of unreduced cytochrome P-450 was reduced to about 10 %. The second phase was thought originally to be due to contamination with a small amount of oxygen, but Gillette (personal communication) has recently expressed the view that it may be due to the presence of a less available form of cytochrome P-450 in the membrane which reacts more slowly with the reductase.

From a variety of experiments that showed the rate of drug metabolism to be more closely related to the rate of cytochrome P-450 reduction than to the total amount of cytochrome P-450 or to the rate of cytochrome c reduction, Gillette's group concluded that NADPH-cytochrome P-450 reductase is rate-limiting in the overall reaction involving microsomal drug metabolism (Gillette and Gram, 1969; Gillette, 1969):

1) Many drugs are metabolized more rapidly by smooth-surfaced microsomes from rabbit liver than by rough-surfaced microsomes (Fouts, 1961; Gram et al., 1967). Holtzman and coworkers (1968) showed that the difference in the metabolism of ethylmorphine by the two kinds of microsomes related to their NADPH-cytochrome P-450 reductase activities rather than to their NADPH-cytochrome c reductase activities or cytochrome P-450 contents. The ratios of ethylmorphine N-demethylase activity, NADPH-cytochrome c reductase activity, NADPH-cytochrome P-450 reductase activity and cytochrome P-450 content in smooth- and rough-surfaced microsomes was 5.65, 2.23, 5.55 and 3.53, respectively.

2) Adrenalectomy of male rats impairs the metabolism of a wide variety of drugs (Remmer, 1958; Kato and Gillette, 1965). Castro and coworkers (Castro et al., 1968; Gillette, 1969) showed that adrenalectomy decreased microsomal N-demethylase, NADPH-cytochrome c reductase and NADPH-cytochrome P-450 reductase activities and that these effects were reversed with cortisone. However, the adrenalectomy induced reduction of cytochrome P-450 content and magnitude of the type I spectral change produced with ethylmorphine were not restored with cortisone. Thus changes were more correlative with drug metabolism and reductase activities than with the other parameters studied.

3) Species variations in hepatic microsomal drug metabolism have long been recognized (Chapter 11). Davies et al. (1969) studied ethylmorphine type I binding, cytochrome P-450 content and NADPH-cytochrome c reductase, NADPH-cytochrome P-450 reductase and ethylmorphine N-demethylase activities in microsomes from mice, rats, rabbits and guinea pigs. They concluded that the considerable variation in ethylmorphine N-demethylation activity observed in the four species more closely related to differences in NADPH-cytochrome P-450 reductase activity than to any of the other microsomal components studied.

Of considerable interest was the observation that type I binding compounds stimulated NADPH-cytochrome P-450 reductase activity whereas type II binding compounds either inhibited or had no effect on the reductase (Gigon et al., 1968, 1969; Gillette and Gram, 1969; Gillette, 1969). Why this should be the case is not understood, but it would seem to support the general rule that type II compounds are less active substrates for the microsomal oxidative systems than type I substances. The activity of NADPH-cytochrome c reductase was not affected by either type I or type II binding compounds. The effects of type I and II compounds on the rate of drug metabolism are not limited to oxidative reactions; the reduction of p-nitrobenzoate is stimulated by type I compounds and inhibited by type II compounds (Sasame and Gillette, 1969; Gillette and Gram, 1969).

NADPH-cytochrome P-450 reductase activities of microsomes from male and female rats were determined with the idea that an explanation might be found for the well known sex difference in drug metabolism in this species (Gigon et al., 1968, 1969). Only a slight sex difference in the reductase activity was found and this was probably due to the small difference in cytochrome P-450 content of the microsomes. However, ethylmorphine (type I compound) caused a much greater stimulation of NADPH-cytochrome P-450 reductase in microsomes from males than it did in microsomes from females. This suggested to the authors that the cytochrome P-450 in microsomes from female rats is less capable of participating in the oxidation of substrates than that in microsomes from male rats.

Nothing is known about NADPH-cytochrome P-450 reductase other than what is known about its activity. The assumption is that NADPH-cytochrome P-450 reductase reflects the activity of NADPH-cytochrome c reductase, or of some other flavoprotein, as it functions as part of the microsomal multi-enzyme hydroxylase complex. Failure to observe parallel activities of NADPH-cytochrome c reductase and NADPH-cytochrome P-450 reductase under a variety of conditions does not eliminate this possibility.

E. Heat Stable, Lipid Factor

Lu and Coon and associates (Lu and Coon, 1968; Coon and Lu, 1969; Lu et al., 1969, 1969a) separated solubilized hepatic microsomes into three fractions containing cytochrome P-450, an NADPH reductase and a heat stable, lipid factor (vide infra). The combination of all three fractions was required for maximal drug-metabolizing activity. The lipid factor was unaffected by heating for 2 hours at 100°C at neutral pH or for 10 minutes at 50°C in 0.1 N HCl or H_2SO_4, but was destroyed by ashing (Lu et al., 1969a). Activity was completely extracted into a few volumes of ether or chloroform at neutral pH. No protein was detectable. Attempts to replace the fraction with the following phospholipid preparations over a wide range of concentrations proved unsuccessful: rat liver lecithin or phosphatidyl ethanolamine, bovine phosphatidyl serine or sphingomyelin, egg yolk lecithin, pig heart phosphatidyl ethanolamine or plasmalogen, or cardiolipin. The possibility should be considered that the lipid factor may act physically in such a way as to provide access of the drug to cytochrome P-450.

IV. PHARMACOLOGIC SIGNIFICANCE OF A COMMON ENZYME SYSTEM FOR DRUG METABOLISM

To perform therapeutically, a drug must produce a transitory effect; only in very special cases is it desired that the action of a drug be permanent. For a drug to produce a temporary effect usually means that it undergo biotransformation. The great majority of drugs in common use exist partly in nonpolar form at body pH; in this form they are almost completely reabsorbed into the circulation by way of the kidney tubule. The oxidations, reductions, hydrolyses, and conjugations that drugs undergo almost invariably result in products which are more polar than their parents; thus, the products are more readily excreted by the kidney. Without these biotransformations, the effects of some drugs would last for months (Brodie et al., 1965), and many others would have to be discarded because of their unreasonably long duration of action. Compounds may not have been designed for therapeutic use with their biotransformation in mind, but frequently biotransformation or its lack determined their degree of acceptability. That drugs, regardless of their myriad structures, should be readily metabolized, seems remarkable when we consider the relatively narrow limits of specificity of enzymes for natural substrates.

Teleologically, the concept of a multitude of enzymes for a multitude of drug substrates is untenable. If drugs, as we know them, were to be developed, a common enzyme system was essential. This is not to say that drugs, as we do not know them, would not have been created, but they would have had to be developed on a much more restricted basis than those which currently stock our pharmacies. A common drug-metabolizing system renders drug metabolism more susceptible to environmental influences (Chapter 13) than would be possible if a large number of enzyme systems were involved. The many known examples of interactions of drugs at the metabolic site to produce mutual stimulatory or inhibitory effects on each other's biotransformation would not be possible without a common metabolizing system.

REFERENCES

Alvares, A. P., Schilling, G., Levin, W., and Kuntzman, R.: Studies on the induction of CO-binding pigments in liver microsomes by phenobarbital and 3-methylcholanthrene. Biochem. Biophys. Res. Commun. *29:* 521–526, 1967.

Alvares, A. P., Schilling, G., Levin, W., and Kuntzman, R.: Alteration of the microsomal hemoprotein by 3-methylcholanthrene: effects of ethionine and actinomycin D. J. Pharmacol. Exp. Ther. *163:* 417–424, 1968.

Anders, M. W. and Mannering, G. J.: Inhibition of drug metabolism. I. Kinetics of the inhibition of the N-demethylation of ethylmorphine by 2-diethylaminoethyl 2,2-diphenylvalerate (SKF 525-A) and related compounds. Mol. Pharmacol. *2:* 319–327, 1966.

Anderson, B. M., Reynolds, M. L., and Anderson, C. D.: Hydrophobic interactions of inhibitors with yeast alcohol dehydrogenase. Biochim. Biophys. Acta *99:* 46–55, 1965.

Appleby, C. A.: A soluble haemoprotein P-450 from nitrogen-fixing Rhizobium bacteroids. Biochim. Biophys. Acta *147:* 399–402, 1967.

Appleby, C. A.: Properties of soluble hemoprotein P-450 purified from *Rhizobium japonicum* bacteroids. In *Structure and Function of Cytochromes*, ed. by K. Okunuki, M. D. Kamen and I. Sekuzu, pp. 666–679, University Park Press, Baltimore, Md., 1968.

Appleby, C. A.: Electron transport systems of *Rhizobium japonicum*. I. Haemoprotein P-450, other CO-reactive pigments, cytochromes and oxidases in bacteroids from N₂-fixing root nodules. Biochim. Biophys. Acta *172:* 71–87, 1969.

Appleby, C. A.: Electron transport systems of *Rhizobium japonicum*. II. Rhizobium haemoglobin, cytochromes and oxidases in free-living (cultured) cells. Biochim. Biophys. Acta *172:* 88–105, 1969a.

Baker, J. R. and Chaykin, S.: The biosynthesis of trimethylamine-N-oxide. J. Biol. Chem. *237:* 1309, 1962.

Brodie, B. B., Axelrod, J., Cooper, J. R.,

Gaudette, L., La Du, B. N., Mitoma, C., and Udenfriend, S.: Detoxication of drugs and other foreign compounds by liver microsomes. Science *121:* 603–604, 1955.

Brodie, B. B., Cosmides, G. J., and Rall, D. P.: Toxicology and the biomedical sciences. Science *148:* 1547–1554, 1965.

Brodie, B. B., Gillette, J. R., and La Du, B. N.: Enzymatic metabolism of drugs and other foreign compounds. Ann. Rev. Biochem. *27:* 427–454, 1958.

Brown, R. R., Miller, J. A., and Miller, E. C.: The metabolism of methylated aminoazo dyes. IV. Dietary factors enhancing demethylation *in vitro*. J. Biol. Chem. *209:* 211–222, 1954.

Cammer, W., Schenkman, J. B., and Estabrook, R. W.: EPR measurements of substrate interaction with cytochrome P-450. Biochem. Biophys. Res. Commun. *23:* 264–268, 1966.

Castro, J. A., Greene, F. E., Gigon, P., Sasame, H., and Gillette, J.: Effect of adrenalectomy on various components of the mixed-function oxygenase system of rat liver microsomes. Fed. Proc. *27:* 350, 1968.

Chaplin, M. D. and Mannering, G. J.: Role of phospholipids in the drug metabolizing system of rat liver microsomes. Fed. Proc. *28:* 484, 1969.

Cleland, W. W.: The kinetics of enzyme-catalyzed reactions with two or more substrates or products. I. Nomenclature and rate equations. Biochim. Biophys. Acta *67:* 104–137, 1963.

Coccia, P. F. and Westerfeld, W. W.: The metabolism of chlorpromazine by liver microsomal enzyme systems. J. Pharmacol. Exp. Ther. *157:* 446–458, 1967.

Conney, A. H.: Pharmacological implications of microsomal enzyme induction. Pharmacol. Rev. *19:* 317–366, 1967.

Conney, A. H., Brown, R. R., Miller, J. A., and Miller, E. C.: The metabolism of methylated aminoazo dyes. VI. Intracellular distribution and properties of the demethylase system. Cancer Res. *17:* 628–633, 1957.

Coon, M. J. and Lu, A. Y. H.: Fatty acid ω-oxidation in a soluble microsomal enzyme system containing P-450. In *Microsomes and Drug Oxidations*, ed. by J. R. Gillette, A. H. Conney, G. J. Cosmides, R. W. Estabrook, J. R. Fouts, and G. J. Mannering, pp. 151–166, Academic Press, New York, 1969.

Cooper, J. R. and Brodie, B. B.: The enzymatic metabolism of hexobarbital (Evipal). J. Pharmacol. Exp. Ther. *114:* 409–417, 1955.

Cooper, D. Y., Estabrook, R. W. and Rosenthal, O.: The stoichiometry of C_{21} hydroxylation of steroids by adrenocortical microsomes. J. Biol. Chem. *238:* 1320–1323, 1963.

Cooper, D. Y., Levin, S., Narasimhulu, S., Rosenthal, O., and Estabrook, R. W.: Photochemical action spectrum of the terminal oxidase of mixed function oxidase systems. Science *147:* 400–402, 1965.

Das, M., Orrenius, S., Ernster, L., and Gnosspelius, Y.: Stereospecificity of certain reduced nicotinamide-adenine dinucleotide phosphate-linked reactions in rat liver microsomes. FEBS Letters *1:* 89–92, 1968.

Davies, D. S., Gigon, P. L., and Gillette, J. R.: Species and sex differences in electron transport systems in liver microsomes and their relationship to ethylmorphine demethylation. Life Sci. *8:* 85–91, 1969.

El Defrawy, S.: Factors effecting changes in components of the hepatic microsomal enzyme system responsible for drug metabolism. Fed. Proc. *26:* 462, 1967.

Ernster, L. and Orrenius, S.: Substrate-induced synthesis of the hydroxylating enzyme system of liver microsomes. Fed. Proc. *24:* 1190–1199, 1965.

Estabrook, R. W. and Cohen, B.: Organization of the microsomal electron transport system. In *Microsomes and Drug Oxidations*, ed. By J. R. Gillette, A. H. Conney, G. J. Cosmides, R. W. Estabrook, J. R. Fouts, and G. J. Mannering, pp. 95–109, Academic Press, New York, 1969.

Estabrook, R. W., Cooper, D. Y., and Rosenthal, O.: The light reversible carbon monoxide inhibition of the steroid C21-hydroxylase system of the adrenal cortex. Biochem. Z. *338:* 741–755, 1963.

Fouts, J. R.: The metabolism of drugs by subfractions of hepatic microsomes. Biochem. Biophys. Res. Commun. *6:* 373–378, 1961.

Fujita, T., Itagaki, E., and Sato, R.: Purification and properties of cytochrome b_1 from *Escherichia coli*. J. Biochem. *53:* 282–290, 1963.

Garfinkel, D.: Studies on pig liver microsomes. I. Enzymic and pigment composition of different microsomal fractions. Arch. Biochem. Biophys. *77:* 493–509, 1958.

Gigon, P. L., Gram, T. E., and Gillette. J, R.: Effect of drug substrates on the reduction of hepatic microsomal cytochrome P-450 by NADPH. Biochem. Biophys. Res. Commun. *31:* 558–562, 1968.

Gigon, P. L., Gram, T. E., and Gillette, J. R.: Studies on the rate of reduction of hepatic microsomal cytochrome P-450 by reduced nicotinamide adenine dinucleotide phosphate: effect of drug substrates. Mol. Pharmacol. *5:* 109–122, 1969.

Gillette, J. R.: Metabolism of drugs and other foreign compounds by enzymatic mechanisms. Progr. Drug Res. *6:* 13–73, 1963.

Gillette, J. R.: Biochemistry of drug oxidation and reduction by enzymes in hepatic endoplasmic reticulum. Advan. Pharmacol. *4:* 219–261, 1966.

Gillette, J. R.: Mechanisms of oxidation by enzymes in the endoplasmic reticulum. In *Biochemical Aspects of Antimetabolites and of Drug Hydroxylation*, Vol. 16 in the Federation of European Biochemical Society Symposia Series, (ed. D. Shugar) Academic Press, New York, pp. 109–124, 1969.

Gillette, J. R., Brodie, B. B., and La Du, B. N.: The oxidation of drugs by liver microsomes: On the role of TPNH and oxygen. J. Pharmacol. Exp. Ther. *119:* 532–540, 1957.

Gillette, J. R., Conney, A. H., Cosmides, G. J., Estabrook, R. W., Fouts, J. R., and Mannering, G. J., Eds. *Microsomes and Drug Oxidations*, Academic Press, New York, 1969.

Gillette, J. R. and Gram, T. E.: Cytochrome P-450 reduction in liver microsomes and its relationship to drug metabolism. In *Microsomes and Drug Oxidations*, ed. by J. R. Gillette, A. H. Conney, G. J. Cosmides, R. W. Estabrook, J. R. Fouts, and G. J. Mannering, pp. 133–149, Academic Press, New York, 1969.

Gillette, J. R., Kamm, J. J., and Sasame, H. A.: Mechanism of p-nitrobenzoate reduction in liver: The possible role of cytochrome P-450 in liver microsomes. Mol. Pharmacol. *4:* 541–548, 1968.

Gnosspelius, Y., Thor, H., and Orrenius, S.: A comparative study on the effects of phenobarbital and 3,4-benzpyrene on the hydroxylating enzyme of rat-liver microsomes. Chem.-Biol. Interactions *1:* 125–137, 1969/70.

Gram, T. E., Rogers, L. A., and Fouts, J. R.: Further studies on the metabolism of drugs by subfractions of hepatic microsomes. J. Pharmacol. Exp. Ther. *155:* 479–493, 1967.

Guarino, A. M., Gram, T. E., Gigon, P. L., Greene, F. E., and Gillette, J. R.: Changes in Michaelis and spectral constants for aniline in hepatic microsomes from phenobarbital-treated rats. Mol. Pharmacol. *5:* 131–136, 1969.

Hamaguchi, K. and Geiduschek, E. P.: The effect of electrolytes on the stability of the deoxyribonucleate helix. J. Am. Chem. Soc. *84:* 1329–1338, 1962.

Hashimoto, Y., Yamano, T., and Mason, H. S.: An electron spin resonance study of microsomal electron transport. J. Biol. Chem. *237:* PC3843–PC3845, 1962.

Hayaishi, O.: Oxygenases. In *International Congress of Biochemistry*, 6th, New York, Proceedings of the Plenary Sessions and the Program, Vol. 33, pp. 31–43, Washington, D. C., 1964.

Hernandez, P. H., Gillette, J. R., and Mazel, P.: Studies on the mechanism of action of mammalian hepatic azoreductase. I. Azoreductase activity of reduced nicotinamide adenine dinucleotide phosphate-cytochrome c reductase. Biochem. Pharmacol. *16:* 1859–1875, 1967.

Hernandez, P. H., Mazel, P., and Gillette, J. R.: Studies on the mechanism of action of mammalian hepatic azoreductase. II. The effects of phenobarbital and 3-methcholanthrene on carbon monoxide sensitive and insensitive azoreductase activities. Biochem. Pharmacol. *16:* 1877–1888, 1967a.

Hildebrandt, A. G. and Estabrook, R. W.: Spectrophotometric studies of cytochrome P-450 of liver microsomes after induction with phenobarbital and 3-methylcholanthrene. In *Microsomes and Drug Oxidations*, ed. by J. R. Gillette, A. H. Conney, G. J. Cosmides, R. W. Estabrook, J. R. Fouts, and G. J. Mannering, pp. 331–347, Academic Press, New York, 1969.

Hildebrandt, A. G., Leibman, K. C., and Estabrook, R. W.: Metyrapone interaction with hepatic microsomal cytochrome P-450 from rats treated with phenobarbital. Biochem. Biophys. Res. Commun. *37:* 477–485, 1969.

Hildebrandt, A., Remmer, H., and Estabrook, R. W.: Cytochrome P-450 of liver microsomes—one pigment or many. Biochem. Biophys. Res. Commun. *30:* 607–612, 1968.

Hofmeister, F.: Zur Lehre von der Wirkung der Salze. Arch. Exp. Pathol. Pharmakol. *24:* 247–260, 1888.

Holtzman, J. L., Gram, T. E., Gigon, P. L., and Gillette, J. R.: The distribution of the components of mixed-function oxidase between the rough and the smooth endoplasmic reticulum of liver cells. Biochem. J. *110:* 407–412, 1968.

Horecker, B. L.: Triphosphopyridine nucleotide-cytochrome c reductase in liver. J. Biol. Chem. *183:* 593–605, 1950.

Ichikawa, Y., Hagihara, B., and Yamano, T.: Magnetic and spectrophotometric properties of the microsomal carbon monoxide binding pigment. Arch. Biochem. Biophys. *120:* 204–213, 1967.

Ichikawa, Y., Uemura, T., and Yamano, T.: The role of the hydrophobic bonding in hemoprotein P-450 and the effect of organic compounds on the conversion of hemoprotein P-450 to hemoprotein P-420. In *Structure and Function of Cytochromes*, ed. by K. Okunuki, M. D. Kamen, and I. Sekuzu, pp. 634–644, University Park Press, Baltimore, Md., 1968.

Ichikawa, Y. and Yamano, T.: Reconversion of detergent- and sulfhydryl reagent-produced P-420 to P-450 by polyols and glutathione. Biochim. Biophys. Acta *131:* 490–497, 1967.

Ichikawa, Y. and Yamano, T.: Preparation and physicochemical properties of functional hemoprotein P-450 from mammalian tissue microsomes. Biochim. Biophys. Acta *200:* 220–240, 1970.

Imai, Y. and Sato, R.: Substrate interaction with hydroxylase system in liver microsomes. Biochem. Biophys. Res. Commun. *22:* 620–626, 1966.

Imai, Y. and Sato, R.: Evidence for two forms of P-450 hemoprotein in microsomal membranes. Biochem. Biophys. Res. Commun. *23:* 5–11, 1966a.

Imai, Y. and Sato, R.: Studies on the substrate interactions with P-450 in drug hydroxylation by liver microsomes. J. Biochem. *62:* 239–249, 1967.

Imai, Y. and Sato, R.: Conversion of P-450 to P-420 by neutral salts and other reagents. European J. Biochem. *1:* 419–426, 1967a.

Ishidate, K., Kawaguchi, K., and Tagawa, K.: Change in P-450 content accompanying aerobic formation of mitochondria in yeast. J. Biochem. *65:* 385–392, 1969a.

Ishidate, K., Kawaguchi, K., Tagawa, K., and Hagihara, B.: Hemoproteins in anaerobically grown yeast cells. J. Biochem. *65:* 375–383, 1969.

Jefcoate, C. R. E. and Gaylor, J. L.: Ligand interactions with hemoprotein P-450. II. Influence of phenobarbital and methylcholanthrene induction processes on P-450 spectra. Biochemistry *8:* 3464–3472, 1969.

Jefcoate, C. R. E., Gaylor, J. L., and Calabrese, R. L.: Ligand interactions with cytochrome P-450. I. Binding of primary amines. Biochemistry *8:* 3455–3463, 1969.

Kamin, H., Masters, B. S. S., Gibson, Q. H., and Williams, C. H., Jr.: Microsomal TPNH-cytochrome c reductase. Fed. Proc. *24:* 1164–1171, 1965.

Katagiri, M., Ganguli, B. N. and Gunsalus, I. C.: A soluble cytochrome P-450 functional in methylene hydroxylation. J. Biol. Chem. *243:* 3543–3546, 1968.

Kato, R. and Gillette, J. R.: Sex differences in the effects of abnormal physiological states on the metabolism of drugs by rat liver microsomes. J. Pharmacol. Exp. Ther. 150: 285–291, 1965.

Kaufman, S.: The enzymatic conversion of phenylalanine to tyrosine. J. Biol. Chem. 226: 511–524, 1957.

Keilin, D. and Hartree, E. F.: Cytochrome and cytochrome oxidase. Proc. Roy. Soc., London, Ser. B, 127: 167–191, 1939.

Kimura, T.: Animal non-heme iron protein as a component of the electron transport system in steroid hydroxylases. In Biogenesis and Action of Steroid Hormones, ed. by R. I. Dorfman, K. Yamasaki, and M. Dorfman, pp. 126–131, Geron-X, Inc., Los Altos, Calif., 1968.

Kimura, T. and Suzuki, K.: Enzymatic reduction of non-heme iron protein (adrenodoxin) by reduced nicotinamide adenine dinucleotide phosphate. Biochem. Biophys. Res. Commun. 20: 373–379, 1965.

Kimura, T. and Suzuki, K.: Components of the electron transport system in adrenal steroid hydroxylase. Isolation and properties of non-heme iron protein (adrenodoxin). J. Biol. Chem. 242: 485–491, 1967.

Kinoshita, T. and Horie, S.: Studies on P-450. III. On the absorption spectrum of P-450 in rabbit liver microsomes. J. Biochem. 61: 26–34, 1967.

Klingenberg, M.: Pigments of rat liver microsomes. Arch. Biochem. Biophys. 75: 376–386, 1958.

Kratz, F. and Staudinger, H.: Spektrale Änderungen von Kaninchenlebermikrosomen durch Cumarin. Hoppe-Seyler's Z. Physiol. Chem. 349: 455–458, 1968.

Kuntzman, R.: Drugs and enzyme induction. Ann. Rev. Pharmacol. 9: 21–36, 1969.

Kuntzman, R., Jacobson, M., Schneidman, K., and Conney, A. H.: Similarities between oxidative drug-metabolizing enzymes and steroid hydroxylases in liver microsomes. J. Pharmacol. Exp. Ther. 146: 280–285, 1964.

Kuntzman, R., Lawrence, D., and Conney, A. H.: Michaelis constants for the hydroxylation of steroid hormones and drugs by rat liver microsomes. Mol. Pharmacol. 1: 163–167, 1965.

Kuntzman, R., Levin, W., Schilling, G., and Alvares, A.: The effects of 3-methylcholanthrene and phenobarbital on liver microsomal hemoproteins and on the hydroxylation of benzpyrene. In Microsomes and Drug Oxidations, ed. by J. R. Gillette, A. H. Conney, G. J. Cosmides, R. W. Estabrook, J. R. Fouts, and G. J. Mannering, pp. 349–369, Academic Press, New York, 1969.

La Du, B. N., Gaudette, L., Trousof, N., and Brodie, B. B.: Enzymatic dealkylation of aminopyrine (Pyramidon) and other alkylamines. J. Biol. Chem. 214: 741–752, 1955.

Leibman, K. C., Hildebrandt, A. G., and Estabrook, R. W.: Spectrophotometric studies of interactions between various substrates in their binding to microsomal cytochrome P-450. Biochem. Biophys. Res. Commun. 36: 789–794, 1969.

Levin, W. and Kuntzman, R.: Studies on the incorporation of δ-aminolevulinic acid into microsomal hemoprotein: Effect of 3-methylcholanthrene and phenobarbital. Life Sci. 8: 305–311, 1969.

Levin, W. and Kuntzman, R.: Biphasic decrease of radioactive hemoprotein from liver microsomal CO-binding particles. Effect of 3-methylcholanthrene. J. Biol. Chem. 244: 3671–3676, 1969a.

Levin, W. and Kuntzman, R.: Biphasic decrease of radioactive hemoprotein from liver microsomal carbon monoxide-binding particles. Effect of phenobarbital and chlordane. Mol. Pharmacol. 5: 499–506, 1969b.

Lu, A. Y. H. and Coon, M. J.: Role of hemoprotein P-450 in fatty acid ω-hydroxylation in a soluble enzyme system from liver microsomes. J. Biol. Chem. 243: 1331–1332, 1968.

Lu, A. Y. H., Junk, K. W., and Coon, M. J.: Resolution of the cytochrome P-450-containing ω-hydroxylation system of liver microsomes into three components. J. Biol. Chem. 244: 3714–3721, 1969a.

Lu, A. Y. H., Strobel, H. W., and Coon, M. J.: Hydroxylation of benzphetamine and other drugs by a solubilized form of cytochrome P-450 from liver microsomes: lipid requirement for drug demethylation. Biochem. Biophys. Res. Commun. 36: 545–551, 1969.

Machinist, J. M., Orme-Johnson, W. H., and Ziegler, D. M.: Microsomal oxidases. II. Properties of a pork liver microsomal N-oxide dealkylase. Biochemistry 5: 2939–2943, 1966.

Maclennan, D. H., Tzagoloff, A., and McConnell, D. G.: The preparation of microsomal electron-transfer complexes. Biochim. Biophys. Acta 131: 59–80, 1967

Mannering, G. J.: Significance of stimulation and inhibition of drug metabolism in pharmacological testing. In Selected Pharmacological Testing Methods, ed. by A. Burger, pp. 51–119, Marcel Dekker, New York, 1968.

Mannering, G. J., Sladek, N. E., Parli, C. J., and Shoeman, D. W.: Formation of a new P-450 hemoprotein after treatment of rats with polycyclic hydrocarbons. In Microsomes and Drug Oxidations, ed. by J. R. Gillette, A. H. Conney, G. J. Cosmides, R. W. Estabrook, J. R. Fouts, and

G. J. Mannering, pp. 303–330, Academic Press, New York, 1969.

Mason, H. S.: Mechanisms of oxygen metabolism. Science *125:* 1185–1188, 1957.

Mason, H. S.: Oxidases. Ann. Rev. Biochem. *34:* 595–634, 1965.

Mason, H. S., North, J. C., and Vanneste, M.: Microsomal mixed-function oxidations: the metabolism of xenobiotics. Fed. Proc. *24:* 1172–1180, 1965.

Mason, H. S., Yamano, T., North, J. C., Hashimoto, Y., and Sakagishi, P.: The structure and oxidase function of liver microsomes. In *Oxidases and Related Redox Systems*, ed. by T. E. King, H. S. Mason, and M. Morrison, Vol. 2, pp. 879–903, John Wiley & Sons, Inc., New York, 1965a.

Masters, B. S. S., Bilimoria, M. H., Kamin, H., and Gibson, Q. H.: The mechanism of 1- and 2-electron transfers catalyzed by reduced triphosphopyridine nucleotide-cytochrome c reductase. J. Biol. Chem. *240:* 4081–4088, 1965a.

Masters, B. S. S., Kamin, H., Gibson, Q. H., and Williams, C. H., Jr.: Studies on the mechanism of microsomal triphosphopyridine nucleotide-cytochrome c reductase. J. Biol. Chem. *240:* 921–931, 1965.

McMahon, R. E. and Sullivan, H. R.: The microsomal hydroxylation of ethylbenzene: Stereochemical, induction and isotopic studies. In *Microsomes and Drug Oxidations*, ed. by J. R. Gillette, A. H. Conney, G. J. Cosmides, R. W. Estabrook, J. R. Fouts, and G. J. Mannering, pp. 239–247, Academic Press, New York, 1969.

Mitani, F. and Horie, S.: Studies on P-450. V. On the substrate-induced spectral change of P-450 solubilized from bovine adrenocortical mitochondria. J. Biochem. *65:* 269–280, 1969.

Miyake, Y., Gaylor, J. L., and Mason, H. S.: Properties of a submicrosomal particle containing P-450 and flavoprotein. J. Biol. Chem. *243:* 5788–5797, 1968.

Miyake, Y., Mori, K., and Yamano, T.: A study of some spectral properties of P-450 in a submicrosomal particle. Arch. Biochem. Biophys. *133:* 318–326, 1969.

Mueller, G. C. and Miller, J. A.: The reductive cleavage of 4-dimethylaminoazobenzene by rat liver: the intracellular distribution of the enzyme system and its requirement for triphosphopyridine nucleotide. J. Biol. Chem. *180:* 1125–1136, 1949.

Mueller, G. C. and Miller, J. A.: The metabolism of methylated aminoazo dyes. II. Oxidative demethylation by rat liver homogenates. J. Biol. Chem. *202:* 579–587, 1953.

Narasimhulu, S., Cooper, D. Y., and Rosenthal, O.: Spectrophotometric properties of a triton-clarified steroid 21-hydroxylase system of adrenocortical microsomes. Life Sci. *4:* 2102–2107, 1965.

Nemethy, G.: Hydrophobic interactions. Angew. Chem. Int. Ed. Engl. *6:* 195–206, 1967.

Nemethy, G. and Scheraga, H. A.: The structure of water and hydrophobic bonding in proteins. III. The thermodynamic properties of hydrophobic bonds in proteins. J. Phys. Chem. *66:* 1773–1789, 1963.

Netter, K. J.: Untersuchungen zur mikrosomalen Napthalinhydroxylierung. Arch. Exp. Pathol. Pharmakol. *262:* 375–387, 1969.

Netter, K. J., Kahl, G.-F., and Magnussen, M. P.: Kinetic experiments on the binding of metyrapone to liver microsomes. Arch. Exp. Pathol. Pharmakol. *265:* 205–215, 1969.

Nilsson, A. and Johnson, B. C.: Cofactor requirements of the O-demethylating liver microsomal enzyme system. Arch. Biochem. Biophys. *101:* 494–498, 1963.

Nishibayashi, H., Omura, T., and Sato, R.: The binding of ethyl isocyanide by hepatic microsomal hemoprotein. Biochim. Biophys. Acta *118:* 651–654, 1966.

Nishibayashi, H., Omura, T., Sato, R., and Estabrook, R. W.: Comments on the absorption spectra of hemoprotein P-450. In *Structure and Function of Cytochromes*, ed. by K. Okunuki, M. D. Kamen, and I. Sekuzu, pp. 658–665, University Park Press, Baltimore, Md., 1968.

Nishibayashi, H. and Sato, R.: Preparation of hepatic microsomal particles containing P-450 as sole heme constituent and absolute spectra of P-450. J. Biochem. *63:* 766–779, 1968.

Omura, T., Narasimhulu, S., and Estabrook, R.: Unpublished observations cited during the discussion of a presentation by R. Sato, T. Omura and H. Nishibayashi. In *Oxidases and Related Redox Systems*, ed. by T. E. King, H. S. Mason, and M. Morrison, Vol. 2, p. 876, John Wiley & Sons, Inc., New York, 1965.

Omura, T., Sanders, E., Estabrook, R. W., Cooper, D. Y., and Rosenthal, O.: Isolation from adrenal cortex of a nonheme iron protein and a flavoprotein functional as a reduced triphosphopyridine nucleotide-cytochrome P-450 reductase. Arch. Biochem. Biophys. *117:* 660–673, 1966.

Omura, T. and Sato, R.: A new cytochrome in liver microsomes. J. Biol. Chem. *237:* 1375–1376, 1962.

Omura, T. and Sato, R.: Fractional solubilization of haemoproteins and partial purification of carbon monoxide-binding cytochrome from liver microsomes. Biochim. Biophys. Acta *71:* 224–226, 1963.

Omura, T. and Sato, R.: The carbon monoxide-binding pigment of liver microsomes. I. Evidence for its hemoprotein nature. J. Biol. Chem. 239: 2370–2378, 1964.

Omura, T. and Sato, R.: The carbon monoxide-binding pigment of liver microsomes. II. Solubilization, purification, and properties. J. Biol. Chem. 239: 2379–2385, 1964a.

Omura, T. and Sato, R.: Unpublished observations cited by Sato et al., 1965.

Omura, T., Sato, R., Cooper, D. Y., Rosenthal, O., and Estabrook, R. W.: Function of cytochrome P-450 of microsomes. Fed. Proc. 24: 1181–1189, 1965a.

Orrenius, S.: Further studies on the induction of the drug-hydroxylating enzyme system of liver microsomes. J. Cell Biol. 26: 725–733, 1965.

Orrenius, S., Berg, A., and Ernster, L.: Effects of trypsin on the electron transport systems of liver microsomes. European J. Biochem. 11: 193–200, 1969.

Orrenius, S. and Ernster, L.: Phenobarbital-induced synthesis of the oxidative demethylating enzymes of rat liver microsomes. Biochem. Biophys. Res. Commun. 16: 60–65, 1964.

Parli, C. J. and Mannering, G. J.: Induction of drug metabolism. IV. Relative abilities of polycyclic hydrocarbons to increase levels of microsomal 3-methyl-4-methylaminoazobenzene N-demethylase activity and cytochrome P_1-450. Mol. Pharmacol. 6: 178–183, 1970.

Phillips, A. H. and Langdon, R. G.: Hepatic triphosphopyridine nucleotide-cytochrome c reductase: Isolation, characterization, and kinetic studies. J. Biol. Chem. 237: 2652–2660, 1962.

Posner, H. S., Mitoma, C., Rothberg, S., and Udenfriend, S.: Enzymic hydroxylation of aromatic compounds. III. Studies on the mechanism of microsomal hydroxylation. Arch. Biochem. Biophys. 94: 280–290, 1961a.

Posner, H. S., Mitoma, C., and Udenfriend, S.: Enzymic hydroxylation of aromatic compounds. II. Further studies of the properties of the microsomal hydroxylating system. Arch. Biochem. Biophys. 94: 269–279, 1961.

Reif, A. E., Brown, R. R., Potter, V. R., Miller, E. C., and Miller, J. A.: Effect of diet on the antimycin titer of mouse liver. J. Biol. Chem. 209: 223–226, 1954.

Remmer, H.: Die Verstarkung der Abbaugeschwindigkeit von Evipan durch Glykocorticoide. Arch. Exp. Pathol. Pharmakol. 233: 184–191, 1958.

Remmer, H. and Merker, H. J.: Drug-induced changes in the liver endoplasmic reticulum: Association with drug-metabo-

lizing enzymes. Science 142: 1657–1658, 1963.

Remmer, H. and Merker, H. J.: Effect of drugs on the formation of smooth endoplasmic reticulum and drug-metabolizing enzymes. Ann. N. Y. Acad. Sci. 123: 79–97, 1965.

Remmer, H., Schenkman, J., Estabrook, R. W., Sasame, H., Gillette, J., Narasimhulu, S., Cooper, D. Y., and Rosenthal, O.: Drug interaction with hepatic microsomal cytochrome. Mol. Pharmacol. 2: 187–190, 1966.

Remmer, H., Schenkman, J. B., and Greim, H.: Spectral investigations on cytochrome P-450. In Microsomes and Drug Oxidations, ed. by J. R. Gillette, A. H. Conney, G. J. Cosmides, R. W. Estabrook, J. R. Fouts, and G. J. Mannering, pp. 371–386, Academic Press, New York, 1969.

Rubin, A., Tephly, T. R., and Mannering, G. J.: Kinetics of drug metabolism by hepatic microsomes. Biochem. Pharmacol. 13: 1007–1016, 1964.

Sasame, H. A.: Unpublished observations, 1964, cited by Gillette, 1966, 1969.

Sasame, H. A. and Gillette, J. R.: Studies on the relationship between the effects of various substances on absorption spectrum of cytochrome P-450 and the reduction of p-nitrobenzoate by mouse liver microsomes. Mol. Pharmacol. 5: 123–130, 1969.

Sato, R., Nishibayashi, H., and Ito, A.: Characterization of two hemoproteins of liver microsomes. In Microsomes and Drug Oxidations, ed. by J. R. Gillette, A. H. Conney, G. J. Cosmides, R. W. Estabrook, J. R. Fouts, and G. J. Mannering, pp. 111–132, Academic Press, New York, 1969.

Sato, R., Omura, T., and Nishibayashi, H.: Carbon monoxide-binding hemoprotein and NADPH-specific flavoprotein in liver microsomes and their roles in microsomal electron transfer. In Oxidases and Related Redox Systems, ed. by T. E. King, H. S. Mason, and M. Morrison, pp. 861–878, John Wiley & Sons, Inc., New York, 1965.

Schenkman, J. B., Ball, J. A., and Estabrook, R. W.: On the use of nicotinamide in assays for microsomal mixed-function oxidase activity. Biochem. Pharmacol. 16: 1071–1081, 1967b.

Schenkman, J. B., Frey, I., Remmer, H., and Estabrook, R. W.: Sex differences in drug metabolism by rat liver microsomes. Mol. Pharmacol. 3: 516–525, 1967a.

Schenkman, J. B., Greim, H., Zange, M., and Remmer, H.: On the problem of possible other forms of cytochrome P-450 in liver microsomes. Biochim. Biophys. Acta 171: 23–31, 1969.

Schenkman, J. B., Remmer, H., and Estabrook, R. W.: Spectral studies of drug interaction with hepatic microsomal cytochrome. Mol. Pharmacol. *3:* 113–123, 1967.

Schenkman, J. B. and Sato, R.: The relationship between the pH-induced spectral change in ferriprotoheme and the substrate-induced spectral change of the hepatic microsomal mixed-function oxidase. Mol. Pharmacol. *4:* 613–621, 1968.

Shoeman, D. W., Chaplin, M. D., and Mannering, G. J.: Induction of drug metabolism. III. Further evidence for the formation of a new P-450 hemoprotein after treatment of rats with 3-methylcholanthrene. Mol. Pharmacol. *5:* 412–419, 1969a.

Shoeman, D. W., Vane, F., and Mannering, G. J.: Differences in the hepatic cytochrome P-420 obtained from normal and 3-methylcholanthrene (MC) treated rats. Fed. Proc. *29:* 738, 1970.

Shoeman, D. W., White, J. G., and Mannering, G. J.: Cytochrome P-420: Tubular aggregates from hepatic microsomes. Science *165:* 1371–1372, 1969.

Sih, C. J.: Enzymatic mechanism of steroid hydroxylation. Science *163:* 1297–1300, 1969.

Sih, C. J., Tsong, Y. Y., and Stein, B.: The roles of reduced nicotinamide-adenine dinucleotide phosphate in steroid hydroxylation. J. Am. Chem. Soc. *90:* 5300–5302, 1968.

Silverman, D. A. and Talalay, P.: Studies on the enzymic hydroxylation of 3,4-benzpyrene. Mol. Pharmacol. *3:* 90–101, 1967.

Sladek, N. E.: Studies on the stimulation of drug metabolism by phenobarbital and polycyclic hydrocarbons. Ph.D. Dissertation, University of Minnesota, 1966.

Sladek, N. E. and Mannering, G. J.: Evidence for a new P-450 hemoprotein in hepatic microsomes from methylcholanthrene treated rats. Biochem. Biophys. Res. Commun. *24:* 668–674, 1966.

Sladek, N. E. and Mannering, G. J.: Induction of drug metabolism. I. Differences in the mechanisms by which polycyclic hydrocarbons and phenobarbital produce their inductive effects on microsomal N-demethylating systems. Mol. Pharmacol. *5:* 174–185, 1969.

Sladek, N. E. and Mannering, G. J.: Induction of drug metabolism. II. Qualitative differences in the microsomal N-demethylating systems stimulated by polycyclic hydrocarbons and by phenobarbital. Mol. Pharmacol. *5:* 186–199, 1969a.

Strittmatter, P. and Velick, S. F.: A microsomal cytochrome reductase specific for diphosphopyridine nucleotide. J. Biol. Chem. *221:* 277–286, 1956.

Suzuki, K. and Kimura, T.: An iron protein as a component of steroid 11β-hydroxylase

complex. Biochem. Biophys. Res. Commun. *19:* 340–345, 1965.

Takesue, Y., Omura, T., and Sato, R.: Unpublished observations cited by Sato et al., 1965.

Tonomura, Y., Sekiya, K., and Imamura, K.: The optical rotary dispersion of myosin A. I. Effect of inorganic salt. J. Biol. Chem. *237:* 3110–3115, 1962.

Trivus, R. H. and Spirtes, M. A.: The stoichiometry of microsomal drug dependent NADPH oxidation. Fed. Proc. *24:* 152, 1965.

Ullrich, V.: On the hydroxylation of cyclohexane in rat liver microsomes. Hoppe-Seyler's Z. Physiol. Chem. *350:* 357–365, 1969.

Von Hippel, P. H. and Wong, K.-Y.: The effect of ions on the kinetics of formation and the stability of the collagen-fold. Biochemistry *1:* 664–674, 1962.

Von Hippel, P. H. and Wong, K.-Y.: Neutral salts: The generality of their effects on the stability of macromolecular conformations. Science *145:* 577–580, 1964.

Von Hippel, P. H. and Wong, K.-Y.: On the conformational stability of globular proteins. The effects of various electrolytes and nonelectrolytes on the thermal ribonuclease transition. J. Biol. Chem. *240:* 3909–3923, 1965.

Warburg, O.: *Heavy Metal Prosthetic Groups and Enzyme Action*, Clarendon Press, Oxford, 1949.

Whysner, J. A., Ramseyer, J., Kazmi, G. M., and Harding, B. W.: Substrate induced spin state changes in cytochrome P-450. Biochem. Biophys. Res. Commun. *36:* 795–801, 1969.

Williams, C. H., Jr. and Kamin, H.: Microsomal triphosphopyridine nucleotide-cytochrome c reductase of liver. J. Biol. Chem. *237:* 587–595, 1962.

Yohro, T. and Horie, S.: Subcellular distribution of P-450 in bovine *corpus luteum.* J. Biochem. *61:* 515–517, 1967.

Ziegler, D. M., Mitchell, C. H., and Jollow, D.: The properties of a purified hepatic microsomal mixed function amine oxidase. In *Microsomes and Drug Oxidations*, ed. by J. R. Gillette, A. H. Conney, G. J. Cosmides, R. W. Estabrook, J. R. Fouts, and G. J. Mannering, pp. 173–188, Academic Press, New York, 1969.

Ziegler, D. M. and Pettit, F. H.: Formation of an intermediate N-oxide in the oxidative demethylation of N,N-dimethylaniline catalyzed by liver microsomes. Biochem. Biophys. Res. Commun. *15:* 188–193, 1964.

Ziegler, D. M. and Pettit, F. H.: Microsomal oxidases. I. The isolation and dialkylarylamine oxygenase activity of pork liver microsomes. Biochemistry *5:* 2932–2938, 1966.

13

Environmental Factors Influencing Drug Metabolism

A. H. CONNEY

I. INTRODUCTION

Studies during the past 15 years have shown that the duration and intensity of action of many drugs in animals depend on the activity of drug-metabolizing enzymes localized in the microsomal fraction of liver homogenate which is derived from the endoplasmic reticulum of the liver cell. Environmental factors play an important role in regulating the activity of drug-metabolizing enzymes in the liver, and the activity of these enzymes can be altered by dietary and nutritional factors, x-irradiation, hormonal changes in the body and by the ingestion of foreign chemicals (Conney and Burns, 1962; Gillette, 1963; Fouts, 1963; Nair and DuBois, 1968). In addition, there are diurnal variations in the rate of drug and steroid hydroxylation (Radzialowski and Bousquet, 1968; Colas et al., 1969), and changes in atmospheric pressure and respiratory oxygen can also influence drug metabolism (Kitagawa, 1968; Merritt and Medina, 1968).

The administration to animals of numerous drugs and environmental chemicals can inhibit or potentiate the pharmacological and toxicological action of other drugs by altering the activity of drug-metabolizing enzymes in liver microsomes, and it appears that this effect also occurs in man. Recent studies have shown that steroid hormones are substrates for the same liver microsomal enzymes that hydroxylate drugs. Accordingly, treatment of animals with inhibitors or stimulators of drug hydroxylation also alter the hydroxylation of steroids.

This chapter describes some of the pharmacological and toxicological implications of the stimulatory and inhibitory effect of foreign chemicals on the metabolism of drugs and steroids in experimental animals and man. Research on the effect of foreign chemicals on the metabolism of drugs and normal body constituents by enzymes in liver microsomes has expanded rapidly during recent years and several reviews have appeared that emphasize various aspects of this problem (Conney and Burns, 1962; Gillette, 1963; Fouts, 1963; Burns, 1964; Remmer and Merker, 1965; Ernster and Orrenius, 1965; Conney, 1967; Conney et al., 1967; Gelboin, 1967; Mannering, 1968; Kuntzman, 1969; Conney, 1969).

II. EFFECT OF ENZYME INDUCTION ON THE DURATION OF DRUG ACTION

The chronic administration of one drug can reduce the pharmacologic activity of another drug by stimulating its metabolic inactivation. Drugs appear to exert

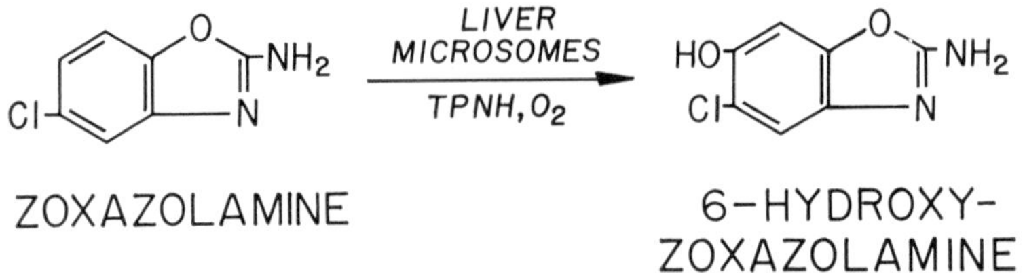

Fig. 13.1. Hydroxylation of zoxazolamine by liver microsomes.

this effect by increasing the amount of drug-metabolizing enzymes in liver microsomes, referred to as "enzyme induction." The mechanisms by which drugs exert this effect are discussed in Chapter 14.

The administration of compounds that stimulate the activity of drug-metabolizing enzymes in liver microsomes markedly decreases the duration of action of a subsequent dose of many drugs, such as zoxazolamine, meprobamate, carisoprodol, diphenylhydantoin and several barbiturates that are metabolized to pharmacologically inactive metabolites. As an example, the liver microsomal enzyme that hydroxylates zoxazolamine was studied in some detail.

Zoxazolamine is a muscle relaxant drug that is hydroxylated in the 6– position by liver microsomes to a pharmacologically inactive metabolite (Fig. 13.1), and any increase in the activity of this enzyme would be expected to shorten the duration of action of zoxazolamine. The stimulatory effect of 3,4-benzpyrene and phenobarbital on zoxazolamine hydroxylase activity in rat liver microsomes is shown in Fig. 13.2. Administration of 3,4-benzpyrene rapidly stimulated zoxazolamine hydroxylase, and maximum enzyme activity was observed within 24 hours. Increased zoxazolamine hydroxylase activity was found 24 hours after starting phenobarbital administration, but maximum stimulation was not obtained until 3–4 days later. In a similar manner, maximum stimulation of the hexobarbital-metabolizing enzyme system in rat liver microsomes was observed after 3–4 days of injections with phenobarbital. The activity of these enzymes returned to control values within several days after withdrawal of drug administration. The increased zoxazolamine hydroxylase activity in liver microsomes of rats pretreated with phenobarbital and 3,4-benzpyrene correlated well with an accelerated rate of metabolism of zoxazolamine *in vivo*. The biological half-life of zoxazolamine was 9 hours in control rats, 48 minutes in phenobarbital-pretreated rats and only 10 minutes in rats pretreated with 3,4-benzpyrene (Fig. 13.3).

Pretreatment of rats with drugs that stimulate zoxazolamine hydroxylase activity shortened the duration of action of zoxazolamine because this drug is metabolized to a pharmacologically inactive metabolite. Control rats given a high dose of zoxazolamine were paralyzed for 730 minutes; rats pretreated for 4 days with phenylbutazone, a weak inducer, were paralyzed for 307 minutes; rats pretreated for 4 days with phenobarbital, a moderately strong inducer, were paralyzed for 102 minutes; and rats pretreated for 1 day with 3,4-benzpyrene, a very strong inducer, were paralyzed for only 17 minutes. Although pretreatment of rats with polycyclic hydrocarbons, such as 3,4-benzpyrene, decreases the pharmacologic action of zoxazolamine by stimulating its metabolism, 3,4-benzpyrene does not decrease the pharmacologic action of hexobarbital or stimulate its metabolism. These results indicate that polycyclic hydrocarbons

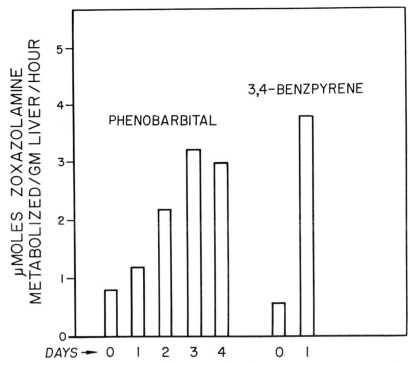

Fig. 13.2. Stimulatory effect of phenobarbital and 3,4-benzpyrene on zoxazolamine hydroxylase activity in rat liver microsomes. Male rats weighing 40g were injected i.p. with either 25 mg/kg of 3,4-benzpyrene once or with 37 mg/kg of sodium phenobarbital twice daily. (From Conney et al., 1960.)

show considerable specificity as enzyme inducers and do not stimulate the activity of all drug-metabolizing enzymes. The relative specificity of polycyclic hydrocarbons and the relative nonspecificity of phenobarbital as enzyme inducers are discussed in more detail elsewhere (Conney, 1967).

More than 200 drugs, insecticides, carcinogens and other chemicals are known to stimulate the activity of drug-metabolizing enzymes in liver microsomes (Conney, 1967; Mannering, 1968). Examples include hypnotics and sedatives, anesthetic gases, central nervous system stimulants, anticonvulsants, tranquilizers, antipsychotic drugs, hypoglycemic agents, anti-inflammatory drugs, muscle relaxants, analgesics, antihistaminics, alkaloids, and steroid hormones. In addition, many chemicals present in man's environment can stimulate the activity of drug-metabolizing enzymes in the liver microsomes of animals, and can markedly alter the duration and intensity of drug action. Examples of such chemicals include polycyclic aromatic hydrocarbons in cigarette smoke, polluted city air and certain cooked foods (Arcos et al., 1961; Conney, 1967; Welch et al., 1969), halogenated hydrocarbon insecticides (Hart et al., 1963; Hart and Fouts, 1965; Conney et al., 1967), urea herbicides (Kinoshita et al., 1966), food preservatives (Gilbert and Goldberg, 1965; Creaven et al., 1966), various dyes used as coloring agents (Radomski, 1961; Levin and Conney, 1967), and caffeine and flavones in foodstuffs (Mitoma et al., 1968; Wattenberg et al., 1968). Cedar chips and other bedding used for the housing of animals are also potent stimulators of

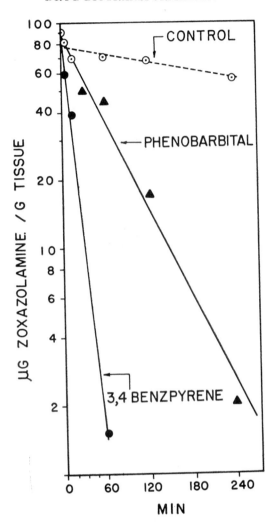

Fig. 13.3. *In vivo* metabolism of zoxazolamine in rats pretreated with phenobarbital or 3,4-benzpyrene. Immature male rats were injected i.p. with 37 mg/kg of sodium phenobarbital twice daily for 4 days or 25 mg/kg of 3,4-benzpyrene 24 hours before an i.p. injection of 100 mg/kg of zoxazolamine. The concentration of zoxazolamine in total body homogenate was measured. (From Conney *et al.*, 1960.)

drug metabolism, and care must be taken in choosing such material for the housing of animals (Ferguson, 1966; Vesell, 1967).

The stimulatory effect of halogenated hydrocarbon insecticides on drug metabolism was observed (Hart and Fouts, 1965) after animal quarters were treated with chlordane. Studies on drug metabolism were disrupted for several weeks, even though insecticide treatment had stopped. Treatment of rodents with many commonly used halogenated hydrocarbon insecticides increases the activity of enzymes in liver microsomes that oxidatively metabolize drugs such as hexobarbital, aminopyrine and chlorpromazine, and the increased enzyme levels compare with a decreased action of hexobarbital. Examples of such insecticides include chlordane, DDT, DDE, methoxychlor, aldrin, endrin, dieldrin, heptachlor and benzene hexachloride. Unlike the halogenated hydrocarbons, several organophosphorus insecticides, when given chronically, inhibit the hydroxylation of drugs and steroids by liver microsomes (Rosenberg and Coon, 1958; Welch *et al.*, 1959; Welch *et al.*, 1967a).

The stimulatory effect of halogenated hydrocarbon insecticides on drug metabolism in rats lasts for several weeks after cessation of exposure, presumably because of the prolonged storage of these compounds in body fat. A single intraperitoneal injection of dieldrin (40 mg/kg) or DDT (200 mg/kg) resulted in a gradual elevation in the metabolism of hexobarbital and acetophenetidin *in vitro* to a maximum of 2–3 times control values in 5–10 days (Ghazal *et al.*, 1964); hexobarbital metabolism was elevated for longer than 65 days and returned to control values by 90 days. Drug metabolism returned toward the control values within 20 days after injection of dieldrin into rats.

Of considerable interest is a species difference with regard to the effect of DDT on drug metabolism. Although chlordane stimulates hexobarbital metabolism in the rat and mouse, DDT and its metabolites stimulate hexobarbital metabolism in the rat, but not in the mouse (Cram and Fouts, 1967). The reason is not known.

The effect of low levels of DDT on drug metabolism in rats was investigated, and feeding as little as 5 ppm of DDT in the diet for 3 months resulted in elevated levels of liver microsomal enzymes that metabolize hexobarbital and aminopyrine (Hart and Fouts, 1965). More recently, Kinoshita *et al.* (1966) found that 1 ppm of DDT in the diet caused significant induction of microsomal enzymes in rats. This level is the same as the permitted level of 1 ppm established in February of 1968 by the Food and Drug Administration for several foods. Studies on the effects of small oral doses of chlordane on the metabolism of drugs in dogs revealed that treatment of dogs with 5 mg/kg of chlordane orally 3 times a week for 5–6 weeks stimulated the metabolism of phenylbutazone, antipyrine and bishydroxycoumarin (Burns *et al.*, 1965; Conney *et al.*, 1967; Welch *et al.*, 1967).

As little as 10 μg of DDT (combined DDT and DDE) per gram of fat is associated with enhanced metabolism of pentobarbital in the rat. Two days after the intraperitoneal administration of DDT, the duration of sleep produced by a dose of pentobarbital was decreased by 25% with 1 mg of DDT per kg and by 50% with 2 mg of DDT per kg, and the corresponding concentrations of DDT in the fat were 9.4 and 15.5 μg/gm (Gerboth and Schwabe, 1964). Since many people have these concentrations of DDT and other halogenated hydrocarbon insecticides in their fat (Durham, 1965; Quinby *et al.*, 1965), it is possible that such persons may have elevated levels of microsomal enzymes that oxidize drugs. Recent observations suggest that individuals occupationally exposed to high levels of DDT and lindane metabolize some drugs more rapidly than the general population, and this is discussed in Section VII.

III. EFFECT OF ENZYME INDUCTION ON DRUG TOXICITY

The levels of drug-metabolizing enzymes in liver are important in acute toxicity studies, and factors which influence the amount of these enzymes may alter drug toxicity. Table 13.1 shows that pretreatment of rats with the potent enzyme inducer, 3-methylcholanthrene, markedly decreases the acute toxicity

TABLE 13.1

Effect of enzyme induction on the acute toxicity of drugs in rats

Pretreatment	Mortality (%)				
	Zoxazolamine[a]	Meproba-mate[b]	Pentobarbital[c]	Strychnine[d]	Schradan[d]
None	100	65	100	70	6
3-Methylcholanthrene	0				
Phenobarbital		0			
Chlorcyclizine			30		
Phenaglycodol				5	81
Thiopental				15	75

[a] Male rats weighing 45–50g were injected intraperitoneally with 20 mg/kg of 3-methylcholanthrene and were given a challenging intraperitoneal dose of zoxazolamine (150 mg/kg) 24 hours later (ten rats in each group).

[b] Male rats weighing 45–50g were injected with 37 mg/kg of sodium phenobarbital intraperitoneally twice daily and were given a challenging dose of meprobamate (250 mg/kg) 16 hours after the last dose (ten rats in each group).

[c] Adult female rats were fed 0.026% chlorcyclizine in the diet for 3 weeks and were given an intraperitoneal dose of pentobarbital (58 mg/kg). (From Thompson et al., 1959.)

[d] Adult female rats were given daily intraperitoneal injections of phenaglycodol (70 mg/kg) or thiopental (20 mg/kg) for 4 days and were given a challenging intraperitoneal dose of strychnine sulfate (1.6 mg/kg) or Schradan (octamethylpyrophosphoramide, 20 mg/kg). (From Kato, 1961.)

of zoxazolamine. All of the control rats were killed by a dose of 150 mg/kg of zoxazolamine, whereas all the rats survived this treatment when pretreated with a single injection of 3-methylcholanthrene 24 hours prior to the high dose of zoxazolamine. Similarly, pretreatment of rats with enzyme inducers decreased the acute toxicity of meprobamate, pentobarbital and strychnine, which are examples of drugs that are converted by microsomal enzymes to less toxic metabolites.

The insecticides Schradan and Guthion are examples of compounds that are relatively non-toxic until they are metabolized by the liver microsomes to active cholinesterase inhibitors. Table 13.1 shows that pretreatment of rats with stimulators of microsomal enzymes markedly increases the toxicity of Schradan. Control animals treated with Schradan had only 6% mortality, while animals given Schradan after pretreatment with the enzyme inducers phenaglycodol or thiopental had a mortality of 75–81%. Similarly, stimulation of the Guthion-metabolizing enzyme with 3-methylcholanthrene increased the lethality of Guthion, whereas inhibition of this enzyme system with SKF 525-A (β-diethylaminoethyldiphenylpropylacetate) decreased the lethality of the insecticide (Murphy and DuBois, 1958).

The chronic administration of drugs not only stimulates the metabolism of other compounds, but in some instances the pharmacological or toxic effect of a drug when given chronically, diminishes, because it stimulates its own metabolism. Examples of drugs that exert this effect in dogs are inclusive of phenylbutazone, tolbutamide, probenecid, chlorcyclizine and hexobarbital. The importance of this effect during chronic toxicity studies is discussed in Chapter 17.

Several examples are known in which enzyme induction blocks chemical carcinogenesis. The potent liver carcinogen, 3'-methyl-4-dimethylaminoazobenzene, did not produce hepatomas when fed to rats simultaneously with 3-methyl-cholanthrene or certain other polycyclic aromatic hydrocarbons (Richardson, et al., 1952; Miller et al., 1958). An explanation followed the finding that the polycyclic hydrocarbons increased the activity of liver microsomal enzymes that metabolize aminoazo dyes to noncarcinogenic products (Conney et al., 1956). The formation of cancers at a variety of sites (liver, ear duct and mammary gland), resulting from the administration of 2-acetyl-aminofluorene, 4-dimethyl-aminostilbene or 9,10-dimethyl-1,2-benzanthracene to rats, is inhibited by the administration of polycyclic hydrocarbons that stimulate the activity of car-cinogen-metabolizing enzymes in liver microsomes (Miller et al., 1958; Huggins et al., 1964; Huggins and Pataki, 1965; Tawfic, 1965). In contrast to the inhibi-tion of chemical carcinogenesis, SKF 525-A, an inhibitor of microsomal enzymes, enhances the carcinogenicity of 9,10-dimethyl-1,2-benzanthracene (Wheatley, 1968).

The ability of enzyme inducers to block chemical carcinogenesis in animals raises the possibility that cancer formation by environmental carcinogens in man might be blocked by suitable nontoxic enzyme inducers. This concept has led to a search for nontoxic chemicals that induce the synthesis of benzpyrene hy-droxylase activity in liver, lung and gastrointestinal tract (Wattenberg, 1966; Wattenberg and Leong, 1965; Wattenberg et al., 1968, 1968a). In some instances, however, carcinogens are formed by the action of microsomal hydroxylases. This occurs for dimethylnitrosamine and 2-acetylaminofluorene. The latter is detoxified by ring hydroxylation to noncarcinogenic metabolites and it is also N-hydroxylated to a potent carcinogen. It is of interest that both metabolic pathways of animals are enhanced by treatment with polycyclic hydrocarbons.

IV. TESTS FOR ENZYME INDUCTION

To determine whether a compound induces drug-metabolizing enzymes, the liver or its fractions from treated animals is assayed for enzyme activity with suitable drugs as substrates. The analysis of cytochrome P-450 has also been used as a test for enzyme induction, since the concentration of this carbon mon-oxide-binding hemoprotein in liver microsomes increases after animals are treated with stimulators of drug-metabolizing enzymes. However, there are exceptions. For instance, 3-methylcholanthrene increases the concentration of cytochrome P-450 in liver microsomes but does not increase hexobarbital metabolism. Recent observations indicate that although 3-methylcholanthrene increases the con-centration of total CO-binding hemoprotein in liver microsomes, this inducer changes the composition of the CO-binding hemoproteins (Sladek and Manner-ing, 1966; Levin and Kuntzman, 1969).

Numerous simple tests have been devised to identify compounds worthy of more detailed study, or to explore enzyme induction in man. They involve meas-urement of the duration of action of standard drugs or the amount of an easily measured drug or metabolite in the blood or urine. Hexobarbital and zoxazola-mine are useful test drugs because duration of action in the body is regulated largely by the levels of liver microsomal enzymes and because most of the in-ducers decrease the duration of action of one or both. It is important to study both test drugs, for both are metabolized more rapidly after treatment of the animal with nonspecific inducers such as phenobarbital. On the other hand, polycyclic aromatic hydrocarbons, such as 3-methylcholanthrene or 3,4-benz-pyrene, accelerate the metabolism of zoxazolamine but not hexobarbital. For this test, the suspected inducer is injected twice daily for 4 days into 50g male rats. On the 5th day a dose of hexobarbital or zoxazolamine is injected and the duration of sleep or paralysis is measured (Conney et al., 1960).

The rate of metabolism of a barbiturate in rats or dogs has been used as a test for the induction of enzymes (Remmer, 1962; Remmer and Siegert, 1964). In dogs, phenylbutazone is present in the plasma at 7 hours after an intraperitoneal injection of 25 mg/kg, and the chronic administration of several inducers of liver microsomal enzymes causes the plasma level of phenylbutazone to be much lower at 7 hours after its administration (Burns et al., 1963; Burns et al., 1965). Antipyrine, a drug that is distributed in body water and does not bind appreciably to plasma proteins, has been used to measure increases and decreases in the rate of drug metabolism. The rate of antipyrine metabolism in dogs, measured by determining blood levels, is accelerated after chronic treatment with several inducers of microsomal enzymes (Cucinell et al., 1965; Welch et al., 1967). In contrast, the rate of metabolism of antipyrine is slowed when dogs are treated chronically with bishydroxycoumarin, an inhibitor of drug metabolism. Remmer and his associates have given Dipyrone to rats dogs, and humans, and they have measured the urinary excretion of its metabolite 4-aminoantipyrine as an indicator of enzyme induction (Remmer, 1962a; Remmer and Siegert, 1964; Siegert, et al., 1964).

Since drugs that stimulate drug metabolism by liver microsomes also stimulate the hydroxylation of steroids in animals and man (Section VI), the measurement of the urinary excretion of the metabolite of cortisol, 6β-hydroxycortisol (in relation to the total 17-hydroxycorticosteroids, which are not changed by the inducers), may be a useful test for the induction of liver microsomal hydroxylases in man.

In rats the urinary excretion of ascorbic acid may be used as an index of enzyme induction. Compounds that increase the activity of microsomal enzymes stimulate the metabolism of glucose and galactose via the glucuronic acid pathway through D-glucuronic acid and L-gulonic acid to ascorbic acid (Burns et al., 1960; Conney et al., 1961). There is a parallel acceleration of the synthesis of D-glucaric acid, and treatment of patients with typical inducers causes the excretion of more D-glucaric acid in the urine (Aarts, 1965). This may prove to be useful as a test for enzyme induction in man.

Examination of the hepatic parenchymal cell under the electron microscope reveals proliferation of the smooth-surfaced endoplasmic reticulum in animals treated with phenobarbital (Remmer and Merker, 1965; Fouts and Rogers, 1965). Other liver microsomal enzyme inducers, such as tolbutamide, nikethamide, chlordane and DDT, also cause a proliferation of the smooth-surfaced endoplasmic reticulum. Chemicals like 3-methylcholanthrene, which stimulate a smaller number of microsomal pathways, have a much smaller effect on the smooth-surfaced endoplasmic reticulum. Electron microscopic examination of the smooth-surfaced endoplasmic reticulum may be a useful index of drug-induced changes in liver microsomal enzyme levels.

V. ENZYME INDUCTION IN NONHEPATIC TISSUES

Studies by Wattenberg and Leong (1962) and Wattenberg et al. (1962), using an extremely sensitive method, demonstrated the presence of 3,4-benzpyrene hydroxylase activity in the kidney, adrenal and small intestine of normal rats. They found that the administration of polycyclic aromatic hydrocarbons caused large increases in benzpyrene hydroxylase activity in the kidney and small intestine and also caused the appearance of activity, previously too low to be detected, in the thyroid, lung and testis. Studies by Dr. R. Welch in our laboratory have shown that treatment of rats with polycyclic hydrocarbons also increases the activity of benzpyrene hydroxylase in the placenta, skin and ovaries. Dietary factors can regulate benzpyrene hydroxylase activity in the gastrointestinal tract, and a 15-fold decrease in benzpyrene hydroxylase activity in duodenal mucosa was observed in rats starved for 72 hours or fed a fat-free diet (Wattenberg et al., 1962).

Over 100 chemicals have been investigated as potential stimulators of benzpyrene hydroxylase activity in liver and small intestine (Wattenberg and Leong, 1965). Several phenothiazine derivatives (chlorpromazine, promazine, phenothiazine, pyrathiazine and thioridazine) increased benzpyrene hydroxylase activity in the gastrointestinal tract and liver. Administration of phenothiazine increases benzpyrene hydroxylase activity in the liver, gastrointestinal tract, kidney, lung, spleen and thymus, but no detectable activity was present in the hearts or brains of control or phenothiazine-treated rats. Administration of several flavones and 2-phenylbenzothiazoles also induced increased benzpyrene hydroxylase activity in the liver and lung (Wattenberg et al., 1968, 1968a). Although benzpyrene hydroxylase activity was present in adrenals from control rats, this activity was not increased by treatment with phenothiazine or 3-methylcholanthrene. Phenobarbital and several other stimulators of hepatic drug metabolism were among the compounds that had little or no effect on benzpyrene hydroxylase activity in the gastrointestinal tract or placenta of the rat. Treatment of rats for several days with phenobarbital did not enhance the activity of pentobarbital oxidase in lung, nitroreductase in kidney, or aminopyrine N-demethylase in kidney, heart, spleen, brain, muscle or lung. Of considerable interest is that, although treatment of rabbits with phenobarbital increased the activity of drug-metabolizing enzymes in the kidney (Uehleke and Greim, 1968), this increase was not observed in the rat.

By treating animals with polycyclic hydrocarbons, several nonhepatic pathways of drug metabolism are stimulated. Application of 3,4-benzpyrene to the skin of rodents increased glucuronide synthesis (Dutton and Stevenson, 1962) and 3,4-benzpyrene hydroxylation (Conney, unpublished observations) by skin homogenate. 3-Methylcholanthrene injections induced the formation of aminoazo dye N-demethylase activity in lung and kidney (Gilman and Conney, 1963) and menadione reductase in the lung (Huggins and Fukunishi, 1964). The presence of inducible N-demethylase, hydroxylase, reductase and glucuronyl transferase activity in nonhepatic tissues suggests that these enzymes, as well as their hepatic counterparts, may play a role in the biotransformation of drugs and other foreign chemicals. Also suggested is that changes in the low activity of these enzymes at or near a receptor may alter the action of drugs and other chemicals that have

TABLE 13.2

Similarities between hepatic hydroxylases that metabolize drugs and steroids

1. Localized in liver microsomes; require TPNH and oxygen for activity.
2. Higher activity in adult male rats than in adult female rats.
3. Little or no sex difference in enzyme activity in mice.
4. Higher activity in male rats than in male mice.
5. Higher activity in adult male rats than in immature male rats.
6. Inhibition *in vitro* by the addition of SKF 525-A or chlorthion.
7. Activity is inhibited by carbon monoxide and the inhibition is reversed by monochromatic light at 450 mμ.
8. Activity is inhibited by the *in vivo* administration of carbon tetrachloride to rats.
9. Activity is increased after chronic treatment of rats with various drugs or halogenated hydrocarbon insecticides.
10. Steroid hormones are competitive inhibitors of drug-metabolizing enzymes.

escaped metabolic conversion by the liver. It is possible that changes in the activity of drug-metabolizing enzymes in the gastrointestinal tract may have importance for the absorption of some drugs that are administered orally, but little experimental work has been done on this topic.

VI. STIMULATORY EFFECT OF DRUGS ON THE METABOLISM OF NORMAL BODY CONSTITUENTS

Many similarities exist between drug and steroid hydroxylases in liver microsomes (Kuntzman *et al.*, 1964), suggesting that drugs and steroids are substrates for the same hydroxylating enzymes (Table 13.2). Treatment of rats with phenobarbital for several days increases the activity of enzymes in liver microsomes that hydroxylate androgens, estrogens, progestational steroids and adrenocortical steroids (Fig. 13.4). The administration of as little as 1 mg/kg of sodium phenobarbital twice daily for 4 days increases significantly the activity of rat liver microsomal enzymes that hydroxylate estradiol and estrone. Interestingly, treatment of rats with phenobarbital does not increase the A-ring reduction of Δ^4-3-ketosteroids by liver microsomes. Several structurally unrelated drugs and insecticides that stimulate drug-metabolizing enzyme activity also stimulate steroid hydroxylase activity. Examples include phenobarbital, diphenylhydantoin, chlorcyclizine, norchlorcyclizine, orphenadrine, phenylbutazone, chlordane, DDT and o,p'-DDD.

The accelerated hydroxylation of steroid hormones by liver microsomal enzymes of rats pretreated with phenobarbital or other drugs is reflected *in vivo* by an accelerated metabolism and altered physiologic action of steroids. The increased progesterone hydroxylase activity induced by phenobarbital is associated with a decrease in the anesthetic action of large doses of progesterone and a lowered concentration of progesterone and its metabolites in the brain and total body of the rat (Conney *et al.*, 1966). Chronic treatment with phenobarbital reduces the anesthetic action of deoxycorticosterone, androsterone and Δ^4-androstene-3,17-dione while accelerating their metabolism by liver microsomes. Treatment of immature male rats with phenobarbital or chlordane for several days prior to an injection of testosterone or testosterone propionate inhibits the growth promoting effect of these androgens on the seminal vesicles (Levin *et al.*, 1969). Phenobarbital and several other drugs inhibit the action of estradiol,

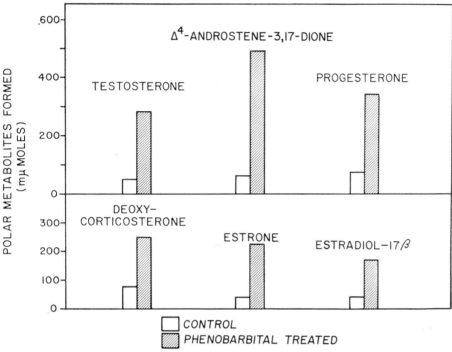

Fig. 13.4. Stimulatory effect of phenobarbital on steroid hydroxylation by rat liver microsomes. Immature rats were injected i.p. with 37 mg/kg of sodium phenobarbital twice daily for 4 days. The animals were killed the following day and microsomes from 330 mg of male rat liver were incubated with 700 mμmoles of testosterone-4-C^{14}, Δ⁴-androstene-3,17-dione-4-C^{14}, progesterone-4-C^{14} or deoxycorticosterone-4-C^{14} for 5 minutes at 37° in the presence of an NADPH-generating system. Microsomes from 330 mg of female rat liver were incubated with 700 mμmoles of estradiol-4-C^{14} or estrone-4-C^{14} for 15 minutes in the presence of an NADPH-generating system. Formation of polar metabolites with the chromatographic mobility of hydroxylated substrate was measured. (From Conney and Klutch, 1963; Conney et al., 1966; Levin et al., 1968.)

estrone and diethylstilbestrol on the rat uterus and stimulate the metabolism of these estrogens in vitro and in vivo (Levin et al., 1968, 1968a; Welch et al., 1968).

Since synthetic estrogens and progestational steroids are widely used as oral contraceptives, the possibility was investigated that the metabolism of these steroids could be increased by stimulators of liver microsomal enzymes. The results obtained indicate that chronic treatment of rats with phenobarbital inhibits the uterotropic action of ethynyl estradiol-3-methyl ether (mestranol), norethindrone and norethynodrel (Levin et al., 1968a). The inhibitory effect of low doses of phenobarbital on the uterotropic action of ethynyl estradiol-3-methyl ether is shown in Table 13.3. The significance of these drug interactions in humans is not known.

Some compounds that stimulate the hydroxylation of steroids by liver microsomes in animals also alter pathways of steroid metabolism in man. Treatment of humans with phenobarbital, N-phenylbarbital, diphenylhydantoin, phenylbutazone or o,p'-DDD markedly stimulates the metabolism of cortisol to 6β-hydroxycortisol, a minor metabolite of cortisol (Werk et al., 1964; Bledsoe et al., 1964; Burstein and Klaiber, 1965; Kuntzman et al., 1966, 1968). These drugs

TABLE 13.3

Inhibitory effect of phenobarbital on the uterotropic action of ethynyl estradiol-3-methyl ether (mestranol)

Daily dose of phenobarbital (mg/kg)	Mestranol	Uterine wet weight (mg)	Inhibition of uterine response (%)
0	—	18.7 ± 0.5	—
0	+	30.2 ± 1.1	—
75	+	19.4 ± 0.3	93
25	+	21.8 ± 0.7	72
5	+	23.8 ± 1.2	56
0.5	+	26.4 ± 1.4	33

Immature female rats were injected intraperitoneally twice daily with sodium pheno-barbital for 4 days. Mestranol (1.0 μg) was given orally on the following day and uterine wet weight was determined 4 hours later. (From Levin *et al.*, 1968a.)

have been shown to stimulate the activity of an enzyme in guinea pig liver microsomes that hydroxylates cortisol in the 6β-position or the activity of microsomal enzymes that oxidize drugs. The stimulatory effect of N-phenyl-barbital and phenylbutazone on the enzyme system in guinea pig liver micro-somes that hydroxylates cortisol in the 6β-position is shown in Figure 13.5, and the stimulatory effect of these drugs on the urinary excretion of 6β-hydroxy-cortisol in man is shown in Figure 13.6. The daily administration of 600 mg of phenylbutazone for 14 days or gradually increasing doses of N-phenylbarbital (300–1200 mg/day) for 33 days caused several-fold increases in the urinary excretion of 6β-hydroxycortisol in man. Since stimulators of liver microsomal

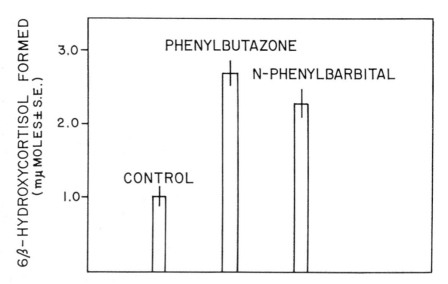

Fig. 13.5. Stimulatory effect of phenylbutazone and N-phenylbarbital on cortisol 6β-hydroxylase acitivity in guinea pig liver microsomes. Adult female guinea pigs were in-jected i.p. with 50 mg/kg of N-phenylbarbital twice daily for 10 days or with 60 mg/kg of phenylbutazone twice daily for 10 days. The guinea pigs were killed the day after the last injection, and microsomes from 666 mg of liver were incubated with 100 mμmoles of cor-tisol-4-C[14] for 30 minutes in the presence of an NADPH-generating system. (From Kuntz-man *et al.*, 1968 and unpublished observations by the same authors.)

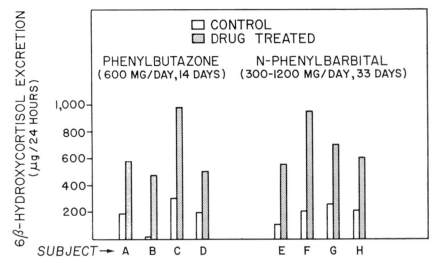

Fig. 13.6. Stimulatory effect of phenylbutazone and N-phenylbarbital on the urinary excretion of 6β-hydroxycortisol in man. (From Kuntzman *et al.*, 1968 and unpublished observations by the same authors.)

hydroxylases increase the urinary excretion of 6β-hydroxycortisol in man, the measurement of this substance in urine deserves additional study as a test for the measurement of man's ability to hydroxylate drugs and steroids.

Of considerable interest, Dr. E. Werk has studied two patients with Cushing's syndrome and has presented evidence that the administration of diphenylhydantoin stimulates the 6β-hydroxylation of cortisol and ameliorates the symptoms of Cushing's syndrome (Werk *et al.*, 1964, 1966). However, insufficient work has been done to determine whether enhanced hydroxylation of steroids can decrease the pharmacological action of these substances in man, and additional studies are needed to evaluate the physiological importance of drug-induced increases in steroid hydroxylation.

The administration of barbiturates to animals enhances the enzymatic glucuronidation of bilirubin by the liver microsomes, stimulates the bile flow and accelerates the *in vivo* metabolism of bilirubin (Catz and Yaffee, 1962; Roberts and Plaa, 1967). These observations suggested that barbiturates might be effective in the treatment of hyperbilirubinemia in man. Interestingly, chronic administration of phenobarbital lowered the serum bilirubin level in patients with chronic intrahepatic cholestasis (Thompson and Williams, 1967) and in some, but not all infants with congenital nonhemolytic jaundice (Crigler and Gold, 1966, 1969; Yaffee *et al.*, 1966; DeLeon *et al.*, 1967). The decrease in plasma concentration of bilirubin in subjects treated with phenobarbital was associated with a decreased half-life of bilirubin (Crigler and Gold, 1969). The effectiveness of phenobarbital in lowering the concentration of serum bilirubin in some infants with congenital nonhemolytic jaundice suggested that these infants did not have a complete genetic block in ability to synthesize the enzymes involved in bilirubin metabolism. This observation is of considerable importance, for it suggests the possibility of treating some "genetic diseases" with a suitable enzyme inducer.

Treatment of pregnant animals with phenobarbital increases the levels of enzymes that metabolize drugs and bilirubin in the newborn, and it appears that

TABLE 13.4
Effect of phenobarbital received during pregnancy on concentration of total serum bilirubin in the human neonate

Day	Serum bilirubin (mg/100 ml)	
	Control	Phenobarbital
1	3.8 ± 0.4	2.1 ± 0.4
2	5.0 ± 0.6	2.5 ± 0.4
3	5.7 ± 0.7	2.2 ± 0.4
4	5.2 ± 0.8	1.8 ± 0.4

Twelve pregnant women were treated with sodium phenobarbital (average dose, 60 mg/day) for 2 weeks or longer prior to delivery. The concentration of total serum bilirubin in their offspring and in 16 control babies were compared during the first 4 days of life. Rh and ABO sensitized and premature babies were excluded. (From Maurer *et al.*, 1968.)

this effect also occurs in humans (Maurer *et al.*, 1968; Trolle, 1968). Administration of 60 mg of phenobarbital to pregnant women daily for 2 weeks or longer before delivery markedly inhibited the transient hyperbilirubinemia that normally occurs in the newborn during the first few days of life (Table 13.4), presumably by stimulating hepatic enzymes that metabolize bilirubin.

Further need for additional investigation was suggested by the studies of Boggs *et al.* (1967). They indicate a positive relationship between increasing levels of neonatal serum bilirubin and the incidence of low motor and/or low mental scores attained at 8 months of age. These relationships do not begin abruptly at the 20 mg% level of serum bilirubin, but may be seen to rise progressively and to become substantial at a concentration of 16–19 mg%. These results suggest a desirability in preventing or decreasing the transient hyperbilirubinemia. Studies on the use of phenobarbital should proceed cautiously, however, since phenobarbital also stimulates the activity of liver microsomal enzymes that metabolize steroid hormones. It is not known whether this effect, if it occurred in the human fetus or neonate, would be harmful.

The induction of liver microsomal enzymes by phenobarbital or other drugs in animals is associated with an increased concentration of cytochrome P-450 and with increased levels of NADPH oxidase and NADPH-cytochrome c reductase in animal liver microsomes. Treatment of animals with drugs that increase the levels of liver microsomal enzymes also increase the activity of hepatic enzymes involved in (1) the incorporation of C^{14}-acetate or C^{14}-mevalonate into cholesterol, (2) the hydroxylation of cholesterol in the 7α-position, (3) the deiodination of thyroxin, (4) the demethylation of the methylated purines, 6-dimethylaminopurine and 6-methylaminopurine, and (5) the synthesis of proteins. The implications of these effects are reviewed elsewhere (Conney, 1967; Kuntzman, 1969).

Cytochrome P-450, a microsomal hemoprotein that binds carbon monoxide when the cytochrome is reduced, is of particular interest because it has been implicated as the terminal oxidase of the enzyme system in liver microsomes that hydroxylates drugs, carcinogens and steroids. Treatment of rats with phenobarbital or 3-methylcholanthrene increases the apparent concentration of cytochrome P-450 in liver microsomes, and recent studies have indicated that the composition of the microsomal hemoprotein found after phenobarbital treatment is not the same as that found in liver microsomes after 3-methylcholanthrene (3-MC) treatment (Sladek and Mannering, 1966; Kuntzman, 1969; Levin and Kuntzman, 1969; Mannering et al., 1969). Carbon monoxide interacts with reduced microsomal hemoprotein obtained from 3-MC-treated rats as expected, but the maximum absorption of this complex was found at 448 mμ instead of at 450 mμ, which is the maximum for the hemoprotein from microsomes of normal or phenobarbital-treated rats. Pretreatment of rats with puromycin, ethionine or actinomycin D prevented the spectral changes in microsomal hemoprotein caused by 3-MC treatment, which suggests that this hydrocarbon changes the composition of microsomal hemoproteins by a mechanism that involves protein synthesis.

Recent studies have shown that treatment of rats with 3-MC lowers the Michaelis constant for the hydroxylation of 3,4-benzpyrene, possibly due to a greater affinity of 3,4-benzpyrene for the hemoprotein preferentially formed in 3-MC-treated rats. Although the V_{max} was increased, the K_m for the hydroxylation of 3,4-benzpyrene and other drugs did not change when rats were treated with phenobarbital..

VII. STIMULATORY EFFECT OF FOREIGN CHEMICALS ON THE METABOLISM OF DRUGS AND CARCINOGENS IN MAN

Phenobarbital and several other drugs that stimulate drug metabolism in animals also exert this effect in man. Examples are summarized in Table 13.5. The chronic administration of phenobarbital to dogs decreases the plasma half-life of diphenylhydantoin, and it appears that phenobarbital also stimulates the metabolism of diphenylhydantoin in man. The plasma levels of diphenylhydantoin were compared in two groups of epileptic patients who received daily, for prolonged periods of time, either 300 mg of diphenylhydantoin alone or in combination with 120 mg of phenobarbital (Table 13.6). The plasma levels of diphenylhydantoin were significantly lower in those patients who received phenobarbital. The stimulation of diphenylhydantoin metabolism by phenobarbital is apparently not a problem in the management of the epileptic patient, since phenobarbital also possesses anticonvulsant activity. However, the simultaneous administration of diphenylhydantoin with drugs that enhance the metabolism of diphenylhydantoin, but lack anticonvulsant activity, may present difficulty.

Treatment of rats with phenobarbital for several days increases the activity of liver microsomal enzymes that metabolize bishydroxycoumarin and warfarin. In accord with these observations, administration of phenobarbital decreases the blood level and anticoagulant activity of coumarin anticoagulants in man. The interactions of enzyme inducers with coumarin anticoagulants are described in Chapter 17.

Alcoholics metabolize tolbutamide more rapidly than non-alcoholics (Kater et al., 1969), and this should be considered when alcoholics are given tolbutamide for the treatment of diabetes. People who ingest alcohol chronically have an increased activity of the hepatic enzyme that metabolizes pentobarbital, whereas the activity of this enzyme system is inhibited by the *in vitro* addition of alcohol to the incubation mixture (Rubin and Lieber, 1968). These observations may explain the increased tolerance of alcoholics to barbiturates and other sedatives

TABLE 13.5

Enzyme induction in man

Stimulator	Enhanced metabolism
Phenobarbital and other barbiturates	Coumarin anticoagulants (Dayton *et al.*, 1961; Cucinell *et al.*, 1965; MacDonald *et al.*, 1969). Diphenylhydantoin (Cucinell *et al.*, 1965). Digitoxin (Jeliffe and Blankenhorn, 1961). Dipyrone (Remmer, 1962). Cortisol (Burstein and Klaiber, 1965). Testosterone (Southren *et al.*, 1969). Bilirubin (Crigler and Gold, 1966, 1969; Yaffee *et al.*, 1966).
Glutethimide	Glutethimide (Schmid *et al.*, 1964). Warfarin (MacDonald *et al.*, 1969). Dipyrone (Remmer, 1962).
Phenylbutazone	Aminopyrine (Chen *et al.*, 1962). Cortisol (Kuntzman *et al.*, 1966).
Chloral hydrate	Bishydroxycoumarin (Cucinell *et al.*, 1966).
Meprobamate	Meprobamate (Douglas *et al.*, 1963).
Ethanol	Pentobarbital (Rubin and Lieber, 1968). Tolbutamide (Kater *et al.*, 1969).
Diethylnicotinamide (Coramine)	Bilirubin (Sereni *et al.*, 1967).
Diphenylhydantoin	Cortisol (Werk *et al.*, 1964).
o,p'-DDD	Cortisol (Bledsoe *et al.*, 1964).
Cigarette smoke	3,4-Benzpyrene (Welch *et al.*, 1969). Aminoazo dyes (Welch *et al.*, 1969). Nicotine (Beckett and Triggs, 1967).
DDT, Lindane	Antipyrine (Kolmodin *et al.*, 1969).

Decreased plasma level was criterion for enhanced metabolism of bilirubin and most drugs. Increased urinary excretion of 6β-hydroxycortisol or polar metabolites of testosterone was used as an index of steroid hydroxylation. Enhanced enzymatic oxidation of pentobarbital by human liver and enhanced metabolism of benzpyrene and aminoazo dye by enzymes in human placenta were used as the criteria for accelerated metabolism of these compounds.

when sober, and the enhanced sensitivity of these individuals to sedatives when inebriated.

A recent study by Kolmodin *et al.* (1969) showed that people exposed to DDT and lindane in a pesticide factory metabolize antipyrine more rapidly than a control population, and it is likely that the factory workers also have enhanced metabolism of other drugs. Additional work is needed to determine how much exposure to DDT and other insecticides is needed to enhance the metabolism of drugs in man.

TABLE 13.6

Effect of phenobarbital administration on plasma levels of diphenylhydantoin in man

Drug treatment	No. of subjects	Plasma level of diphenylhydantoin (mg/L)
Diphenylhydantoin (300 mg)	10	11.4 ± 1.6 (S.E.)
Diphenylhydantoin (300 mg) + Phenobarbital (120 mg)	9	3.5 ± 0.7 (S.E.)

Epileptic patients received drugs chronically for at least two months. (From Cucinell *et al.*, 1965.) (S.E. = standard error.)

Since people are exposed to low levels of 3,4-benzpyrene and other carcinogenic hydrocarbons in certain smoked and cooked foods, polluted city air, soil, tobacco smoke and in tars, mineral oils, pitches and soots, it is important to learn the levels of carcinogen-metabolizing enzymes in the human population. Also important is to determine whether chronic exposure to environmental carcinogens, such as polycyclic hydrocarbons, increases the levels of enzymes that detoxify these and other foreign chemicals. The presence of 3,4-benzpyrene and other polycyclic hydrocarbons in cigarette smoke may stimulate the hydroxylation of 3,4-benzpyrene in man, and recent studies have demonstrated a stimulatory effect of cigarette smoking on benzpyrene hydroxylase activity in the human placenta—a readily obtainable human tissue. Little or no benzpyrene hydroxylase activity was observed in human placentas obtained after childbirth from nonsmokers, but this enzyme was found in placentas obtained from women who smoked 10–40 cigarettes a day (Welch *et al.*, 1969). In several individuals smoking the same number of cigarettes, placental benzpyrene hydroxylase activity varied 25-fold. The variability is of considerable interest, for the poor inducibility of benzpyrene hydroxylase in some people exposed to polycyclic hydrocarbons may reflect an abnormal carcinogenic risk in these individuals. Cigarette smoking enhances the *in vivo* metabolism of nicotine in man (Beckett and Triggs, 1967), an effect which may explain the tolerance to nicotine in smokers. Since polycyclic aromatic hydrocarbons and nicotine enhance the metabolism of some drugs in animals (Conney, 1967), it would be of interest to determine if cigarette smoking alters the metabolism and action of these drugs in man.

VIII. INHIBITORY EFFECT OF FOREIGN CHEMICALS ON DRUG AND STEROID METABOLISM

A. Animal Studies

Fifteen years ago, J. Axelrod, B. B. Brodie and their associates and the Smith Kline and French Laboratories found that rodents treated with SKF 525-A (β-diethyl-aminoethyldiphenylpropylacetate) 40–60 minutes before receiving a dose of hexobarbital slept 5 times longer than animals that received hexobarbital alone. This important observation was explained by an inhibitory effect of SKF 525-A on liver microsomal enzymes that metabolize hexobarbital to pharmacologically inactive products. The addition of SKF 525-A to rat liver homogenate inhibits the side chain oxidation of hexobarbital, pentobarbital and secobarbital, the N-dealkylation of aminopyrine, ephedrine, meperidine and dibenamine, the

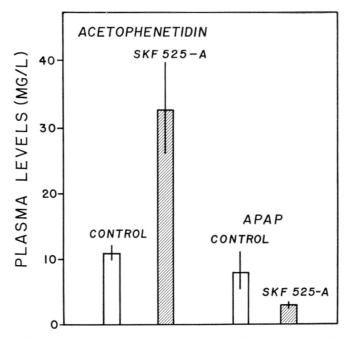

Fig. 13.7. Inhibitory effect of SKF 525-A on acetophenetidin metabolism. Plasma levels of acetophenetidin and N-acetyl-p-aminophenol (APAP) were determined three hours after an intraperitoneal injection of 200 mg/kg of acetophenetidin. Open bars represent values for control rats and solid bars represent values for rats injected intraperitoneally with 35 mg/kg of SKF 525-A forty minutes prior to acetophenetidin administration. (From Conney *et al.*, 1966a.)

O-dealkylation of codeine and acetophenetidin and the deamination of amphetamine. These observations were reflected *in vivo* by increased half-lives of hexobarbital, pentobarbital, meperidine, ephedrine, aminopyrine and acetophenetidin in animals given SKF 525-A shortly before administration of the test drug (Fig. 13.7).

Animals that received SKF 525-A had considerably higher plasma levels of acetophenetidin three hours after a dose of the drug than did the control rats. In accord with these results, the plasma levels of the major metabolite of acetophenetidin, N-acetyl-p-aminophenol, were lower in the treated rats than in the control rats. Inhibition of acetophenetidin metabolism resulted in a significant prolongation of the drug's antipyretic action, suggesting that acetophentidin does not require metabolism to N-acetyl-p-aminophenol to exert its antipyretic action. The use of enzyme inhibition and enzyme induction as a procedure for determining whether the parent compound or a metabolite is responsible for the pharmacological action of a drug is a useful concept in pharmacology, (Conney *et al.*, 1966a) a concept discussed elsewhere.

Many drugs inhibit the metabolic detoxification of other drugs and thus cause an increased pharmacologic response (reviewed by Gillette, 1963, 1966; Mannering, 1968). The metabolism of pentobarbital and meprobamate was inhibited by chlorcyclizine, glutethimide, phenaglycodol, imipramine and phenylisopropylhydrazine during the first 30 minutes after administration to rats (Kato *et al.*, 1964); ethylmorphine and codeine inhibited the metabolism of hexobarbital by

TABLE 13.7

Effect of SKF 525-A and desmethylimipramine on the uterotropic action of estrone

Pretreatment	Estrone	Uterine wet weight	Picograms per uterus	% Increase
Saline	—	18.4 ± 0.3	—	—
	+	20.3 ± 0.9	7.9 ± 0.6	—
SKF 525-A (25 mg/kg)	—	19.5 ± 0.3	—	—
	+	25.0 ± 0.7	15.3 ± 1.9	94
DMI (15 mg/kg)	—	19.0 ± 0.7	—	—
	+	26.3 ± 1.1	17.7 ± 4.3	124

Immature female rats were injected i.p. with SKF 525-A or desmethylimipramine (DMI) and 0.1 μg of estrone-6,7-H³ was injected i.p. 30 minutes later. Rats were killed 4 hours after the dose of estrone, and the uteri were removed and weighed. Radioactivity in the uterus was determined. Each value represents the average and standard error from 6–7 animals.

rats *in vivo* (Rubin *et al.*, 1964); and desmethylimipramine potentiated the action of amphetamine by inhibiting its metabolism (Sulser *et al.*, 1966; Consolo *et al.*, 1967). The available evidence suggests that the short-lasting inhibitory effect of one drug on the metabolism of another drug results from the inhibitor acting as an alternative substrate for drug-metabolizing enzymes (Mannering, 1968).

Some compounds which inhibit the metabolism of a drug for 1–6 hours after a single dose may stimulate the metabolism of the same drug 12–24 hours later or after chronic administration (Serrone and Fujimoto, 1962; Kato *et al.*, 1964). For instance, an acute dose of SKF 525-A inhibits the metabolism of hexobarbital and prolongs its hypnotic action for several hours. However, when SKF 525-A is given chronically to rats, the metabolism of the barbiturate is accelerated and its hypnotic action drastically reduced. Other examples of compounds that either inhibit or stimulate the metabolism of drugs by enzymes in liver microsomes depending on whether they are given acutely or chronically include chlorcyclizine, phenylbutazone and glutethimide. Several drugs, when given chronically, inhibit the metabolism of other drugs. Examples include chloramphenicol, phenyramidol, p-aminosalicylic acid, meperidine, morphine, chlorthion and carbon tetrachloride.

Inhibitors of drug-metabolizing enzymes in liver microsomes also inhibit steroid metabolism, and this effect can potentiate the action of steroids in animals. The effect of SKF 525-A and desmethylimipramine on the uterotropic action of estrone was studied by Mr. W. Levin and Dr. R. Welch in our laboratory, and it is seen in Table 13.7 that these inhibitors of drug metabolism potentiate the uterotropic action of estrone. SKF 525-A also inhibits the metabolism of cortisol to polar compounds and potentiates the induction of hepatic tyrosine transaminase by cortisol in the rat (Kupfer and Peets, 1967).

Pretreatment of rats with carbon tetrachloride impairs the oxidation of hexobarbital, aminopyrine, ethyl morphine and the reduction of p-nitrobenzoic acid by liver microsomes. This effect is associated with a decreased concentration of cytochrome P-450 in the liver microsomes (Dingell and Heimberg, 1968; Sasame *et al.*, 1968). The activity of drug-metabolizing enzymes declined to about 10% of normal within 8 hours after the administration of carbon tetrachloride, and enzyme activity remained at low levels 24 hours after the dose. Enzyme activity gradually returned to the control value during the next 7 days.

TABLE 13.8

Inhibitory effect of carbon tetrachloride on the metabolism of estradiol-17β and estrone by rat liver microsomes

Treatment	Estradiol metabolized (mμmoles)	Estrone metabolized (mμmoles)
Control	42 ± 3	144 ± 5
CCl₄	7 ± 1	32 ± 7

Immature female rats were given 0.67 ml/kg of carbon tetrachloride orally 24 hours prior to sacrifice. Microsomes equivalent to 333 mg of liver were incubated for 15 minutes with 700 mμmoles of estradiol-4-C^{14} or estrone-4-C^{14} and an NADPH-generating system. Each value represents the mean and standard error of 3 values, where each value was obtained with the pooled livers from 3 rats.

TABLE 13.9

Effect of carbon tetrachloride pretreatment on the action of estradiol-17β and estrone on the uterus

Estrogen administered	CCl₄	Uterine wet weight (mg)	Picogram equivalents per uterus
—	—	18.7 ± 0.6	
—	+	19.7 ± 0.7	
Estradiol	—	22.9 ± 1.0	22.0 ± 1.6
Estradiol	+	28.2 ± 0.9	44.7 ± 4.5
Estrone	—	21.8 ± 0.2	7.7 ± 1.9
Estrone	+	26.2 ± 1.2	44.6 ± 3.7

Immature female rats were given 0.67 ml/kg of carbon tetrachloride orally, and 0.02 μg of estradiol-6,7-H^3 or 0.1 μg of estrone-6,7-H^3 was injected i.p. 24 hours later. All rats were killed 4 hours after the administration of estrogen. The uteri were weighed and radioactivity in the uterus was quantified. The results are expressed as the average and standard error obtained from 8 rats.

Carbon tetrachloride also inhibits the hydroxylation of steroid hormones. Pretreatment of rats markedly inhibited the microsomal metabolism of estrone and estradiol (Table 13.8). The inhibitory effect of carbon tetrachloride on the metabolism of estrogens *in vitro* is reflected *in vivo* by an enhanced uterotropic action of estradiol and estrone in animals. (Table 13.9).

B. Human Studies

Although the inhibitory effect of drugs on drug metabolism is well documented in laboratory animals, it was only recently recognized that one drug can inhibit the metabolism of a second drug in man. Phenylbutazone, sulfaphenazole, phenyramidol and bishydroxycoumarin inhibit the metabolic inactivation of tolbutamide in man, an effect that can cause profound hypoglycemia. The half-life of tolbutamide was increased 4-fold when a subject was given sulfaphenazole (Christensen *et al.*, 1963) and the half-life of tolbutamide was increased 2.5- and 3.5-fold in human subjects treated with phenyramidol or bishydroxycoumarin, respectively (Solomon and Schrogie, 1967). The combined administration of bishydroxycoumarin and diphenylhydantoin has resulted in toxicity, explained by an inhibitory effect of bishydroxycoumarin on the metabolism of diphenylhydantoin (Hansen *et al.*, 1966).

Phenyramidol inhibits the metabolism of bishydroxycoumarin in the mouse, rabbit and man, an inhibition which reflected a more intense pharmacologic action of the anticoagulant (Solomon and Schrogie, 1966). This effect must be considered in human therapy, or serious hemorrhage may ensue. The potentiation of the action of coumarin anticoagulants by phenylbutazone results from displacement of the anticoagulant from binding sites on plasma protein (Aggeler et al., 1967), thus increasing the amount of free coumarin available for interaction with receptor sites in the liver. Sulfonamides, salicylates and other acidic drugs, all strongly bound to plasma protein, may also enhance the action of coumarin anticoagulants by displacing them from plasma proteins rather than influencing metabolism directly.

Some drugs inhibit the metabolism of other drugs by nonmicrosomal pathways, the case for monoamine oxidase inhibitors. Many reports have shown that patients treated with a monoamine oxidase inhibitor, such as tranylcypromine or iproniazid, are unusually sensitive to a subsequent dose of sympathomimetic amines, which are metabolized by this enzyme. Indeed, severe hypertensive reactions have occurred when patients treated with monoamine oxidase inhibitors have ingested cheese or other foods with a high tyramine content. Allopurinol, a xanthine oxidase inhibitor used for the treatment of gout, inhibits the metabolism of 6-mercaptopurine, azathioprine and other drugs that are metabolized by xanthine oxidase. A serious drug interaction was recently observed when a patient on allopurinol therapy for gout received azathioprine to block the immune response for a heart transplant. Because metabolism of the drug was inhibited by allopurinol, symptoms of overdosage with azathioprine occurred. Fortunately, this drug interaction was recognized and the patient recovered.

Acknowledgments

Some of the studies described here were supported by Research Contract No. PH 43-65-1066 from the Pharmacology-Toxicology Programs, National Institute of General Medical Sciences, National Institutes of Health.

REFERENCES

Aarts, E. M.: Evidence for the function of D-glucaric acid as an indicator for drug-induced enhanced metabolism through the glucuronic acid pathway in man. Biochem. Pharmacol. 14: 359–363, 1965.

Aggeler, P. M., O'Reilly, R. A., Leong, L., and Kowitz, P. E.: Potentiation of anticoagulant effect of warfarin by phenylbutazone. New Eng. J. Med. 276: 496–501, 1967.

Arcos, J. C., Conney, A. H., and Buu-Hoi, N. P.: Induction of microsomal enzyme synthesis by polycyclic aromatic hydrocarbons of different molecular sizes. J. Biol. Chem. 236: 1291–1296, 1961.

Beckett, A. H. and Triggs, E. J.: Enzyme induction in man caused by smoking. Nature 216: 587, 1967.

Bledsoe, T., Island, D. P., Ney, R. L., and Liddle, G. W.: An effect of o,p'-DDD on the extra-adrenal metabolism of cortisol in man. J. Clin. Endocrinol. 24: 1303–1311, 1964.

Boggs, T. R., Jr., Hardy, J. B., and Frazier, T. M.: Correlation of neonatal serum total bilirubin concentrations and developmental status at age eight months. A preliminary report from the collaborative project. J. Pediat. 71: 553–560, 1967.

Burns, J J.: Implications of enzyme induction for drug therapy. Amer. J. Med. 37: 327–331, 1964.

Burns, J. J., Conney, A. H., Dayton, P. G., Evans, C., Martin, G. R., and Taller, D.: Observations on the drug-induced synthesis of D-glucuronic, L-gluonic and L-ascorbic acids in rats. J. Pharmacol. Exp. Ther. 129: 132–138, 1960.

Burns, J. J., Conney, A. H., and Koster, R.: Stimulatory effect of chronic drug administration on drug-metabolizing enzymes in liver microsomes. Ann. N. Y. Acad. Sci. 104: 881–893, 1963.

Burns, J. J., Cucinell, S. A., Koster, R., and Conney, A. H.: Application of drug metabolism to drug toxicity studies. Ann. N. Y. Acad. Sci. *123:* 273–286, 1965.

Burstein, S. and Klaiber, E. L.: Phenobarbital-induced increase in 6β-hydroxycortisol excretion: clue to its significance in human urine. J. Clin. Endocrinol. *25:* 293–296, 1965.

Catz, C. and Yaffee, S. J.: Pharmacological modification of bilirubin conjugation in the newborn. Amer. J. Dis. Child. *104:* 516–517, 1962.

Chen, W., Vrindten, P. A., Dayton, P. G., and Burns, J. J.: Accelerated aminopyrine metabolism in human subjects pretreated with phenylbutazone. Life Sci. *1:* 35–42, 1962.

Christensen, L. K., Hansen, J. M., and Kristensen, M.: Sulphaphenazole-induced hypoglycaemic attacks in tolbutamide-treated diabetics. Lancet *2:* 1298–1301, 1963.

Colas, A., Gregonis, D., and Moir, N.: Daily rhythms in the hydroxylation of 3β-hydroxyandrost-5-en-17-one by rat liver microsomes. Endocrinol. *84:* 165–167, 1969.

Conney, A. H.: Pharmacological implications of microsomal enzyme induction. Pharmacol. Rev. *19:* 317–366, 1967.

Conney, A. H.: Drug metabolism and therapeutics. N. Eng. J. Med. *280:* 653–660, 1969.

Conney, A. H., Bray, G. A., Evans, C., and Burns, J. J.: Metabolic interactions between L-ascorbic acid and drugs. Ann. N. Y. Acad. Sci. *92:* 115–127, 1961.

Conney, A. H. and Burns, J. J.: Factors influencing drug metabolism. Advances Pharmacol. *1:* 31–58, 1962.

Conney, A. H., Davidson, C., Gastel, R., and Burns, J. J.: Adaptive increases in drug-metabolizing enzymes induced by phenobarbital and other drugs. J. Pharmacol. Exp. Ther. *130:* 1–8, 1960.

Conney, A. H., Jacobson, M., Levin, W., Schneidman, K., and Kuntzman, R.: Decreased central depressant effect of progesterone and other steroids in rats pretreated with drugs and insecticides. J. Pharmacol. Exp. Ther. *154:* 310–318, 1966.

Conney, A. H. and Klutch, A.: Increased activity of androgen hydroxylases in liver microsomes of rats pretreated with phenobarbital and other drugs. J. Biol. Chem. *238:* 1611–1617, 1963.

Conney, A. H., Miller, E. C., and Miller, J. A.: The metabolism of methylated aminoazo dyes V. Evidence for induction of enzyme synthesis in the rat by 3-methylcholanthrene. Cancer Res. *16:* 450–459, 1956.

Conney, A. H., Sansur, M., Soroko, F., Koster, R., and Burns, J. J.: Enzyme induction and inhibition in studies on the pharmacological actions of acetophenetidin. J. Pharmacol. Exp. Ther. *151:* 133–138, 1966a.

Conney, A. H., Welch, R. M., Kuntzman, R., and Burns, J. J.: Effects of pesticides on drug and steroid metabolism. Clin. Pharmacol. Ther. *8:* 2–10, 1967.

Consolo, S., Dolfini, E., Garattini, S., and Valzelli, L.: Desipramine and amphetamine metabolism. J. Pharm. Pharmacol. *19:* 253–256, 1967.

Cram, R. L. and Fouts, J. R.: The influence of DDT and gamma-chlordane on the metabolism of hexobarbital and zoxazolamine in two mouse strains. Biochem. Pharmacol. *16:* 1001–1006, 1967.

Creaven, P. J., Davies, W. H., and Williams, R. T.: The effect of butylated hydroxytoluene, butylated hydroxyanisole and octyl gallate upon liver weight and biphenyl 4-hydroxylase activity in the rat. J. Pharm. Pharmacol. *18:* 485–489, 1966.

Crigler, J. F., Jr. and Gold, N. I.: Sodium phenobarbital-induced decrease in serum bilirubin in an infant with congenital nonhemolytic jaundice and kernicterus. J. Clin. Invest. *45:* 998–999, 1966.

Crigler, J. F., Jr. and Gold, N. I.: Effect of sodium phenobarbital on bilirubin metabolism in an infant with congenital, nonhemolytic, unconjugated hyperbilirubinemia and kernicterus. J. Clin. Invest. *48:* 42–55, 1969.

Cucinell, S. A., Conney, A. H., Sansur, M., and Burns, J. J.: Drug interactions in man: 1. Lowering effect of phenobarbital on plasma levels of bishydroxycoumarin (Dicumarol) and diphenylhydantoin (Dilantin). Clin. Pharmacol. Ther. *6:* 420–429, 1965.

Cucinell, S. A., Odessky, L., Weiss, M., and Dayton, P. G.: The effect of chloral hydrate on bishydroxycoumarin metabolism. J.A.M.A. *197:* 366–368, 1966.

Dayton, P. G., Tarcan, Y., Chenkin, T., and Weiner, M.: The influence of barbiturates on coumarin plasma levels and prothrombin response. J. Clin. Invest. *40:* 1797 1802, 1961.

DeLeon, A., Gartner, L. M., and Arias, I. M.: The effect of phenobarbital on hyperbilirubinemia in glucuronyl transferase-deficient rats. J. Lab. Clin. Med. *70:* 273–278, 1967.

Dingell, J. V. and Heimberg, M.: The effects of aliphatic halogenated hydrocarbons on hepatic drug metabolism. Biochem. Pharmacol. *17:* 1269–1278, 1968.

Douglas, J. F., Ludwig, B. J., and Smith, N.: Studies on the metabolism of meprobamate. Proc. Soc. Exp. Biol. Med. *112:* 436–438, 1963.

Durham, W. F.: Pesticide exposure levels in

man and animals. Arch. Environ. Health *10:* 842–846, 1965.

Dutton, G. J. and Stevenson, I. H.: The stimulation by 3,4-benzpyrene of glucuronide synthesis in skin. Biochim. Biophys. Acta *58:* 633–634, 1962.

Ernster, L. and Orrenius, S.: Substrate-induced synthesis of the hydroxylating enzyme system of liver microsomes. Fed. Proc. *24:* 1190–1199. 1965.

Ferguson, H. C.: Effect of red cedar chip bedding on hexobarbital and pentobarbital sleep time. J. Pharm. Sci. *55:* 1142–1143, 1966.

Fouts, J. R.: Factors influencing the metabolism of drugs in liver microsomes. Ann. N. Y. Acad. Sci. *104:* 875–880, 1963.

Fouts, J. R. and Rogers, L. A.: Morphological changes in the liver accompanying stimulation of microsomal drug-metabolizing enzyme activity by phenobarbital, chlordane, benzpyrene or methylcholanthrene in rats. J. Pharmacol. Exp. Ther. *147:* 112–119, 1965.

Gelboin, H. V.: Carcinogens, enzyme induction and gene action. Adv. Cancer Res. *10:* 1–81, 1967.

Gerboth, G. and Schwabe, U.: Einfluss von gewebsgespeichertem DDT auf die Wirkung von Pharmaka. Arch. Exp. Pathol. Pharmakol. *246:* 469–483, 1964.

Ghazal, A., Koransky, W., Portig, J., Vohland, H. W., and Klempau, I.: Beschleunigung von Entgiftungsreaktionen durch verschiedene Insecticide. Arch. Exp. Pathol. Pharmakol. *249:* 1–10, 1964.

Gilbert, D. and Golberg, L.: Liver weight and microsomal processing (drug metabolizing) enzymes in rats treated with butylated hydroxytoluene or butylated hydroxyanisole. Biochem. J. *97:* 28P, 1965.

Gillette, J. R.: Metabolism of drugs and other foreign compounds by enzymatic mechanisms. Prog. Drug Res. *6:* 11–73, 1963.

Gillette, J. R.: Biochemistry of drug oxidation and reduction by enzymes in hepatic endoplasmic reticulum. Adv. Pharmacol. *4:* 219–261, 1966.

Gilman, A. G. and Conney, A. H.: The induction of aminoazo dye N-demethylase in nonhepatic tissues by 3-methylcholanthrene. Biochem. Pharmacol. *12:* 591–593, 1963.

Hansen, J. M., Kristensen, M., Skovsted, L., and Christensen, L. K.: Dicumarol-induced diphenylhydantoin intoxication. Lancet *2:* 265–266, 1966.

Hart, L. G. and Fouts, J. R.: Further studies on the stimulation of hepatic microsomal drug-metabolizing enzymes by DDT and its analogs. Arch. Exp. Pathol. Pharmakol. *249:* 486–500, 1965.

Hart, L. G., Shultice, R. W., and Fouts,

J. R.: Stimulatory effects of chlordane on hepatic microsomal drug metabolism in the rat. Toxicol. Appl. Pharmacol. *5:* 371–386, 1963.

Huggins, C. and Fukunishi, R.: Induced protection of adrenal cortex against 7,12-dimethylbenz(α)anthracene. Influence of ethionine. Induction of menadione reductase. Incorporation of thymidine-H³. J. Exp. Med. *119:* 923–942, 1964.

Huggins, C., Grand, L. C., and Fukunishi, R.: Aromatic influences on the yields of mammary cancers following administration of 7,12-dimethylbenz(α)anthracene. Proc. Nat. Acad. Sci. USA *51:* 737–742, 1964.

Huggins, C. and Pataki, J.: Aromatic azo derivatives preventing mammary cancer and adrenal injury from 7,12-dimethylbenz(α)anthracene. Proc. Nat. Acad. Sci. USA *53:* 791–796, 1965.

Jelliffe, R. W. and Blankenhorn, D. H.: Effect of phenobarbital on digitoxin metabolism. Clin. Res. *14:* 160, 1961.

Kater, R. M. H., Tobon, F., and Iber, F. L.: Increased rate of tolbutamide metabolism in alcoholic patients. J.A.M.A. *207:* 363–365, 1969.

Kato, R.: Modifications of the toxicity of strychnine and octomethylpyrophosphoramide (OMPA) induced by pretreatment with phenaglycodol and thiopental. Arzneimittel-Forsch. *11:* 797–798, 1961.

Kato, R., Chiesara, E. and Vassanelli, P.: Further studies on the inhibition and stimulation of microsomal drug-metabolizing enzymes of rat liver by various compounds. Biochem. Pharmacol. *13:* 69–83, 1964.

Kinoshita, F. K., Frawley, J. P., and DuBois, K. P.: Effects of subacute administration of some pesticides on microsomal enzyme systems. Toxicol. Appl. Pharmacol. *8:* 345–346, 1966.

Kinoshita, F. K., Frawley, J. P., and DuBois, K. P.: Quantitative measurement of induction of hepatic microsomal enzymes by various dietary levels of DDT and Toxaphene in rats. Toxicol. Appl. Pharmacol. *9:* 505–513, 1966.

Kitagawa, H.: Studies on drug metabolism. I. Effect of respiratory oxygen on the duration of pentobarbital-induced sleep. Chem. Pharm. Bull. *16:* 1589–1592, 1968.

Kolmodin, B., Azarnoff, D. L., and Sjoqvist, F.: Effect of environmental factors on drug metabolism: Decreased plasma half life of antipyrine in workers exposed to chlorinated insecticides. J. Clin. Pharmacol. Ther., *10:* 638–642, 1969.

Kuntzman, R.: Drugs and enzyme induction. Ann. Rev. Pharmacol. *9:* 21–36, 1969.

Kuntzman, R., Jacobson, M., and Conney, A. H.: Effect of phenylbutazone on cortisol metabolism in man. Pharmacologist *8:* 195, 1966.

Kuntzman, R., Jacobson, M., Levin, W., and Conney, A. H.: Stimulatory effect of N-phenylbarbital (phetharbital) on cortisol hydroxylation in man. Biochem. Pharmacol. *17:* 565–571, 1968.

Kuntzman, R., Jacobson, M., Schneidman, K, and Conney, A. H.: Similarities between oxidative drug-metabolizing enzymes and steroid hydroxylases in liver microsomes. J. Pharmacol. Exp. Ther. *146:* 280–285, 1964.

Kupfer, D. and Peets, L.: Potentiation of cortisol induction of hepatic tyrosine transaminase by β-diethylaminoethyl diphenylpropylacetate. Nature *215:* 637–638, 1967.

Levin, W. and Conney, A. H.: Stimulatory effect of polycyclic hydrocarbons and aromatic azo derivatives on the metabolism of 7,12-dimethylbenz(α)anthracene. Cancer Res. *27:* 1931–1938, 1967.

Levin, W. and Kuntzman, R.: Biphasic decrease in radioactive hemoprotein from rat liver CO-binding particles: Effect of 3-methylcholanthrene. J. Biol. Chem. *244:* 3671–3676, 1969.

Levin, W., Welch, R. M., and Conney, A. H.: Effect of phenobarbital and other drugs on the metabolism and uterotropic action of estradiol-17β and estrone. J. Pharmacol. Exp. Ther. *159:* 362–371, 1968.

Levin, W., Welch, R. M., and Conney, A. H.: Decreased uterotropic potency of oral contraceptives in rats pretreated with phenobarbital. Endocrinol. *83:* 149–156, 1968a.

Levin, W., Welch, R. M., and Conney, A. H.: Inhibitory effect of phenobarbital or chlordane pretreatment on the androgen-induced increase in seminal vesicle weight in the rat. Steroids *13:* 155–161, 1969.

MacDonald, M. G., Robinson, D. S., Sylwester, D., and Jaffe, J. J.: The effects of phenobarbital, chloral betaine and glutethimide administration on warfarin plasma levels and hypoprothrombinemic responses in man. Clin. Pharmacol. Ther. *10:* 80–84, 1969.

Mannering, G. J.: Significance of stimulation and inhibition of drug metabolism. In *Selected Pharmacological Testing Methods.* Ed. Alfred Burger, pp. 51–119, Marcel Dekker, New York, 1968.

Mannering, G. J., Sladek, N. E., Parli, C. J., and Shoeman, D. W.: Formation of a new P-450 hemoprotein after treatment of rats with polycyclic hydrocarbons. In *Microsomes and Drug Oxidations.* Ed. J. R. Gillette, A. H. Conney, G. J. Cosmides, R. W. Estabrook, J. R. Fouts, and G. J. Mannering, pp. 303–330, Academic Press, New York, 1969.

Maurer, H. M., Wolff, J. A., Finster, M., Poppers, P. J., Pantuck, E., Kuntzman, R., and Conney, A. H.: Reduction in concentration of total serum bilirubin in offspring of women treated with phenobarbitone during pregnancy. Lancet *2:* 122–124, 1968.

Merritt, J. H. and Medina, M. A.: Altitude-induced alterations in drug action and metabolism. Life. Sci. *7:* 1163–1169, 1968.

Miller, E. C., Miller, J. A., Brown, R. R., and MacDonald, J. C.: On the protective action of certain polycyclic aromatic hydrocarbons against carcinogenesis by aminoazo dyes and 2-acetylaminofluorene. Cancer Res. *18:* 469–477, 1958.

Mitoma, C., Sorich, T. J., and Neubauer, S. E.: The effect of caffeine on drug metabolism. Life Sci. *7:* 145–151, 1968.

Murphy, S. D. and DuBois, K. P.: The influence of various factors on the enzymatic conversion of organic thiophosphates to anticholinesterase agents. J. Pharmacol. Exp. Ther. *124:* 194–202, 1958.

Nair, V. and DuBois, K. P.: Prenatal and early postnatal exposure to environmental toxicants. Chicago Medical School Quarterly, *27:* 75–89, 1968.

Quinby, G. E., Hayes, W. J., Jr., Armstrong, J. F., and Durham, W. F.: DDT storage in the U.S. population. J.A.M.A. *191:* 175–179, 1965.

Radomski, J. L.: The absorption, fate and excretion of citrus Red No. 2 (2,5-dimethoxyphenyl-azo-2-naphthol) and external D and C No. 14 (1-xylylazo-2-naphthol). J. Pharmacol. Exp. Ther. *134:* 100–109, 1961.

Radzialowski, F. M. and Bousquet, W. F.: Daily rhythmic variation in hepatic drug metabolism in the rat and mouse. J. Pharmacol. Exp. Ther. *163:* 229–238, 1968.

Remmer, H.: Drugs as activators of drug enzymes. *Proc. 1st Inter. Pharmacol. Mtg.,* Stockholm, vol. 6, pp. 235–249, MacMillan, New York, 1962.

Remmer, H.: Drug tolerance. In *Ciba Foundation Symposium on Enzymes and Drug Action.* ed. by J. L. Mongar and A. V. S. DeReuck, pp. 276–298, Little Brown, Boston, 1962a.

Remmer, H. and Merker, H. J.: Effect of drugs on the formation of smooth endoplasmic reticulum and drug-metabolizing enzymes. Ann. N. Y. Acad. Sci. *123:* 79–97, 1965.

Remmer, H. und Siegert, M.: Beschleunigter Arzneimittelabbau durch Enzyminduktion beim Hunde nach Behandlung mit Phenobarbital. Arch. Exp. Pathol. Pharmakol. *247:* 522–543, 1964.

Richardson, H. L., Stier, A. R., and Borsos-Nachtnebel, E.: Liver tumor inhibition and adrenal histologic responses in rats to which 3′-methyl-4-dimethylaminoazobenzene and 20-methylcholanthrene were simultaneously administered. Cancer Res. *12:* 356–361, 1952.

Roberts, R. J. and Plaa, G. L.: Effect of phenobarbital on the excretion of an exogenous bilirubin load. Biochem. Pharmacol. *16:* 827–835, 1967.

Rosenberg, P. and Coon, J. M.: Increase of hexobarbital sleeping time by certain anticholinesterases. Proc. Soc. Exp. Biol. Med. *98:* 650–652, 1958.

Rubin, A., Tephly, T. R., and Mannering, G. J.: Inhibition of hexobarbital metabolism by ethylmorphine and codeine in the rat. Biochem. Pharmacol. *13:* 1053–1057, 1964.

Rubin, E. and Lieber, C. S.: Hepatic microsomal enzymes in man and rat: induction and inhibition by ethanol. Science *162:* 690–691, 1968.

Sasame, H. A., Castro, J. A., and Gillette, J. R.: Studies on the destruction of liver microsomal cytochrome P-450 by carbon tetrachloride administration. Biochem. Pharmacol. *17:* 1759–1768, 1968.

Schmid, K., Cornu, F., Imhof, P., und Keberle, H.: Die biochemische Deutung der Gewöhnung an Schlafmittel. Schweiz. Med. Wochensch. *94:* 235–240, 1964.

Sereni, F., Perletti, L. and Marini, A.: Influence of diethylnicotinamide on the concentration of serum bilirubin of newborn infants. Pediat. *40:* 446–449, 1967.

Serrone, D. M. and Fujimoto, J. M.: The effect of certain inhibitors in producing shortening of hexobarbital action. Biochem. Pharmacol. *11:* 609–615, 1962.

Siegert, M., Alsleben, B., Liebenschutz, W., und Remmer, H.: Unterschiede in der mikrosomalen Oxydation und Acetylierung von Arzneimitteln bei verschiedenen Arten und Rassen. Arch. Exp. Pathol. Pharmakol. *247:* 509–521, 1964.

Sladek, N. E. and Mannering, G. J.: Evidence for a new P-450 hemoprotein in hepatic microsomes from methylcholanthrene-treated rats. Biochem. Biophys. Res. Commun. *24:* 668–674, 1966.

Solomon, H. M. and Schrogie, J. J.: Effect of phenyramidol on the metabolism of bishydroxycoumarin. J. Pharmacol. Exp. Ther. *154:* 660–666, 1966.

Solomon, H. M. and Schrogie, J. J.: Effect of phenyramidol and bishydroxycoumarin on the metabolism of tolbutamide in human subjects. Metabolism *16:* 1029–1033, 1967.

Southren, A. L., Gordon, G. G., Tochimoto, S., Krikun, E., Krieger, D., Jacobson, M., and Kuntzman, R.: Effect of N-phenylbarbital (phetharbital) on the metabolism of testosterone and cortisol in man. J. Clin. Endocrinol. *29:* 251–256, 1969.

Sulser, F., Owens, M. L., and Dingell, J. V.: On the mechanism of amphetamine po-

tentiation by desipramine (DMI). Life Sci. *5:* 2005–2010, 1966.

Tawfic, H. N.: Studies on ear duct tumors in rats. Part II. Inhibitory effect of methylcholanthrene and 1,2-benzanthracene on tumor formation by 4-dimethylaminostilbene. Acta Pathol. Jap. *15:* 255–259, 1965.

Thompson, I. D., Dolowy, W. C., and Cole, W. H.: Development of a resistance to sodium pentobarbital in rats fed on a diet containing chlorcyclizine hydrochloride. J. Pharmacol. Exp. Ther. *127:* 164–166, 1959.

Thompson, R. P. H. and Williams, R.: Treatment of chronic intrahepatic cholestasis with phenobarbitone. Lancet *2:* 646–648, 1967.

Trolle, D.: Decrease of total serum bilirubin concentration in newborn infants after phenobarbitone treatment. Lancet *2:* 705–708, 1968.

Uehleke, H. und Greim, H.: Stimulierung der Oxydation von Fremdstoffen in Nierenmikrosomen durch Phenobarbital. Arch. Pharmakol. Exp. Pathol. *261:* 152–161, 1968.

Vesell, E. S.: Induction of drug-metabolizing enzymes in liver microsomes of mice and rats by softwood bedding. Science *157:* 1057–1058, 1967.

Wattenberg, L. W.: Chemoprophylaxis of carcinogenesis: A review. Cancer Res. *26:* 1520–1526, 1966.

Wattenberg, L. W. and Leong, J. L.: Histochemical demonstration of reduced pyridine nucleotide dependent polycyclic hydrocarbon-metabolizing systems. J. Histochem. Cytochem. *10:* 412–420, 1962.

Wattenberg, L. W. and Leong, J. L.: Effects of phenothiazines on protective systems against polycyclic hydrocarbons. Cancer Res. *25:* 365–370, 1965.

Wattenberg, L. W., Leong, J. L., and Strand, P. J.: Benzpyrene hydroxylase activity in the gastrointestinal tract. Cancer Res. *22:* 1120–1125, 1962.

Wattenberg, L. W., Page, M. A., and Leong, J. L.: Induction of increased benzpyrene hydroxylase activity by flavones and related compounds. Cancer Res. *28:* 934–937, 1968.

Wattenberg, L. W., Page, M. A., and Leong, J. L.: Induction of increased benzpyrene hydroxylase activity by 2-phenylbenzothiazoles and related compounds. Cancer Res. *28:* 2539–2544, 1968a.

Welch, R. M., Harrison, Y. E., and Burns, J. J.: Implications of enzyme induction in drug toxicity studies. Toxicol. Appl. Pharmacol. *10:* 340–351, 1967.

Welch, R. M., Harrison, Y., Gommi, B. W., Poppers, P. J., Finster, M., and Conney, A. H.: Stimulatory effect of cigarette smoking on the hydroxylation of 3,4-

benzpyrene and the N-demethylation of 3-methyl-4-monomethylaminoazobenzene by enzymes in human placenta. Clin. Pharmacol. Ther. *10:* 100–109, 1969.

Welch, R. M., Levin, W., and Conney, A. H.: Insecticide inhibition and stimulation of steroid hydroxylases in rat liver. J. Pharmacol. Exp. Ther., *155:* 167–173, 1967a.

Welch, R. M., Levin, W., and Conney, A. H.: Stimulatory effect of phenobarbital on the metabolism *in vivo* of estradiol-17β and estrone in the rat. J. Pharmacol. Exp. Ther. *160:* 171–178, 1968.

Welch, R. M., Rosenberg, P., and Coon, J. M.: Inhibition of hexobarbital metabolism by chlorthion (p-nitro-m-chlorophenyldimethylthionophosphate). The Pharmacologist *1:* 64, 1959.

Werk, E. E., Jr., MacGee, J., and Sholiton, L. J.: Effect of diphenylhydantoin on cortisol metabolism in man. J. Clin. Invest. *43:* 1824–1835, 1964.

Werk, E. E., Jr., Sholiton, L. J., and Olinger, C. P.: Amelioration of nontumorous Cushing's syndrome by diphenylhydantoin. 2nd Int. Congress Hormonal Steroids, Milan, Abstracts, Int. Congr. Ser. No. III, Excerpta Medica Foundation, p. 301, New York, 1966.

Wheatley, D. N.: Enhancement and inhibition of the induction by 7,12-dimethylbenz(α)anthracene of mammary tumors in female Sprague-Dawley rats. Brit. J. Cancer *22:* 787–797, 1968.

Yaffee, S. J., Levy, G., Matsuzawa, T., and Baliah, T.: Enhancement of glucuronide conjugating capacity in a hyperbilirubinemic infant due to apparent enzyme induction by phenobarbital. New Eng. J. Med. *275:* 1461–1466, 1966.

14

Mechanisms of Induction of Drug Metabolism Enzymes

H. V. GELBOIN

I. INTRODUCTION

A large segment of this review concerns the changes induced by polycyclic hydrocarbons and drugs on the level of certain enzyme activities and the mechanism of these changes. It is, therefore, important to summarize briefly some of the factors which may affect the observed activity of an enzyme system.

Enzyme control mechanisms may be classified into two broad categories. Firstly, there are those factors that affect the enzymatic activity of specific protein molecules, and secondly, those factors that regulate the amount of enzyme protein. In respect to the former, the activity of an enzyme may be affected by the concentration of either substrate or product. A prime example of substrate inhibition is the inhibitory effect of high levels of acetylcholine on acetylcholinesterase (Nachmanson and Wilson, 1945). Typical product inhibition is exemplified by the inhibition of hexokinase by its reaction product, glucose-6-phosphate (Crane and Sols, 1953). The latter may be an example of an "isosteric inhibition." The inhibitor is sterically related to the substrate or cofactor and competes with either of the latter for the catalytic site on the enzyme. Thus, isosteric inhibition may take place if the tissue preparation contains a compound which competes with substrate or cofactor for the catalytic site on the enzyme.

Other enzyme controls may involve either a stimulation or inhibition of the enzyme by an "allosteric" modification. In this type of inhibition or activation, the molecule modifying enzyme activity is not a steric analog of the substrate but rather exerts its effect on the enzyme by binding to a site other than the binding site of the substrate. Feedback inhibition, in which a distal product of a metabolic pathway inhibits an early enzyme in the pathway, is an example of this type of inhibition. A typical example of an enzyme modified in this way is aspartate transcarbamylase which catalyzes an early step in pyrimidine synthesis and which is inhibited by one of the end products of pyrimidine biosynthesis, cytidine triphosphate (Gerhardt and Pardee, 1962). Another example of alteration of enzyme activity which is not related to an altered protein amount is the activation of the digestive enzymes. These are prime examples of inactive enzymes which are activated subsequent to their synthesis (Neurath and Dixon, 1957). The zymogens are converted to the active enzyme form by structural modification, and this type of activation can easily mimic enzyme induction, *i.e.*, an increased rate of *de novo* synthesis of enzyme protein.

Other cases of activation and inactivation are those that occur through an association and dissociation of peptide subunits of an enzyme. This has been called "molecular conversion" by Monod and Jacob (1961). Phosphorylase is inactivated when phosphate is split from the enzyme by a phosphatase (Wosilait and Sutherland, 1956). This inactivation apparently occurs because the enzyme is split into two subunits. Phosphorylation of the protein reverses this process and activates the enzyme. Epinephrine and glucagon stimulate the activity of phosphorylase by increasing the formation of cyclic 3',5'-adenylate which increases the activity of the enzyme that phosphorylates the subunits (Rall and Sutherland, 1961).

The amount of enzyme protein may be regulated by factors affecting either or both the rate of enzyme synthesis or the rate of enzyme degradation. The term "enzyme induction" has been specifically used to describe the process which increases the rate of synthesis of an enzyme relative to its normal rate of synthesis in the uninduced organism. Enzyme repression is the process in which the rate of enzyme synthesis is decreased relative to the normal rate. In many of the studies in mammalian systems the terms "induction" and "repression" are used to explain an increase or decrease in enzyme activity but where enzyme protein amount has actually not been determined.

In many of the reports cited in this review, a rigorous demonstration of an increase in the amount of enzyme protein has not been established. For the purpose of this review the terms "enzyme induction" and "enzyme repression" will be used, although direct evidence for "induction" or "repression" are often lacking.

Berlin and Schimke (1965) have pointed out the importance of both enzyme synthesis and degradation in many studies on enzyme induction. Thus, a stabilization of an enzyme which prevents its degradation may mimic enzyme induction. Examples of this are the ten-fold increase in thymidylate kinase activity when thymidine is administered. This increase is not due to an increased rate of enzyme synthesis, *i.e.*, to enzyme induction, but rather to a thymidine stabilization of thymidine kinase (Bojarski and Hiatt, 1960). Also, tryptophan administration increases tryptophan pyrrolase activity by increasing its affinity for a cofactor hematin (Feigelson and Greengard, 1962) which stabilizes the enzyme and prevents its degradation (Schimke *et al.*, 1964). Thus, in the absence of tryptophan, the enzyme has a half-life of about three hours; in its presence enzyme degradation is not detectable.

Another example of enzyme stabilization mimicking enzyme induction is the two-fold increase in rat liver arginase when the rats are deprived of food for six days. During this time, however, the rate of arginase synthesis is constant while the degradation of the enzyme is halted. On changing from a high to a low protein diet the rate of degradation is increased and the rate of synthesis decreased. This mimics but is not true enzyme repression, which can be defined as a decrease in the rate of enzyme synthesis (Schimke, 1964).

II. EFFECTS OF POLYCYCLIC HYDROCARBONS ON PROTEIN SYNTHESIS

A single *in vivo* administration of certain polycyclic hydrocarbons and drugs to rats increases a large number of liver microsomal enzyme activities. This phenomenon and types of enzymes involved has been discussed in several broad reviews (Gillette, 1963; Conney, 1967; Gelboin, 1967). Among the many enzyme systems which are enhanced by polycyclic hydrocarbons are N-demethylation (Conney et al., 1956; Conney et al., 1959; Decken and Hultin, 1960), O-demethylation (Henderson and Mazel, 1964), S-demethylation (Henderson and Mazel, 1964), aromatic ring C- and N-hydroxylation (Conney et al., 1959; Dao and Yogo, 1964; Gillette, 1963; Cramer et al., 1960), reduction of the azo linkage and aminoazo dyes (Conney et al., 1956; Conney et al., 1959; Jervell et al., 1965; Decken and Hultin, 1960), the glucuronide conjugation of hydroxy compounds (Inscoe and Axelrod, 1960), and various components of the microsomal electron transport enzymes (Conney, 1967; Ernster & Orrenius, 1965). Many of the latter enzyme systems are also enhanced by a variety of drugs of different types and of varied clinical use.

The literature reveals that almost all of the enzyme activities increased by hydrocarbon or drug pretreatment that have been localized intracellularly have been found in the microsomal fraction. Certain other "inducible" enzymes of rat liver such as tryptophan pyrrolase, serine dehydrase, and arginase are not significantly affected by treatment of the rat with hydrocarbons or drugs. Although a large number of compounds of different molecular types may increase the same enzyme system, there are a number of enzymes which are increased by one class of compound and not another; e.g., microsomal androgen hydroxylases, although inducible by phenobarbital, are not affected by 3,4-benzpyrene (BP) treatment. In contrast, the enzyme system that hydroxylates 3,4-benzpyrene is induced by pretreatment with either BP or phenobarbital. Thus, the profile of enzyme systems induced by a particular compound may be unique.

In other cases, however, two inducers may increase a similar profile of enzymes. An explanation for these differences and for the molecular basis of hydrocarbon or drug-induced alterations in enzyme activity must await knowledge in several areas. Questions must be answered concerning the transport and availability of the inducer to its initial cellular site of action as well as to the nature of the receptor. Other problems are that of the metabolic conversion of an inactive administered compound to an active form, and finally, there is the question of the mechanism of the induction process.

Arcos et al. (1961) showed that many polycyclic hydrocarbons increase liver size, with a proportionate increase in total liver protein. Within four days after the administration of methylcholanthrene (MC), naphthacene, or anthanthrene there was a 20 to 30 % increase in liver protein content. Although MC increased total protein content of the liver, it did not change the amount of protein per gram of liver. On the other hand, the administration of phenobarbital and related drugs caused an increase in both the total liver protein and in the amount of protein per gram of wet weight of liver. Conney et al. (1960) and Conney and Gilman (1963) have found that phenobarbital, chlorcyclizine, orphenadrine, or phenylbutazone caused increases in microsomal protein per gram of wet liver ranging from 22 to 39 %.

Orrenius et al. (1965) reported an increase in both protein and RNA content of the microsomes of liver treated with phenobarbital for a 120-hour period. The latter investigators fractionated the microsomes and reported an increase in both the agranular and granular endoplasmic reticulum 120 hours after the rats were treated with phenobarbital. The phenobarbital effect was considerably greater in the agranular endoplasmic reticulum where a two-fold increase was observed; the granular endoplasmic reticulum increased only 20% upon phenobarbital treatment. These results are consistent with the reports from several laboratories of a proliferative effect of phenobarbital on the agranular endoplasmic reticulum. Thus, Remmer and Merker (1963) and Fouts and Rogers (1965) have demonstrated by electron microscopy an increased content of the agranular endoplasmic reticulum of liver after rats or rabbits were treated with phenobarbital.

The studies demonstrating an increased protein content, a proliferation of the agranular endoplasmic reticulum, and an induction of a variety of microsomal enzymes, raises the question as to the effect of polycyclic hydrocarbons and drugs on the protein synthesizing systems of the microsomes. Kato *et al.* (1965) studied the effect of phenobarbital on the *in vivo* incorporation of C^{14}-leucine into the various subcellular fractions of rat liver. This study (Kato *et al.*, 1965) showed that phenobarbital affected only the rate of incorporation of amino acid into the microsomal fractions. The proteins from a highly purified nuclear fraction, mitochondria, or the soluble fraction of the cell sap showed a similar incorporation rate in control and in phenobarbital-treated rats.

Microsomes, however, from phenobarbital-treated rats showed approximately a 25% increase in the incorporation of C^{14}-leucine. This increase was observed both in the deoxycholate-soluble proteins of the microsomes, that is, in the lipoprotein component as well as in the ribosomal components of rat liver microsomes. Decken and Hultin (1960) reported an increase of 22% in the *in vitro* incorporation of C^{14}-leucine into microsomal protein. Gelboin and Sokoloff (1961, 1964) using different types of *in vitro* amino acid incorporating systems found a 60% and 30% increase in leucine C^{14} incorporation *in vitro* after the rats were pretreated with MC.

The increased incorporation of DL-leucine C^{14} *in vitro* observed at 15 minutes incubation in preparations from MC-treated rats appeared not to be due to any possible preservative effect by the MC pretreatment. Thus, both the initial rate of leucine incorporation and the total amount of amino acid incorporated at 30 minutes was higher in the preparation from the MC-treated rats. Pretreatment of the rats with phenobarbital causes a 163% increase in the leucine C^{14} incorporation. Gelboin and Sokoloff (1961) also observed the stimulatory effect of MC when SRNA-leucine C^{14} or SRNA-proline C^{14} were used as a precursor in place of the free amino acid. This result suggests that at least part of the stimulatory effect of MC on amino acid incorporation is not due to soluble factors which may influence the formation of SRNA-bound amino acid. In a subsequent study, Gelboin and Sokoloff (1964) found evidence for increased levels of GTP in rat liver supernatant of animals treated with MC. Supernatant from MC-treated rats was more effective in supporting microsomal amino acid incorporation than rat liver supernatant fluid from control rats.

Gelboin (1964) and Kato *et al.* (1965, 1966) have examined the mechanism of the MC and phenobarbital stimulation of protein synthesis. They used techniques which enabled them to examine amino acid incorporation directed by endogenous messenger RNA and that directed solely by a synthetic messenger RNA polyuridylic acid. The microsomal incorporating system can be operationally described as consisting of two parts, the messenger RNA and the microsomal amino acid incorporation site, *i.e.*, the microsomal RNA protein complex on which messenger RNA "programs" amino acid incorporation. Preincubation of the microsomes in the presence of an energy source, GTP and Mg^{+2}, removes phenylalanine incorporating activity, normally directed by messenger RNA. Phenylalanine incorporation can then be restored by the addition of poly-uridylic acid.

The rate of loss of messenger RNA activity during preincubation of the microsomes from MC- or PB-treated rats parallels the loss of activity observed in the initially less active microsomes from normal rats. The results showing similar rates of loss of messenger RNA activity suggest that the increased incorporation in microsomes from MC- or PB-treated microsomes is not due to an MC-induced inhibition of the loss of endogenous messenger RNA activity or to an MC-induced stabilization of the microsomal bound messenger RNA.

The latter studies (Gelboin and Sokoloff, 1964 and Kato et al., 1965, 1966) showed that with the nonpreincubated microsomes, i.e., those containing endogenous RNA, the addition of polyuridylic acid-stimulated incorporation to the same extent in microsomes from control and MC-treated rats. This suggests that the number of messenger-free binding sites for poly-U is not affected by MC treatment. However, after the removal of endogenous messenger RNA activity, the addition of polyuridylic stimulated phenylalanine incorporation to a greater extent in the preparation from MC- and PB-treated rats than in normal preparations. This suggests that after preincubation there are more messenger RNA-free microsomal sites for the binding of polyuridylic acid in the preparations from MC- and PB-treated rats than there are in the microsomes from normal rats. Also, with no preincubation, the addition of 100 μg of polyuridylic acid was sufficient to saturate the binding sites of microsomes from normal and MC-treated rats. After preincubation, however, 100 μg was sufficient to saturate the active sites of the normal microsomes but was insufficient to saturate the active sites of the microsomes from MC-treated rats. If one assumes that the newly available sites are those that were previously occupied by the released messenger RNA, then the results are interpreted to mean that the MC microsomes contained, prior to preincubation, a greater amount of messenger RNA and, hence, upon preincubation more active sites became available in the MC preparation than in the normal preparation.

Kato et al. (1965, 1966) found that phenobarbital caused similar but quantitatively greater differences than MC in the microsomal protein synthesizing activity. Microsomes from PB-treated rats are almost twice as responsive to the addition of polyuridylic acid. Thus, microsomes from phenobarbital-treated rats are more active in endogenous L-(^{14}C) phenylalanine incorporation, and after the removal of endogenous messenger RNA are much more sensitive than control microsomes to polyuridylic acid-directed L-(^{14}C)phenylalanine incorporation. This is likely due to a phenobarbital-induced increase in both the endogenous microsomal messenger RNA content and the total number of microsomal binding sites for messenger RNA.

In further examining this effect, Kato et al. (1965, 1966) found the increased activity of microsomes from phenobarbital-treated rats in respect to both endogenous mRNA-directed polyuridylic and directed phenylalanine incorporation was not observed in the ribosomes isolated from the same experimental animals. Figure 14.1, from Kato et al. (1966), shows that with nonpreincubated microsomes, L-(^{14}C)phenylalanine incorporation remains constant at two levels of

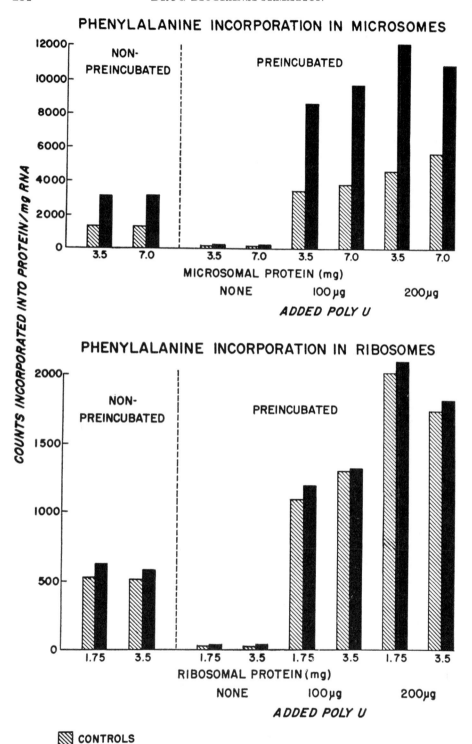

Fig. 14.1. L-[^{14}C]-phenylalanine incorporation in nonpreincubated microsomal and ribosomal preparations from control and phenobarbital-treated rats. (Kato *et al.*, 1966.)

added microsomes and in each case the microsomes from phenobarbital-treated rats are about twice as active as controls. After preincubation, however, both control and phenobarbital microsomes are inactive unless polyuridylic acid is added to the system. With the addition of either 100 μg or 200 μg of polyuridylic acid the phenobarbital microsomes are about twice as active as the control preparations. The lower half of the chart shows a similar experiment performed with ribosomes isolated from the same group of rats. Although there are marked differences in microsomal L-(^{14}C)phenylalanine incorporation, there is only a negligible difference between ribosomes from control and phenobarbital-treated rats. This is true when L-(^{14}C)phenylalanine incorporation is directed either by endogenous messenger RNA or by polyuridylic acid. Hence, the factors responsible for the stimulatory activity of phenobarbital are removed by desoxycholate treatment during the preparation of the ribosomes and are likely components of the endoplasmic reticulum.

Siefert et al. (1968) examined the effect of phenobarbital in vivo administration on the in vitro phenylalanine incorporating activity of isolated ribosomes. Within 5 hours after phenobarbital treatment, ribosomes showed an increased phenylalanine incorporation; at 17 hours the activity of microsomes and membrane-bound ribosomes diminished. These authors also found that the sensitivity of microsomes to added synthetic messenger RNA was 40% greater when isolated from phenobarbital-treated rats. They also found that the ribosomal fraction from phenobarbital-treated rats contained a greater number of more rapidly sedimenting polysomal components. They suggest that phenobarbital increases the number of ribosomal binding sites for mRNA attachment.

Gelboin (1964) found that actinomycin D not only inhibited the MC induction of benzpyrene hydroxylase but also prevented the MC-induced changes in microsomal protein synthesis. Thus, the MC-induced changes in microsomal amino acid incorporation appear dependent on RNA synthesis. The changes in gross protein synthesis parallel the increase in microsomal enzyme activity. They probably comprise changes in the rates of synthesis of many proteins. This is true since the microsomal enzymes comprise a relatively small number of the total cell proteins and even marked changes in their rates of synthesis could not account for the gross changes in protein synthesis.

III. EFFECT OF INDUCERS ON THE TURNOVER AND ACTIVITY OF MICROSOMAL PROTEINS

Jick and Shuster (1966) have investigated the turnover of microsomal induced NADPH cytochrome c reductase and microsomal protein in the livers of mice treated with phenobarbital. Figure 14.2 shows a phenobarbital-induced increase in the incorporation of L-leucine into microsomal NADPH cytochrome c reductase. Figure 14.3 shows that phenobarbital markedly inhibits the loss of radioactivity from prelabelled NADPH cytochrome c reductase. The half-life of in vivo loss of radioactivity from enzyme protein averaged 2.8 days in control mice; however, they detected no loss of radioactivity from the purified enzyme in phenobarbital-treated mice. Jick and Shuster concluded from the studies that phenobarbital causes both an increase in the rate of synthesis and a decreased rate of breakdown of microsomal NADPH cytochrome c reductase.

Kuriyama et al., (1969) have also examined the effect of phenobarbital on the synthesis and degradation of total microsomal proteins and two enzymes of the

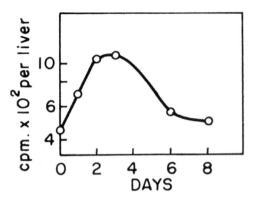

Fig. 14.2. Effect of phenobarbital treatment on the incorporation of L-leucine into microsomal NADPH-cytochrome c reductase. Mice received injections twice daily of sodium phenobarbital, 75 mg/kg, or 0.9% NaCl. At various times one group of 4 control mice and one group of phenobarbital-treated mice were injected with 20 μC of L-leucine-^{3}H. The mice were killed 90 min after the injection of labeled leucine. Treatment was stopped after 4 days. Each *point* is the average value based on 2 separate isolations of enzyme from the pooled steapsin digest obtained from the livers of two mice. (Jick and Shuster, 1966.)

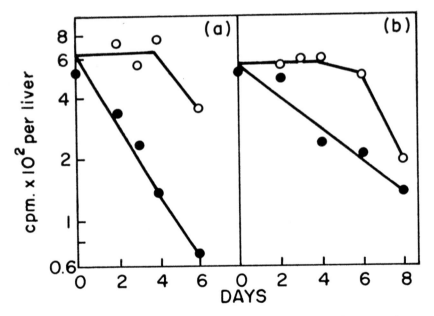

Fig. 14.3. The loss of radioactivity from prelabeled NADPH-cytochrome c reductase in mice treated with phenobarbital. a, treatment was begun 24 hr after the injection of 25 μC of L-leucine-^{3}H. Mice received injections twice daily of sodium phenobarbital, 75 mg/kg, or of 0.25 ml of 0.9% NaCl. Each *point* is the average value based on two separate isolations of enzyme from the pooled steapsin digests obtained from the livers of two or three mice. ×- - - -×, enzyme from control animals; ○- - - -○, enzyme from phenobarbital-treated mice. b, conditions were the same as those in a except that treatment was stopped after 4 days. Each *point* is based on two separate isolations of enzyme from the pooled steapsin digests obtained from the livers of two mice. (Jick and Shuster, 1966.)

microsomal endoplasmic reticulum, NADPH-cytochrome c reductase and cytochrome b_5. The two enzymes were isolated and purified, and the effect of phenobarbital on the synthesis and degradation of the enzymes was determined with both C^{14}-leucine and C^{14}-guanidino-labeled arginine. Figure 14.4 shows that a single administration of phenobarbital induced a prompt increase in the rate of total microsomal protein and NADPH-cytochrome c reductase synthesis but did not effect the rate of cytochrome b_5 synthesis. They also found that the induced

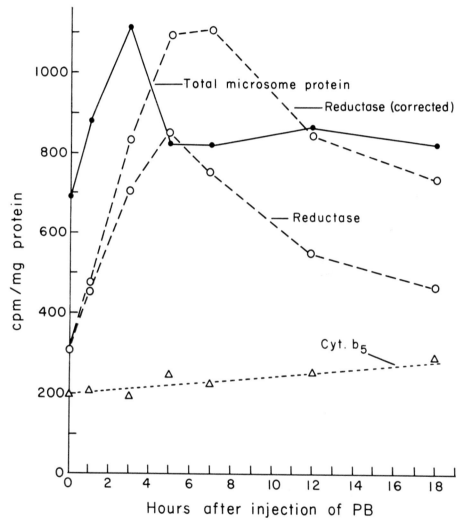

Fig. 14.4. Change in the rates of synthesis of cytochrome b_5, reductase, and total proteins of washed microsomes. At 1, 3, 5, 7, 12, and 18 hrs after the i.v. PB injection, DL-leucine-1-C^{14} (5 μC/100 g body weight) was injected intravenously, and the animals killed after 40 min. At each time point, the livers of three rats were pooled for the preparation of washed microsomes and for the separation and purification of microsomal enzymes. The raw data for the reductase were corrected for concurrent changes in microsomal enzyme content by multiplying the corresponding specific radioactivities by the ratio; enzyme content in the microsomes of PB-treated rats/enzyme content in the microsomes of control rats. (Kuriyama et al., 1969.)

reductase was both chromatographically and immunochemically identical to the enzyme normally found in the liver. When repeated phenobarbital doses were given, the increases in NADPH-cytochrome c reductase amount were greater and there was a moderate rise in cytochrome b_5 content. Both of these effects seem to be the result of a drastic reduction in the rates of enzyme degradation.

Thus, in addition to increasing the rate of NADPH cytochrome c reductase synthesis, phenobarbital also drastically reduces its rate of degradation. It also appears that the increase in cytochrome b_5 content is in part due to a reduction in its rate of degradation. Figure 14.5 shows that in the presence of phenobarbital there is essentially no loss of radioactivity from purified cytochrome b_5 or cytochrome c reductase. These data are in agreement with those of Jick and Shuster (1966).

Upon cessation of phenobarbital treatment there is a progressive reduction in NADPH cytochrome c reductase amount which seems to be due to an increased rate of degradation during its continued synthesis. However, when leucine-C^{14} is used, the marked difference in enzyme turnover between normal and phenobarbital-treated animals may be due to a more efficient reutilization of the labeled amino acid (Loftfield and Harris, 1956; Gan and Jeffay, 1967). In order to mini-

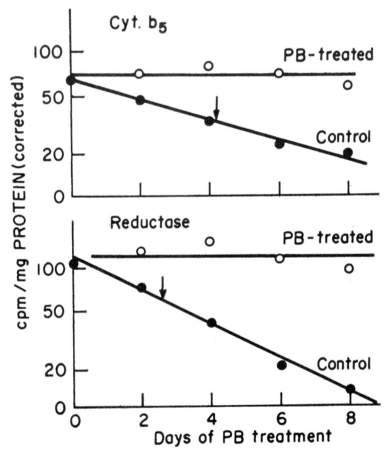

Fig. 14.5. Decay of specific radioactivities of cytochrome b_5 and NADPH-cytochrome c reductase in normal and PB-treated rats. (Kuriyama et al., 1969.)

mize this possibility, Kuriyama *et al.* also performed their studies with C^{14}-guanidino-L-arginine as the radioactive amino acid. This amino acid is not significantly reutilized because of its rapid degradation through the urea cycle (Swick and Hande, 1956; Swick, 1958; Schimke, 1964; Stephen and Waterlow, 1966). These investigators, however, found similar results with the guanidino-labeled arginine as with leucine indicating that the apparent differences in the rates of synthesis and degradation after phenobarbital treatment were not due largely to an altered reutilization of free amino acids (Ernster and Orrenius, 1965).

Kuriyama *et al.* also found that phenobarbital inhibited the loss of radioactivity from total microsomal protein. These results can be compared to the studies reported by Schimke, *et al.* (1968), who found that phenobarbital only prevented the loss of radioactivity from microsomes when leucine-H^3 was used as the radioactive precursor and not when guanidino-C^{14} arginine was used. The difference in half-life of the proteins from control and PB-treated rats was only from 2.1 days to 2.3 days. Thus, the work of Kuriyama, *et al.* (1969), Schimke *et al.* (1968) and Jick and Shuster (1966) all agree that phenobarbital stimulates the synthesis of microsomal NADPH-cytochrome c reductase. The results of Kuriyama *et al.*, and Jick and Shuster also conclude that phenobarbital inhibits the degradation rate of microsomal proteins. Schimke *et al.* (1968), however, reported no effect of phenobarbital on the rate of degradation.

Kuriyama *et al.* also found that the phenobarbital induced increase in the rate of incorporation of amino acid into total microsomal membrane protein was an earlier event than the increase in the rate of reductase synthesis. The protein preparation they found was labeled at a faster rate and contained approximately 50 % of the original microsomal protein. The authors suggest that this fraction may reflect a phenobarbital-induced synthesis of a "primary membrane" which may precede the synthesis of the phenobarbital-induced enzymes which may be then deposited on the primary membrane.

Schimke *et al.* (1968) have also approached the problem of microsomal membrane synthesis and the effect of phenobarbital by the use of a double-labeling technique in which one amino acid, labeled with H^3, is administered to control rats, and the identical amino acid, labeled with C^{14}, is administered to phenobarbital-treated rats. Figure 14.6 shows that the ratio of H^3 to C^{14} in different endoplasmic reticulum proteins varies to a marked extent. Although this technique has not afforded an identification of each protein, it clearly shows that phenobarbital effects the synthesis of the various microsomal proteins in rather different degrees. Thus, if phenobarbital increased the rate of synthesis of all proteins to the same extent, the ratio of H^3 to C^{14} of the various fractions would be the same. These results suggest that phenobarbital increases the synthesis of some but not all proteins of the endoplasmic reticulum. The double-labeling technique introduced by Schimke *et al.* (1968) may be of use in further clarifying the selectivity and mode of action of phenobarbital.

Several investigators have suggested the involvement of heme synthesis in the formation of microsomal cytochromes as a regulating factor in the formation of the microsomal cytochromes (Granick, 1966). The biosynthetic pathway of heme involves the condensation of glycine and succinyl CoA in the presence of δ-aminolevulinic acid synthetase and pyridoxal phosphate to form δ-aminolevulinic acid (ALA).

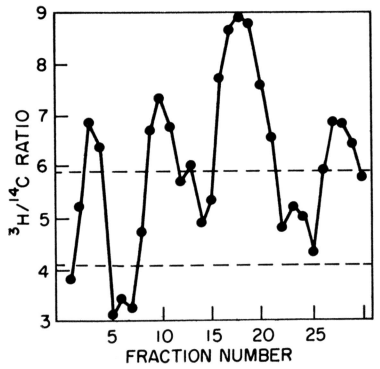

Fig. 14.6. Effect of phenobarbital on differential synthesis of endoplasmic reticulum proteins. One rat was treated with phenobarbital (60 mg/kg i.p. daily) for 4 days and then received ^{3}H-leucine (100 μc). A second rat received saline injections for 4 days and then received ^{14}C-leucine (20 μc). Both rats were sacrificed 4 hr later; 8×10^6 hepatocytes were prepared from each liver (Howard *et al.*, 1967) combined and smooth endoplasmic reticulum was prepared and chromatographed. The results are given as ^{3}H/^{14}C ratios in fractions of solubilized membrane protein after gradient elution from DEAE-cellulose. The broken lines represent the 99% tolerance limits of the mean in the control experiment with a P value of 0.01. In another control experiment, in which each of two animals first received phenobarbital for 4 days, and then received separately ^{3}H and ^{14}C-leucine, and a combined smooth endoplasmic reticulum preparation was studied, similar confidence limits for ^{3}H/^{14}C ratios were found (Schimke *et al.*, 1968.)

The ALA synthetase is a mitochondrial enzyme and is thought to be the rate-limiting step in heme biosynthesis (Granick, 1966; Granick and Urata, 1963; Granick, 1963; Tschudy *et al.*, 1965). Since ALA synthetase has a relatively short half-life of 60 to 70 minutes (Marver, *et al.*, 1966), its induction and repression may be significant to the changed activities of certain microsomal enzymes. Marver (1968) has reported a rapid increase of ALA synthetase within several hours after phenobarbital was administered. He suggests that the increase in this activity provides the additional heme required for the drug-induced increases of microsomal cytochromes. Marver also reports that phenobarbital stimulates Fe^{59} incorporation into microsomes and that the administration of heme largely prevents the increase in cytochrome P-450 induced by phenobarbital.

Heme administration also prevents the stimulation of phospholipid synthesis, and the increase in NADPH cytochrome *c* reductase, aminopyrine N-demethylase and hexobarbital oxidase induced by phenobarbital. Since hematin is also a known repressor of heme biosynthesis, the suggestion is that heme biosynthesis plays an important role in the induction of microsomal enzymes. It is possible, however, that the receptor sites for the inducer may be microsomal heme proteins, and that administered hematin may compete with the normal receptor site for the inducer. Marver's data suggests that heme synthesis is required for the production of increased amounts of microsomal cytochromes. It is not certain, however, whether heme biosynthesis is also necessary for the early larger rises in certain enzymes, e.g., the aryl hydrocarbon hydroxylases. These increases are observed in tissue culture within one hour (Nebert and Gelboin, 1968a) and *in vivo* within four to five hours after hydrocarbon administration. The work of Marver, however, suggests a role for ALA synthetase regulation and heme biosynthesis in microsomal enzyme induction. Whether the role is initial or concomitant to the general increase in microsomal cytochromes remains to be determined.

Levin and Kuntzman (1969) have also found that phenobarbital administration stimulates the synthesis of microsomal hemo-proteins as measured by either Fe^{59} incorporation, or either glycine or δ-aminolevulinic acid (ALA) incorporation into a microsomal fraction containing heme protein. They reported no effect of PB or MC pretreatment on the incorporation of ALA into "CO-binding microsomal particles." They did, however, report that the rate of loss of radioactivity from the "particle" was decreased by MC treatment. In these studies it would be important to characterize the nature of the radioactivity in the particle. The authors suggest that this is evidence for an MC induction of a second hemoprotein moiety or a change in the composition of the CO-binding particles.

Several investigators have reported a drug induced shift in the absorption spectra of CO-binding pigments in liver microsomes. This shift after MC administration is not observed after phenobarbital is given and involves a change in absorption maximum from 450 mμ to between 445 and 448 mμ.

Hildebrandt et al. (1968) and Schenkman et al. (1969) have discussed the problem of the possible forms of cytochrome P-450 and have suggested that the P-450 exists only in two forms, that of the native enzyme and that of an enzyme-substrate complex. Kuntzman et al. (1968) have reported that ethionine and actinomycin D prevents the MC induced shift to 448 from 450, suggesting a role for RNA and protein synthesis in the shift. These authors suggest that the inhibitor studies indicate that MC stimulates the synthesis of a heme protein which is different from P-450. In other studies, Schenkman and Sato (1968) found that the addition of substrates alters the absolute spectrum of the cytochrome P-450 and that the spectrum of the P-450 induced by the polycyclic hydrocarbon appears similar to the heme protein in the presence of substrate. They conclude that the P-450 exists in only two forms, that of the native enzyme and that of the enzyme substrate complex.

Studies by Sladek and Mannering (1969a; 1969b) have also indicated that the mechanism by which polycyclic hydrocarbons and phenobarbital produce their inductive effects on microsomal N-demethylating systems are different, and that the microsomal N-demethylation stimulated by polycyclic hydrocarbons is also different than that stimulated by phenobarbital. These studies also suggest the possibility of different forms of the enzyme or of two different enzyme systems for N-demethylation.

Studies by Gurtoo et al. (1968) and Alvares et al. (1968) have shown that pretreatment with benzpyrene alters the kinetic behavior of microsomal aryl hydrocarbon hydroxylase. These alterations may be due to allosteric conversion of the control enzyme to a different form or may be due to the induced synthesis of a new and different hydroxylase.

The changes in the spectral properties of microsomal cytochromes and the kinetic behavior of microsomal hydroxylase after pretreatment of the animal with MC may be due to several possibilities. The MC may indeed induce the synthesis of an entirely new enzyme. If the microsomes contained more of this enzyme they would exhibit different spectral and kinetic behavior. Another possibility is that the control enzyme is converted to a different form which exhibits different kinetic behavior and shows changed spectral characteristics. Either of the above mechanisms may require RNA and protein synthesis, the first for the direct synthesis of the new enzyme, and the second mechanism requiring the synthesis of a protein needed for the allosteric conversion of the pre-existing enzyme.

Studies from Orrenius' laboratory (Ernster and Orrenius, 1965; Orrenius et al., 1965; Orrenius and Ericsson, 1966) suggested that phenobarbital increases the synthesis of phospholipid in liver endoplasmic reticulum, since they found a 2- and 6-fold greater specific activity of $P^{32}PO_4$ in microsomal phospholipid. Holtzman and Gillette (1968) have suggested that part of this difference was due to a change in the specific activity of the phosphate pools and to a decrease in the catabolism of microsomal phospholipid. The increased synthesis, however, was not observed in female rats. Thus, it appears that microsomal phospholipid synthesis is stimulated during enzyme induction in male rats and microsomal phospholipid catabolism is reduced by the phenobarbital in both male and female rats.

The involvement of phospholipid catabolism in microsomal enzyme induction is an area which is just beginning to be explored and may be highly relevant and central to the induction process. At this time it is difficult to assess the role of the reported alterations in phospholipid metabolism in microsomal enzyme induction.

IV. EFFECTS OF INHIBITORS ON THE INDUCTION OF ENZYME ACTIVITIES IN VIVO

A. Enzyme Induction In Vivo

Ethionine has been found to block protein synthesis by being incorporated in S-adenosyl-ethionine and thereby preventing the synthesis of ATP (Villa-Trevino et al., 1963). The prevention of protein synthesis by this inhibitor, therefore, is complex and may occur at different levels, such as amino acid activation, messenger RNA or transfer RNA synthesis, or polypeptide synthesis. Thus, inhibition of enzyme induction by ethionine does not precisely localize the inhibited steps of the gene-action system. Ethionine completely inhibits the induction of aminoazo dye N-demethylase activity by MC (Conney et al., 1956). Ethionine had no effect on the levels of this enzyme in control rats, and the simultaneous administration of methionine completely reversed the inhibitory effect of ethionine on the induction. Ethionine also inhibited the induction of DAB reductase.

Conney et al. (1957) obtained similar results when they examined the effect of ethionine on the induction of benzpyrene hydroxylase by MC pretreatment. Ethionine completely prevented the induction, and the inhibition was not observed when methionine was given simultaneously. In another study, Cramer et al. (1960) found that ethionine completely inhibited the MC induction of acetylaminofluorene hydroxylation. The inhibition was reversed by methionine.

Puromycin blocks protein synthesis at the microsomal level by preventing the transfer of soluble RNA-bound amino acid into polypeptide chains (Yarmolinsky and de la Haba (1959)).

Gelboin and Blackburn (1963) examined the effect of puromycin on the MC induction of benzpyrene hydroxylase in liver, kidney, small intestine, and lungs. To avoid the problem of chronic toxicity of the inhibitor these investigators used a short 7-hour period of induction. Puromycin completely inhibited the MC-induced increase in activity in liver, kidney, and small intestine. In lung the stimulatory effect of MC was inhibited by 50%. Orrenius et al. (1965) reported that puromycin prevented the phenobarbital-induced increase in N-demethylation, TPNH cytochrome c reductase activity, and the CO-binding pigment of the microsomes. Conney and Gilman (1963) reported a complete inhibition by puromycin of the increase in aminoazo dye N-demethylase induced by either MC or phenobarbital. Puromycin given simultaneously with either MC or phenobarbital completely prevented the increase in enzyme activity. Puromycin alone had no effect on enzyme activity.

Jervell et al. (1965) have reported that MC-inducible DAB reductase is also increased in rats by starvation. The induction by starvation is prevented by the simultaneous administration of either puromycin or ethionine but not by actinomycin D. This enzyme appears to have a shorter half-life than that suggested by the studies of Conney (1965) for aminoazo dye N-demethylase. The administration of puromycin 10 hours after the start of the fast decrease the level of enzyme so that it returned to its normal level within 48 hours. These investigators suggest that carbohydrate represses rat liver DAB reductase formation.

In each case reported, puromycin was found to be an effective inhibitor of polycyclic hydrocarbon or phenobarbital-induced enzyme activity. The question arises as to the dependence of new enzyme synthesis on newly-formed messenger RNA. The induction may require activation of specific genes producing induction specific RNAs or may involve the activation of stable messenger RNAs at the microsomal or translational level. To examine this aspect of the problem, several investigators, Gelboin and Blackburn (1963) and Conney (1965) have used actinomycin D, an inhibitor of DNA-dependent RNA synthesis (Reich et al., 1961; Tamaoki and Mueller, 1962; Merits, 1963; and Korner and Munro, 1963) on the drug-induced enzyme synthesis.

Gelboin and Blackburn (1963) examined the effect of actinomycin on the MC induction of benzpyrene hydroxylase in liver, lung, kidney, and small intestine. During a 7-hour period of induction and a 9-hour period of exposure to actinomycin, the inhibitor was found to prevent completely the induction of benzpyrene hydroxylase in liver and small intestine and to prevent partially the induction of this enzyme activity in kidney and lungs. It is possible that in liver and small intestine the messenger RNA for this enzyme is rapidly turning over, and a blockage or increase of enzyme synthesis depends on newly synthesized messenger RNA. On the other hand, the failure of actinomycin D to completely block the MC induction in kidney and small intestine may reflect either an inability of the inhibitor to reach its site of action in adequate concentration or alternatively the stability of the messenger RNA for these enzymes may be greater in kidney and lung, and the induction process may take place at least in part at the level of microsomal translation.

Conney (1965) reported that actinomycin D inhibited the MC-induction of aminoazo dye N-demethylase in the livers of male rats. Actinomycin D also prevented the MC-induced increase in rat liver DAB reductase activity and in the phenobarbital-induced increase in the microsomal content of CO-binding pigment (Jervell et al., 1965 and Orrenius et al., 1965). There have been no reports of failure of actinomycin D to prevent induction of microsomal enzymes by methylcholanthrene or by phenobarbital. Jervell et al. (1965), however, reported that actinomycin failed to prevent the increase in DAB reductase activity induced by starvation. This suggests that there may be a second mechanism by which microsomal enzymes can be induced which is independent of DNA-dependent RNA synthesis.

The stimulatory effect of polycyclic hydrocarbons and drugs on certain liver microsomal enzymes appears not to be mediated through the endocrine system, since the stimulation of at least the aryl hydrocarbon hydroxylase is observed in adrenalectomized and hypophysectomized rats.

B. Enzyme Induction in Isolated Perfused Rat Liver

Juchau et al. (1965) have shown that microsomal BP hydroxylase is induced in isolated induced perfused rat liver when 3,4-benzpyrene is added to the perfusing medium. Maximal enzyme induction was obtained after $6\frac{1}{2}$ hours of perfusion and the degree of stimulation at that time was 2- to 3-fold over the control values. These studies and those on the induction of aryl hydrocarbon hydroxylase in cell cultures (Nebert and Gelboin, 1968b) demonstrate that the inducer can act directly on the target tissue and its action as an inducer does not require the concomitant functioning of the endocrine system. Hormonal influences, however, are not entirely ruled out in the isolated perfused liver since endogenous levels of hormones would be expected to be present in the liver. Cell culture studies utilizing individual tissues in continuing culture for several weeks would be expected to dilute out any endogenous hormone. In these cells grown in culture for several weeks the aryl hydrocarbon hydroxylase is inducible. Thus, the studies of Juchau et al. (1965), and Nebert and Gelboin (1968b) demonstrate that the inducer acts directly on the target tissue.

V. ENZYME INDUCTION IN CELL CULTURE

Insightful information on the mechanism of regulation of gene action and enzyme induction and repression has come from studies with microorganisms. It seems that cell culture would offer unique opportunities for the study of microsomal enzyme induction. Recently, the induction of microsomal aryl hydrocarbon hydroxylase in hamster embryo cell culture has been reported and has yielded some new information on the properties of aryl hydrocarbon hydroxylase and its mechanism of induction (Alfred and Gelboin, 1967; Nebert and Gelboin, 1968a, 1968b). Upon addition of a polycyclic hydrocarbon to the medium, the aryl hydroxylase rises after a lag of about 35 minutes. The rise continues linearly from 12 to 16 hours. Upon removal of the inducer from the medium, the enzyme level declines rapidly.

Figure 14.7 shows some characteristics of the enzyme induction system. This figure should be read only vertically. The enzyme is inducible in cells derived from whole mouse, hamster, or rat embryos. The hydroxylase is also inducible in cells obtained by microdissection from embryonic lung, small intestine, liver, and limb. The inducibility in these tissues is as great as that observed with cells from whole embryos; this suggests that a relatively large proportion of the total cell population is being induced. Optimal induction was observed in cells sub-

Inducibility	Species (embryo)	Origin of cell	Gestational age	Number of subcultures
High	Hamster Mouse	Lung Small intestine Liver	14 days	2–5
Moderate	Rat	Limb	12 days	6
Low	Chick Guinea Pig	Brain	9 days	>6

Fig. 14.7. Characteristics of the aryl hydroxylase induction system. (Gelboin, 1968.)

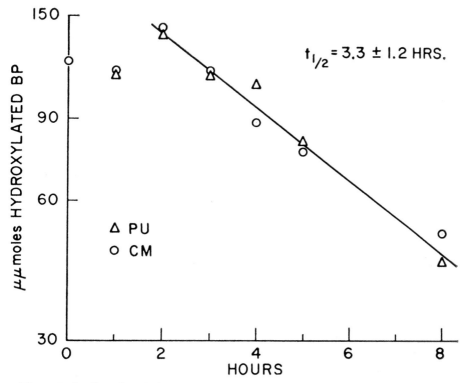

Fig. 14.8. Semilog plot of the rate of decay of previously induced aryl hydroxylase activity. The effects of 60 μM puromycin (PU) and of fresh control medium alone (CM) were not significantly different. (Nebert and Gelboin, 1968b.)

cultured 2 to 6 times. Cells subcultured 11 times were about 50 % as inducible as secondary cultures. The enzyme system activity and its inducibility varied considerably in different established cell lines.

A. Estimation of Half-life of Induced Aryl Hydroxylase Activity

Figure 14.8 shows the rate of decay of previously induced aryl hydroxylase activity when inducer is replaced with fresh control medium or when puromycin is added. The half-life of the induced microsomal hydroxylase system was 3.3 ± 1.2 hours; this value does not include the 2- or 3-hour lag period preceding the decline in enzyme activity. In rat liver microsomal membranes, the half-lives of various components *in vivo* ranged from 75 to 113 hours, with total membrane lipids having 10 to 30 % shorter half-lives (Omura, *et al.*, 1967).

B. Effects of Metabolic Inhibitors on Inducible Aryl Hydroxylase

Figure 14.9 shows the effects of three metabolic inhibitors on aryl hydroxylase induction. The addition of BA to the medium produced a 9-fold increase in enzymatic activity in 4 hours. The addition of actinomycin D, puromycin, or cycloheximide in combination with the inducer completely prevented the hydroxylase induction. The complete block of induction by actinomycin D indicates a requirement for DNA-dependent RNA synthesis for the induction of microsomal aryl hydroxylase activity. Concomitant analysis of RNA synthesis during this 4-hour experiment showed that actinomycin D inhibited at least 90 % of ^{3}H-uridine incorporation into RNA.

That the induction process requires protein synthesis is indicated by the complete prevention of the increase in hydroxylase activity by puromycin and cycloheximide. Although these data do not show an increase in enzyme protein nor rule out an activation of pre-existing enzyme, they do show the requirement of protein synthesis for the increased enzyme activity. Puromycin and cycloheximide inhibited ^{14}C-protein hydrolysate incorporation into cellular protein by at least 95 %.

Figure 14.10 depicts the effects of actinomycin D and puromycin, alone or in combination with the inducer, BA, on aryl hydroxylase activity in cells which had been induced for the preceding 24 hours by BA. Enzyme activity continued to increase at a linear rate in cells exposed to additional inducer. The presence of actinomycin D, with or without the hydrocarbon inducer, produced a greater increase in hydroxylase activity during the initial 4 hours than that observed with BA alone.

The addition of puromycin prevented the increased stimulation of hydroxylase activity by actinomycin D, with and without inducer. The lack of sensitivity to actinomycin D inhibition has been found during glucocorticoid induction of tyrosine-α-ketoglutarate transaminase in hepatoms tissue culture cells (Tomkins, *et al.*, 1965; Thompson *et al.*, 1966; and Peterkofsky and Tomkins, 1967) and has been interpreted as resulting from the inhibition of the synthesis of a labile cytoplasmic translation repressor by relatively high concentrations of actinomycin D. A similar hypothesis has been proposed for the actinomycin D prolongation of the induction of thymidine kinase, which occurs after pox virus infection of HeLa cells (McAuslan, 1963).

Following the addition of puromycin, with or without inducer, or the replace-

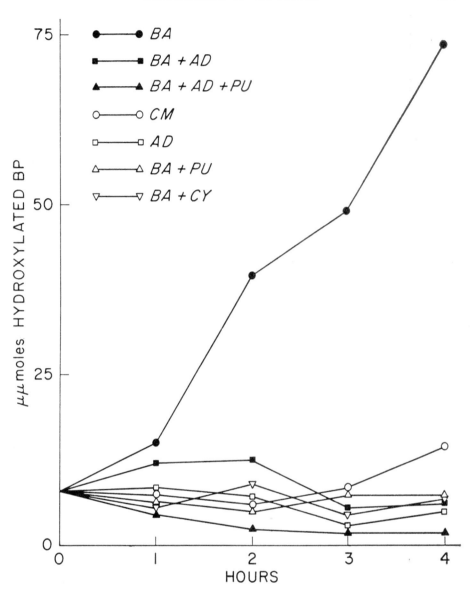

Fig. 14.9. The effects of 0.4 μM actinomycin D (AD), 60 μM puromycin (PU) and 3.5 μM cycloheximide (CY) on aryl hydroxylase induction by 13 μM BA. The responses to inducer alone (BA) and control medium alone (CM) are also illustrated. The antibiotics and the inducer were added simultaneously. When puromycin or cycloheximide was added alone to cells in control medium, no effect on hydroxylase activity was found. At these concentrations of antibiotics, actinomycin D prevented more than 90% of RNA synthesis, and puromycin and cycloheximide prevented more than 95% of protein synthesis. (Nebert and Gelboin, 1968b.) (BA = benzanthracene.)

ment of BA with fresh control medium, aryl hydroxylase activity in the previously induced cells generally remained nearly the same for three hours, after which a first order decay rate ensued. The insensitivity to puromycin for several hours may be due to the assembly of already synthesized components of the hy-

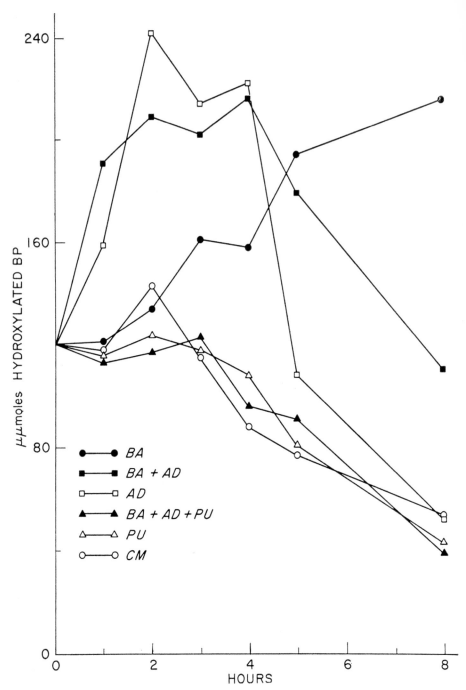

Fig. 14.10. The effects of 0.4 μM actinomycin D (AD), 60 μM puromycin (PU) and control medium (CM) on hydroxylase activity of previously induced cells. The cultures had been treated with 13 μM BA for 25 hours, at which time the medium of all dishes was replaced with fresh medium containing the indicated additions. Concomitant experiments to determine the degree of inhibition of RNA and protein synthesis were carried out. Actinomycin D prevented 75% of ^{3}H-uridine incorporation into perchloric acid-precipitable residue in the initial 15 min following its addition; there was 80% inhibition in the second 15-min period, more than 90% inhibition from 30 to 90 min, and 95 to 98% during the remaining $6\frac{1}{2}$ hr. Puromycin blocked 90% of the ^{14}C-protein hydrolysate incorporation into trichloracetic acid-precipitable protein in the initial 15 min following its addition and 95 to 99% of incorporation during the remaining $7\frac{3}{4}$ hr. (Nebert and Gelboin, 1968b.)

droxylase system. Such a response has been reported for the conversion of sub-units to active carbamyl phosphate synthetase in tadpole liver mitochondrial fractions (Tatibana and Cohen, 1965). A similar delay before the decline of aryl hydroxylase activity was seen when the hydrocarbon inducer was replaced with fresh control medium. This observation suggests that during this period either the induction process is continuing because of the presence of residual amounts of BA or the hydroxylase is being assembled into membrane from previously synthesized precursors.

C. A Translation-independent Phase of Aryl Hydrocarbon Hydroxylase Induction (Nebert and Gelboin, 1970)

The development of insensitivity to actinomycin D inhibition indicates that the early phases of induction involve the synthesis of an induction specific RNA which accumulates and thereby permits the induction process to become inde-pendent of RNA synthesis. Two important questions are whether this RNA can accumulate in the absence of protein synthesis or translation, and can translation occur in the absence of inducer, *i.e.* if the inducer is operating at the level of RNA synthesis, can the translation proceed without the inducer after the RNA is synthesized.

Figure 14.11 shows that the presence of cycloheximide, during a 10-hour period in which the cells are treated with BA, completely prevented the normal rise in aryl hydrocarbon hydroxylase activity. Removal of the cycloheximide-containing medium and replacement by BA-containing medium produced an immediate linear increase in the microsomal enzyme activity, indicating the effective re-versal of the block in protein synthesis. Whether the cycloheximide and BA was replaced with inducer-free medium or with BA-containing medium, an identical rise in hydroxylase activity was observed for at least the first 6 hours. The rise in aryl hydrocarbon hydroxylase activity was prevented during the second 10-hour period if cycloheximide continued to be present. In cells treated initially with cycloheximide without BA, the enzyme level did not rise when the cyclo-heximide-containing medium was replaced with fresh control medium. Thus, these data suggest that the translation step can occur in the absence of inducer, once the induction-specific RNA has been synthesized.

A second question is whether the induction-specific RNA can be synthesized in the absence of protein synthesis or translation. Figure 14.12 demonstrates the effect of high levels of actinomycin D on hydroxylase activity in cells pre-viously treated with BA plus cycloheximide. The addition of actinomycin D, with or without inducer, to cells previously treated with BA plus cycloheximide, stimulated aryl hydrocarbon hydroxylase activity to a greater extent than did BA alone, or control medium alone. The continued presence of cycloheximide prevented the actinomycin D effect, indicating that the marked stimulation by actinomycin D requires protein synthesis. Therefore, these results show that, in the presence of inducer and an essentially complete block of protein synthesis the cells still pass from an actinomycin D sensitivity to an actinomycin D in-sensitivity. If this transition represents the synthesis of an induction-specific RNA, one can conclude that the RNA species can be synthesized in the absence of translation. Also, these data suggest that the inducer is operating at a level independent of translation.

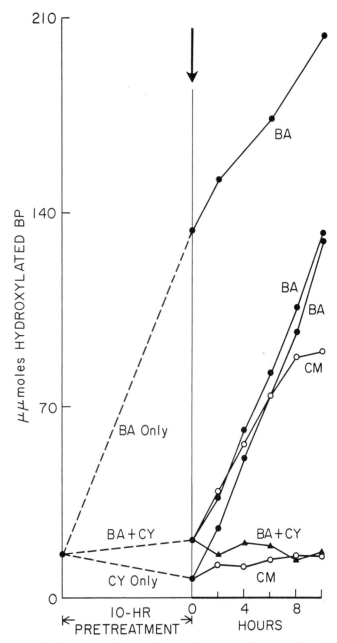

Fig. 14.11. Aryl hydrocarbon hydroxylase activity in cells exposed to 13 μM inducer (BA), or control medium (CM), following previous treatment with BA, or 3.5 μM cycloheximide (CY), or both. The heavy arrow depicts where the pretreatment medium was removed from all dishes, the surface of the cell layer was washed once with 4 ml of Dulbecco's isotonic phosphate buffer, and fresh medium containing the indicated additions was added. In those cells previously exposed to cycloheximide, protein synthesis returned to 100% of normal within the first 30-min period following removal of the inhibitor. (Nebert and Gelboin, 1970.)

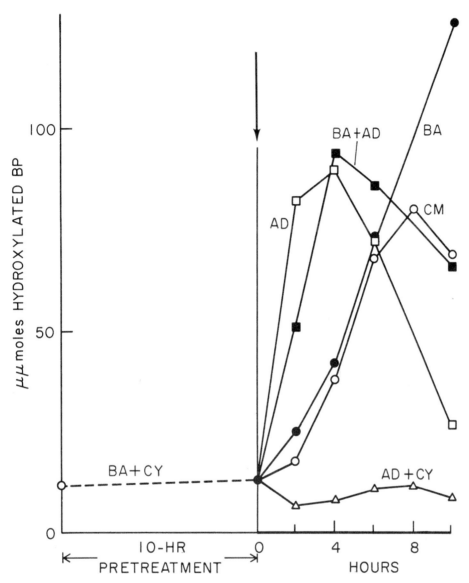

Fig. 14.12. The effects of 0.40 μM actinomycin D (AD), 13 μM inducer (BA), control medium alone (CM), and 3.5 μM cycloheximide (CY) on aryl hydrocarbon hydroxylase activity in cells previously treated with inducer plus cycloheximide. (Nebert and Gelboin, 1970.)

Results of studies in cell culture have suggested the following sequence of events in microsomal enzyme induction. Firstly, upon addition of the inducer to the culture medium, it is rapidly incorporated within several minutes into the cell. This has been found by the use of radioactive inducer and fluorescence microscopy (Miller and Gelboin, unpublished observations). After incorporation, there appears a rapid interaction between inducer and receptor site which is then followed by a period of RNA synthesis. This stage of enzyme induction involving RNA synthesis is sensitive to actinomycin-D inhibition. This early RNA synthesis phase is independent of translation, since it occurs in the presence of inhibitors of protein synthesis.

The next stage is the protein synthesis stage which is sensitive to inhibitors of protein synthesis. This stage can proceed in the absence of the RNA synthesis stage and can occur in the presence of actinomycin D. This stage seems to be the polymerization of amino acid into polypeptide chains.

The next step appears to be an assembly process of the newly-made polypeptide chains. This is independent of protein synthesis and may persist for up to two hours. This entire process results in the appearance of increased levels of aryl hydrocarbon hydroxylase. The specific protein, which is made and assembled in the microsomes, may be either the hydroxylase or another protein which may activate by an allosteric mechanism an inactive form of the hydroxylase. All of these events appear before there are gross changes in either protein or RNA synthesis. This suggests that the RNA and protein, which are required to be synthesized, are very small percentages of total cell RNA and protein and that many of the gross changes of RNA and protein synthesis may be subsequent to, and parallel, but not directly responsible for, the appearance of the early increases on enzyme level.

VI. THE EFFECT OF INDUCERS ON RNA METABOLISM

Loeb and Gelboin (1964) and Hishizawa et al. (1964) reported an increased orotic acid incorporation into RNA after MC treatment. Jervell et al. (1965) obtained the same results using liver slices. The latter determined the specific activities of acid-soluble uridine nucleotides in the preparation from MC-treated rats and found them greater than that of the control rats. They pointed out, however, that the higher specific activities of the acid-soluble uridine nucleotides from the MC-treated rats did not account for the greater increase in the specific activity of the RNA. The above investigators suggest that the increased specific activity of the RNA indicates an MC-induced increase in the rate of RNA synthesis. This conclusion must be viewed with caution, since the intracellular and intranuclear pool size of precursors of RNA, as well as the rate of degradation of RNA, may markedly affect the specific activity of the RNA. Bresnick et al. (1966) reported a failure to detect increased orotic acid incorporation after MC pretreatment. The latter did not investigate the specific activity of the RNA precursors.

An accumulation of RNA in the nuclei of MC-treated rats may be expected if MC increases the rate of nuclear RNA synthesis and does not concomitantly increase the rate of RNA degradation or the transfer of RNA out of the nucleus. Loeb and Gelboin (1963, 1964) reported that MC has no effect on the amount of DNA per gram of wet liver; also, 4 hours after MC treatment the RNA content of isolated nuclei was the same as in the controls. However, 16 hours after MC treatment they found a significant increase in the amount of nuclear RNA. In 4 experiments, there was a 15 to 50% increase in the RNA content of the isolated nuclei as shown by an increase in the RNA to DNA ratio.

Loeb and Gelboin (1964) reported that the sedimentation profile of nuclear RNA from control and MC-treated animals was grossly similar. These findings were confirmed by Bresnick et al. (1966). Normal nuclear RNA showed three peaks of RNA which corresponded to 33S, 19S, and 6S (Svedberg units). The stimulatory effect of MC on orotic acid incorporation was unequal in the various RNA fractions analyzed but was largest in the 9S to 23S region. This area corresponds roughly to some of the RNA fractions reported to have the greater amount of activity in stimulating the incorporation of amino acids into protein in a cell-free E. coli system.

Loeb and Gelboin (1964) tested the nuclear RNA obtained from normal and MC-treated rats for its activity in directing the incorporation of L-phenylalanine-(U)-C^{14} into protein in the cell-free E. coli system of Matthaei and Nirenberg (1961). In this system, isolated nuclear RNA had 5–10 times the stimulatory activity of microsomal RNA isolated by a similar procedure. Soluble RNA showed no activity. The nuclear RNA from the MC-treated rats was more active than were equivalent amounts of RNA obtained from normal rats. Thus, at each of the three levels of added RNA, the MC preparation was from 29 to 57 % more active.

Holland et al. (1966) have shown that heated ribosomal RNA as well as DNA is able to act as template in the incorporation of amino acids in an E. coli system. These results suggest the possibility that the increased template activity may not be due to a greater number of messenger RNA molecules but may be due to an MC-induced alteration in the physical state of the RNA.

Gelboin, Wortham and Wilson (1967) found that 3 hours after MC treatment and 20 hours after PB treatment there was a 30–50 % increase in RNA polymerase activity of rat liver nuclei.

Madix and Bresnick (1967) have reported a methylcholanthrene stimulation in the template activity of chromatin isolated from the liver of rats pretreated with MC for 16 hours. Thus, in both the studies with isolated nuclei and isolated chromatin, MC appears to increase template activity. The increase is not observed when isolated DNA is used as a template and there is no effect of MC on the melting temperature of DNA isolated from rat liver.

Bresnick et al. (1968) reported changes in cytoplasmic RNA after the administration of 3-methylcholanthrene. These changes were observed by 3 hours after MC was administered and involved an increased incorporation of a nucleic acid precursor to a 45S cytoplasmic particle in the liver of MC-treated rats. This effect was also observed in adrenalectomized rats. These authors also suggest that MC increased the turnover of ribosomal RNA and suggest a possible role of ribosomal RNA in the microsomal enzyme induction. It is possible that this change in ribosomal RNA synthesis is related to the increased amino acid incorporating ability in microsomes from drug-treated rats.

Thus, the various studies on the effect of MC on nuclear RNA metabolism have shown that: (1) MC causes an increase in the uptake of orotic acid into nuclear RNA which suggests increased RNA synthesis; (2) MC increases the amount of RNA in liver cell nuclei; (3) RNA isolated from the liver cell nuclei of MC-treated rats has greater stimulatory activity in an E. coli phenylalanine-incorporating system; and (4) the administration of MC in vivo stimulates RNA polymerase activity of either isolated liver nuclei or isolated chromatin. These effects of MC suggest an alteration in genetic transcription.

Table 14.1 shows a summary of the various effects of methylcholanthrene (MC) and phenobarbital (PB) on various aspects of nuclear and microsomal metabolism.

TABLE 14.1

Summary of effects of methylcholanthrene or phenobarbital on gene-action system

Microsomes	Nucleus

Increase of:
1. Specific enzymes and protein (MC, PB)
2. Amino acid incorporation (MC, PB)
   a. More mRNA (PB)
   b. More sensitive to added mRNA (PB)
3. Effects prevented by:
   a. Puromycin (MC, PB)
   b. Actinomycin-D (MC, PB)
   c. Ethionine (MC, PB)
Inhibition of:
1. NADPH cytochrome c reductase degradation (PB)
2. b_5 degradation (PB)
Changes in:
1. Spectral properties of P-450 (MC)
2. Phospholipid metabolism (MC)
3. Kinetic behavior of hydroxylase (MC)
	Increase of:
	1. Orotic acid-^{14}C incorporation into RNA (MC)
	2. RNA/DNA ratio (MC)
	3. Messenger RNA content (MC)
	4. Stimulation of RNA polymerase (MC, PB)

REFERENCES

Alfred, L. J. and Gelboin, H. V.: Benzpyrene hydroxylase induction by polycyclic hydrocarbons in hamster embryonic cells grown *in vitro*. Science *157:* 75–76, 1967.

Alvares, A. P., Schilling, G. R., and Kuntzman, R.: Differences in the kinetics of benzpyrene hydroxylation by hepatic drug-metabolizing enzymes from phenobarbital and 3-methylcholanthrene-treated rats. Biochem. Biophys. Res. Comm. *30:* 588–593, 1968.

Arcos, J. S., Conney, A. H., and Buu-Hoi, N. P.: Induction of microsomal enzyme synthesis by polycyclic aromatic hydrocarbons of different molecular sizes. J. Biol. Chem. *236:* 1291–1296, 1961.

Berlin, C. M. and Schimke, R. T.: Influence of turnover rates on the responses of enzymes to cortisone. Molec. Pharmacol. *1:* 149–156, 1965.

Bojarski, T. B. and Hiatt, H. H.: Stabilization of thymidylate kinase activity by thymidylate and by thymidine. Nature *188:* 1112–1114, 1960.

Bresnick, E., Brand, R., and Knight, J. A.: Ribonucleic acid biosynthesis in methylcholanthrene-treated rats. Biochim. Biophys. Acta *114:* 227–233, 1966.

Bresnick, E., Synerholm, M. E., and Tizard, G. T.: Changes in liver cytoplasmic RNA after administration of 3-methyl-cholanthrene. Mol. Pharmacol. *4:* 218–223, 1968.

Conney, A. H.: Enzyme induction and drug toxicity. In: Proc. 2nd Intl. Pharmacol. Mtg., Prague, Vol. *4:* pp. 277–297 (Pergamon, N.Y.) 1965.

Conney, A. H.: Pharmacological implications of microsomal enzyme induction. Pharmacol. Rev. *19:* 317–366, 1967.

Conney, A. H., Davison, C., Gastel, R. and Burns, J. J.: Adaptive increases in drug-metabolizing enzymes induced by phenobarbital and other drugs. J. Pharmacol. Exp. Ther. *130:* 1–8, 1960.

Conney, A. H., Gillette, J. R., Inscoe, J. K., Trams, E. G. and Posner, H. S.: 3,4-Benzpyrene-induced synthesis of liver microsomal enzymes which metabolize foreign compounds. Science *130:* 1478–1479, 1959.

Conney, A. H. and Gilman, A. G.: Puromycin inhibition of enzyme induction by 3-methylcholanthrene and phenobarbital. J. Biol. Chem. *238:* 3682–3685, 1963.

Conney, A. H., Miller, E. C., and Miller, J. A.: The metabolism of methylated aminoazo dyes. V. Evidence for induction of enzyme synthesis in the rat by 3-methylcholanthrene. Cancer Res. *16:* 450–459, 1956.

Conney, A. H., Miller, E. C. and Miller, J. A.: Substrate-induced synthesis and other properties of benzpyrene hydroxylase in rat liver. J. Biol. Chem. *228:* 753–766, 1957.

Cramer, J. W., Miller, J. A., and Miller, E. C.: The hydroxylation of the carcinogen 2-acetylaminofluorene by rat liver: Stimulation by pretreatment *in vivo* with 3-methylcholanthrene. J. Biol. Chem. *235:* 250–256, 1960.

Crane, R. K. and Sols, A.: The association of hexokinase with particulate fractions of brain and other tissue homogenates. J. Biol. Chem. *203:* 273–292, 1953.

Dao, T. L. and Yogo, H.: Effects of polynuclear aromatic hydrocarbons on benzpyrene hydroxylase activity in rats. Proc. Soc. Exp. Biol. Med. *116:* 1048–1050, 1964.

Decken, von der, A. and Hultin, T.: Inductive effects of 3-methylcholanthrene on enzyme activities and amino acid incorporation capacity of rat liver microsomes. Arch. Biochem. Biophys. *90:* 201–207, 1960.

Ernster, L. and Orrenius, S.: Substrate-induced synthesis of the hydroxylating enzyme system of liver microsomes. Fed. Proc. *24:* 1190–1199, 1965.

Feigelson, P. and Greengard, O.: Regulation of liver tryptophan pyrrolase activity. J. Biol. Chem. *237:* 1908–1913, 1962.

Fouts, J. R. and Rogers, L. A.: Morphological changes in the liver accompanying stimulation of microsomal drug metabolizing enzyme activity by phenobarbital, chlordane, benzpyrene or methylcholanthrene in rats. J. Pharmacol. Exp. Ther. *147:* 112–119, 1965.

Gan, J. C. and Jeffay, H.: Origins and metabolism of the intracellular amino acid pools in rat liver and muscle. Biochim. Biophys. Acta *148:* 448–459, 1967.

Gelboin, H. V.: Studies on the mechanism of methylcholanthrene induction of enzyme activities. II. Stimulation of microsomal and ribosomal amino acid incorporation: The effects of polyuridylic acid and actinomycin D. Biochim. Biophys. Acta *91:* 130–144, 1964.

Gelboin, H. V.: Carcinogens, enzyme induction and gene action. Adv. in Cancer Res. *10:* 1–81, 1967.

Gelboin, H. V.: Effect of carcinogens on gene action. Monograph of 22nd Annual Symp. on Fundamental Cancer Research, Univ. of Texas, M. D. Anderson Hosp., Houston, Texas, March, 1968.

Gelboin, H. V. and Blackburn, N.: Stimulatory effect of 3-methylcholanthrene on microsomal amino acid incorporation and benzpyrene hydroxylase activity and its inhibition of actinomycin D. Biochim. Biophys. Acta *72:* 657–660, 1963.

Gelboin, H. V. and Sokoloff, L.: The effects of 3-methylcholanthrene and phenobarbital on amino acid incorporation into protein. Science *134:* 611–612, 1961.

Gelboin, H. V. and Sokoloff, L.: Studies on the mechanism of methylcholanthrene induction of enzyme activities of rat liver. Biochim. Biophys. Acta *91:* 122–129, 1964.

Gelboin, H. V., Wortham, J. J., and Wilson, R. G.: 3-Methylcholanthrene and pheno-

barbital stimulation of rat liver RNA polymerase. Nature (London) *214:* 281–283, 1967.

Gerhardt, J. C. and Pardee, A. B.: The enzymology of control by feedback inhibition. J. Biol. Chem. *237:* 891–896, 1962.

Gillette, J. R.: Metabolism of drugs and other foreign compounds by enzymatic mechanisms. Prog. Drug Res. *6:* 11–73, 1963.

Granick, S.: Induction of the synthesis of δ-aminolevulinic acid synthetase in liver parenchyma cells in culture by chemicals that induce acute porphyria. J. Biol. Chem. *238:* PC2247–2249, 1963.

Granick, S.: The induction *in vitro* of the synthesis of δ-aminolevulinic acid synthetase in chemical porphyria: A response to certain drugs, sex hormones, and foreign chemicals. J. Biol. Chem. *241:* 1359–1375, 1966.

Granick, S. and Urata, G.: Increase in activity of δ-amino-levulinic acid synthetase in liver mitochondria induced by feeding of 3,5-dicarbethoxy-1,4-dihydrocollidine. J. Biol. Chem. *238:* 821–827, 1963.

Gurtoo, H. L., Campbell, T. C., Webb, R. E., and Plowman, K. M.: Effect of aflatoxin and benzpyrene pretreatment upon the kinetics of benzpyrene hydroxylase. Biochem. Biophys. Res. Comm. *31:* 588–595, 1968.

Henderson, J. F. and Mazel, P.: Studies of the induction of microsomal S-, N- and O-demethylases. Biochem. Pharmacol. *13:* 1471–1474, 1964.

Hildebrandt, A., Remmer, H., and Estabrook, R. W.: Cytochrome P-450 of liver microsomes—one pigment or many. Biochem. Biophys. Res. Comm. *30:* 607–612, 1968.

Hishizawa, T., Otsuka, H., and Terayama, H.: Metabolic behavior of nucleic acids in subcellular fractions from liver of rats treated with methylcholanthrene. J. Biochem. (Tokyo) *56:* 97–100, 1964.

Holland, J. J., Clayton, A. B., and McCarthy, B. J.: Stimulation of protein synthesis *in vitro* by partially degraded ribosomal ribonucleic acid and transfer ribonucleic acid. Biochem. *5:* 358–365, 1966.

Holtzman, J. L. and Gillette, J. R.: The effect of phenobarbital on the turnover of microsomal phospholipid in male and female rats. J. Biol. Chem. *243:* 3020–3028, 1968.

Howard, R. B., Christiansen, A. K., Gibbs, F. A., and Pesch, L.: The enzymatic preparation of isolated intact parenchymal cells from rat liver. J. Cell Biol. *35:* 675–684, 1967.

Inscoe, J. K. and Axelrod, J.: Some factors

affecting glucuronide formation *in vitro*. J. Pharmacol. Exp. Ther. *129:* 128–131, 1960.

Jervell, K. F., Christoffersen, T., and Morland, J.: Studies on the 3-methylcholanthrene induction and carbohydrate repression of rat liver dimethylaminoazobenzene reductase. Arch. Biochem. *111:* 15–22, 1965.

Jick, H. and Shuster, L.: The turnover of microsomal reduced nicotinamide adenine dinucleotide phosphate-cytochrome *c* reductase in the livers of mice treated with phenobarbital. J. Biol. Chem. *241:* 5366–5369, 1966.

Juchau, M. R., Cram, R. L., Plaa, G. L., and Fouts, J. R.: The induction of benzypyrene hydroxylase in the isolated perfused rat liver. Biochem. Pharmacol. *14:* 473–482, 1965.

Kato, R., Jondorf, W. R., Loeb, L. A., Ben, T., and Gelboin, H. V.: Studies on the mechanism of drug induced microsomal enzyme activities. V. Phenobarbital stimulation of endogenous messenger RNA and polyuridylic acid-directed L-[^{14}C]-phenylalanine incorporation. Mol. Pharmacol. *2:* 171–186, 1966.

Kato, R., Loeb, L. and Gelboin, H. V.: Microsome-specific stimulation by phenobarbital of amino acid incorporation *in vivo*. Biochem. Pharmacol. *14:* 1164–1166, 1965.

Korner, A. and Munro, A.: Actinomycin inhibition of *in vitro* protein synthesis in rat liver. J. Biochem. Biophys. Res. Comm. *11:* 235–238, 1963.

Kuntzman, R., Levin, W., Jacobson, M. and Conney, A. H.: Studies on microsomal hydroxylation and the demonstration of a new carbon monoxide binding pigment in liver microsomes. Life Sciences *7:* 215–224, 1968.

Kuriyama, Y., Omura, T., Siekevitz, P. and Palade, G. E.: Effect of phenobarbital on the synthesis and degradation of the protein components of rat liver microsomal membranes. J. Biol. Chem. *244:* 2017–2026, 1969.

Levin, W. and Kuntzman, R.: Studies on the incorporation of δ-aminolevulinic acid into microsomal hemoprotein: effect of 3-methylcholanthrene and phenobarbital. Life Sciences *8:* 305–311, 1969.

Loeb, L. A. and Gelboin, H. V.: Stimulation of amino-acid incorporation by nuclear ribonucleic acid from normal and methylcholanthrene-treated rats. Nature (London) *199:* 809–810, 1963.

Loeb, L. A. and Gelboin, H. V.: Methylcholanthrene-induced changes in rat liver nuclear RNA. Proc. Natl. Acad. Sci. U.S.A. *52:* 1219–1226, 1964.

Loftfield, R. B. and Harris, A. H.: Partici-

pation of free amino acids in protein synthesis. J. Biol. Chem. *219:* 151–159, 1956.

Madix, J. C. and Bresnick, E.: Increased efficacy of liver chromatin as a template for RNA synthesis after administration of 3-methylcholanthrene. Biochem. Biophys. Res. Comm. *28:* 445–452, 1967.

Marver, H. S.: The role of heme in the synthesis and repression of microsomal protein. Proc. Mtg. of Intl. Symposium on Microsomes and Drug Oxidation, Bethesda, Md., Feb., 1968.

Marver, H. S., Collins, A., Tschudy, D. P., and Rechcigl, M., Jr.: δ-Aminolevulinic acid synthetase. J. Biol. Chem. *241:* 4323–4329, 1966.

Matthaei, J. H. and Nirenberg, M. W.: Characteristics and stabilization of DNAase-sensitive protein synthesis in *E. coli* extracts. Proc. Natl. Acad. Sci. U.S.A. *47:* 1580–1588, 1961.

McAuslan, B. R.: The induction and repression of thymidine kinase in the poxvirus-infected HeLa cell. Virology *21:* 383–389, 1963.

Merits, I.: Actinomycin inhibition of RNA synthesis in rat liver. Biochem. Biophys. Res. Comm. *10:* 254–259, 1963.

Miller, J. and Gelboin, H. V.: Unpublished observations.

Monod, J. and Jacob, F.: Teleonomic mechanism in cellular metabolism, growth and differentiation. Cold Spring Harbor Symp. *28:* 389–401, 1961.

Nachmanson, D. and Wilson, I. B.: Studies on cholinesterase I. On the specificity of the enzyme in nerve tissue. J. Biol. Chem. *158:* 653–666, 1945.

Nebert, D. W. and Gelboin, H. V.: Substrate-inducible aryl hydroxylase in mammalian cell culture: I. Assay and properties of induced enzyme. J. Biol. Chem. *243:* 6242–6249, 1968a.

Nebert, D. W. and Gelboin, H. V.: Substrate-inducible microsomal aryl hydroxylase in mammalian cell culture. II. Cellular responses during enzyme induction. J. Biol. Chem. *243:* 6250–6261, 1968b.

Nebert, D. W. and Gelboin, H. V.: The role of RNA and protein synthesis in microsomal aryl hydrocarbon hydroxylase induction in cell culture: the independence of transcription and translation. J. Biol. Chem. *245:* 160–168, 1970.

Neurath, H. and Dixon, G. H.: Structure and activation of trypsinogen and chymotrypsinogen. Fed. Proc. *16:* 791–801, 1957.

Omura, T., Siekevitz, P., and Palade, G. E.: Turnover of constituents of the endoplasmic reticulum membranes of rat hepatocytes. J. Biol. Chem. *242:* 2389–2396, 1967.

Orrenius, S., Ericsson, J. L. E., and Ernster, L.: Phenobarbital-induced synthesis of the microsomal drug-metabolizing enzyme system and its relationship to the proliferation of endoplasmic membranes. A morphological and biochemical study. J. Cell Biol. 25: 627–639, 1965.

Orrenius, S. and Ericsson, J. L. E.: Enzyme-membrane relationship in phenobarbital induction of synthesis of drug-metabolizing enzyme system and proliferation of endoplasmic membranes. J. Cell Biol. 28: 181–198, 1966.

Peterkofsky, B. and Tomkins, G. M.: Effect of inhibitors of nucleic acid synthesis on steroid-mediated induction of tyrosine aminotransferase in hepatoma cell cultures. J. Mol. Biol. 30: 49–61, 1967.

Rall, T. W. and Sutherland, E. W.: The regulatory role of adenosine-3',5'-phosphate. Cold Spring Harbor Symp. Quant. Biol. 26: 347–354, 1961.

Reich, E., Franklin, R. M., Shaktin, A. J., and Tatum, E. L.: Effect of actinomycin D on cellular nucleic acid synthesis and virus production. Science 134: 556–557, 1961.

Remmer, H. and Merker, H. J.: Drug-induced changes in the liver endoplasmic reticulum: Association with drug-metabolizing enzymes. Science 142: 1657–1658, 1963.

Schenkman, J. B. and Sato, R.: The relationship between the pH-induced spectral change in ferriprotoheme and the substrate-induced spectral change of the microsomal mixed-function oxidase. Mol. Pharmacol. 4: 613–620, 1968.

Schenkman, J. B., Grain, H., Zange, M., and Remmer, H.: On the problem of possible other forms of cytochrome P-450 in liver microsomes. Biochim. Biophys. Acta 171: 23–31, 1969.

Schimke, R. T.: The importance of both synthesis and degradation in the control of arginase levels in rat liver. J. Biol. Chem. 239: 3808–3817, 1964.

Schimke, R. T., Ganschow, R., Doyle, D., and Arias, I. M.: Regulation of protein turnover in mammalian tissues. Fed. Proc. 27: 1223–1230, 1968.

Schimke, R. T., Sweeney, E. W. and Berlin, C. M.: An analysis of the kinetics of rat liver tryptophan pyrrolase induction: The significance of both enzyme synthesis and degradation. Biochim. Biophys. Res. Comm. 15: 214–219, 1964.

Siefert, von J., Greim, H., and Chandra, P.: Die wirkung von phenobarbital auf die ribosomenfraktionen der rattenleber. Hoppe-Seyler's Z. Physiol. Chem. 349: 1179–1184, 1968.

Sladek, N. E. and Mannering, G. J.: In-duction of drug metabolism. I. Differences in the mechanisms by which polycyclic hydrocarbons and phenobarbital produce their inductive effects on microsomal N-demethylating systems. Mol. Pharmacol. 5: 174–185, 1969a.

Sladek, N. E. and Mannering, G. J.: Induction of drug metabolism II. Qualitative differences in the microsomal N-demethylating systems stimulated by polycyclic hydrocarbons and by phenobarbital. Mol. Pharmacol. 5: 186–199, 1969b.

Stephen, J. M. L. and Waterlow, J. C.: Use of carbon-14-labelled arginine to measure the catabolic rate of serum and liver proteins and the extent of amino-acid recycling. Nature 211: 978–980, 1966.

Swick, R. W.: Measurement of protein turnover in rat liver. J. Biol. Chem. 231: 751–764, 1958.

Swick, R. W. and Hande, D. T.: The distribution of fixed carbon in amino acids. J. Biol. Chem. 218: 577–585, 1956.

Tamaoki, T. and Mueller, G. C.: Synthesis of nuclear and cytoplasmic RNA of HeLa cells and the effect of actinomycin D. Biochem. Biophys. Res. Comm. 9: 451–454, 1962.

Tatibana, M. and Cohen, P. P.: Formation and conversion of macromolecular precursor(s) in the biosynthesis of carbamyl phosphate synthetase. Proc. Natl. Acad. Sci. U.S.A. 53: 104–111, 1965.

Thompson, E. B., Tomkins, G. M., and Curran, J. F.: Induction of tyrosine α-ketoglutarate transaminase by steroid hormones in a newly established tissue culture cell line. Proc. Natl. Acad. Sci. U.S.A. 56: 296–303, 1966.

Tomkins, G. M., Garren, L. D., Howell, R. R., and Peterkofsky, B.: The regulation of enzyme synthesis by steroid hormones: The role of translation. J. Cell Comp. Physiol. 66: 137–151, 1965.

Tschudy, D. P., Perlroth, M. G., Marver, H. S., Collins, A. and Hunter, G., Jr.: Acute intermittent porphyria: The first "overproduction disease" localized to a specific enzyme. Proc. Natl. Acad. Sci. U.S.A. 53: 841–847, 1965.

Villa-Trevino, S., Shull, K. H. and Farber, E.: The role of adenosine triphosphate deficiency in ethionine-induced inhibition of protein synthesis. J. Biol. Chem. 238: 1757–1763, 1963.

Wosilait, W. D., and Sutherland, E. W.: The relationship of epinephrine and glucagon to liver phosphorylase. J. Biol. Chem. 218: 469–481, 1956.

Yarmolinsky, M. B. and de la Haba, G. L.: Inhibition by puromycin of amino acid incorporation into protein. Proc. Natl. Acad. Sci. U.S.A. 45: 1721–1729, 1959.

15

Genetic Factors Modifying Drug Metabolism and Drug Response

BERT N. LA DU

I. INTRODUCTION

Man's ability to dispose of drugs given for therapeutic purposes and his capacity to detoxify foreign chemicals in his food and environment depend upon the unusual properties of special detoxication enzyme systems present in his liver and other organs. These protective systems have become better understood in recent years, particularly those localized in the liver microsomes which catalyze so many types of drug transformations.

In the course of the investigations on drug metabolism and drug disposition in man, it has been noted that there are often rather striking individual differences in the response to drugs and in the ability to metabolize and dispose of drugs. Some of the person-to-person differences are due to environmental factors (Conney, 1967), but some have clearly demonstrated to be genetically determined. The scientific study of genetic factors which account for individual differences in drug metabolism and in drug response is called *pharmacogenetics*. It is a relatively new area of pharmacological investigation, and it requires the application of biochemical, physiological, pathological and immunological techniques as well as genetic and pharmacological methodology. Pharmacogenetic studies will provide new information about the genetic determinants of drug action and drug metabolism, and the results will find many practical applications in therapeutics and clinical toxicology.

In the following sections a selected number of pharmacogenetic examples will be described to illustrate the diversity of conditions that have been discovered. In essentially every example the application of drug metabolism methods in the evaluation of genetic factors will be apparent. In most of them, it will be obvious that further studies are needed by investigators with experience in drug metabolism methodology and in biochemical pharmacology to make further advances; and, in some instances, identify more precisely the nature of the inherited defect.

II. DETECTION OF PHARMACOGENETIC CONDITIONS

It is important to review briefly how new pharmacogenetic conditions are discovered and what steps are taken to investigate unusual drug effects that may be caused by genetic mutations. An observation that a patient has an unexpected drug response, or appears to metabolize a drug in an unusual way, has been the way most pharmacogenetic studies were initiated. Since drugs are rarely excreted entirely in an unchanged form, and most drugs either undergo structural modifications by metabolic transformation (as oxidations, reductions, hydrolysis) or by conjugation reactions, it is to be expected that the enzymes catalyzing these reactions will be different in some individuals due to genetic mutations. Quantitative and qualitative differences in the enzymes can affect drug metabolism in many ways; the clinician may observe that a drug is unusually potent in a particular patient, or a drug may produce signs of overdosage toxicity when given in the usual way. Either of these findings could result from a limited capacity of the patient to dispose of the drug because of an inherited deficiency of one of the drug metabolism enzymes.

If the pharmacological effects of the drug and adverse symptoms (overdose toxicity) are known to be well correlated with particular plasma concentrations of the drug, it should be relatively easy to determine whether the patient really has an increased sensitivity to the agent and reacts to low concentrations the way most people do at higher blood levels. He is more likely to show a normal response at the appropriate tissue concentrations but develop higher levels than expected due to faulty metabolism.

Of course, a genetic mutation could also increase the quantity of a drug enzyme, or change the structure of the enzyme in such a way that it would be a more efficient catalyst than normal. These patients would appear to be resistant to the drug and require larger doses than normal to achieve therapeutically effective blood and tissue concentrations.

Inherited differences in proteins of drug receptors could account for individual differences in drug sensitivity or drug resistance, but such alterations are much less likely to account for unusual drug effects than genetic mutations that modify the enzymes concerned with drug metabolism.

Careful, detailed studies of the affected patients and their close relatives should establish the basis for the abnormal drug reaction and whether the condition is present in other family members. This approach is very much like that used to study a new "inborn error of metabolism." In many ways, the inherited pharmacogenetic conditions are analogous to hereditary metabolic disorders except that the substrate is a drug rather than a nutritional metabolite.

Another way new pharmacogenetic conditions can be detected is to conduct a survey in a sample population and look for either a distinct subpopulation or for individuals with an unusual response. The test to be carried out with each subject could theoretically be a complicated study of drug metabolism *in vivo*, or it might be a simple assay *in vitro* on a blood or urine sample. There are many practical reasons why population surveys have not been favored as a means to find new pharmacogenetic markers; the expense, ethical considerations, the special screening methodology and work force required, all are serious limitations. The method to be used for typing or classifying each subject is of particular importance. The sample population study by Evans *et al.* (1960) (discussed in Section IIB, below) is useful as a reference. These workers carefully determined the best time to make a single determination of the blood isoniazid concentration after an oral dose of the drug and obtain a reasonable index of the rate of isoniazid metabolism. The resulting data (isoniazid levels 6 hours after drug administration) clearly established bimodality even though only about 250 people were tested. The isoniazid polymorphism is unusual in that about half of the population is slow (and half fast) in acetylating isoniazid. The sample population thus included adequate numbers of individuals from both subpopulations, but if the slow acetylator phenotype represented only a few percent of the population, this group might have been more difficult to identify. The test conditions they developed were well designed to obtain the information needed, and the dose and timing of the blood sample were selected to be optimal for this purpose. It is interesting to note that if they had measured the isoniazid concentration in the blood at 2 hours rather than at 6 hours, they would have found a continuous, unimodal curve (Knight *et al.*, 1959).

If a population survey shows a bimodal or multimodal distribution, the subpopulations may be distinct because of genetic differences, and various genetic hypotheses can be proposed and tested by family studies and pedigree analyses. A continuous, unimodal distribution curve, however, does not necessarily mean that the variation in response is due to environmental factors; genetic factors, particularly if several genes are involved, may give effects in combination which result in a curve that appears to be a normal (Gaussian) distribution.

Population surveys and studies of individual cases (and their families) are used in pharmacogenetics in order to reach ultimately the same objectives. These aims are: to evaluate the contribution of hereditary factors; to determine the mode of inheritance (dominant or recessive; sex-linked or autosomal-linked) in order to understand the biochemical basis of the variation; to establish the frequency of the unusual genes in the population as well as the number of allelic genes involved; and to evaluate the clinical importance of the pharmacogenetic variation. Most of the pharmacogenetic conditions studied to date are characterized by rather striking drug effects, differing from the normal response in very obvious ways. These include the hemolysis of red blood cells, methemoglobinemia, or prolonged muscular paralysis. It can be expected that many more pharmacogenetic differences exist in man which produce less pronounced effects, but are, nevertheless, important in determining the wide individual variation in therapeutic effectiveness and toxicity thresholds in the population. Future investigations in pharmacogenetics will demonstrate the importance of these more common, but less dramatic, variations.

It should be noted that carefully conducted studies with a small series of identical and fraternal twins make it possible to determine whether an observed variation in drug response can be attributed primarily to genetic or environmental factors. In 1957, twin studies by Bönicke and Lisboa (1957) indicated that genetic factors largely accounted for the wide individual differences in the rate of acetylation of isoniazid. More recently, Vesell and Page (1968a–c) have shown that genetic factors are primarily responsible for the wide variation in the rate of metabolism of antipyrine, dicumarol and phenybutazone (as measured by the rate of decline of the drug concentrations in plasma) (Table 15.1). Studies on twins by Alexanderson *et al.* (1969) indicate that most of the variability of nortriptyline metabolism is genetically determined. Statistical analysis of the variation within pairs of identical twins compared with the variation within pairs of fraternal twins gives an index of the relative contribution of genetic versus environmental factors (Osborne and DeGeorge, 1959). Obviously, such data do not indicate how many genes are involved nor how they are transmitted

TABLE 15.1

Plasma half-lives of dicumarol, antipyrine and phenylbutazone in identical and fraternal twins[a]

			Identical twins						Fraternal twins		
Twin	Age	Sex	Dicumarol Hours	Antipyrine Hours	Phenyl-butazone Days	Twin	Age	Sex	Dicumarol Hours	n tipy rine Hours	Phenyl-butazone Days
HeM	48	M	25.0	11.3	1.9	AM	21	F	45.0	15.1	7.3
HoM	48	M	25.0	11.3	2.1	SM	21	M	22.0	6.3	3.6
DT	43	F	55.5	10.3	2.8	DL	36	F	46.5	7.2	2.3
UW	43	F	55.5	9.6	2.9	DS	36	F	51.0	15.0	3.3
JG	22	M	36.0	11.5	2.8	SA	33	F	34.5	5.1	2.1
PG	22	M	34.0	11.5	2.8	FM	33	F	27.5	12.5	1.2
JaT	44	M	74.0	14.9	4.0	JaH	24	F	7.0	12.0	2.6
JaT	44	M	72.0	14.9	4.0	JeH	24	F	19.0	6.0	2.3
CJ	55	F	41.0	6.9	3.2	FD	48	M	24.5	14.7	2.8
FJ	55	F	42.5	7.1	2.9	PD	48	M	38.0	9.3	3.5
GeL	45	M	72.0	12.3	3.9	LD	21	F	67.0	8.2	2.9
GuL	45	M	69.0	12.8	4.1	LW	21	F	72.0	6.9	3.0
DH	26	F	46.0	11.0	2.6	EK	31	F	40.5	7.7	1.9
DW	26	F	44.0	11.0	2.6	RK	31	M	35.0	7.3	2.1

[a] From Vesell and Page (1968a-c).

and expressed. They do furnish evidence that the observed individual variation in drug metabolism is due to the particular genetic constitution of each individual.

III. INHERITED VARIATIONS IN DRUG METABOLISM ENZYMES

A. Serum Cholinesterase Variants and Succinylcholine Sensitivity

After succinylcholine was introduced as a muscle relaxant agent and was placed in general use, it was noted that an occasional patient reacted abnormally to the drug. These patients were given the usual dose of succinylcholine but they remained paralyzed for a much longer time than expected and had to be given artificial respiration for hours because of the prolonged paralysis of the respiratory muscles.

Succinylcholine contains two ester groups (two molecules of choline are combined in ester linkage *via* the two acidic groups of succinic acid) and hydrolysis of one ester linkage gives the products, choline and succinylmonocholine, an inactive metabolite. Succinylcholine hydrolysis is catalyzed by serum cholinesterase (pseudocholinesterase) and it was, at first, suspected that the patients showing the unusual sensitivity to the drug must be deficient in their serum esterase. Tests were made on their serum for cholinesterase activity, but these showed the activity to be normal or only moderately reduced. Careful studies were then undertaken by Kalow and his associates in the late 1950's to investigate the properties of the serum cholinesterase of succinylcholine-sensitive patients.

Qualitative differences were found in the "atypical" cholinesterase of succinylcholine-sensitive individuals (Kalow and Davies, 1958; Kalow, 1960). The atypical esterase had a lower affinity for choline-ester substrates and it was a less efficient catalyst in hydrolyzing succinylcholine at low concentrations of the drug substrate, as would occur in the serum of patients receiving the drug. The

TABLE 15.2

Hereditary variants of serum cholinesterase in man and succinylcholine sensitivity[a]

Type of Esterase	Esterase Characteristics				Homozygote Characteristics		
	Relative Activity (%)	Dibucaine No.	Fluoride No.	Remarks	Genotype	Frequency	Response to Succinylcholine
Normal (usual)	100	80	60	Normal	$E_1^u E_1^u$	96:100	Normal
Atypical (dibucaine resistant)	50	20	20	Decreased affinity for cholinesters and inhibitors such as dibucaine	$E_1^a E_1^a$	1:2500	Prolonged
Fluoride resistant	55	65	30	Decreased affinity for cholinesters and fluoride	$E_1^f E_1^f$	Very rare	Prolonged
Silent	0–5	—	—	Very low or no detectable activity	$E_1^s E_1^s$	1:100,000	Prolonged
C_5^+	130	—	—	30% more activity than C_5^-	E_2^+	(10:100 are of the E_2^+ phenotype)	Significance uncertain; may increase hydrolysis
Cynthiana	200–300	80	60	2–3 times more activity than $E_1^u E_1^u$	unknown	Very rare	Shortened

[a] After Kalow (1965); supplemented by information on Cynthiana variant after Neitlich (1966) and Yoshida and Motulsky (1969); and on Silent by Altland and Goedde (1970).

atypical esterase was also less susceptible to dibucaine inhibition and other esterase inhibitors than normal serum cholinesterase. A spectrophotometric test was developed by Kalow and Genest (1957) which included dibucaine as an inhibitor and benzoylcholine was the substrate. This test made it possible to identify the type of esterase present in test sera. The dibucaine concentration selected $(1 \times 10^{-5}$ M) produced about 80% inhibition of normal esterase (dibucaine number = 80) and 20% inhibition of the atypical esterase (dibucaine number = 20). The dibucaine inhibition test could also be used to detect heterozygous carriers of the trait; their serum cholinesterase was inhibited by about 60% (dibucaine number = 60). Heterozygous carriers have a mixture in approximately equal concentrations of normal and atypical cholinesterases in their blood. Family studies and serum analyses provided convincing evidence that the individuals with atypical esterase had inherited a rare gene from both parents, and their unusual sensitivity to succinylcholine was due to the abnormal type of esterase in their blood. Kalow and Gunn (1959) found that about 3.8% of the Canadian population were heterozygous carriers of the atypical esterase gene and 1:2820 was homozygous for the atypicl esterase gene.

Several other variant forms of serum cholinesterase have been discovered more recently that also affect the response to succinylcholine (Table 15.2). However, the atypical (dibucaine resistant) type continues to be the variant form found most frequently in patients who have shown prolonged responses to succinylcholine. The fluoride resistant variant resembles the dibucaine resistant type since it also has a lower affinity for choline-esters. It is detected by taking advantage of its lower affinity for fluoride than normal esterase. The fluoride resistant variant is less inhibited than normal esterase by fluoride, and a standard assay has been developed (Harris and Whittaker, 1961) which gives "fluoride numbers." The combination of dibucaine inhibition and fluoride inhibition tests makes it possible to distinguish several distinct cholinesterase phenotypes (Table 15.2).

Another esterase variant of interest is determined by the "silent" gene. Individuals homozygous for this gene have essentially no detectable serum cholinesterase activity (Kattamis, et al., 1967; Altland and Goedde, 1970). Although they lack serum esterase, they show no unusual signs or symptoms and apparently have no disturbance in intermediary metabolism. Their enzymatic deficiency is expressed only by an exaggerated response to succinylcholine if they should receive the drug.

A very rare but unusual type of serum cholinesterase is called the Cynthiana variant (Neitlich, 1966; Yoshida and Motulsky, 1969). Affected individuals have nearly three times as much serum cholinesterase activity as normal, and they hydrolyze succinylcholine very rapidly. The drug is destroyed so quickly that these individuals are *resistant*, rather than sensitive, to the drug. The nature of the genetic mutation is not known; it appears that more enzyme (with normal characteristics) is synthesized, rather than an enzyme variant that is an unusually efficient catalyst, with a higher than normal turnover number (Yoshida and Motulsky, 1969).

One genetic locus, E_1, determines the type of serum cholinesterase each person inherits, and the four allelic genes at that locus (*normal* or *usual*, *dibucaine resistant*, *fluoride resistant* and *silent*) permit many genotypic combinations.

Practically, it can be said that succinylcholine sensitivity is to be expected only in those individuals with no normal esterase; heterozygous people have one-half the usual concentration of normal enzyme, and this is sufficient to protect them adequately.

Another locus, E_2, affects the characteristics of the serum cholinesterase but it is less important than E_1. E_2 determines whether serum contains an extra esterase component, C_5 which can be identified by starch gel and paper electrophoresis (Harris et al., 1962). About 10% of the people are C_5^+ and they have about 25% more serum cholinesterase activity than C_5^- people.

The level of serum cholinesterase activity in the general population with the normal (or usual) type of enzyme varies considerably from person to person, and the rate of succinylcholine hydrolysis in this group shows wide individual variations for this reason. The rare variant forms of the esterase extend the limits at both ends of the scale; little or no significant activity in people homozygous for the silent allele, and unusually high activity in individuals with the Cynthiana variant. The significance of the wide spectrum of serum cholinesterase activity has been demonstrated by its importance in succinylcholine hydrolysis. In fact, this has been the main stimulus to study the genetic variations and the frequency of the variant forms of the enzyme in the population. Less is known about the significance of the esterase in the hydrolysis of the other drugs containing ester groups. The local anesthetic, procaine, and a number of structural analogues of procaine are also hydrolyzed by serum cholinesterase (Kalow, 1952). It has been suggested that a major portion of the procaine absorbed is hydrolyzed in the blood by this esterase (Brodie et al., 1948). Aspirin is also hydrolyzed in human serum by cholinesterase in vitro, but it has not been established whether aspirin is hydrolyzed mainly in the blood, or in the tissues. There is no evidence that a deficiency of serum cholinesterase would affect the distribution or metabolism of the drug.

B. Slow and Rapid Acetylation of Isoniazid

The main route of metabolism of isoniazid (INH) in man is its conjugation with acetyl coenzyme A to form acetyl-INH. The reaction is catalyzed by an N-acetyltransferase in the liver. The acetylated drug can be excreted by the kidney more efficiently than INH, and the biological half-life of the drug in the body depends upon how rapidly the drug can be acetylated.

Soon after isoniazid was introduced as an antitubercular agent in the 1950's, it was noticed that individuals differed widely in their rates of INH metabolism, whether measured by the rate of disappearance of the drug from the plasma or by the ratio of free drug to acetylated drug excreted in the urine.

Evans et al. (1960) measured the concentration of INH in the blood of 267 individuals 6 hours after they received a standard dose (9.8 mg/Kg) and plotted the data as a frequency distribution histogram (Fig. 15.1). There was bimodality, with a mean for one subpopulation at approximately 1 μg/ml, and a mean for the other subpopulation between 4 and 5 μg/ml. The subpopulations were designated "rapid inactivators" and "slow inactivators," and they were assumed to represent 2 distinct phenotypes. Several family pedigrees were analyzed according to this classification and a reasonable genetic hypothesis was developed. It was assumed that the rate of INH acetylation was determined by 2 autosomal

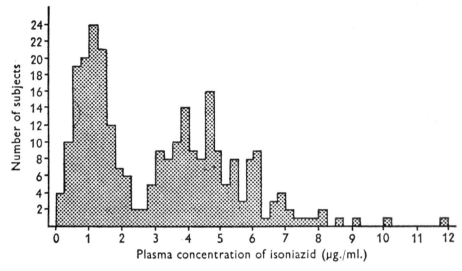

Fig. 15.1. Plasma concentrations of isoniazid 6 hours after oral administration of the drug to 267 members of 53 families (from Evans *et al.*, 1960).

genes at one locus, and that slow acetylators were homozygous for the recessive allele (rr), and rapid acetylators were either RR or Rr. Evans *et al.* (1960) calculated the gene frequencies from their sample population using the incidence of the slow inactivators (52.2%) as a measure of r^2; the resulting gene frequencies were $R = 0.277$, and $r = 0.723$. Further tests of the genetic hypothesis were then made by predicting the number of children of each phenotype (rapid or slow) that would be expected from parental matings representing the three possible phenotypic combinations (*rapid* × *rapid, rapid* × *slow*, and *slow* × *slow*) (Table 15.3). The numbers of children of each phenotype found agreed very closely with the expected numbers, and the genetic hypothesis was supported by these results.

The recessive gene is present in an unusually high frequency (0.723), and over

TABLE 15.3

Rapid and slow inactivators of isoniazid in children from parents of each phenotypic combination[a]

Phenotypic Matings	No. of Matings	No. of Children	Number of Children of Each Phenotype			
			Rapid		Slow	
			Expected	Observed	Expected	Observed
S × S	16	51	0	0	51	51
R × S	24	70	40.62	42	29.36	28
R × R	13	38	31.30	31	6.68	7
	53	159		73		86

[a] From Evans *et al.*, 1960, modified by Kalow, 1962. The hypothesis is made that slow-inactivator persons are homozygous for a recessive allele.

[b] S, Slow inactivator; R, rapid inactivator.

half of the people are slow acetylators of INH. There is no obvious advantage in being a slow acetylator, and no selective advantage has been suggested which might explain the gene frequencies observed. The acetylation polymorphism does not seem to influence the outcome of tuberculosis treatment, nor the development of isoniazid-resistant tubercle bacilli (Evans, 1968).

Slow inactivators of isoniazid have less N-acetyltransferase in their liver than rapid inactivators, but the characteristics of the enzymes isolated and purified from human liver of both phenotypes seem to be identical (Jenne, 1965; Weber, 1971). The quantitative difference suggests that slow acetylators synthesize the enzyme more slowly or it is destroyed more rapidly. Careful studies are in progress to look for qualitative differences in the "rapid" and "slow" enzyme, since structural differences might cause the slow enzyme to be more unstable.

One might presume that the enzyme has a natural substrate, and expect that it would be metabolized at different rates in slow and rapid acetylators. This would be a clue to the importance of the rapid or slow phenotypes. However, no natural substrate (or substrates) of the liver N-acetyltransferase has been identified.

Human liver N-acetyltransferase catalyzes the acetylation of a number of drugs in addition to isoniazid. Some of these are listed in Table 15.4. The list is not complete; other drugs that are acetylated in the body may properly belong in the table. Whether or not they should be included is difficult to decide because other drug N-acetyltransferases exist. Unless the drug shows a polymorphism in its acetylation rate like INH does, it is uncertain that the drug is a substrate for the isoniazid N-acetyltransferase. Sulfamethazine acetylation meets this very well; in fact, this sulfonamide can be used like isoniazid to type people as rapid or slow acetylators (Evans and White, 1964; Evans, 1969).

As might be expected, slow acetylators of isoniazid are more likely to develop

TABLE 15.4

Some drugs inactivated by acetylation in man

Group I. Drugs believed to be acetylated by INH N-acetyltransferase

Isoniazid (INH)
Sulfamethazine
Hydralazine (Apresoline)
Diaminodiphenylsulfone (Dapsone)
Phenelzine (Nardil)[a]

Group II. Drugs acetylated, but importance of INH N-acetyltransferase polymorphism uncertain

Sulfamethoxypyridazine
Sulfisoxazole (Gantrisin)
Sulfadiazine

Group III. Drugs believed to be acetylated mainly by systems other than the INH N-acetyltransferase system

p-Aminosalicylic Acid
p-Aminobenzoic Acid
Sulfanilamide

[a] Evidence, still incomplete, suggests that phenelzine is acetylated by this system (Evans *et al.*, 1965).

a cumulative toxicity to the drug. The principle toxicity to isoniazid is a peripheral neuritis (Hughes *et al.*, 1954; Devadatta *et al.*, 1960) but this adverse effect can be prevented by giving extra pyridoxine to the patients, and the vitamin does not alter the antitubercular activity of INH. Evans *et al.* (1965) found toxic symptoms from phenelzine to be more common in patients slow in acetylation, and a lupus erythematosus-like reaction from hydralazine is more likely to occur in slow acetylators (Perry *et al.*, 1967). It appears that slow acetylation of these drugs contributes in some way to their potential toxicity, but the high incidence of slow acetylators in the population and relatively low frequency of these toxic reactions suggest that additional factors we do not yet understand are involved in these reactions.

Since the peripheral neuritis associated with isoniazid accumulation can be prevented by feeding extra pyridoxine, it might appear there is no practical reason to determine a patient's acetylator phenotype, or be concerned about the high concentrations of INH in patients receiving this drug. An interesting type of drug-drug interaction in patients treated with INH and diphenylhydantoin is described in the following section, which illustrates why the patient's acetylation phenotype is useful information and of practical value.

C. Slow Metabolism of Diphenylhydantoin (Dilantin)

Diphenylhydantoin is poorly excreted by the kidney, and removal of the drug from the body depends upon its metabolism to a more water-soluble derivative, 5-phenyl-5′p-hydroxyphenylhydantoin, which has a *para* hydroxyl group on one of the phenyl rings. The hydroxylated derivative is conjugated with glucuronic acid and excreted in the urine.

Diphenylhydantoin is hydroxylated by an enzyme system in the microsomal fraction of liver cells. It is one of many drugs metabolized by oxidative reactions (hydroxylation, dealkylation and deamination) in liver microsomes that require oxygen, NADPH and a special electron transport system that includes cytochrome P-450 (Gillette, 1966). It is not known how many distinct drug metabolism enzymes there are in the microsomes, but genetic mutations might alter their activity and change the individual's capacity to metabolize one or more drugs.

Kutt *et al.* (1964) found a reduced ability to hydroxylate diphenylhydantoin in several members of a family through a patient who developed overdose toxicity symptoms when given the usual doses of the drug. The patient accumulated the drug and was found to have higher blood concentrations than expected, and he excreted much less of the hydroxylated metabolite in the urine than normal. Two relatives of the patient were found to have a similar limited ability to hydroxylate diphenylhydantoin, and the familial incidence suggests that the metabolic defect is inherited. Presumably, the defective system is the microsomal hydroxylase, but evidence for this conclusion by direct enzymatic tests *in vitro* has not been obtained. It is possible that another type of inherited defect accounts for the findings. Diphenylhydantoin, like many other drugs (Conney, 1967), has the property of accelerating its own rate of metabolism upon repeated administration. Perhaps these individuals have a hereditary deficiency which prevents the usual increase in microsomal enzyme activity (enzyme induction) so that the activity remains at its basal level. It is evident, however, that the reduced capacity of the affected individuals to metabolize diphenylhydantoin requires that lower doses of the drug be given to maintain therapeutic tissue concentrations and avoid overdosage toxic reactions. Kutt has also found a few patients who metabolize diphenylhydantoin much more rapidly than usual, but it is uncertain whether they have inherited a more efficient microsomal hydroxylase or have a greater capacity for enzyme induction with repeated doses of the drug.

Kutt *et al.* (1966) noted that some patients given both diphenylhydantoin and isoniazid in the usual doses developed signs of diphenylhydantoin overdosage (nystagmus, ataxia and drowsiness) when receiving both drugs. Since these patients had not shown signs of diphenylhydantoin overdosage previously, it was clear that isoniazid had reduced the tolerance to diphenylhydantoin. Kutt *et al.* (1968) obtained experimental evidence that isoniazid is an inhibitor of diphenylhydantoin metabolism (hydroxylation) from studies with rat liver microsomes *in vitro*. It is reasonable to assume that isoniazid acts as an inhibitor of diphenylhydantoin hydroxylation by liver microsomes in these patients.

More recently, Kutt *et al.* (1970) have established that the patients most likely to show intolerance to diphenylhydantoin when receiving both drugs are those who are the slowest acetylators of isoniazid (Fig. 15.2). Thus, an interesting type of drug-drug interaction appears to result from the genetically determined slow acetylation trait, when these drugs are given together.

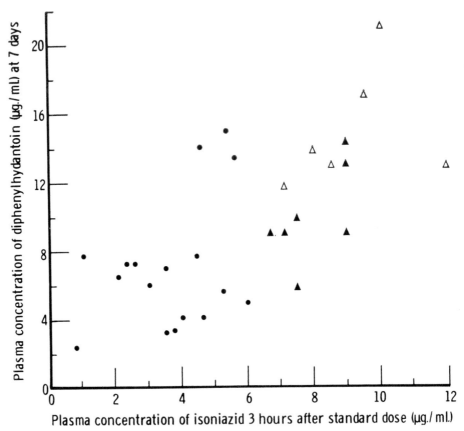

Fig. 15.2. Relationship between diphenylhydantoin concentration at 7 days and the rate of isoniazid metabolism in patients receiving both drugs (from Kutt *et al.*, 1970).

D. Acetophenetidin and Methemoglobinemia

Shahidi (1968) discovered an unusual reaction to acetophenetidin in 2 sisters in a Swiss family. Severe hemolysis and methemoglobinemia developed if either sister were given 2 to 5 grams of the drug. At times the methemoglobin level reached 50% and hemolysis was so extensive that blood transfusions were required for the younger sister. The symptoms were not attributed to the drug at first because they seemed to occur spontaneously at irregular intervals and they appeared while the patient was in the hospital, under close supervision. The patient (the younger sister) denied taking any drugs, but Shahidi examined the urine carefully for unusual compounds and found abnormal substances which suggested that a phenetidin-like compound must have been taken. Finally, he was able to obtain the admission that the attacks had been induced by acetophenetidin taken secretly by the patient.

The usual metabolic fate of acetophenetidin in man is O-dealkylation (O-deethylation) in the liver to N-acetyl-p-aminophenol. The hydroxyl group is then conjugated to form glucuronide and sulfate derivatives (Fig. 15.3). Shahidi concluded that the two sisters were deficient in the liver microsomal enzyme required to catalyze the O-dealkylation reaction. If this pathway were not available, the drug would be metabolized by an alternative pathway that ordinarily is a minor route of metabolism for acetophenetidin. The presence of appreciable amounts of 2-hydroxyphenetidin in the urine of these patients suggested that the drug was deacylated and then hydroxylated. The resulting o-aminophenol metabolite is known to be a toxic compound, as it causes hemolysis and methemoglobinemia. The diversion of the drug to the alternative metabolic pathway which includes a toxic metabolite appears to explain the unusual clinical symptoms from acetophenetidin in the sisters.

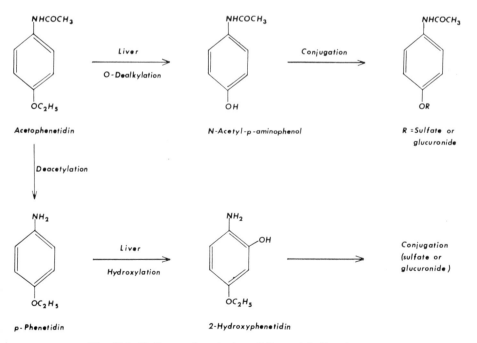

Fig. 15.3. Pathway of acetophenetidin metabolism in man

It is of interest that both the main pathway (O-dealkylation) and the minor pathway (hydroxylation to 2-hydroxyphenetidin) are oxidative reactions catalyzed by enzymes in liver microsomes. If a genetic mutation causes a deficiency of the microsomal O-dealkylation enzyme system, it must be a rather specific deficiency that spares the microsomal hydroxylase system. Further studies would be of interest, particularly a direct assay of these enzymes by *in vitro* techniques, to see whether this hypothesis is correct.

Shahidi (1968) found that the administration of phenobarbital for several days followed by a small dose of acetophenetidin to the younger sister resulted in an accentuated degree of hemolysis and methemoglobin formation. Phenobarbital is known to induce the liver microsomal drug metabolism enzymes, but the patient's enzymatic deficiency was not corrected by phenobarbital induction. In fact, phenobarbital probably induced the microsomal hydroxylase, and thus increased the production of the toxic metabolite.

IV. HEREDITARY METABOLIC DISORDERS WHICH MODIFY DRUG EFFECTS—GLUCOSE-6-PHOSPHATE DEHYDROGENASE (G6PD) DEFICIENCIES AND PRIMAQUINE SENSITIVITY

Unusual reactions to drugs may be inherited without the hereditary trait being directly associated with the metabolism or disposition of the offending drugs; for example, an inborn error may affect the internal environment of cells or tissues in such a way that drugs produce unusual effects in the abnormal environment. There are a number of inherited enzymatic deficiencies of the red blood cells that are compensated for under ordinary circumstances. They confer unusual susceptibility to adverse drug effects if certain drugs are given (Peters, 1968). The best known examples are the variety of deficiences of erythrocyte glucose-6-phosphate dehydrogenase. At least 80 distinct variant forms of the dehydrogenase have been identified (Motulsky, 1971). All of these variants do not cause hemolysis with primaquine and other drugs; Kirkman (1968) has pointed out that, in general, those variants with activity less than 30 % of the normal value are the ones regularly associated with hemolytic reactions to drugs. The mechanism which accounts for red cell hemolysis is not known, although it is clear that the reduced level of G6PD activity makes these cells less efficient in generating NADPH, the reduced cofactor for glutathione reductase. An adequate supply of glutathione seems to be critical for maintaining the integrity of the erythrocyte membrane; G6PD deficient cells show a reduction in their glutathione concentration when they are incubated with acetylphenylhydrazine (Beutler *et al.*, 1955), and drug-sensitive individuals can be recognized by this simple *in vitro* test.

A variety of drugs and chemicals cause red cell hemolysis in individuals deficient in G6PD. A selected number of these agents are listed in Table 15.5. Males are more likely to show the enzymatic deficiency and drug sensitivity than females, since the gene determining the characteristics of G6PD is carried on the X chromosome. In a population of American Negroes surveyed by Childs *et al.* (1958), about 15 % of the males had drug-sensitive cells by the glutathione stability test of Beutler (1957), and 1.6 % of the females were classified as "reactors" (Table 15.6). The inheritance is thus sex-linked without dominance. The X chromosome of the males can be *normal* or *defective* and two male genotypes "reactor" or "normal" are expected; females are classified into three groups;

TABLE 15.5

Drugs and other agents that can cause clinically significant hemolysis in glucose-6-PO₄ dehydrogenase deficient individuals

Acetanilid: 3.6 g	Nitrofurazone (Furacin): 1.5 g[a]
Phenylhydrazine: 30 mg	Nitrofurantoin (Furadantin): 400 mg
Sulfanilamide: 3.6 g	Furazolidone: 400 mg
Sulfacetamide	Furaltodone (Altofur): 1.0 g
Sulfapyridine: 4.0 g	Quinidine: 0.8 g[a]
Sulfamethoxypyridazine (Kynex): 2.0 g	Primaquine: 30 mg
Salicylazosulfapyridine (Azulfidine): 6.8 g	Pamaquine: 30 mg
Thiazolsulfone	Pentaquine
Diaminodiphenylsulfone: 200 mg	Quinocide: 30 mg
Trinitrotoluene[a]	Naphthalene
	Neosalvarson: 600 mg
	Fava Beans

[a] Hemolysis observed principally in Caucasians.
From Kirkman (1968).

TABLE 15.6

Distribution of glutathione stability values in erythrocytes from randomly selected negro males and females[a]

	Genotype[b]	Expected Frequency		Observed Occurrence[c]	
				Number	Frequency
Females					
Normal	AA	p²	.742	172	.935
Intermediate	Aa	2pq	.239	9	.049
Reactor	aa	q²	.019	3	.016
				184	
Males					
Normal	AY	p	.864	120	.833
Intermediate	—	—	0	3	.021
Reactor	aY	q	.136	21	.146
				144	

[a] Calculated on the assumption of sex-linked inheritance without dominance, frequency of 0.136 (q) for the reactor gene and a frequency of 0.864 (p = 1 − q) (after Childs *et al.*, 1958).

[b] A, normal X chromosome; a, chromosome with gene causing primaquine sensitivity.

[c] The glutathione stability test fails to discriminate well between normals and intermediates. More reliable tests to detect heterozygous G6PD deficiency are now available as discussed by Prins (1970).

"normal," "intermediate" or "reactor," depending on the presence of two normal X chromosomes, one normal and one defective, and two defective X chromosomes, respectively.

V. HEREDITARY DEFICIENCY OF DRUG-ACTIVATING ENZYMES—HYPOXANTHINE-GUANINE PHOSPHORIBOSYLTRANSFERASE

Some drugs are administered in an inactive form and must be metabolized to pharmacologically active derivatives by specific enzyme systems *in vivo*. An inherited deficiency of a drug-activating enzyme would be a pharmacogenetic condition in which drug ineffectiveness is inherited.

Allopurinol is used to treat patients with hyperuricemia. It is useful because it has two effects; 1) it acts directly as an inhibitor of xanthine oxidase, and this reduces the formation of uric acid at the expense of more xanthine and hypoxanthine, but these purines are more soluble; 2) it also reduces the rate of purine biosynthesis by a "feedback inhibition" of an early step of purine synthesis, the synthesis of phosphoribosylamine (Fig. 15.4) (Seegmiller et al., 1967).

In order to act as a "feedback inhibitor," allopurinol must be metabolized to an active derivative, the corresponding nucleotide. This transformation of allopurinol requires phosphoribosylpyrophosphate (PRPP), and the enzyme, hypoxanthine-guanine phosphoribosyltransferase (H-G-PRT). The latter enzyme is deficient in patients with the Lesch-Nyhan syndrome and in some adult patients with gout. It has been proposed that these patients have hyperuricemia because they are unable to convert guanine to guanylic acid and hypoxanthine to inosinic acid, and that these nucleotides normally act as "feedback" inhibitors to regulate the early step of purine synthesis (Fig. 15.4).

As would be expected, allopurinol inhibits xanthine oxidase in these patients, but it is ineffective in reducing purine biosynthesis. These patients also are unresponsive to some of the other purine antimetabolites which require a similar conversion to their nucleotides by H-G-PRT to be active. These drugs include: 6-thioguanine, 6-mercaptopurine, 8-azaguanine and azathioprine (Kelley et al., 1969). One should not expect these drugs to produce their usual antineoplastic effects in patients deficient in hypoxanthine-guanine phosphoribosyltransferase.

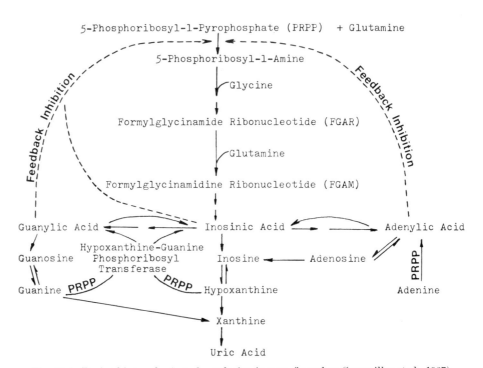

Fig. 15.4. Purine biosynthesis and regulation in man (based on Seegmiller et al., 1967).

VI. HEREDITARY RESISTANCE TO COUMARIN ANTICOAGULANTS

A very unusual type of pharmacogenetic condition in man is the hereditary resistance to the coumarin anticoagulant drugs described by O'Reilly et al. (1964). They noted that a 73-year-old man who was given warfarin following a myocardial infarction showed no anticoagulant response to the usual dose of the drug. The dosage was gradually increased and a prothrombin response was finally achieved, but it required 145 mg per day. Since the mean daily dose of warfarin needed to maintain patients adequately is 6.8 ± 2.8 mg (O'Reilly et al., 1968), this patient required approximately 20 times the usual dose. O'Reilly et al. (1964) found that the patient did not metabolize warfarin faster than normal, and there were no other unusual differences in the binding of the drug to plasma proteins or in the physiological distribution of warfarin. Other family members were tested and six of them in three generations had a similar resistance to warfarin (Fig. 15.5), one of these was an identical twin of the propositus. O'Reilly and Aggeler (1965) concluded from the pedigree that coumarin resistance was inherited as an autosomal mendelian dominant trait.

Resistant individuals were found to show another characteristic, an unusual sensitivity to the antidotal effects of vitamin K. This sensitivity was also calculated to be about 20 times that observed in other patients. These findings have been interpreted by O'Reilly et al. (1968) to mean that an enzyme or a receptor site involved in the synthesis of the clotting factors II, VII, IX and X has been modified by genetic mutation in some way to alter its affinity for both coumarin anticoagulants and vitamin K.

O'Reilly (1970) has reported on a second large kindred with coumarin resistance in 4 generations. Detailed biochemical investigations on the resistant individuals gave very similar results to those from the first kindred.

The variation in response of members of the second kindred was studied by determining the reduction in prothrombin-complex activity after a single dose of warfarin. The distribution of responses is shown in Figure 15.6. The mean responses for the coumarin-resistant subjects and the normal relatives are sepa-

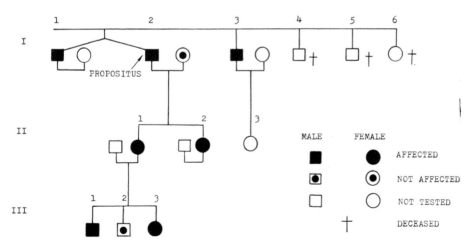

Fig. 15.5. Pedigree of family M. with hereditary resistance to coumarin anticoagulant drugs (redrawn from O'Reilly and Aggeler, 1965).

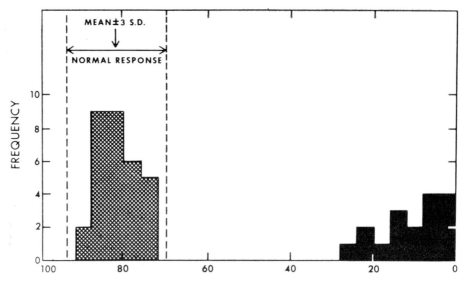

REDUCTION OF PROTHROMBIN ACTIVITY AT 48 HOURS (%)

Fig. 15.6. Reduction of prothrombin-complex activity 48 hours after a single dose of warfarin in family McC. and normal subjects. The 32 members with a normal response are indicated by the cross hatched bars, the 18 members with coumarin resistance by the black bars. (From O'Reilly, 1970.)

rated by 18 standard deviations, and the test is very well suited for classification of the family members.

Coumarin resistance is the first clearly established example of an inherited resistance to a drug, in man.

VII. OTHER HEREDITARY DISORDERS WITH ALTERED DRUG EFFECTS

If the definition of pharmacogenetics were extended to include all hereditary traits which modify drug effects by direct, indirect or unknown mechanisms, a very large number of additional hereditary disorders and inherited conditions should be discussed. Obviously, this is impossible, but it would be arbitrary and undesirable to limit the field to those conditions which are exclusively disturbances revealed by abnormal drug effects, with no signs of their presence otherwise. Those interested in the relationship between hereditary variations in man and unusual drug effects will want to read some of the literature references given below and the general references which follow.

Inherited variations in the structure of hemoglobin, for example, may predispose a patient to undesirable drug effects, such as methemoglobinemia and hemolysis. Anesthesia is a potential hazard for patients with sickle cell hemoglobin since hypoxia may cause intravascular sickling followed by infarction (Motulsky and Stamatoyannopoulos, 1968).

Malignant hyperthermia with muscular rigidity is a rare but dangerous complication associated with anesthesia which is inherited. The etiology of this condition is unknown. Frequently a combination of halothane and succinylcholine was used, but this was not always the case. Some patients had malignant hyperthermia and rigidity, others had hyperthermia without rigidity; evidently the group is not homogeneous (Britt and Kalow, 1968). Kalow *et al.* (1970) have suggested that patients subject to muscle rigidity may have an abnormality in intracellular calcium metabolism, based upon studies with skeletal muscle biopsies for patients with this disorder.

Other hereditary diseases in which drugs produce characteristic unusual or exaggerated effects include mongolism, familial dysautonomia, subaortic stenosis, glaucoma, and a variety of red blood cell enzymatic deficiencies. These, and others are discussed in Kalow's book on pharmacogenetics (Kalow, 1962) and in several more recent conferences and general reviews (Clarke *et al.*, 1968; Evans, 1968; Peters, 1968; Szeinberg and Sheba, 1968; La Du, 1969; Vesell, 1969).

REFERENCES

Alexanderson, B., Price-Evans, D. A. and Sjöqvist, F.: Steady-state plasma levels of nortriptyline in twins: influence of genetic factors and drug therapy. Brit. Med. J. *4:* 764–768, 1969.

Altland, K., and Goedde, H. W.: Heterogeneity in the silent gene phenotype of pseudocholinesterase of human serum. Biochem. Genet. *4:* 321–338, 1970.

Beutler, E.: The glutathione instability of drug-sensitive red cells: a new method for the *in vitro* detection of drug sensitivity. J. Lab. Clin. Med. *49:* 84–95, 1957.

Beutler, E., Dern, R. J. and Alving, A. S.: The hemolytic effect of primaquine VI. An *in vitro* test for sensitivity of erythrocytes to primaquine. J. Lab. Clin. Med. *45:* 40–50, 1955.

Bönicke, R., and Lisboa, B. P.: Uber die Erbbedingtheit der intraindividuellen Konstanz der Isoniazidausscheidung beim Menschen. (Untersuchungen an eineügen und zwillingen.) Naturwissenschaften *44:* 314, 1957.

Britt, B. A. and Kalow, W.: Hyperridigity and hyperthermia associated with anesthesia. Ann. N.Y. Acad. Sci. *151:* 947–957, 1968.

Brodie, B. B., Lief, P. A. and Poet, R.: The fate of procaine in man following its intravenous administration and methods for the estimation of procaine and diethylaminoethanol. J. Pharmacol. Exp. Therap. *94:* 359–366, 1948.

Childs, B., Zinkham, W., Browne, E. A., Kimbro, E. L. and Torbert, J. V.: A genetic study of a defect in glutathione metabolism of the erythrocyte. Bull. Johns Hopkins Hosp. *102:* 21–37, 1958.

Clarke, C. A., Price-Evans, D. A., Harris, R., McConnell, R. B. and Woodrow, J. C.: Genetics in medicine: a review Part II Pharmacogenetics. Quart. J. Med. New Series *XXXVII:* 183–219, 1968.

Conney, A. H.: Pharmacological implications of microsomal enzyme induction. Pharmacol. Rev. *19:* 317–366, 1967.

Devadatta, S., Gangadharam, P. R. J., Andrews, R. H., Fox, W., Ramakrushnan, C. V., Selkon, J. B. and Velu, S.: Peripheral neuritis due to isoniazid. Bull. World Health Org. *23:* 587–598, 1960.

Evans, D. A. P.: Clinical pharmacogenetics. In *Recent Advances in Medicine*, ed. by D. N. Baron, N. Compston, and A. M. Dawson, pp. 203–242, J. & A. Churchill Ltd., London, 1968, 15th Ed.

Evans, D. A. P.: An improved and simplified method of detecting the acetylator phenotype. J. Med. Genet. *6:* 405–407, 1969.

Evans, D. A. P., Davison, K. and Pratt, R. T. C.: The influence of acetylator phenotype on the effects of treating depression with phenelzine. Clin. Pharmacol. Therap. *6:* 430–435, 1965.

Evans, D. A. P., Manley, K. A. and McKusick, V. C.: Genetic control of isoniazid metabolism in man. Brit. Med. J. *2:* 485–491, 1960.

Evans, D. A. P. and White, T. A.: Human acetylation polymorphism. J. Lab. Clin. Med. *63:* 394–404, 1964.

Gillette, J. R.: Biochemistry of drug oxidation and reduction by enzymes in hepatic endoplasmic reticulum. Adv. Pharmacol. *4:* 219–261, 1966.

Harris, H., Hopkinson, D. A. and Robson, E. B.: Two dimensional electrophoresis of pseudocholinesterase components in normal human serum. Nature, Lond. *196:* 1296–1298, 1962.

Harris, H., and Whittaker, M.: Differential inhibition of human serum cholinesterase with fluoride. Recognition of two new phenotypes. Nature *191:* 496–498, 1961.

Hughes, H. B., Biehl, J., Jones, A. P. and Schmidt, L. H.: Metabolism of isoniazid in man as related to the occurrence of peripheral neuritis. Amer. Rev. of Tuberc. *70:* 266–273, 1954.

Jenne, J. W.: Partial purification and properties of the isoniazid transacetylase in human liver. Its relationship to the acetylation of p-aminosalicylic acid. J. Clin. Invest. *44:* 1992–2002, 1965.

Kalow, W.: Hydrolysis of local anesthetics by human serum cholinesterase. J. Pharmacol. Exp. Therap. *104:* 122–134, 1952.

Kalow, W.: Cholinesterase types. In Ciba Foundation Symp. *Biochemistry of Human Genetics.* Little, Brown, Boston, pp. 39–59, 1960.

Kalow, W.: *Pharmacogenetics. Heredity and the response to drugs.* W. B. Saunders, Philadelphia, London, 1962.

Kalow, W.: Contribution of hereditary factors to the response to drugs. Fed. Proc. *24:* 1259–1265, 1965.

Kalow, W. and Davies, R. O.: The activity of various esterase inhibitors toward atypical human serum cholinesterase. Biochem. Pharmacol. *1:* 183–192, 1958.

Kalow, W., and Genest, K.: A method for the detection of atypical forms of human serum cholinesterase. Determination of dibucaine numbers. Can. J. Biochem. Physiol. *35:* 339–346, 1957.

Kalow, W., and Gunn, D. R.: Some statistical data on atypical cholinesterase of human serum. Ann. Human Genet. *23:* 239–250, 1959.

Kalow, W., Britt, B. A., Terreau, M. E. and Haist, C.: Metabolic error of muscle metabolism after recovery from malignant hyperthermia. Lancet *II:* 895–898, 1970.

Kattamis, C., Davies, D. and Lehmann, H.: The silent serum cholinesterase gene. Acta Genet. *17:* 299–303, 1967.

Kelley, W. N., Green, M. L., Rosenbloom, F. M., Henderson, J. F. and Seegmiller, J. E.: Hypoxanthine-Guanine phosphoribosyltransferase deficiency in gout. Ann. Int. Med. *70:* 155–206, 1969.

Kirkman, H. N.: Glucose-6-phosphate dehydrogenase variants and drug-induced hemolysis. Ann. N.Y. Acad. Sci. *151:* 753–764, 1968.

Knight, R. A., Selin, M. J. and Harris, H. W.: Genetic factors influencing isoniazid blood levels in humans. 18th Conference Chemother. Tuberc. *18:* 52–58, 1959.

Kutt, H., Wolk, M., Scherman, R. and McDowell, F.: Insufficient parahydroxylation as a cause of diphenylhydantoin toxicity. Neurol. *14:* 542–548, 1964.

Kutt, H., Winters, W., and McDowell, F. H.: Depression of parahydroxylation of diphenylhydantoin by antituberculosis chemotherapy. Neurol. *16:* 594–602, 1966.

Kutt, H., Verebely, K. and McDowell, F.: Inhibition of diphenylhydantoin metabolism in rats and in rat liver microsomes by antitubercular drugs. Neurol. *18:* 706–710, 1968.

Kutt, H., Brennan, R., Dehejia, H. and Verebely, K.: Diphenylhydantoin intoxication. A complication of isoniazid therapy. Am. Rev. of Resp. Dis. *101:* 377–383, 1970.

La Du, B. N.: Pharmacogenetics. Med. Clin. of N. Amer. *53:* 839–855, 1969.

Motulsky, A. G., and Stamatoyannopoulos, G.: Drugs, anesthesia and abnormal hemoglobins. Ann. N.Y. Acad. Sci. *151:* 808–821, 1968.

Motulsky, A. G., Yoshida, A. and Stamatoyannopoulos, G.: Glucose-6-phosphate dehydrogenase variants. Ann. N.Y. Acad. Sci., *179:* 636-643, 1971.

Neitlich, H. W.: Increased plasma cholinesterase activity and succinyl-choline resistance: a genetic variant. J. Clin. Invest. *45:* 380–387, 1966.

O'Reilly, R. A.: The second reported kindred with hereditary resistance to oral anticoagulant drugs. New Eng. J. Med. *282:* 1448–1451, 1970.

O'Reilly, R. A., and Aggeler, P. M.: Coumarin anticoagulant drugs: hereditary resistance in man. Fed. Proc. *24:* 1266–1273, 1965.

O'Reilly, R. A., Aggeler, P. M., Hoag, M. S., Leong, L. S. and Kropatkin, M. L.: Hereditary transmission of exceptional resistance to coumarin anticoagulant drugs. The first reported kindred. New Eng. J. Med. *271:* 809–815, 1964.

O'Reilly, R. A., Pool, J. G. and Aggeler, P. M.: Hereditary resistance to coumarin anticoagulant drugs in man and rat. Ann. N.Y. Acad. Sci. *151:* 913–931, 1968.

Osborne, R. H., and DeGeorge, F. V.: *Genetic Basis of Morphological Variation, an Evaluation and Application of the Twin Study Method.* Harvard University Press, Cambridge, Massachusetts, 1959.

Perry, H. M., Jr., Sakamoto, A. and Tan, E. M.: Relationship of acetylating enzyme to hydralazine toxicity. J. Lab. Clin. Med. *70:* 1020–1021, 1967.

Peters, J. H.: Genetic factors in relation to drugs. Ann. Rev. Pharmacol. *8:* 427–452, 1968.

Prins, H. K.: The detection of heterozygous G6PD deficiency similarity between glutathione deficiency and G6PD deficiency. Humangenetik *9:* 254–255, 1970.

Seegmiller, J. E., Rosenbloom, F. M. and Kelley, W. N.: Enzyme defect associated with a sex-linked human neurological disorder and excessive purine synthesis. Science *155:* 1682–1984, 1967.

Shahidi, N. T.: Acetophenetidin-induced methemoglobinemia. Ann. N.Y. Acad. Sci. *151:* 822–832, 1968.

Szeinberg, A., and Sheba, Ch.: Pharmacogenetics. Israel J. Med. Sci. *4:* 488–493, 1968.

Vesell, E.: Recent progress in pharmacogenetics. Adv. in Pharmacol. Chemotherapy *7:* 1–52, 1969.

Vesell, E. S., and Page, J. G.: Genetic control of drug levels in man: antipyrine. Science *161:* 72–73, 1968a.

Vesell, E. S., and Page, J. G.: Genetic control of dicumarol levels in man. J. Clin. Invest. *47:* 2657–2663, 1968b.

Vesell, E. S., and Page, J. G.: Genetic control of drug levels in man: phenylbutazone. Science *159:* 1479–1480, 1968c.

Weber, W. W.: Acetylating, deacetylating and amino acid conjugating enzymes. *In* Handbuch der Exp. Pharmakologie *28:* In Press.

Yoshida, A., and Motulsky, A. G.: A pseudocholinesterase variant (E cynthiana) associated with elevated plasma enzyme activity. Am. J. Human Genetics *21:* 486–498, 1969.

GENERAL REFERENCES

Kalow, W.: *Pharmacogenetics, Heredity and the Response to Drugs.* W. B. Saunders Co., Philadelphia, 1962. (Book on Pharmacogenetics.)

Kalow, W. and other contributors: Experimental and Clinical Aspects of Pharmacogenetics. Fed. Proc. *24:* 1259–1292, 1965. (Symposium on Pharmacogenetics.)

La Du, B. N. and Kalow, W., Eds., Pharmacogenetics. Ann. N.Y. Acad. Sci. *151:* 691–1001, 1968. (Conference on Pharmacogenetics.)

Goedde, H.: Pharmacogenetics. 2. International Titisee Workship. Humangenetik *9:* 197–280, 1970. (Conference on Pharmacogenetics.)

16

The Value of Determining the Plasma
Concentration of Drugs in Animals and Man

BERNARD B. BRODIE
WATSON D. REID

I. DRUG TOXICITY: GENERAL CONSIDERATIONS

The preceding chapters testify that pharmacology is emerging as a quantitative science able to take advantage of methodological advances in many disciplines to determine the biological action of chemical agents in terms of physiological and biochemical principles. In recent years, however, the number and variety of chemicals that affect man have increased at an enormous rate and have created a public health problem of major proportions. In addition to drugs, which have become increasingly potent and administered over extended periods of time, we are confronted with a profusion of chemicals in the form of air and water pollutants, herbicides, pesticides, cosmetics and food additives.

Today, pharmacology faces a great challenge to develop unifying and simplifying generalizations to accelerate the application of its new discoveries to clinical therapeutics, drug development, and control of environmental hazards. In this chapter we shall review some general principles of toxicology which have evolved during the past two decades and attempt to suggest certain approaches and areas of future research which may lead to further advances in the development of new drugs and in clinical therapeutics. Since the clinical use of a great number of potentially efficacious drugs is limited or prohibited by their toxic effects, it is of utmost importance for pharmacologists and clinicians alike to understand, insofar as is possible, the mechanisms of adverse reactions to drugs.

A drug may produce toxicity either through excessive or undesired physiological actions or by cytotoxic chemical reactions with components of tissue cells. Drug hazards of the former type may be understood from the nature of the physiological control systems on which drugs act. With a ganglionic blocking agent, orthostatic syncope would exemplify the desired blockade of sympathetic ganglia displayed to excess and paralytic ileus of the unwanted blockade of parasympathetic ganglia. Overdosage with chlorpromazine would result in tremors and, with a barbiturate, respiratory arrest. Similarly, antitumor drugs may interrupt biochemical processes essential both to normal and neoplastic cells. In contrast, the second type of toxicity is not closely related to the physiological actions of the drug and involves structural or biochemical damage to the cell. Examples of this cytotoxicity include such drug-induced diseases as drug allergies, blood dyscrasias, hepatotoxicity, nephrotoxicity, drug-induced lupus erythematosis, teratogenic effects and possibly even some forms of behavioral toxicity. We shall consider only the first category of toxic reactions in this chapter.

II. SCREENING DRUGS FOR EXCESSIVE OR UNDESIRED ACTIONS ON PHYSIOLOGICAL CONTROL SYSTEMS

A. Projection of Animal Data to Man

The screening of drugs for potential therapeutic and toxic effects is generally carried out in laboratory animals, such as mice, rats, rabbits, dogs and cats, and it is on data obtained with these animals that the decision to test the drug in man usually depends. The great difficulty in our system of drug development is the vast species variation in the therapeutic or toxic effects of chemical substances.

The projection of animal data directly to man should not be made on the assumption that the same dose of drug (in mg/kg) will attain the same concentration at drug receptors in man as in animals. In the past, the large variations among species in the response to a drug usually were attributed to differences in the sensitivity of receptor sites. In recent years, however, this view has been revised at least in part by the discovery that variation in drug metabolism within and between species is the rule rather than the exception; hence variations in response are more often due to differences in amounts of unbound drug available to sites of action. A crucial problem in pharmacology currently being investigated in several laboratories is to determine the extent to which drug metabolism accounts for species variability in response.

B. Drugs That Act Reversibly

With reversibly acting compounds, the reaction

$$D + R \; \underset{k_2}{\overset{k_1}{\rightleftharpoons}} \; DR$$

rapidly reaches an equilibrium where the rate at which the drug-receptor complex is formed ($k_1[D][R]$) equals the rate at which it is dissociated ($k_2[DR]$). In general, the drug in plasma water is in dynamic equilibrium with that attached to the receptors; in other words the rate constants of association (k_1) and dissociation (k_2) are so rapid that changes in drug concentration in plasma water will be paralleled by changes in the number of drug-receptor complexes and in the intensity of response. It is important to appreciate that the amount of drug complexed with receptors depends not only on the first order rate constants k_1 and k_2, but on the concentration of unbound drug in plasma.

It is fortunate that the majority of drugs used clinically are reversibly acting compounds, because this fact provides an opportunity to derive a wealth of useful information about toxicity of those agents from kinetic studies of their concentrations in plasma. The two most important applications of measuring drug levels in plasma are 1) to provide a rational basis for the extrapolation of toxicity studies in animals to man in the screening for new drugs, and 2) to promote the safety and efficacy of drugs in clinical use by relating toxic and therapeutic effects to plasma levels in patients.

C. Drugs That Act Nonreversibly

With some drugs, the quantity of active agent attached to receptors is not related to the plasma level. The drug (D) reacts covalently with the receptors (R) to form a drug receptor complex (DR),

$$D + R \rightarrow DR$$

and the complex persists long after the drug disappears from the rest of the body. Nonreversible ("hit-and-run") drugs are usually chemically reactive and rapidly metabolized, in some cases nonenzymatically. Their effects are not related to the plasma level at a given moment but to the level over a short period of time. Hence, their effects are usually more intense after high levels of short duration than after low levels of long duration.

For some nonreversibly acting drugs, such as reserpine, which probably do not form covalent bonds, it is presumed that

$$D + R \; \underset{k_2 \text{ slow}}{\overset{k_1 \text{ rapid}}{\rightleftharpoons}} \; DR$$

i.e. the rate constant of dissociation (k_2) is slow relative to the rate constant of association (k_1) and therefore the drug remains fixed to receptors while it disappears elsewhere from the body.

These nonreversibly acting agents are inherently dangerous: 1) Their action is persistent and the rate of recovery may vary in relation to the rate at which the receptor is reformed. For example, monoamine oxidase inhibitors act for a shorter time in mice than in larger animals species (Spector *et al.*, 1960). 2) Although nonreversibly acting drugs do not accumulate, their effects do and hence plasma levels are not a guide to drug therapy.

Monoamine oxidase inhibitors, dicumarol and reserpine present common clinical problems in that their effects are cumulative although their levels are not. It is of historical interest that dicumarol was isolated as the bleeding factor in spoiled sweet clover disease by a biochemist, Link (1943), who realizing that the effects of the drug far outlasted its presence in the body suggested that the "poison" might have clinical value, provided the prothrombin time was used as a guide to therapy. In the early days of reserpine, a number of elderly patients treated for hypertension ended up in mental hospitals because physicians were unaware that such small daily doses could induce "endogenous" depression.

Simple kinetic studies in animals will disclose whether a new drug acts nonreversibly. Drugs that act nonreversibly in animals will also act nonreversibly in man and are likely to elicit untoward effects unless handled with care.

D. Importance of Plasma Concentrations of Drugs

Central to an understanding of a drug's toxicity is the question of whether or not its therapeutic and toxic effects are related to its concentration in plasma. It may be assumed that the pharmacological response will be determined by the quantity of the agent that is fixed to the drug receptors. Although this quantity cannot be determined directly, the concentration of the drug in plasma may be assayed, and hence it is important to know whether changes in the plasma concentration of drug are reflected by changes in the amount of drug at effector sites.

It should be pointed out that many reports still refer to the blood level and force the reader to guess whether the author really means blood level or has merely carelessly used this term as a synonym for plasma level. Kinetically, the blood level is not a good index of the amount of drug attached to receptor sites. For example, quinacrine is highly localized in leukocytes; hence, changes in whole blood concentration are more apt to reflect changes in leukocyte count than in amounts of drug at receptors (Shannon *et al.*, 1944).

A therapeutic agent may be inactive itself but its biotransformation may lead to a formation of an active product. In this case, the response will be related to the plasma level of active product rather than to the level of the administered drug. Whenever a time-response study shows that a drug reaction is clearly unrelated in time to the plasma level, the possibility must be considered that a metabolic product might mediate the action of the drug. A study of such relationships has disclosed a number of new therapeutic agents (Brodie, 1964). Drug-induced lesions may also be mediated through a metabolite.

III. SPECIES DIFFERENCES IN DRUG ACTION

A. Evolution of Enzymes Which Metabolize Drugs

Since drug metabolism is such a major variable in comparative pharmacology, it is pertinent to ask why therapeutic agents are metabolized at all. A clue to this question is provided by the structure of the kidney. Foreign organic compounds flow down tubules lined with a membrane with lipoidal characteristics. Compounds that have a high lipid solubility will be almost completely reabsorbed while lipid insoluble substances will pass through into the urine. The kidney is so poorly equipped to excrete liposoluble substances that highly liposoluble drugs, such as thiopental or quinacrine, would have a half-life of about 100 years if the body lacked the means of making these substances less lipid soluble. With some notable exceptions the metabolism of a drug generally renders it less liposoluble. Drug-metabolizing enzymes are not the usual enzymes of intermediary metabolism, but were developed in evolution to permit the organism to dispose of liposoluble substances—hydrocarbons, alkaloids, terpenes, and sterols—ingested in food which would accumulate to enormous levels if they were not converted to excretable derivatives. One might speculate that new drugs are metabolized because they simulate classes of foreign organic compounds to which animals have always been exposed (Brodie and Maickel, 1962).

The phylogenetic development of these microsomal enzymes may be considered in terms of the water requirements of terrestrial animals. The failure of the kidney to handle liposoluble compounds poses no problem to fish since these substances rapidly diffuse through the lipoidal gills. Correspondingly, many aquatic animals have a poor capacity to oxidize drugs or convert them to glucuronides or ethereal sulfates. Before animals could live permanently on land, another way to dispose of liposoluble impurities in food had to be evolved, or they would finally accumulate to toxic levels. The problem was solved by the development of nonspecific enzymes which convert liposoluble compounds to polar derivatives, which are excretable by the kidney. Looking at the problem in this way, the capacity of an animal to metabolize drugs might depend on the foreign compounds with which the species was faced several million years ago.

B. Use of Plasma Levels to Overcome Species Differences in Drug Response

Large species differences in drug response are associated with drugs, especially the liposoluble substances that undergo extensive metabolism. The failure to recognize species differences in rates of drug metabolism may lead to the accumulation of toxic concentrations of the therapeutic agent and produce signs of clinical toxicity since rates of metabolism are often slower in man than in animals. However, dependable predictions of activity are possible for drugs whose metabolism shows marked differences in various species if drug responses are related to plasma levels rather than dosage. This point is illustrated by the examples given below.

Despite a 50-fold difference in duration of action and rates of metabolism of barbiturates, various animal species and man recover from these drugs at similar plasma levels. In addition, variations in the effects of these drugs caused by strain and sex differences in rat are circumvented if the measurement of activity is based on plasma levels (Quinn et al., 1955). Another dramatic example of the close relationships between plasma level and drug effect is provided by the compound (ICI-33828).

$$CH_2 = CH \cdot CH \cdot NH \cdot CS \cdot NH \cdot NH \cdot CS \cdot NH \cdot CH_3$$
$$| $$
$$CH_3$$

This compound inhibits pituitary gonadotropic function at vastly different doses in various species. Despite a 200-fold variation in daily dosage, each species, including man, shows an inhibitory response to the same plasma concentration of 3 μg/ml (Duncan, 1963). Likewise, phenylbutazone exerts antirheumatic effects in man at a daily oral dose of about 10 mg/kg (Burns, 1962), compared to the repeated intramuscular doses of 100 mg/kg required to protect against glycerol-induced inflammation in the rabbit's eye. In each instance the plasma levels are 100–150 μg/ml (Yourish et al., 1955). The marked difference in dosage reflects the fact that the biologic half life of phenylbutazone is 3 hours in the rabbit and 70 hours in man.

In man and dog the oral dose of N-isopropylmethoxamine that blocks the epinephrine-induced output of free fatty acids is about 10 mg/kg and plasma levels are 3–6 mg/liter. In mouse and rat the drug elicits no effects in oral doses up to 400 mg/kg since it is metabolized so rapidly that plasma levels do not rise above 0.5 mg/liter. In the isolated adipose tissue of rats and dogs the antilipolytic effects of the drug are equally effective (Burns, 1965). Similarly, in the case of phenacetin 200 mg/kg given orally to rats produces an antipyretic effect against yeast-induced hyperthermia persisting for 4 hr at which time the plasma levels of drug plus its active metabolite N-acetyl-p-aminophenol are about 19 μg/ml (Conney et al., 1966). Similar levels are also produced in man 3 hr after a single oral dose of 1.2 g (i.e. about 20 mg/kg) of phenacetin (Brodie and Axelrod, 1949).

Recently it was observed that Sprague-Dawley rats at the NIH are not as sensitive to the sedative effects of hexobarbital as they were a few years ago. Hypnosis from 100 mg/kg of hexobarbital now last 20 minutes compared to 90 minutes 4 years ago. However, the plasma levels of the drug indicate that the present NIH rats metabolize the drugs much more rapidly than did their forebears, but the sensitivity of the receptors is unchanged. The increased rate of drug metabolism is the result of bedding the rats on red cedar (instead of hardwood) sawdust which elevates the activity of hexobarbital oxidase, aniline hydroxylase and morphine N-demethylase in hepatic microsomes of mice and rats (Vesell, 1968).

C. Some Historical Examples of Consequences of Failing to Determine Plasma Levels

A screening program to find a barbiturate that would be rapidly metabolized in the body led to an extremely unstable drug in dogs. This thiobarbiturate proved to be the longest lasting barbiturate of all time in man (Brodie, 1964). In the case of meperidine, the failure to observe tolerance and addiction in dogs led to the erroneous belief that the drug was nonaddictive in man. How such an error arose is evident from the half-life of the drug which is a few minutes in dogs compared with 4 hours in man (Burns et al., 1955). These experiments in the dogs only proved that one cannot become tolerant or addicted to a drug that is not there! In horses an odd situation occurred with procaine. Race horses who had received a procaine block for leg injuries often won their races—sore feet and all, since the drug is so stable in horses it acts like a central stimulant (Brodie, 1964). Finally, there was the tragic example of chloramphenicol which was thought to elicit a special disease that kills the newborn when actually it was metabolized so slowly that the children died of overdosage (Weiss et al., 1960).

IV. IMPORTANCE OF PLASMA LEVELS IN DRUG SCREENING

A. Difficulties in Finding an Animal Model

Two decades ago, when the field of drug metabolism was in its infancy, it was hoped that an animal species close to man in metabolizing drugs would be discovered. This hope was kindled by observations that a number of medicinal agents elicit pharmacological effects of equal intensity in various mammalian species, including man. The similarity is most readily observed with compounds that are not metabolized (usually highly lipid-insoluble drugs) and which are mainly eliminated from the body through the kidney, a process that is not particularly different from one animal to another. For example, the parenteral dose of tubocurarine to produce a 90–100% neuromuscular block varies between 1 and 5 mg/kg in 9 species, including man (Zaimis, 1953), and the effects of about 300 ganglionic blocking agents, all quaternary ammonium compounds, vary by only 100–200% in 5 species of animals (Nador, 1960). Likewise, in dogs and man tolazoline has the same biological half-life and equal activity as an adrenergic blocking agent (Brodie et al., 1952). However, isopropylmethoxamine has almost no adrenergic blocking activity in rats, which metabolize it at an amazingly rapid rate compared with cats and dogs, which metabolize it slowly (Burns, 1965).

The effects of the thiazide diuretics on kidney function are quantitatively similar in animals and man (Berliner, 1965). However, the diuretic ethacrynic acid—a liposoluble agent whose action is terminated by metabolic breakdown rather than excretion—is much less active in rat, guinea pig, and monkey than in rabbit, dog, or man (Beyer et al., 1965), suggesting that the variability in response could be due to differences in metabolism. Unfortunately, studies on the

metabolism of ethacrynic acid have been hampered by the instability of its conjugates with glutathione (J. E. Baer, personal communication), and species
differences in the excretion of metabolites have not yet been detected (Beyer
et al., 1965). The available evidence suggests there are inherent differences between
responsive and unresponsive species in the reactivity of ethacrynic acid receptor
sites (Zins *et al.*, 1968).

The above findings indicate that a number of drugs not subject to metabolic
transformation have similar activities in various mammalian species. However,
although the hope of finding an animal species close to man persists, recent
studies in comparative pharmacology indicate that the possibility of finding such
a species is extremely remote. Considering the evolution of drug-metabolizing
enzymes, it is not surprising that the activity of a particular enzyme is vastly
different from one species to another and that some species completely lack a
particular enzyme. Thus, the cat is unable to convert phenols to glucuronides
(Robinson and Williams, 1958), and dogs do not acetylate primary amines
(Muenzen *et al.*, 1926). The cat is generally deficient in drug-metabolizing enzymes; chlorpromazine (Gothelf and Karczmar, 1963), diphenylhydantoin
(Firemark *et al.*, 1963), or desipramine (Dingell *et al.*, 1964), given in single doses,
persist in the body for days.

Furthermore, the relative importance of multiple pathways of drug metabolism may vary from ones species to another. Thus, ephedrine can undergo
N-demethylation, hydroxylation, or deamination (Axelrod, 1953). Deamination
is the major route in the rabbit, but in the dog and rat this reaction is virtually
absent. In the dog demethylation is a major pathway, while in the rat hydroxylation is an important route. In monkeys, the patterns of metabolism of certain
drugs may be similar to those in man (R. T. Williams, personal communication),
but the very great differences in the rates of metabolism severely limit the usefulness of primates as models for drug screening. Furthermore, the relative importance of different pathways of drug metabolism may vary greatly in new and
old world monkeys. In other species, such as mice and rats, there also exists considerable strain (Jay, 1955) and sex (Gillette, 1967) differences in response to
drugs.

B. Screening Tests in Animals May Fail to Detect Clinically Useful Drugs

The fact that foreign organic compounds tend to be metabolized more slowly
in man than in animals raises the possibility that drugs rejected on the basis of
being inactive in animals might prove to be useful therapeutic agents if tested
in man. The following are examples of drugs that would not have been discovered
by animal screening: Oxyphenbutazone is metabolized so quickly in animals
that it could not have been discovered by tests formerly used. In fact, according
to its half-life in the dog, about 30 minutes, the drug should have been discarded
forthwith (Burns, 1962). The relatively short half-life of phenylbutazone in
animals has already been mentioned. The potent antirheumatic action of this
drug turned up quite by chance when it was used as a solubilizing agent for the
parenteral injection of aminopyrine (Gsell and Muller, 1950). Imipramine, a
mild tranquilizing agent in animals, would not have been disclosed as a potential
antidepressant (counteraction and reversal of reserpine syndrome) in rabbits or

mice, since these animals fail to convert the drug in appreciable amounts to the active metabolite desipramine (Dingell et al., 1964; Brodie, 1965). Likewise, desipramine would not have been evident as an antidepressant agent in rabbits and mice, since these animals inactivate the drug too rapidly (Dingell et al., 1964).

From these results it may be concluded that the action of a number of drugs would have been difficult to disclose by the usual screening procedures because of their rapid biotransformation in animals. The studies described in this report suggest that considerable data obtained by studies of drugs in animals are readily transferable to man if the results are expressed in terms of plasma levels. But these levels should not be expected to explain all differences in drug responses between animals and man. For one thing, pharmacological end points in man are often quite different from those in animals. For example, it is difficult to compare the effects of chlorpromazine in man and rat, since their behavior is expressed quite differently. Again, target sites might be equally responsive to a drug, but the net effects may be different. Thus, a primary action of reserpine in brain appears to be impairment of monoamine storage processes (cf. Reid and Brodie, 1968), but the net effects might also depend on the relative turnover rates of these amines. Environmental factors may also affect drug responses. Thus, amphetamine toxicity is increased by exciting stimuli (Gunn and Gurd, 1940). Likewise, the action of a convulsant is facilitated by light or noise (Gastaut and Hunter, 1950). Despite these observations, the biological effects of drugs will be much more closely related to the plasma or tissue level than to dose.

C. Measurement of Plasma Levels in Patients

In recent years it has become evident that individual variability in drug metabolism influences the action of therapeutic agents in man and that a common cause of drug intolerance rises from "overdosage" due to patient-to-patient variability in rates of drug metabolism. Individual differences in metabolism are most prominent with liposoluble drugs, such as dicumarol and tromexan, which show a tenfold or more variation among patients (Burns et al., 1953; Weiner et al., 1950); a similarly wide variability in plasma drug levels occurs in psychiatric patients treated with chlorpromazine (Curry, 1968, Curry and Marshall, 1968). Other drugs metabolized at widely variable rates are diphenylhydantoin, isoniazid, amidopyrine, antipyrine and quinidine.

D. Drug Screening in Man

How can a clinical pharmacologist be expected to evaluate accurately a drug if, unknown to him, the plasma level progressively accumulates or oscillates between that which is ineffective and toxic? Early information about the physiological disposition of a drug in man is needed to develop dosage schedules which will improve the efficiency of screening and reduce the danger of overdosage. The administration of a drug in a single small dosage based on only a limited amount of animal toxicity is safe in experienced hands. With the development of highly sensitive analytical procedures, it may be possible to study the physiologic disposition of a drug after doses of only a few milligrams. These preliminary results might be sufficient to decide if a drug should be abandoned because its absorption is inadequate or its disappearance from the body is too rapid. Such early information would be of great value in disclosing which of a series of drugs have a suitable physiological disposition to warrant further study.

Shannon (1945) was the first to show that a major variable in the clinical screening of antimalarials was the individual rate of drug metabolism and that this variable may be circumvented by relating drug effects to plasma levels. These studies showed that the antimalarial effects of the cinchona alkaloids, quinacrine, and many other agents were found to be highly correlated with plasma levels but not with dosage. By relating effects to plasma levels, only a few patients were needed to gain a definitive assay of activity, compared with the large numbers that would have been required if effects had been related to dosage.

In these studies the disease process itself was not a variable, since reproducible strains of malaria were used. The argument for correlating therapeutic effects with plasma levels would be more convincing if it could be demonstrated in a more variable disease—mental disease, for example. Preliminary studies with desipramine suggest that the precise control of plasma levels may be important in facilitating the screening of psychiatric drugs and increasing their effectiveness. Hammer and Sjoqvist (1967) have given desipramine in a dose of 25 mg every 8 hours to 15 patients. Their preliminary results are as follows: 1) desipramine accumulated in the body for periods varying from 1 to 16 days, the peak plasma levels ranging from 10 to 275 μg/liter and the biological half-life of the drug, determined from the slope of the decline in plasma level after discontinuing the medication, from a few hours to more than 2 days; 2) individual patients showed the same rate of drug inactivation when given the drug a month later; 3) disturbing side effects, including dizziness and orthostatic hypotension, occurred only in the three patients in whom plasma levels exceeded 100 mg/liter; 4) the plasma levels of desipramine were reduced by 50 % in a patient treated with phenobarbital (100 mg a day for 24 days). Studies are now in progress to relate the therapeutic effects to the plasma level of the drug.

E. Rational Regimen of Therapy

Detailed information about the physiological disposition of drugs in man must be readily available to help clinicians prescribe dosage schedules which will provide optimal efficacy and minimal risk of toxicity. The time is approaching when it may be necessary to calculate regimens for certain drugs for each individual patient. As drugs become more effective and similar in structure to natural substances, they also become more toxic. If this trend continues, it will be difficult to take advantage of the more potent and effective agents unless dosage schedules are individualized according to the biological half-life. It must be emphasized, however, that such dosage regimens would be valid only for drugs whose therapeutic effects are related to the plasma level and would not apply to "hit-and-run" drugs, such as reserpine, alkylating agents, and monoamine oxidase inhibitors.

Recently, Jelliffe (1968) has devised a practical regimen for digoxin therapy based on simple pharmacological kinetics. After absorption from the gastrointestinal tract, digoxin declines exponentially in plasma, urine, myocardium, liver and kidney with a half-life of about 1.6 days, corresponding to a loss of 35 % the total body store of glycoside per day. Assuming the patient was given the proper loading dose, which depends upon the volume of distribution, he will require a daily maintenance dose equal to 35% of the loading dose in order to maintain the steady-state level of digoxin. On this regimen the total body level of digoxin (which correlates well with the level in myocardium) will vary by no more than 35%. To attain a steady-state level by administering only a daily maintenance dose of digoxin without a loading dose would require about 5 half-lives of the drug.

Since renal function is the major determinant of the half-life of digoxin, one can correlate the daily maintenance dose, expressed as a percent of the loading dose, with the creatinine clearance (or blood urea nitrogen). Thus, in anuric patients the maintenance dose will be 14% of the loading dose instead of the 35% in patients with a normal creatinine clearance of 105 ml/min. The half-times of H^3-digoxin measured in 10 patients fell within ± 2 standard deviations of the half-times predicted from the patients' creatinine clearance. Thus, in the case of digoxin, the creatinine clearance may be used as a first approximation of the plasma level to regulate dosages of a drug which often produces toxicity in patients with wide fluctuations in renal function. In the relatively small number of patients treated by this method, the incidence of digoxin toxicity has been reduced by approximately two-thirds (R. W. Jelliffe, personal communication).

These results underline the importance of placing a greater reliance upon plasma levels rather than on pharmacological response alone as a guide to a more enlightened approach to drug therapy. Similar pharmacokinetics describe the plasma level of the antibiotic kanamycin in man (Orme and Cutler, 1969). The same kinetic principles illustrated by digoxin also apply to drugs which undergo extensive metabolism rather than excretion, although somewhat greater difficulties may be encountered with the latter due to the large number of factors which may influence the activity of microsomal enzyme systems.

V. CONCLUSION

The prediction of untoward responses from animal studies still remains a crucial problem. Although there are vast individual and species variations in the metabolism of a large number of pharmacodynamic agents, in many instances the pharmacological responses are similar for equal plasma levels of drug. This suggests that receptors for this type of drug may be quite similar in various mammalian species. The practical implications of this concept point to a greater reliance upon plasma levels rather than pharmacological response alone as a guide to a more enlightened approach to drug therapy in man and to screening tests in animals.

REFERENCES

Axelrod, J.: Studies on sympathomimetic amines. I. The biotransformation and physiological disposition of l-ephedrine and l-norepinephrine. J. Pharmacol. Exp. Ther. *109:* 62–73, 1953.

Berliner, R. W.: Evaluation of new drugs affecting the kidney. In *Proceedings of the Second International Pharmacological Meeting*, ed. by E. Zaimis, vol. 8, pp. 123–128, Pergamon Press, Oxford, 1965.

Beyer, K. H., Baer, J. E., Michaelson, J. K., and Russo, H. E.: Renotropic charac-teristics of ethacrynic acid: a phenoxy-acetic saluretic-diuretic agent. J. Pharma-col. Exp. Ther. *147:* 1–22, 1965.

Brodie, B. B.: Distribution and fate of drugs; therapeutic implications. In *Absorption and Distribution of Drugs*, ed. by T. B. Binns, pp. 199–251, Williams & Wilkins, Baltimore, 1964.

Brodie, B. B.: Some ideas on the mode of action of imipramine type antidepres-sants. In *The Scientific Basis of Drug Therapy in Psychiatry*, ed. by J. Marks and C. M. B. Pare, pp. 127–146, Pergamon Press, New York, 1965.

Brodie, B. B., Aronow, L., and Axelrod, J.: The fate of benzazoline (Priscoline) in dog and man and a method for its estimation in biological material. J. Pharmacol. Exp. Ther. *106:* 200–207, 1952.

Brodie, B. B. and Axelrod, J.: The fate of acetophenetidin (phenacetin) in man and methods for the estimation of acetophenetidin and its metabolites in biological material. J. Pharmacol. Exp. Ther. *97:* 58–67, 1949.

Brodie, B. B. and Maickel, R. P.: Comparative biochemistry of drug metabolism. In *Proceedings of the First International Pharmacological Meeting*, ed. by B. B. Brodie and E. G. Erdos, vol. 6, pp. 299–324, Pergamon Press, Oxford, 1962.

Burns, J. J.: Species differences and individual variation in drug metabolism. In *Proceedings of the First International Pharmacological Meeting*, ed. by B. B. Brodie, and E. G. Erdos, vol. 6, pp. 277–288, Pergamon Press, Oxford, 1962.

Burns, J. J.: Value of metabolic studies in the evaluation of new drugs in man. In *Evaluation of New Drugs in Man*, ed. by E. Zaimis, pp 21–30, Pergamon Press, Oxford, 1965.

Burns, J. J., Berger, B. L., Lief, P. A., Woolack, A., Papper, E. M., and Brodie, B. B.: The physiological disposition and fate of meperidine (Demerol) in man and a method for its estimation in plasma. J. Pharmacol. Exp. Ther. *114:* 289–298, 1955.

Burns, J. J., Weiner, M., Simson, G., and Brodie, B. B.: The biotransformation of ethyl biscoumacatate (Tromexan) in man, rabbit and dog. J. Pharmacol. Exp. Ther. *108:* 33–41, 1953.

Conney, A. H., Sanbur, M., Soroko, F., Koster, R., and Burns, J. J.: Enzyme induction and inhibition in studies on the pharmacological actions of acetophenetidin. J. Pharmacol. Exp. Ther. *151:* 133–138, 1966.

Curry, S. H.: Determination of nanogram quantities of chlorpromazine and some of its metabolites in plasma using gas-liquid chromatography with an electron-capture detector. Anal. Chem. *40:* 1251–1255, 1968.

Curry, S. H. and Marshall, J. H. L.: Plasma levels of chlorpromazine and some of its relatively non-polar metabolites in psychiatric patients. Life Sci. *7:* 9–17, 1968.

Dingell, J. V., Sulser, F., and Gillette, J. R.: Species differences in the metabolism of imipramine and desmethylimipramine (DMI). J. Pharmacol. Exp. Ther. *143:* 14–22, 1964.

Duncan, W. A. M.: The importance of metabolism studies in relation to drug toxicity. A general review. Proc. Eur. Soc. Study Drug. Toxicity *2:* 67–72, 1963.

Firemark, H., Barlow, C. W., and Roth, L. J.: The entry accumulation and binding of diphenylhydantoin-2-C[14] in brain. Studies on adult, immature and hypercapnic cats. Int. J. Neuropharmacol. *2:* 25–38, 1963.

Gastaut, H. and Hunter, J.: An experimental study of the mechanism of photic activation in idiopathic epilepsy. Electroencephalogr. Clin. Neurophysiol. *2:* 263–287, 1950.

Gillette, J. R.: Individually different responses to drugs according to age, sex functional or pathologic state. In *Ciba Foundation Symposium on Drug Responses in Man*, ed. by G. E. W. Wolstenholme and R. Porter, pp. 24–49, J. &. A. Churchill Ltd., London, 1967.

Gothelf, B. and Karczmar, A. G.: Distribution of intravenously administered chlorpromazine in cat tissues. Int. J. Neuropharmacol. *2:* 39–49, 1963.

Gsell, O. and Muller, W.: Parenterale Pyramidon-Pyrazolidin-Therapie von Rheumatismus und Infekten mittels Irgrapyrin. Schweiz. Med. Wochenschr. *80:* 310–316, 1950.

Gunn, J. A. and Gurd, M. R.: The action of some amines related to adrenaline. Cyclohexylalkylamines. J. Physiol. (London) *97:* 453–470, 1940.

Hammer, W. and Sjoqvist, F.: Plasma level of monomethyl tricyclic antidepressants during treatment with imipramine-like compounds. Life Sci. *6:* 1895–1903, 1967.

Jay, G. E.: Variation in response of various mouse strains to hexobarbital (Evipal). Proc. Soc. Exp. Biol. Med. *90:* 378–380, 1955.

Jelliffe, R. W.: An improved method for digoxin therapy. Ann. Intern. Med. *69:* 703–718, 1968.

Kalow, H.: Esterase action. In *Proceedings of the First International Pharmacological Meeting*, ed. by B. B. Brodie and E. G. Erdos, vol. 6, pp. 137–147, Pergamon Press, Oxford, 1962.

Link, K. P.: The anticoagulant from spoiled sweet clover hay. Harvey Lect. *39:* 162–216, 1943/44.

Muenzen, J. B., Cerecedo, L. R., and Sherwin, C. D.: Comparative metabolism of certain aromatic acids. VIII. Acetylation of amino compounds. J. Biol. Chem. *67:* 469–476, 1926.

Nador, K.: Ganglienblocker. Fortschr. Arzneimittelforsch. *2:* 297–416, 1960.

Orme, B. M. and Cutler, R. E.: The relationship between kanamycin pharmacokinetics distribution and renal function. Clin. Pharmacol. Therap. *10:* 543–550, 1969.

Quinn, G. P., Axelrod, J., and Brodie, B. B.: Species, strain and sex differences in metabolism of hexobarbitone, amido-pyrine, antipyrine and aniline. Biochem. Pharmacol. *1:* 152–159, 1958.

Reid, W. D. and Brodie, B. B.: Mode and site of action of tranquilizers. In *The Mind as a Tissue,* ed. by C. Rupp, pp. 87–122, Hoeber Medical Division, Harper and Row, New York, 1968.

Robinson, D. and Williams, R. T.: Do cats form glucuronides? Biochem. J. *68:* 23P, 1958.

Shannon, J. A.: The study of antimalarials and antimalarial activity in the human malarias. Harvey Lect. Ser. *41:* 43–89, 1945/46.

Shannon, J. A., Earle, D. P., Brodie, B. B., Taggart, J. V., and Berliner, R. W.: The pharmacological basis for the rational use of atabrine in the treatment of malaria. J. Pharmacol. Exp. Ther. *81:* 307–330, 1944.

Spector, S., Shore, P. A., and Brodie, B. B.: Biochemical and pharmacological effects of the monoamine oxidase inhibitors iproniazid 1-phenyl-2-hydrazinopropane (JB516) and 1-phenyl-3-hydrazinobutane (JB835). J. Pharmacol. Exp. Ther. *128:* 15–21, 1960.

Vesell, E. S.: Factors altering the responsiveness of mice to hexobarbital. Pharmacology *1:* 81–97, 1968.

Weiner, M., Shapiro, S., Axelrod, J., Cooper, J. R., and Brodie, B. B.: The physiological disposition of Dicumarol in man. J. Pharmacol. Exp. Ther. *99:* 409–420, 1950.

Weiss, C. F., Glazko, A. J., and Weston, J. K.: Chloramphenicol in the newborn infant. A physiologic explanation of its toxicity when given in excess doses. New Engl. J. Med. *262:* 787–794, 1960.

Yourish, N., Paton, B., Brodie, B. B., and Burns, J. J.: Effect of phenylbutazone (Butazolidin) on experimentally induced ocular inflammation. A.M.A. Arch. Ophthalmol. *53:* 264–266, 1955.

Zaimis, E. J.: Motor end-plate differences as a determining factor in the mode of action of neuromuscular blocking substances. J. Physiol. (London) *122:* 238–251, 1953.

Zins, G. R., Walk, R. A., Guesin, R. E., and Ross, C. R.: The diuretic activity of ethacrynic acid in rats. J. Pharmacol. Exp. Ther. *163:* 210–215, 1968.

17

Application of Metabolic and Disposition Studies in Development and Evaluation of Drugs

JOHN J. BURNS

I. INTRODUCTION

The importance of drug metabolism and disposition studies in understanding the action of drugs has been stressed elsewhere in this volume. Genetic factors account for interspecies and intraspecies differences in drug metabolism. Knowledge of drug metabolic pathways furnishes information on active and toxic metabolites. The stage of an animal's development determines the distribution and metabolism of drugs. The administration of drugs and other foreign chemicals stimulates or inhibits the metabolism of many drugs. The importance of these and other factors in the development and evaluation of drugs will be discussed in this chapter.

II. SPECIES DIFFERENCES

Species differences in response to drugs must be considered in the extrapolation to man of pharmacological and toxicological data obtained in experimental animals. The most important factor which explains species differences appears to be the variation in the rate and pattern of drug metabolism in different animals, but differences may exist in renal and biliary excretion, binding to plasma proteins, tissue distribution and response of the drug at its "receptor site."

Large differences in effective dosage between man and laboratory animals do not necessarily reflect a different sensitivity of the human target organ to the drug, but may depend on differences in the rate and pattern of drug metabolism. This implies that a given pharmacological effect might appear at a plasma concentration which is similar for all mammals, even though the dose required to produce the concentration may vary greatly from species to species. Observations with the muscle relaxant, carisoprodol, support this argument (Gillette, 1965). A 200 mg/kg intraperitoneal dose of the drug showed marked differences in duration of action (loss of righting reflex) which was 10 hours in cats, 5 hours in rabbits, 1.5 hours in rats and 0.2 hours in mice. Despite the marked differences in duration of action, essentially the same plasma concentration was found on recovery from the drug's pharmacological effect.

Studies with the anti-inflammatory agent, phenylbutazone, have pointed out in a striking way the importance of differences in drug metabolism among species

TABLE 17.1

Species differences in the metabolism of phenylbutazone

Species	Half-life
	hours
Man	72
Monkey	8
Dog	6
Rabbit	3
Rat	6
Guinea Pig	5
Horse	6

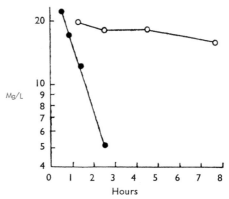

Fig. 17.1 Plasma levels of 5-allyl-5(2-bromo-2-cyclohexenyl)-2-barbituric acid in man (○) and dog (●).

(Burns *et al.*, 1960). Phenylbutazone is metabolized in man at a very slow rate with a half-life averaging 3 days (Table 17.1). However, in the monkey, dog, rabbit, rat and guinea pig, the drug is metabolized at a very rapid rate (half-life, 3–6 hours). Knowledge of the rapid rate of metabolism of phenylbutazone in the horse is of practical importance in view of the fairly wide use of the drug in the treatment of arthritic conditions in racehorses.

Information on the marked species differences in the metabolism of phenylbutazone has made it possible to demonstrate the drugs' anti-inflammatory and sodium-retaining effects in experimental animals. Phenylbutazone exerts an anti-inflammatory effect in patients with rheumatoid arthritis comparable to cortisone and, like the steroid, is capable of blocking the inflammatory effect produced by glycerin injected into the anterior chamber of the rabbit eye. However, in order to show this effect in the rabbit, it was necessary to take into account the fact that the drug is metabolized much more rapidly in this species than in man (Table 17.1). When phenylbutazone was administered intramuscularly to the rabbit in a dose of 100 mg/kg every 8 hours, plasma levels ranged from 100–175 mg/liter which are comparable to those obtained in humans receiving a total daily dose of about 10 mg/kg. Similarly, in order to demonstrate sodium retention with phenylbutazone in the rat, it was also necessary to administer the drug at a high dosage (150 mg/kg, orally) to achieve plasma levels of the same order as those which caused sodium retention in man.

A striking species difference was noted in the metabolism of the experimental oxybarbiturate derivative, 5-allyl-5(2-bromo-2-cyclohexenyl)-2-barbituric acid (Burns, 1962). In the dog this drug disappeared at a very rapid rate (half-life, less than 1 hour) and it had a fleeting duration of anesthetic action. However, when the drug was given to man, it disappeared at an extremely slow rate and its effects persisted for many hours (Fig. 17.1). Thus, studies in the dog did not predict the anesthetic properties of the drug in man.

Species differences have also been observed in the rate of metabolism of meperidine. The drug is metabolized in man at a rate of about 17 % per hour, whereas other species inactivate meperidine much more rapidly. The dog metabolizes meperidine at a rate of about 70 % per hour (Fig. 17.2) and the rat and mouse at even higher rates. This species difference, if also true for other analgesics, ac-

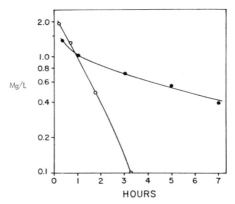

Fig. 17.2 Plasma levels of meperidine in man (●, 1.5 mg/kg, i.v.) and dog (○, 10 mg/kg, i.v.).

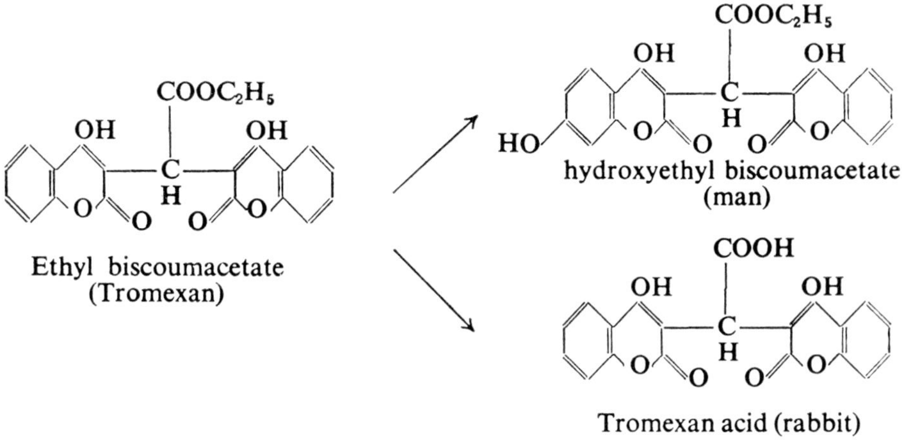

Ethyl biscoumacetate
(Tromexan)

hydroxyethyl biscoumacetate
(man)

Tromexan acid (rabbit)

Fig. 17.3 Pathway of metabolism of ethyl biscoumacetate (Tromexan) in man and rabbit.

counts for the difference in the interpretation of analgesic activity, toxicity, and addiction liability in terms of potential usefulness in man.

Ethyl biscoumacetate (Tromexan) is metabolized in man via hydroxylation to form a 7-hydroxy derivative that lacks anticoagulant activity (Fig. 17.3). However, in the rabbit, the drug is metabolized by de-esterification to a different inactive product. Despite the differences in metabolic pathways, man and rabbit metabolize the drug rapidly with a biological half-life of about 2 hours and, in both species, it exerts a brief anticoagulant effect. The dog, on the other hand, metabolizes ethyl biscoumacetate very slowly, so slowly in fact that pharmacologic studies of the drug in the dog would have given little indication of its short action in man.

Species differences have also been observed in the metabolic fate of the analgesic drug, N-acetyl-p-aminophenol (Welch et al., 1966). In man and dog, the drug is mainly excreted in the urine as a glucuronide conjugate (Table 17.2). However, no glucuronide of the drug was detected in the urine of cats. The failure of the cat to form glucuronides can be explained by the absence of the necessary liver enzyme required for the conjugation reaction. This may be the basis for the unusual sensitivity of the cat to N-acetyl-p-aminophenol.

TABLE 17.2

Metabolism of N-acetyl-p-aminophenol (APAP) in different animal species

Species	% of APAP dose in urine		
	Total Conjugates by acid hydrolysis	APAP glucuronide	APAP sulfate
Man	90	58	4.4
Dog	78	54	4.1
Cat	78	<3	<2

TABLE 17.3

Comparative half-life of drugs in various species

	Man hr.	Rhesus Monkey hr.	Dog hr.
Phenylbutazone	72	8	6
Oxyphenbutazone	72	8	0.5
Antipyrine	12	1.8	1.7
Meperidine	5.5	1.2	0.9

It has been common in recent years to consider that studies of drugs in monkeys may predict metabolic disposition in man better than parallel studies in other laboratory animals. However, this view has been questioned since, in many instances, metabolic data obtained in the monkey have been of no better predictive value in man than those of the dog (Miller, 1968). It was shown that the rhesus monkey and the dog metabolize phenylbutazone, meperidine and antipyrine much more rapidly than does man (Table 17.3). However, the metabolism in man of sulfadimethoxine could not have been predicted from its metabolism in any common laboratory animals, but it could have been if certain species of monkey had been used. (Bridges *et al.*, 1968). Sulfadimethoxine is mainly acetylated in the rabbit, guinea pig and rat, but in man and monkey (*Macaca mulatta*) the major urinary metabolite is a water soluble N'-glucuronide.

III. INDIVIDUAL DIFFERENCES

Marked individual variations exist in the metabolism of drugs which are handled primarily by enzymes in liver microsomes. Because of this variability some patients metabolize a drug so rapidly that therapeutically effective blood and tissue levels are not achieved while others metabolize the same drug so slowly as to result in toxic effects. For this reason, it is usually difficult to predict a clinical response to a given dose of a drug in any one person.

Considerable individual differences have been noted in the metabolism of the anticoagulant drugs, bishydroxycoumarin (Dicumarol) and ethylbiscoumacetate (Tromexan) (Burns, 1962). For bishydroxycoumarin, this may vary from a biological half-life of 7–100 hours. Similarly, the rate of metabolism of ethylbiscoumacetate varies widely in different patients (Fig. 17.4). In some subjects, drug levels remain elevated for more than 8 hours, while in others negligible levels were reached within 3 hours. The wide individual differences in the metabolism of these coumarin anticoagulants can explain why it is difficult to predict the dosage needed in patients to obtain a desired prothrombin response.

Marked variations have been observed in the metabolism of phenylbutazone in man. Following the administration of an intramuscular 800 mg dose of the drug to different subjects, rates of metabolic transformation were observed ranging from a biological half-life of $1\frac{1}{2}$ to 6 days. In view of this, the plateau plasma level of phenylbutazone which was achieved after 4 days of dosage of 800 mg daily ranged in different individuals from 60 to 150 mg/liter (Fig. 17.5).

Individual variations in the metabolism of diphenylhydantoin are an important consideration for adequate therapy with the drug in epilepsy. Patients re-

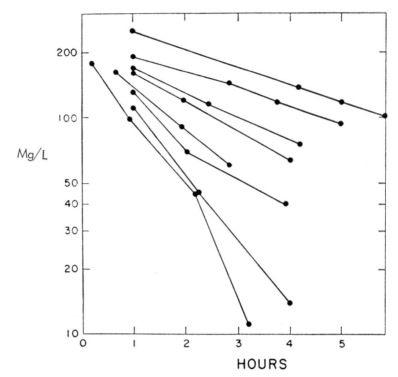

Fig. 17.4 Plasma levels of biscoumacetate after the intravenous administration of 20 mg/kg to various human subjects.

ceiving the same dose of the drug have plasma concentrations which ranged from 2.5 to over 40 mg/liter (Loeser, 1961). Increased incidence of side effects is observed in patients with high plasma levels and inadequate therapy may occur in those with low levels.

Genetic factors play an important role in explaining individual differences in drug metabolism. Evidence for this has come from comparative studies in identical and fraternal twins with bishydroxycoumarin, phenylbutazone, and antipyrine (Vesell and Page, 1968). Marked variability was also observed in the metabolism of antipyrine and hexobarbital among several inbred strains, but uniform metabolism was observed for individual mice of a given strain (Quinn *et al.*, 1958). A discussion of the genetic factors which control the metabolism of drugs is given in Chapter 15.

IV. METABOLIC FATE

Metabolic studies have led to the discovery of new drugs with a variety of therapeutic actions. Not only have some drugs been shown to owe their activity to metabolic products, but knowledge of drug metabolism has furnished the medicinal chemists with clues to new compounds which have more desirable absorption, excretion, metabolism, and tissue distribution characteristics. Present knowledge of metabolic pathways often permits the medicinal chemist to predict what metabolites may be formed from a drug. Examples will be given in this section which demonstrate how metabolic studies can be useful in the development and evaluation of drugs.

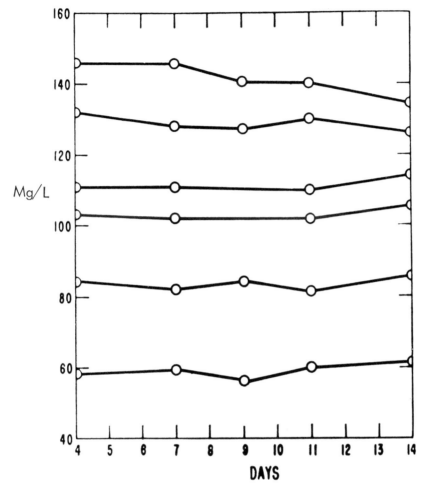

Fig. 17.5 Plasma levels of phenylbutazone after oral administration of 800 mg/day of the drug. Time indicates period from first day of drug administration.

A. Phenylbutazone

Metabolic data have been of considerable importance in understanding the action of phenylbutazone. The drug is metabolized slowly in man to two metabolites which accounts for some of its pharmacologic activity (Fig. 17.6) (Burns *et al.*, 1960). Metabolite I, which is formed by hydroxylation in the benzene ring, possesses the anti-inflammatory and sodium-retaining effect of the parent drug, whereas Metabolite II, which is formed by hydroxylation in the butyl side chain, accounts for the uricosuric effect of phenylbutazone. Metabolite I, now known as oxyphenbutazone, has been introduced as a new drug for the treatment of arthritis and gout. The observation that substitution in the side chain of phenylbutazone resulted in enhanced uricosuric activity led to the discovery of several other agents which have this action. One of these drugs, sulfinpyrazone, is a potent uricosuric agent for the therapy of gout.

Marked differences were observed in the biological half-life of various phenylbutazone analogs as determined by measuring the plasma levels after intra-

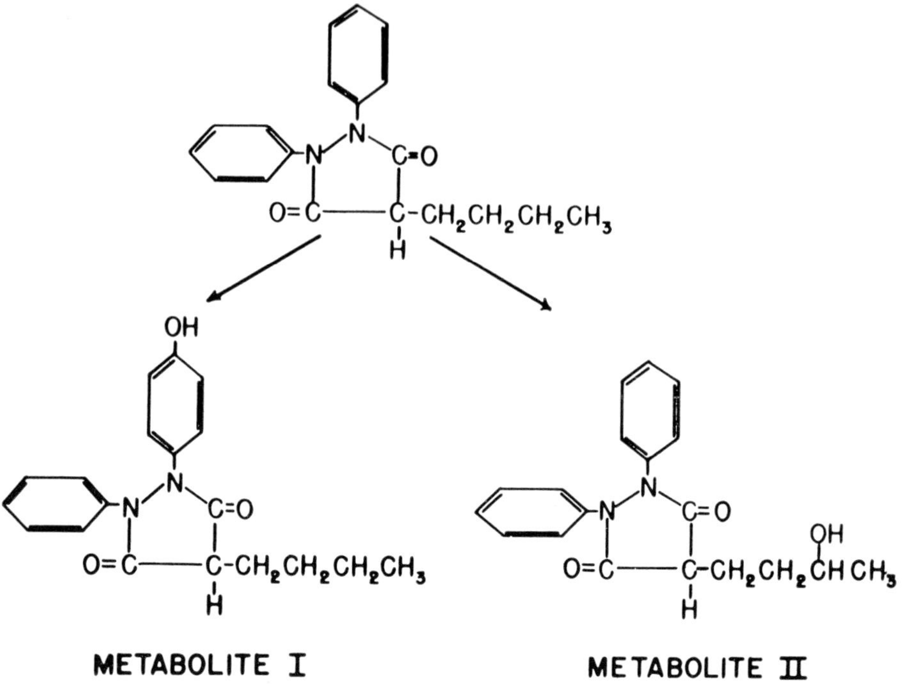

METABOLITE I   **METABOLITE II**

Fig. 17.6 Metabolism of phenylbutazone in man.

venous administration of 600 mg doses of the drug to human subjects (Table 17.4). It will be noted that the compounds disappear with a half-life varying from 3 days for phenylbutazone to 1 hour for G-32567. The striking difference in the rate of disappearance of two phenylbutazone analogs that possess similar chemical structures is shown by the data in Fig. 17.7.

The knowledge of how phenylbutazone and its analogs are metabolized has been of considerable importance in establishing proper dosage schedules for their evaluation in the treatment of arthritis and gout. A rapidly disappearing drug like G-32567 needed to be given at frequent intervals throughout the day to achieve similar plasma levels obtained with much smaller doses of phenylbutazone. In general, slow metabolism of a drug is an advantage since it allows more even control of therapy. However, it has a disadvantage in that if a serious toxicity develops, the drug remains in the body for a considerable time.

B. Zoxazolamine

The metabolism of the muscle-relaxant drug, zoxazolamine, was investigated in man (Burns *et al.*, 1958). Following the administration of zoxazolamine, no unchanged drug was detected in the urine of these subjects, but evidence was found for the urinary excretion of a metabolite in which the amino group of zoxazolamine was replaced by a hydroxyl group (Fig. 17.8). This metabolite, identified as chlorzoxazone, possesses muscle-relaxant activity and was subsequently introduced as a new drug. The major route of metabolism of zoxazolamine and chlorzoxazone in man is by hydroxylation at the 6-position as indicated in Figure 17.8. In early metabolic isolation studies, it was found that samples of urine from zoxazolamine-treated human subjects contained crystals of a sub-

TABLE 17.4

Rate of disappearance of phenylbutazone analogues in man

COMPOUND	R^1	R^2	R^3	HALF LIFE (HR.)
PHENYLBUTAZONE	H	H	$CH_2CH_2CH_2CH_3$	72
METABOLITE I	OH	H	$CH_2CH_2CH_2CH_3$	72
G-15235	CH_3	CH_3	$CH_2CH_2CH_2CH_3$	24
G-28234	NO_2	H	$CH_2CH_2CH_2CH_3$	20
METABOLITE II	H	H	$CH_2CH_2\overset{OH}{C}HCH_3$	8
SULFINPYRAZONE	H	H	$CH_2CH_2-\overset{O}{\overset{\|}{S}}-\bigcirc$	2
G-32567	$\overset{O}{\underset{O}{\overset{\|}{\underset{\|}{S}}}}-CH_3$	$\overset{O}{\underset{O}{\overset{\|}{\underset{\|}{S}}}}-CH_3$	$CH_2CH_2CH_2CH_3$	1

stance originally believed to be a hydroxyl metabolite of zoxazolamine. However, upon further investigation, this compound was identified as uric acid. This serendipitous observation furnished the first clue to the potent uricosuric effect of zoxazolamine which led to its use in the treatment of chronic gout.

C. Acetophenetidine

The major route for the metabolism of acetophenetidine involves ether cleavage to form N-acetyl-p-aminophenol (acetaminophen) which has been thought to be solely responsible for the analgesic activity of acetophenetidine (Fig. 17.9). However, this view has been questioned by recent experiments which show that acetophenetidine has analgesic activity in rats even when its metabolism to N-acetyl-p-aminophenol was inhibited (Conney et al., 1966). Acetophenetidine and acetaminophen are both converted to a slight extent to deacetylated products which are presumably responsible for the small amount of methemoglobinemia produced by these drugs in man.

Recent studies have shown that about 1% of a dose of acetophenetidine to man, dog and cat is excreted in urine as the glucuronide of 2-hydroxy acetophenetidine. Despite the considerable effort required, it is important to identify minor metabolites of a drug since they may be responsible for some of the drug's

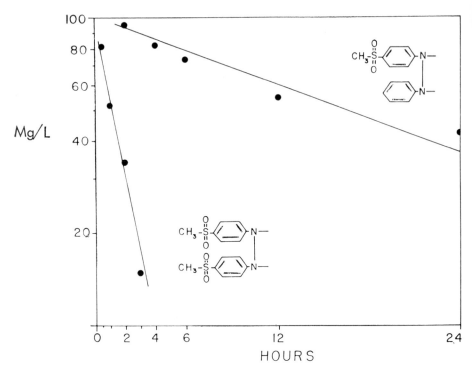

Fig. 17.7 Metabolism of two closely related phenylbutazone analogs in man.

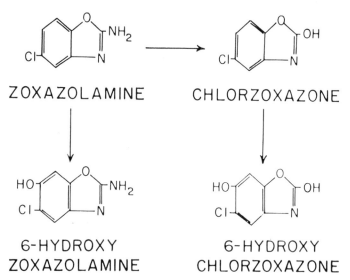

Fig. 17.8 Metabolism of zoxazolamine and chlorzoxazone in man.

pharmacologic and toxicologic actions. In this case, 2-hydroxy acetophenetidine lacks analgesic activity and does not possess any unusual toxicity.

D. Meperidine

Meperidine is inactivated in man by pathways involving both demethylation and hydrolysis (Fig. 17.10) (Burns *et al.*, 1955; Plotnikoff *et al.*, 1952). The drug

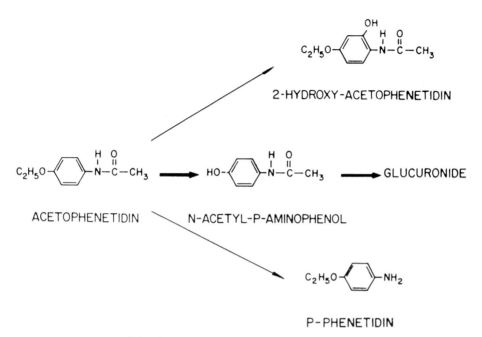

Fig. 17.9 Metabolism of acetophenetidin.

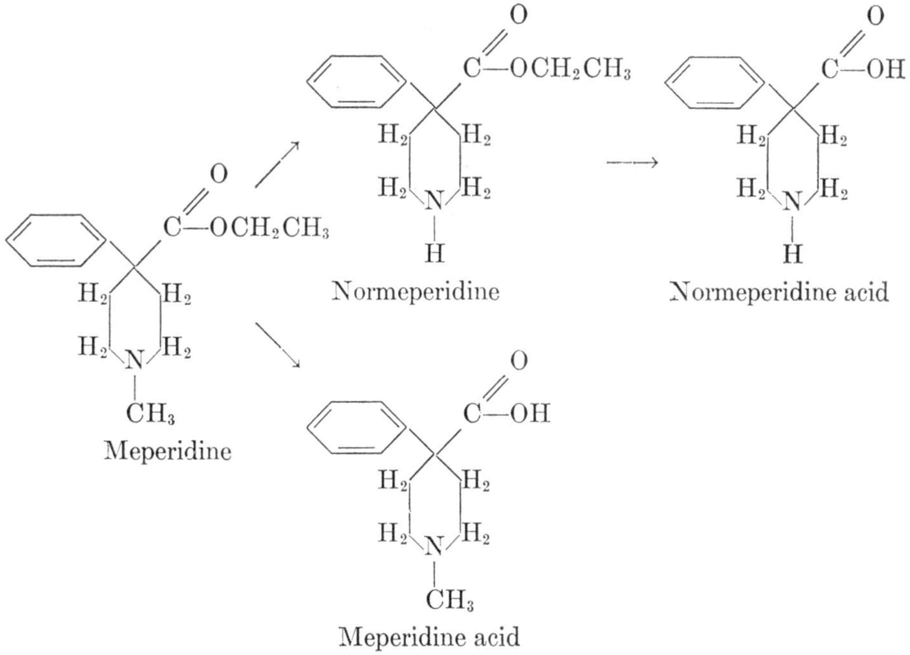

Fig. 17.10 Metabolism of meperidine in man.

is metabolized in man with a biologic half-life of about 3 to 4 hours, though this may vary in different individuals by as much as 100%. The relatively short half-life of meperidine explains the frequency with which the drug must be given to maintain relief of pain. Patients who have established tolerance to meperidine

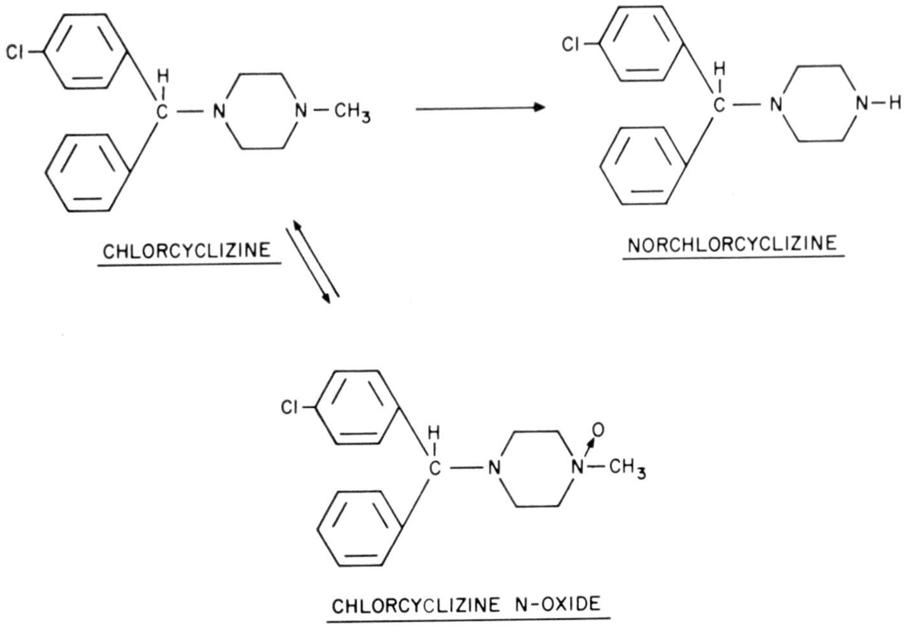

Fig. 17.11 Metabolism of chlorcyclizine.

metabolize the drug in the same way as non-tolerant individuals. It is probable, therefore, that in the development of tolerance to meperidine, the body has not acquired an increased capacity for its inactivation but rather that cellular adaptation must play a major role.

E. Chlorcyclizine

The antihistaminic, chlorcyclizine, is inactivated by demethylation to norchlorcyclizine (Fig. 17.11) (Kuntzman *et al.*, 1967). This metabolic reaction is of interest since norchlorcyclizine is retained in humans for at least 20 days after termination of therapy. Chlorcyclizine is also metabolized to an N-oxide which represents a new mechanism for inactivation of antihistaminic drugs.

Marked differences were observed in the rate of metabolism of the demethylated metabolites of chlorcyclizine and cyclizine, compounds which differ only by a chloro group in the para position of one of the benzene rings. Norchlorcyclizine is metabolized in man with a biological half-life of about 6 days, whereas norcyclizine has a half-life of less than 1 day. The slower rate of metabolism of norchlorcyclizine appears to result from its more marked affinity for plasma and tissue proteins than is observed for norcyclizine. The results in Table 17.5 show the greater binding of norchlorcyclizine to rat lung homogenate than that observed for norcyclizine. As has been reported for other basic drugs, such as imipramine and chlorpromazine, chlorcyclizine and cyclizine give very low plasma levels since they are both markedly localized in tissue, particularly lung (Fig. 17.12).

F. Coumarin Anticoagulants

Although bishydroxycoumarin and ethyl biscoumacetate have similar chemical structures, they differ considerably in the duration of their anticoagulant

TABLE 17.5

Binding of norchlorcyclizine and norcyclizine by rat lung homogenate

% Homogenate	% Bound	
	Norchlorcyclizine	Norcyclizine
20	92	71
10	86	54
5	78	40
2.5	69	31
1.25	58	18
0.625	36	8

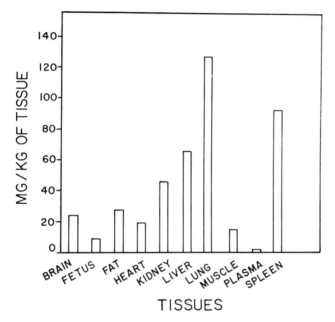

Fig. 17.12 Distribution of cyclizine and its metabolite, norcyclizine, 4 hr after a 25 mg/k intraperitoneal dose of cyclizine hydrochloride to a 15-day pregnant rat.

action (Weiner *et al.*, 1953). Bishydroxycoumarin is so slowly metabolized in man (half-life, 60 hours) that its anticoagulant effect is prolonged and dosage can usually be scheduled once daily and sometimes at less frequent intervals; however, ethyl biscoumacetate is rapidly metabolized (half-life, 2½ hours) and its effects last only a short time. The rapidity by which ethyl biscoumacetate is metabolized necessitates frequent determination of prothrombin time for control of therapy.

Bishydroxycoumarin and ethyl biscoumacetate are localized chiefly in the plasma compartment because of their high affinity for plasma proteins. In fact, an inactive derivative of the latter drug, Tromexan acid, is so markedly bound to plasma proteins that it has been used to estimate plasma volume (Fig. 17.13). The plasma volume obtained by the use of this compound agrees well with the value determined by the Evans blue procedure and that calculated indirectly from the distribution of labeled red blood cells.

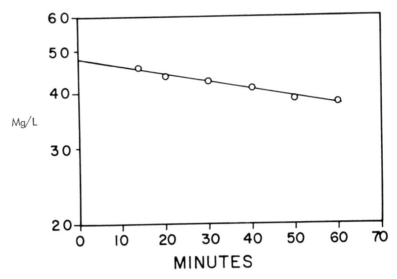

Fig. 17.13 Determination of plasma volume in a patient from plasma concentrations of tromexan acid (150 mg, i.v.). Plasma volume from tromexan acid, 3.02 L; Evans Blue, 2.96 L; ^{32}P-labeled RBC, 3.25 L.

TABLE 17.6

Distribution of N-methyl thiopental at various times in dogs

Times (hrs)	3	6	24	48	72
Dose (mg/Kg)	40	40	40	120	120
*Plasma	2.9	2.0	0.5	1.0	0.5
Liver	7.3	<2.0	<2.0	—	—
Brain	5.0	<2.0	<2.0	—	—
Muscle	8.9	<2.0	<2.0	—	—
Fat	71	93	47	87	21

* Concentrations in mg/Kg.

G. Barbiturates

The importance of fat localization of thiopental in determining its anesthetic properties has been discussed in Chapter 3. Introduction of an N-methyl group into thiopental results in a derivative which has an even more pronounced affinity for body fat (Papper *et al.*, 1955). Within 6 hours after a dose of N-methyl thiopental in dogs, the concentration of the drug in fat is 40 times the plasma concentration and, at 48 hours, appreciable drug is present in fat when the concentration in the rest of the body is negligible (Table 17.6).

Although thiopental differs only from pentobarbital by the replacement of a sulfur for an oxygen, thiopental has a much shorter action than pentobarbital as an intravenous anesthetic (Brodie *et al.*, 1953). When thiopental is administered intravenously to patients, the plasma levels fall off rapidly and then decline at a slower rate (Fig. 17.14). However, the plasma levels of pentobarbital fall off initially to a lesser extent, but subsequently the levels decline at about the same slow rate as for thiopental. The difference between the two drugs can be

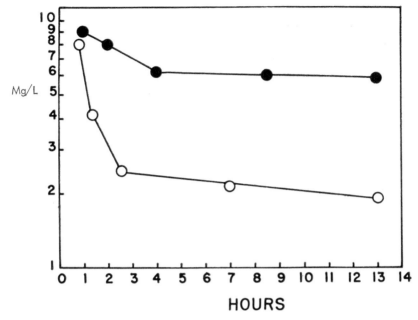

Fig. 17.14 Pentobarbital (●) and thiopental (○) plasma levels in same individual after 0.75 gms, i.v., in 7 min.

explained by the fact that thiopental is more markedly localized than pentobarbital in fat and this accounts for the faster initial decline in plasma levels. Accordingly, thiopental is short-acting since levels quickly fall below the hypnotic level, and this does not happen with the longer acting pentobarbital.

V. ENZYME INDUCTION

Administration of many drugs and other chemicals can lead to a marked increase in their own metabolism or that of a subsequent dose of another drug. As pointed out in Chapters 13 and 14, drugs exert this effect by inducing the synthesis of drug-metabolizing enzymes in liver microsomes. Enzyme induction is important for the interpretation of the results of chronic toxicity tests and explains unexpected drug interactions which occur in patients.

A. Chronic Toxicity Tests

Chronic adminsitration of drugs to dogs stimulates the drug's metabolism; some examples are given in Figure 17.15. In these experiments a test dose of the drug was given to the dog and plasma levels were measured. After chronic dosage (one to three months) with the drug, the same test dose was given again and plasma levels were measured as before. The plasma level of each drug was substantially depressed after chronic treatment, reflecting an increase in the activity of the drug-metabolizing enzymes.

To evaluate the importance of enzyme induction in chronic toxicity tests, further studies (Welch et al., 1967) were carried out with several of the drugs mentioned in Figure 17.15. A dog was given 50 mg/kg of phenylbutazone twice daily for 20 days and plasma levels of the drug were determined 4 hours after the morning dose (Table 17.7). It will be noted that, initially, plasma levels of

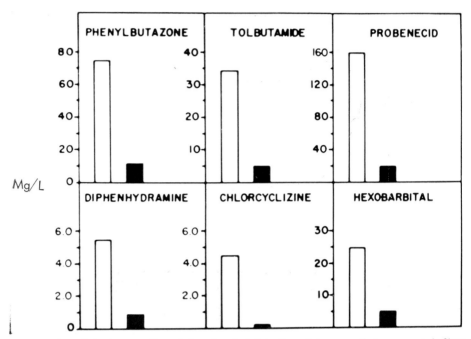

Fig. 17.15 Stimulatory effect of chronic administration of drugs on their own metabolism in dogs. Open bars represent plasma levels before chronic dosage and solid bars represent plasma levels after chronic dosage.

TABLE 17.7

Chronic treatment of dogs with phenylbutazone

Day	Daily Dose mg/kg	Plasma Level mg/L	Side Effects		
			Bloody Stool	Vomiting	Anorexia
1	100	102	—	—	—
2	100	—	+	+	—
3	100	—	+	+	+
4	100	71	+	+	+
5–7	100	—	—	—	—
8	100	28	—	—	—
9–19	100	—	—	—	—
20	100	30	—	—	—
21	200	60	—	—	—
22	200	—	—	—	—
23	300	120	—	+	+
24–29	300	—	±	+	±
30	300	59	—	+	±

phenylbutazone were high but they fell off considerably by the 8th day. Side effects were observed for the first 4 days but they disappeared thereafter. An attempt was then made to increase the dosage of phenylbutazone in order to restore the initial high plasma levels. When the total daily dosage of the drug was increased from 100–200 mg/kg and then to 300 mg/kg, plasma levels returned to the initial high levels by the 23rd day. Side effects of the drug again occurred when the dosage was increased threefold over the original dose. Even

TABLE 17.8

Stimulatory effect of chronic chlorcyclizine administration on its own metabolism in dogs

Day	Daily Oral Dose mg/Kg	Plasma Levels (mg/L)*	
		Chlorcyclizine	Nor-Chlorcyclizine
1–7	10	4.5 ± 1.7	trace
63	15	trace	8.3 ± 2.0
125	20	trace	1.8 ± 0.3

* Average values on 3 dogs.

at this high dosage, plasma level of the drug again fell off indicating the difficulty of overcoming the drug's enzyme inductive effect.

A similar chronic study was also carried out with tolbutamide in the dog. Marked reduction in plasma levels of the drug occurred after the dog received 100 mg/kg for 12 days. When the dosage of the drug was increased gradually to 300 mg/kg over a period of 10 days, plasma levels increased but did not achieve the initial values. At this high dosage of the drug, side effects occurred and the dog died on the 23rd day.

The results obtained in the studies with phenylbutazone and tolbutamide point out the difficulties in adjusting dosage of a drug to overcome the effect of enzyme induction; this was particularly manifested in the case of tolbutamide. Although the dosage of the drug was increased threefold, it was difficult to achieve the initial plasma levels. Serious toxicity developed at the highest dosage level of tolbutamide, which presumably resulted from the increased formation of metabolic products of the drug.

Accumulation of a metabolite was demonstrated after chronic administration of chlorcyclizine to dogs (Table 17.8). Dogs were given oral doses of 10 mg/kg daily of chlorcyclizine and samples of plasma were analyzed for chlorcyclizine and its demethylated metabolite, norchlorcyclizine. During the first 3 days of administration, the drug present in plasma at 24 hours after each dose was mainly chlorcyclizine. Chronic administration of the drug was continued and the daily dosage was gradually increased from 10 mg/kg to 20 mg/kg. Analysis of plasma carried out after two or four months chronic drug treatment revealed that chlorcyclizine was now present in only trace amounts at 24 hours after each dose, whereas norchlorcyclizine was found in significant amounts.

A good example of the importance of enzyme induction for carrying out chronic toxicity tests in rats is given in Fig. 17.16 (Welch *et al.*, 1967). Treatment of rats with a 75 mg/kg intraperitoneal dose of phenylbutazone twice daily for 14 days results in a sharp increase in the drug's own metabolism. This is shown by the reduced plasma levels of the drug which are observed at 14 days compared to the high levels found initially. When phenylbutazone was given to rats in a dosage of 150 mg/kg intraperitoneally, 65 % of the rats developed gastrointestinal ulceration within 24 hours. However, no ulcers were observed when the same dosage was given to rats which were treated chronically with phenylbutazone or with phenobarbital, which also stimulates the metabolism of phenylbutazone.

Enzyme induction has important implications in carrying out drug toxicity tests. The ability of drugs to stimulate their own metabolism upon chronic administration may explain the common observation that drugs become less toxic

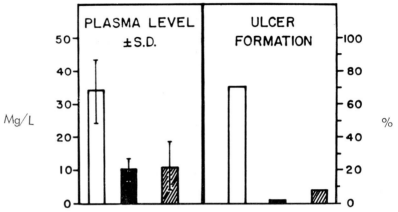

Fig. 17.16 Effect of drug pretreatment in rats on gastric ulcer formation induced by phenylbutazone. Three groups of 12 adult female rats were injected daily (i.p.) for 14 days with either saline (□), 75 mg/kg of phenobarbital (▨), or 75 mg/kg of phenylbutazone twice a day (■). On day 16 all rats received phenylbutazone (75 mg/kg i.p.) twice a day . Plasma phenylbutazone levels (left) and incidence of gastric ulcer formation, in % of total rats, were determined 24 hr later on each group of 12 rats.

during the course of long-term chronic studies in rats and dogs. The significance of enzyme induction to overall design of toxicity studies will have to await further experiences that correlate altered drug metabolism with drug toxicity.

B. Drug Interactions

With recent advances in pharmacotherapy, many patients are receiving several potent drugs simultaneously. During one hospitalization, ten different drugs may be given to the average patient. In the past few years, investigators have uncovered many instances in which one drug may profoundly modify the action of another (Conney, 1967). In these drug interactions, the effect of a drug vital to the patient's therapy may be prevented or, conversely, the action of one agent may be intensified by another to produce an unexpected adverse reaction. Many examples have now been reported of the ability of drugs to stimulate the metabolism of drugs and steroids in man (Conney, 1967).

Administration of phenobarbital to patients receiving bishydroxycoumarin decreases the plasma level of this drug and antagonizes its anticoagulant action. This effect has been attributed to the ability of the barbiturate to increase the metabolism of bishydroxycoumarin by enzymes in liver microsomes. The inhibitory effect of phenobarbital on the action of bishydroxycoumarin was observed in a patient who was treated chronically with 75 mg/day of the anticoagulant (Fig. 17.17). When the patient received phenobarbital daily for four weeks, in addition to bishydroxycoumarin, there was a substantial lowering of the plasma level of bishydroxycoumarin and a decrease in the anticoagulant activity. Upon discontinuing phenobarbital, the plasma level of bishydroxycoumarin and the prothrombin time returned to their original values. A similar effect on plasma level of bishydroxycoumarin and prothrombin time was observed when phenobarbital was again administered.

Experiments were carried out in dogs to investigate the interactions of phenobarbital with bishydroxycoumarin that can occur in man (Welch et al., 1969).

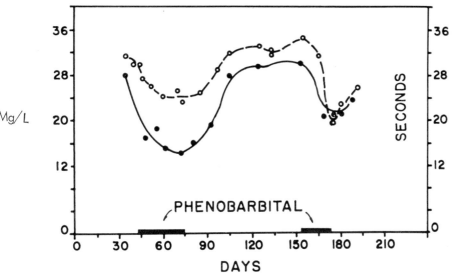

Fig. 17.17 Effect of 60 mg phenobarbital on plasma levels (●) of bishydroxycoumarin (Dicumarol, 75 mg/day) and prothrombin response (○) in a human subject.

Dogs were treated orally with 1 mg/kg of bishydroxycoumarin every other day for 39–44 days, and a constant prothrombin time and plasma level of the drug were obtained (Fig. 17.18). When the dogs were given 10 mg/kg of phenobarbital daily, in addition to bishydroxycoumarin, the prothrombin time fell to a normal value of 5 seconds and the anticoagulant drug was no longer detected in the plasma. Although the dose of bishydroxycoumarin was then increased seven-fold, the prothrombin time and plasma level of the drug were only slightly elevated. At this time, phenobarbital treatment was stopped but administration of of bishydroxycoumarin was continued. The plasma level of bishydroxycoumarin increased markedly 10–15 days after discontinuing phenobarbital treatment and all dogs developed severe hemorrhages.

These effects can be explained by a stimulatory effect of the barbiturates on the metabolism of bishydroxycoumarin. However, when another enzyme inducer, phenylbutazone, was given under the same conditions as phenobarbital, it initially potentiated and then antagonized the anticoagulant activity of bishydroxy-coumarin (Fig. 17.19). This observation can be explained by phenylbutazone displacing bishydroxycoumarin from binding sites on plasma protein followed by its subsequent stimulatory effect on the metabolism of the coumarin anticoagulant. Reports have recently appeared which indicate that phenylbutazone and other drugs which displace a coumarin anticoagulant from its binding to plasma protein, can potentiate their action in man.

Since phenobarbital and possibly other barbiturates significantly antagonize the effect of coumarin anticoagulants in patients, the dose of anticoagulant is often increased to maintain proper therapy. However, if phenobarbital administration is stopped, the rate of metabolism of the coumarin decreases and enhanced anticoagulant activity results with the possibility of hemorrhage occurring. Unfortunately, serious side effects have resulted from this type of interaction. These observations point out that combined therapy with a coumarin anticoagulant

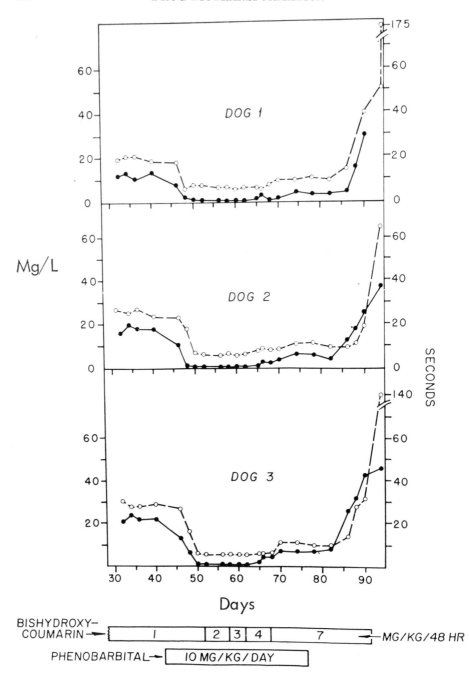

Fig. 17.18 Plasma levels of bishydroxycoumarin (●) and prothrombin time (○) before, during, and after treatment of dogs with phenobarbital.

and a stimulator of drug metabolism can be hazardous if the enzyme stimulator is withdrawn and therapy with the anticoagulant is continued without an appropriate decrease in dose. The studies in the dog given here point out a suitable animal model for the investigation of potentially dangerous interactions of drugs with coumarin anticoagulants.

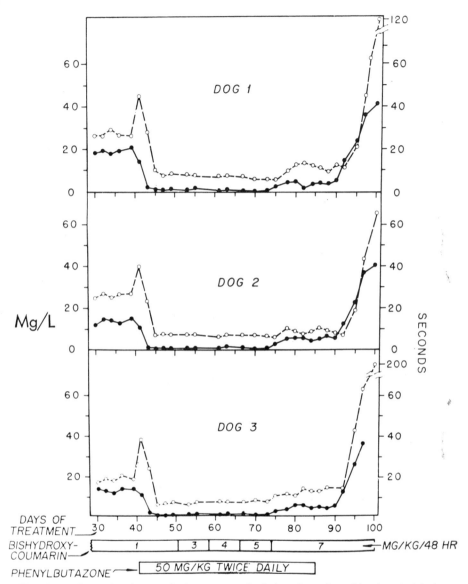

Fig. 17.19 Plasma levels of bishydroxycoumarin (●) and prothrombin time (○) before, during, and after treatment of dogs with phenylbutazone.

C. Tests for Enzyme Induction

Since enzyme induction has been shown to affect the pharmacologic and toxicologic action of a drug during chronic administration, methods are needed to determine whether exposure of animals to foreign compounds, such as drugs and insecticides, can cause an increase in the activity of the hepatic drug-metabolizing enzymes. Measurement of the half-life of a representative drug, such as antipyrine, appears to be a good index of whether or not enzyme induction results from drug administration (Welch *et al.*, 1967). An increase in the rate of metabolism of antipyrine was noted in dogs and monkeys receiving phenobarbital (Fig. 17.20) and in dogs receiving chlordane (Fig. 17.21.)

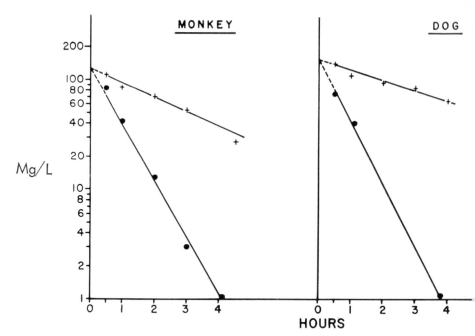

Fig. 17.20 Stimulatory effect of phenobarbital on antipyrine metabolism as measured by rate of decrease of plasma levels of antipyrine. Antipyrine (100 mg/kg) was administered intravenously and plasma half-life determined. One week later the dogs were treated orally with 10 mg/kg of phenobarbital daily for 21 days. The half-life of antipyrine was repeated 24 hr after the last dose of drug. The monkey was treated in a similar way with antipyrine (100 mg/kg i.v.) and then pretreated with phenobarbital (10 mg/kg i.m.) daily for 21 days before another test dose of antipyrine. Control values, (+); phenobarbital pretreated animals (●).

The enzyme inductive properties of a drug can also be demonstrated by determining the effect on one or more of the following (Conney, 1967; Mannering, 1968): (1) duration of action of hexobarbital and zoxazolamine; (2) activity of drug-metabolizing enzymes in liver microsomes, as measured *in vitro;* (3) urinary excretion of natural substrates, such as ascorbic acid, D-glucaric acid and 6β-hydroxycortisol; (4) amount of cytochrome P-450 in hepatic microsomes; (5) changes in hepatic endoplasmic reticulum (as viewed by the electron microscope).

VI. DRUG METABOLISM AND DISPOSITION IN FETUS

The emotionally charged situation following the recognition of the thalidomide-induced malformations created an atmosphere which stimulated governmental regulatory agencies throughout the world to institute requirements for animal studies in an attempt to prevent a recurrence. Teratological studies with thalidomide in various species of animals produced diverse results which made evident the dilemma facing the scientific community.

The difference in teratogenicity of thalidomide in various animal species may be due to interspecies differences in the absorption and metabolism of the dog. After oral administration of thalidomide in daily doses ranging from 25–200 mg/kg, the drug was found to be markedly teratogenic in rabbits, but only slightly so in rats (Schumacher *et al.*, 1968). Although there is virtually no differ-

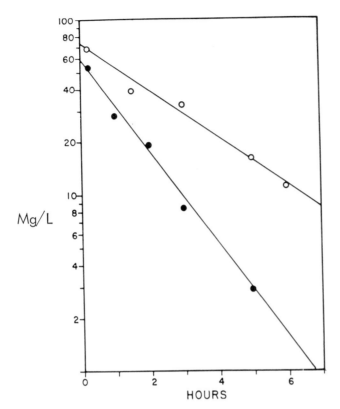

Fig. 17.21 Stimulatory effect of chlordane (5 mg/kg, p.o., 3 times weekly for 6 weeks) on antipyrine metabolism (100 mg/kg i.v.) in the dog. Rate of decrease of plasma levels of antipyrine is shown for dogs before chlordane treatment (○) and after such treatment (●).

ence in the biological half-life of the drug in the rabbit and rat, there are differences in the apparent rate of absorption of thalidomide, the rate of its conversion to metabolites in liver and the rate of the excretion of its metabolites.

Metabolic studies have been helpful in explaining the teratogenic effects of drugs in animals. For instance, it is possible that thalidomide owes its teratogenic effects through conversion to monocarboxylic acid metabolites which are formed from the drug after its passage into the fetus (Keberle et al., 1965). The polarity of these metabolites is such that they are only slowly released from the fetal membranes; therefore, they tend to accumulate in larger quantities than thalidomide itself.

The teratogenic effects observed after administration of large doses of chlorcyclizine to pregnant rats are due to formation of its major metabolite, norchlorcyclizine (King et al., 1965). The teratogenic effects induced by large doses of the structurally related drug, meclizine, can also be accounted for by its metabolism to norchlorcyclizine. Initially it was thought that the antihistaminic properties of chlorcyclizine and meclizine were responsible for their teratogenic effects. However, this cannot be the case since the active teratogenic metabolite for both drugs, norchlorcyclizine, lacks antihistaminic activity.

Although large doses of chlorcyclizine and meclizine can induce malformations in laboratory animals, no evidence of harm to the human fetus has been reported despite the wide use of these drugs over the past fifteen years. This fact points out the difficulty in drawing conclusions from animal teratology studies relative to possible risk in the pregnant female.

The importance of enzyme induction in carrying out teratological studies has been reported (King et al., 1965). When chlorcyclizine was administered to rats at an oral dosage of 50 mg/kg daily from the 10th to 15th day of pregnancy, a high incidence of cleft palates was observed. However, when the rats were given the same daily dosage of the drug from the first through the fifteenth day of pregnancy, the incidence of malformations was markedly reduced. Further studies showed that the actual compound which induced this teratological effect was the demethylated metabolite, norchlorcyclizine, which was present in the fetus in appreciable amounts when the parent drug was given from the 10th to the 15th day. However, when chlorcyclizine was given from the 1st through the 15th day of pregnancy, the metabolism of the parent drug and its demethylated metabolite was stimulated. Thus, the level of norchlorcyclizine in the fetus at the critical period of pregnancy was below that required to cause the malformation.

The inhibitor of drug metabolizing enzymes, SKF-525A has been used to investigate the teratogenic effect of chlorcyclizine in rats (Posner et al., 1967). When SKF-525A was given together with chlorcyclizine to pregnant rats, the concentration of norchlorcyclizine was markedly reduced in the fetus. In accord with these biochemical results, SKF-525A administration significantly antagonized the teratogenic effect of chlorcyclizine. Thus, these results further confirm that norchlorcyclizine is responsible for the teratogenic effect of chlorcyclizine.

VII. IMPAIRED DRUG METABOLISM IN THE NEWBORN

The newborn infant is more sensitive than adults to many drugs and, for this reason, obstetricians and pediatricians exert great care in administering drugs to the newborn or to an expectant mother during childbirth. The passage of drugs across the placenta after giving compounds such as barbiturates and morphine to the mother may occasionally produce anoxia and even death in the newborn. An explanation for the sensitivity of infants to drugs came from the finding that newborn animals lack the liver microsomal enzyme systems for the metabolism of many drugs, such as hexobarbital, aminopyrine, acetophenetidine, acetanilide, l-amphetamine, and chlorpromazine (Fouts and Adamson, 1959; Jondorf et al., 1959).

Impaired drug metabolism in the newborn results in prolonged duration of drug action. Newborn mice treated with 10 mg/kg of hexobarbital slept more than 6 hours, whereas adult mice treated with 10 times this dose of barbiturate slept less than one hour.

The sensitivity of newborn humans to chloramphenicol therapy has resulted in serious toxicity or death when infants were treated with dosages of antibiotic easily tolerated by adults. This effect of chloramphenicol in the newborn has been called the "gray baby syndrome" and can be explained by prolonged and elevated blood levels of chloramphenicol (Weiss et al., 1960). Other examples of low rates of drug metabolism in the newborn infant include the impaired conjugation of N-acetyl-p-aminophenol with glucuronic acid (Vest and Rossier, 1963) and the acetylation of sulfonamides (Fichter and Curtis, 1955).

Treatment of newborn animals with drugs can cause a rapid increase in drug-metabolizing enzyme activity and can also increase the level of glucuronyl transferase in liver microsomes. Treatment of newborn rabbits with phenobarbital for 3–4 days markedly stimulated the activity of liver enzyme systems that metabolize hexobarbital and aminopyrine (Hart *et al.*, 1962), and treatment of expectant mother rabbits with phenobarbital markedly increased the activity of the hexobarbital- and aminopyrine-metabolizing systems in the newborn. Treatment of pregnant rats with chloroquine, or chlorcyclizine, stimulated bilirubin glucuronide formation in the newborn (Arias *et al.*, 1963). Barbiturate treatment also stimulates the liver enzyme that conjugates bilirubin (Catz and Yaffee, 1962). Further studies are indicated to determine whether the detoxification of drugs or bilirubin conjugation can be accelerated in the newborn by careful treatment of pregnant women or newborn infants with drugs that induce the synthesis of hepatic enzymes involved in the conjugation of bilirubin or the detoxification of drugs.

VIII. INVESTIGATION OF NEW DRUGS

Although many aspects of drug metabolism and disposition discussed in this chapter can be applied to the evaluation of a new drug, it must be decided how much of such work is meaningful at each stage in the investigation of a new drug. The nature of the studies depends on the type of drug, the stage of its development, and its intended clinical use. The need for such data in the evaluations of drug safety has been emphasized by the Food and Drug Administration (Goldenthal, 1968). Although specific requirements cannot be given for the types of metabolic studies to be carried out in the investigation of a new drug, certain recommendations have been presented by a WHO Scientific Group (WHO Report, 1966) and by the Committee on Problems of Drug Safety of the Drug Research Board, National Academy of Sciences-National Research Council (1969).

Prior to investigating the drug in man, acute and subacute toxicity studies (one to three months) are carried out in two or more species. In order to evaluate gastrointestinal absorption, plasma concentrations are obtained after oral and parenteral administration in those species selected for subacute toxicity tests (usually rat and dog).

Comparative studies on the rate of metabolism and excretion of the drug may be required to explain significant differences in its pharmacologic and toxicologic actions among species. This can most readily be done by measuring the rate of decline of plasma concentration after administration of drug. As has been pointed out in Chapter 3, some drugs give high plasma concentration because of localization in the plasma compartment, whereas others may give low or insignificant plasma concentration because of extensive tissue distribution. The possibility that a relationship exists between plasma concentration of the drug and its pharmacologic action is determined. A lack of relationship suggests that (1) drug acts through a metabolite, (2) plasma concentration is not proportional to concentration at "receptor site," or (3) drug acts indirectly by triggering an effect which no longer depends on the presence of the drug.

Plasma concentrations of drugs are measured during chronic toxicity studies to determine whether the drug accumulates on repeated administration, or whether enzyme induction occurs with a resulting fall-off of the amount of drug in the animal. If the drug or its metabolite accumulates on repeated administrations, toxicity may increase whereas if enzyme induction occurs, toxicity may fall off or disappear completely.

Detailed studies on the metabolism and disposition of a new drug are usually not carried out prior to its investigation in man, unless evidence is obtained for a major active metabolite or one that has a reasonable persistence in the body. The possibility of species differences must always be considered in deciding how many metabolic studies are necessary at this stage of investigation.

Clinical pharmacologic studies should give as much information as possible to facilitate further investigations with the drug. Knowledge of the rate of absorption, metabolism, and excretion of the drug suggests proper dosage schedules to show safety and efficacy in clinical trials. For many drugs, the ability to measure plasma concentrations in man is limited by the lack of a sufficiently sensitive and specific method. Newer physical techniques, such as gas chromatography, mass spectrometry, and radioactive isotope derivatives, allow detection of extremely small amounts of drugs and their metabolites in plasma and urine. Results obtained by measuring plasma concentrations may explain individual differences in drug response observed in the course of preliminary efficacy studies. Some patients may metabolize or excrete a drug so rapidly that adequate plasma concentration cannot be obtained, whereas others may metabolize or excrete the same drug so slowly as to produce high plasma levels and adverse effects.

Metabolic data obtained in the course of clinical pharmacologic studies should aid in the design of the additional chronic toxicity and pharmacologic tests required for further investigation of the drug. It would be preferable to select the species for chronic toxicity studies (six months or more) which have similar rate and pattern of metabolism as man. Although this may not be possible for most drugs, knowledge of species differences can still aid in the design and interpretation of pharmacologic and toxicologic studies in animals.

Upon completion of the detailed pharmacologic and toxicologic studies, the new drug is administered to a larger number of patients to evaluate its safety and efficacy. Further studies are carried out at this stage on metabolism, protein binding, enzyme induction and inhibition, drug interactions, and placental transfer. In general, the effort expended to study the metabolism of a new drug should be decided on the basis of how such information can be usefully applied to ensure safe and effective use. Upon completion of sufficient clinical studies, a New Drug Application is submitted to the Food and Drug Administration which includes all chemical, biological and clinical data obtained with the drug.

Investigations usually continue on a new drug even after approval of a New Drug Application. Certain adverse effects may not be discovered until the drug has been widely used. This is particularly the case for adverse effects which result from genetic factors or drug interactions. As has been pointed out in this and other chapters of this volume, metabolic studies are very important in explaining many of these adverse reactions.

REFERENCES

Arias, I. M., Gartner, L., Furman, M., and Wolfson, S.: Effect of several drugs and chemicals on hepatic glucuronide forma- tion in newborn rats. Proc. Soc. Exp. Biol. Med. *112:* 1037–1040, 1963.

Bridges, J. W., Kibby, M. R., Walker, S. R., and Williams, R. T.: Species differences in the metabolism of sulphadimethoxine. Biochem. J. *109:* 851–856, 1968.

Brodie, B. B., Burns, J. J., Mark, L. C., Lief, P. A., Bernstein, E., and Papper, E. M.: The fate of pentobarbital in man and dog and a method for its estimation in biological material. J. Pharmacol. Exp. Ther. *109:* 26–34, 1953.

Burns, J. J.: Species differences and individual variations in drug metabolism. In *Proc. First International Pharmacology Meeting*, Stockholm, Vol. 6, pp. 277–287, The Macmillan Company, New York, 1962.

Burns, J. J., Berger, B. L., Lief, P. A., Wollack, A., Papper, E. M., and Brodie, B. B.: The physiological disposition and fate of meperidine (Demerol) in man and a method for its estimation in plasma. J. Pharmacol. Exp. Ther. *114:* 289–298, 1955.

Burns, J. J., Cucinell, S. A., Koster, R., and Conney, A. H.: Application of drug metabolism to drug toxicity studies. Ann. N. Y. Acad. Sci. *123:* 273–286, 1965.

Burns, J. J., Yü, T. F., Berger, L., and Gutman, A. B.: Zoxazolamine: Physiological disposition, uricosuric properties. Amer. J. Med. *25:* 401–408, 1958.

Burns, J. J., Yü, T. F., Dayton, P. G., Gutman, A. B., and Brodie, B. B.: Biochemical pharmacological considerations of phenylbutazone and its analogues. Ann. N. Y. Acad. Sci. *86:* 253–262, 1960.

Catz, C. and Yaffee, S. J.: Pharmacological modification of bilirubin conjugation in the newborn. Amer. J. Dis. Child. *104:* 516–517, 1962.

Conney, A. H.: Pharmacological implications of microsomal enzyme induction. Pharmacol. Rev. *19:* 317–366, 1967.

Conney, A. H., Sansur, M., Soroko, F., Koster, R., and Burns, J. J.: Enzyme induction and inhibition in studies on the pharmacological actions of acetophenetidin. J. Pharmacol. Exp. Ther. *151:* 133–138, 1966.

Fichter, E. G. and Curtis, J. A.: Sulfonamide administration in newborn and premature infants. Amer. J. Dis. Child. *90:* 596–597, 1955.

Fouts, J. R. and Adamson, R. H.: Drug metabolism in the newborn rabbit. Science *129:* 897–898, 1959.

Gillette, J. R.: Drug toxicity as a result of interference with physiological control mechanisms. Ann. N. Y. Acad. Sci. *123:* 42–54, 1965.

Goldenthal, E. I.: Current views on safety evaluation of drugs. FDA Papers *2*(4): 13–18, May 1968.

Hart, L. G., Adamson, R. H., Dixon, R. L., and Fouts, J. R.: Stimulation of hepatic microsomal drug metabolism in the newborn and fetal rabbit. J. Pharmacol. Exp. Ther. *137:* 103–106, 1962.

Jondorf, W. R., Maickel, R. P., and Brodie, B. B.: Inability of newborn mice and guinea pigs to metabolize drugs. Biochem. Pharmacol. *1:* 352–354, 1959.

Keberle, H., Loustalot, P., Mallon, R. K., Faigle, J. W., and Schmid, K.: Biochemical effects of drugs on the mammalian conceptus. Ann. N. Y. Acad. Sci. *123:* 252–262, 1965.

King, C. T. G., Weaver, S. A., and Narrod, S. A.: Antihistamines and teratogenicity in the rat. J. Pharmacol. Exp. Ther. *147:* 391–398, 1965.

Kuntzman, R., Phillips, A., Tsai, I., Klutch, A., and Burns, J. J.: N-oxide formation: A new route for inactivation of the antihistaminic chlorcyclizine. J. Pharmacol. Exp. Ther. *155:* 337–344, 1967.

Loeser, E. W., Jr.: Studies on the metabolism of diphenylhydantoin (Dilantin). Neurology *11:* 424–429, 1961.

Mannering, G. J.: Significance of stimulation and inhibition of drug metabolism in pharmacological testing. In Burger, A., ed., *Selected Pharmacological Testing Methods*, pp. 51–119, Marcel Dekker Inc., New York, 1968.

Miller, C. O., ed., *Conference on Nonhuman Primate Toxicology*, Washington, D. C., U. S. Government Printing Office, 1968.

Papper, E. M., Peterson, R. C., Burns, J. J., Bernstein, E., Lief, P., and Brodie, B. B.: Physiological disposition of certain N-alkyl thiobarbiturates. Anesthesiology *16:* 544–550, 1955.

Plotnikoff, N. P., Elliott, H. W., and Way, E. L.: The metabolism of N-C^{14}H$_3$ labeled meperidine. J. Pharmacol. Exp. Ther. *104:* 377–386, 1952.

Posner, H. S., Graves, A., King, C. T. G., and Wilk, A.: Experimental alteration of the metabolism of chlorcyclizine and the incidence of cleft palate in rats. J. Pharmacol. Exp. Ther. *155:* 494–505, 1967.

Quinn, G. P., Axelrod, J., and Brodie, B. B.: Species, strain and sex differences in metabolism of hexobarbitone, amidopyridine, antipyrine and aniline. Biochem. Pharmacol *1:* 152–159, 1958.

Report of Drug Research Board, Committee on Problems of Drug Safety, National Academy of Sciences-National Research Council: Application of metabolic data to the evaluation of drugs. Clin. Pharmacol. Ther. *10*(5): 607–634, 1969.

Schumacher, H., Blake, D. A., and Gillette, J. R.: Disposition of thalidomide in rabbits and rats. J. Pharmacol. Exp. Ther. *160:* 201–211, 1968.

Vesell, E. S. and Page, J. G.: Genetic control of dicumarol levels in man. J. Clin. Invest. *47:* 2657–2663, 1968.

Vest, M. F. and Rossier, R.: Detoxification in the newborn: The ability of the newborn infant to form conjugates with glucuronic acid, glycine, acetate and glutathione. Ann. N. Y. Acad. Sci. *111:* 183–198, 1963.

Weiner, M., Simson, G., Burns, J. J., Steele, J. M., and Brodie, B. B.: The control of prothrombin activity with Tromexan therapy. Amer. J. Med. *14:* 689–693, 1953.

Weiss, C. F., Glazko, A. J., and Weston, J. K.: Chloramphenicol in the newborn infant. A physiologic explanation of its toxicity when given in excessive doses. New England J. Med. *262:* 787–794, 1960.

Welch, R. M., Conney, A. H., and Burns, J. J.: The metabolism of acetophenetidin and N-acetyl-*p*-aminophenol in the cat. Biochem. Pharmacol. *15:* 521–531, 1966.

Welch, R. M., Harrison, Y. E., and Burns, J. J.: Implications of enzyme induction in drug toxicity studies. Toxic. Appl. Pharmacol. *10:* 340–351, 1967.

Welch, R. M., Harrison, Y. E., Conney, A. H. and Burns, J. J.: An experimental model in dogs for studying interactions of drugs with bishydroxycoumarin. Clin. Pharmacol. Ther. *10*(6): 817–825, 1969.

World Health Organization Scientific Group: Principles for pre-clinical testing of drug safety. WHO Technical Report Series No. 341, Geneva, World Health Organization, 1966.

PART Three

TECHNIQUES FOR STUDYING DRUG BIOTRANS-FORMATION

18

Techniques for Studying Drug Disposition *in Vivo*

ANTHONY TREVOR
MALCOLM ROWLAND
E. LEONG WAY

I. INTRODUCTION

Drug disposition by definition summarizes the complex manner in which a pharmacological agent is handled by the body and so encompasses its absorption, distribution, metabolism, and excretion. In the preceding chapters of this volume, discussion is mainly centered around the individual processes which together make up drug disposition and the documented importance of this area in understanding the nature of the intensity and duration of action of pharmacological agents. Such considerations are the "raison d'etre" of drug disposition studies. The present chapter has an introductory function with respect to *in vivo* considerations pertinent to such studies. Also covered here in some detail are certain techniques not mentioned elsewhere, including practical considerations of solvent extraction methods and the application of relatively simple spectroscopic methods to drug analysis. Subsequent chapters in this section introduce the fundamental principles of various well-used techniques and illustrate the advantages and limitations by reference to practical examples.

II. CONSIDERATIONS PERTINENT TO DRUG DISPOSITION STUDIES

A. Scope and Objectives

While *in vitro* studies are necessary in order to understand the intimate details of any given process, ultimately such information must be extrapolated to the intact animal or man. In many instances information derived from such *in vitro* studies is only of limited predictive value, since it is often difficult to reconcile these findings with experimental observations in the intact animal. The problem is well illustrated by the relation of N-demethylation of narcotic analgetics to the development of tolerance, which has been critically reviewed (Way and Adler, 1962; Way, 1968). Although reduction in the morphine and demethylating activity of liver microsomal enzymes during tolerance development has been documented in a number of *in vitro* investigations, studies in intact animal, including man, indicate no decrease in the N-demethylation of morphine and in some species an increased ability to demethylate narcotic analgetics (Adler, 1967).

In vivo investigations present certain problems to the investigator. The most obvious of these are the choice of experimental animal, drug dosage schedules and the mode of administration, together with the appropriate times of sampling body fluids in tissues in order to obtain relevant information relating to drug disposition. Decisions regarding such matters are necessarily influenced by the aims and objectives of a proposed study, and it is of interest to comment briefly on the range and variety that these may exhibit. Perhaps the simplest objective relates to compliance with FDA regulations concerning new drugs and in this respect guidelines, albeit somewhat arbitrary, have been established (Lehman *et al.*, 1955; Lehman, 1959; Goldenthal, 1968). Here, information concerning the sites of localization of a drug and length of time it remains in the body is deemed essential. Of course, mandatory investigations of drug disposition in an animal similar to man have inherent complications that may influence *in vivo* considerations and there is some doubt that the charge itself is conceptually sound.

The difficulties of extrapolation of animal data to man has stimulated the search for "model" animals from which drug disposition information may be more easily interpreted. The aims of such studies are similar to those of any comparative investigation and hence pose different problems with respect to considerations of choice of animal species, dosage and mode of administration. In some cases, a proposed investigation of drug disposition may represent an ancillary or complementary study designed to elucidate a pharmacologic question related to potency (e.g., active metabolite) or toxicity. In this event, *in vivo* considerations will be more limited and in most cases relate directly to conditions comparable to pharmacodynamic studies. As a final illustration, the underlying motivation may relate more directly to drug design, in which disposition data is anticipated to have predictive value in terms of potential changes in potency and duration of action resulting from molecular modification. Such diversity in the objectives of anticipated drug disposition studies forces consideration of *in vivo* aspects in the present context to be of a somewhat general nature. However, certain emphasis is given to considerations relevant to pharmacokinetic investigations, since these are of particular interest to the authors.

Independent of the rate of drug administration or the animal to be used, the most fundamental objective is the same; namely, that the drug should reach its site of action at a sufficiently high concentration to elicit a pharmacological response. Most drugs are presumed to interact reversibly with their receptors implying an equilibrium between amount bound and that free in the surrounding biophase, the tissue fluids. Tissue concentrations of a drug are in most cases related to that in the circulating blood and accordingly a rise or fall in blood concentration will generally result in changes in pharmacological response. Pharmacokinetic investigations address themselves to the measurement of concentrations of drugs and the establishment of appropriate mathematical models to describe such data, with the aim of correlating these with temporal changes in pharmacological response. Comprehensive appreciation of what occurs following drug administration to either man or animals is possible only when pharmacokinetic analyses complement pharmacodynamic studies. A complete pharmacokinetic study is restricted in the human by the limited ability to sample tissues, with the exception of blood, urine, feces, and occasionally bile, and it is, therefore, necessary to undertake such investigations in animals.

B. Choice of Animal Species

Interspecies differences in drug response may be the result of both pharmacodynamic and physiologic disposition factors. Species variations in the fate of drugs have been demonstrated quite clearly with respect to metabolism. The fact that such differences do exist is of importance in view of the limitations imposed on the extrapolation of data from species to species, particularly from experimental animal to man. Consequently, preliminary considerations regarding selection of a particular species for disposition studies are usually influenced by both the practical requirements of the experiment and by assessment of the degree of permissible extrapolation that the resulting data will afford.

The more practical aspects of a proposed study, such as the number and cost of animals and their suitability for investigation of a particular system, can impose severe limitations on the choice of species. Indeed, such factors have been and continue to be the primary considerations in the selection of the rat as the most commonly employed laboratory animal in drug disposition investigations. Interestingly enough, such a selection is often more reflex than purely involuntary. If economic factors are a primary consideration, the possibility of utilizing a less costly animal species such as the mouse, by investing a little effort in improving the sensitivity of analytical methods, should not be ignored. Conversely, when analytical sensitivity is a limiting factor in, for example, studies on plasma decay of a drug, consideration should be given to the use of a larger and more costly animal species which will permit serial sampling. Such a choice may be more economical in the final analysis since more readily interpretable data may be provided with a comparatively small number of animals. However, it is not our intent to challenge the selection of animal choice from the standpoint of the limited predictability that is afforded by any particular species. Documentation of such issues pertaining to species variation appears elsewhere in this volume. It may be of greater value to comment on those features of drug disposition which appear to be similar, at least qualitatively, in most mammalian species and those aspects which, when different, still remain of predictive value.

Investigation of species variations in drug absorption have usually concerned comparison in the rate and extent of entry of the drug into the blood via the gastrointestinal tract, since the oral mode of administration is most commonly employed in clinical situations. Physiological factors influencing oral absorption (cf., Chapter 2) include transit time, gastrointestinal pH, presence of food, microbial flora together with the blood supply to and metabolic enzymes in the gastrointestinal wall. In addition, drug action itself (e.g., vasoconstriction, local irritation) can influence absorption as well as other aspects of disposition. Since the interplay between such factors can be anticipated to vary considerably between species, it is not surprising that dramatic differences have been demonstrated to exist in the oral absorption of certain compounds (Rall, 1968). The choice of a ruminant such as the sheep or cow, or even the rabbit for studies involving gastrointestinal absorption is particularly illsuited for the extrapolation of resulting data to carnivorous animals such as man. However, there is some suggestion that species variations in gastrointestinal absorption are less apparent in the case of more lipid soluble compounds. This is evidenced by the classic investigations of Hogben *et al.*, (1957) and Schanker *et al.*, (1957) on gastric clearance and more recent comparative studies on the absorption of barbiturates (Hume et al., 1968).

Certain generalizations may also be made concerning drug distribution. While the blood flow to a particular organ is one factor influencing the rate and extent of drug uptake, other factors relating to the properties of the drug, e.g., lipid solubility, molecular size, degree of ionization at physiological pH, also play a predominant role. The entry of various lipid insoluble or ionized drugs into the brain of most mammalian species is limited and quite comparable (Cserr, 1967), although age can play a decisive role particularly with respect to brain uptake of certain drugs (Kupferberg and Way, 1963; Way et al., 1965).

Most drugs are relatively weak organic bases or acids that are partly dissociated at physiologic pH. As has been discussed in Chapters 1 to 3, biologic membranes are more permeable to the unionized drug and relatively impermeable to the ionized species. Hence, the distribution of basic and acidic drugs becomes in part a function of blood pH (Wadell and Butler, 1957). Most organic bases after being absorbed rapidly leave the blood and localize in high concentrations in parenchymatous or reticulo-endothelial tissues (Way, 1953). Organs such as the lungs, spleen, liver and kidneys generally exhibit, within a few minutes after absorption, drug concentrations considerably in excess of those present in the blood. Brain, skeletal muscle, and other tissues also have the ability to concentrate organic bases, but to a much lesser degree. In contrast, organic acidic compounds such as salicylates, sulfonamides, p-aminosalicylic acid, probenecid, etc., are not taken up so avidly by such tissues and exhibit higher plasma concentrations than bases.

This distributive difference is accountable in numerous ways, each partially contributing to the overall effect. Many acidic compounds are largely in the anionic form at blood pH and generally have limited ability to penetrate cells, thereby tending to distribute extracellularly. Also, many are polar molecules and uptake into lipoidal tissue, e.g., brain and fat, is not favored. On the other hand, with basic drugs significant amounts exist at pH 7.4 in the undissociated form which favors cell penetration and allows their combination with anionic receptor sites within the cell, possibly nucleic acids (Way and Adler, 1962). Although the most prevalent plasma protein, albumin, has a net negative charge at physiological pH, many acids are more significantly bound to this macromolecule than bases, further increasing the plasma concentrations of acids (Goldstein et al., 1968).

Species variations in drug binding to plasma proteins is well documented (Anton, 1960; Rolinson and Sutherland, 1965), and the documented findings permit predictions that in general such interactions will be much more extensive in man than in other animals. Also, in almost all species investigated, moderately lipophilic drugs interact extensively with plasma albumin and highly lipophilic compounds are found to localize in fat tissues (cf., Chapter 3). The latter generalization is well illustrated by the ubiquitous and disconcerting occurrence of DDT in animal tissue fat. As a corollary, drugs that concentrate extravascularly, e.g., bases, pesticides, etc., have low amounts in the blood and consequently tend to be removed slowly from the body, particularly if renal tubular reabsorption is also characteristic. Hence, if metabolism of such compounds does not occur, their elimination would indeed be prolonged.

Comparative aspects of drug metabolism have been reviewed quite recently by a number of authors (Conney, 1967; Parke, 1968; Williams, 1967) as well as in Chapter 11. One can expect marked interspecies differences in the metabolic fate of drugs particularly if they are susceptible to microsomal enzyme systems. Indeed, it has been suggested that if one could exclude the variability of microsomal drug metabolism there would be reasonably good consistency between species in terms of drug disposition (Rall, 1968). Quantitative differences may be attributed in part to the level of activity of such microsomal enzyme systems in various species. However, it should be kept in mind that the rate of blood flow to various organs including the liver may contribute significantly to species differences in drug metabolism rates.

In general, the smaller the animal, the higher the cardiac output per unit of body surface area or weight. Hence, the liver of small animals may receive more blood and could metabolize more drug per unit time, even if there was little difference in the overall activity of microsomal enzymes per kilogram body weight. Differences can also be attributed to a relatively complete deficiency of certain drug metabolizing enzyme systems in certain animals. Classic examples are the inability of the dog to acetylate and the lack of the glucuronide conjugating system in the cat. More generalized and rapid metabolic reactions, such as hydrolyses, appear to hold qualitatively for most mammalian species. For example, the ability to hydrolyze heroin rapidly is a phenomenon shared by many mammals and the metabolic pathway for heroin in most, if not all species, is very similar (Way *et al.*, 1965). However, quantitative differences in hydrolytic reactions, for example, plasma cholinesterase activity, are well documented both between and within species (Kalow, 1967).

The excretion of drugs by different species has received limited attention with the exception of the notable variations between mammalian and non-mammalian species with respect to renal elimination. It would appear that the tubular reabsorption of lipophilic substances is a general phenomenon among the commonly employed laboratory animals. Since urinary pH influences excretion, particularly of weak acids and bases, it may be of predictive value to appreciate that herbivores usually excrete an alkaline urine and carnivores an acid urine. As discussed in Chapter 8, an elevated pH favors the excretion of acidic substances and the converse holds for basic drugs.

Extrarenal mechanisms for the excretion of drugs are discussed in Chapter 9. Although interspecies studies on biliary excretion have been limited, it is suggested that little variation exists in the handling of small aromatic molecules by this route (Abou-el-Makerem *et al.*, 1966). It may be of relevance to add that a correlation between polarity and biliary excretion is suggested since the most likely candidates for this pathway are organic acids ionized at physiological pH and bases containing highly polar groupings. From a more practical standpoint, it is important to note that where biliary excretion is of significance, the rat differs from many species including man, by lacking a gall bladder. Consequently, liberation of drugs into the gastrointestinal contents is continuous in the case of this animal.

C. Mode of Administration

Having made a judgment regarding the selection of animal species for study, the prospective investigator next turns his attention to decisions regarding mode of administration. Naturally such considerations are again influenced by the objectives of the study, but certain general observations appear relevant. In the interest of facilitating extrapolation of data from laboratory animals to man, it has frequently been assumed that the mode of administration adopted should be similar to that employed therapeutically. As pointed out earlier, with the oral route, one is immediately confronted with the problem of the marked species variation in the gastrointestinal absorption of many compounds. In addition, there are some practical difficulties to be considered with respect to oral administration of drugs to laboratory animals. Addition of the drug to the normal food or water supply can create enormous variability in terms of quantification of dose and time of administration. Alternatively, the use of feeding tubes, while potentially traumatic to both investigator and animal, is a more efficient means of assuring consistency with respect to the quantitative and temporal aspects of dosage. In oral absorption studies it is common practice to restrict food intake for 12 to 24 hours before drug administration to diminish possible interactions. Generally this is satisfactory; however, in certain species this procedure does not guarantee the absence of materials from the gastrointestinal tract. For example, large boluses can still be found in the stomach of the rabbit after a day of fasting (Chiou et al., 1969).

Parenteral administration is naturally preferred in studies involving drugs that are only poorly absorbed from the gastrointestinal system, or when interest is directed towards disposition events other than the oral absorption process. In standard pharmacokinetic studies intravenous administration, by virtue of its predictability, is the most favored route. While it may be technically difficult to administer a drug intravenously to the smaller laboratory animal, it is generally worth the time to develop techniques allowing this mode of administration. With practice, injection via the tail vein of the mouse or small rat can be accomplished efficiently and reproducibly. The problem of drug solubility is not insurmountable, since many acidic or basic drugs can be readily converted to more soluble salt forms. Even less soluble neutral compounds can often be dissolved in a water miscible nontoxic organic solvent such as propylene glycol or the low molecular weight polyethylene glycols. Despite the predictability of the intravenous mode, it is important to note that its use does not free the investigator entirely from obligations to consider absorption processes in view of the possibility of enterohepatic circulation of the drug.

Alternative parenteral modes require more caution with regard to the interpretation of kinetic information, but are often more convenient and almost as predictable as intravenous administration. The subcutaneous mode has been found useful in our own studies involving the administration of organic basic drugs to small animals. In addition, although intraperitoneal administration is used infrequently at the therapeutic level, it should not be discounted completely since it is easy and often provides rapid predictable plasma levels, especially if the drug is less susceptible to metabolic degradation. Under special circumstances direct injection of the drug into the central nervous system may be required. With the possible exception of the mouse, such procedures in unanesthetized animals necessitate implantation and permanent mounting of a cannula in a specific area of the brain. For such procedures, it would be prudent to seek the cooperation of a neuropharmacologist.

Occasionally, a drug may precipitate at the site of administration or may be given in such a form, e.g., sparingly soluble materials, such that rate of solution controls the rate of drug elimination from the body. In such cases erroneous information regarding the intrinsic speed of drug removal from the species is obtained. It is also important to appreciate that with the intraperitoneal or oral routes, most of the administered drug passes through the liver, and in the event of extensive hepatic metabolism only small quantities of the drug may appear in the blood (Boyes *et al.*, 1970). In such cases it may well be necessary to administer much higher doses than it would initially be apparent from intravenous studies. Clearly any such differences in dose required to produce a particular pharmacologic response via different routes of administration, are of predictive value in terms of disposition events.

D. Posological Considerations

Logically the dose of a drug used in disposition studies should be of the same order of magnitude as that required to produce the desired pharmacodynamic or therapeutic effect. In many cases dosage has been based on a kilogram per body weight basis, but there is some indication that it may be more appropriately based on a surface area measurement (Freireich *et al.*, 1966), since the latter more closely relates to the size of target and metabolizing organs. While animals differ greatly in rate of drug elimination, they exhibit quite marked similarities in distribution. Hence, an intravenous dose to a variety of animals, based on body surface area, may be anticipated to produce a closer correlation of the pharmacologic response between species, provided that each species has the same sensitivity to the drug in question. In the event of marked differences in sensitivity, it may be advisable to employ equipotent doses.

Administration by other routes, involving elimination simultaneously with absorption, will naturally effect the dose necessary to produce a given response. In general, smaller animals are able to eliminate drugs more rapidly and consequently require proportionately higher doses when a drug is administered other than by the intravenous route. Many drugs are eliminated by an apparent monoexponential function, which means that the fraction of a drug lost per unit time is the same at any point in its elimination. When this is the case, it is readily demonstrated that the duration of drug effect is related to the logarithm of the dose rather than dose itself, so that with increasing doses, the duration does not increase linearly (Levy, 1968).

In disposition studies, limitations in analytical sensitivity often encourage the practice of administering relatively large doses of a drug to an animal. This increases the likelihood of encountering saturation effects and altered disposition by pharmacologic action at such high doses. Dose dependent phenomena involving limited capacity process have been documented for all aspects of disposition including gastrointestinal absorption and metabolism, protein binding, liver microsomal enzyme activity and renal tubular and biliary transport (Levy, 1968). When such effects occur, the rate of drug elimination becomes independent of dose and may become reasonably constant (zero order elimination). Hence, the decline of the drug in the body will no longer be monoexponential and will exhibit a more complex function, changing with increasing dose. By the same token, excessive doses will also influence the ratio of metabolites produced and can alter distribution patterns of a drug. The problem can be alleviated if disposition studies are carried out at more than one dose level, one or more of which should be commensurate with the proposed therapeutic dosage range.

In certain cases it may be necessary to administer drugs to animals on a repeated basis as, for example, in chronic toxicity studies or investigations assessing drug induced stimulation of enzyme activity. In many cases, pharmacological response in a variety of animals can be shown to occur at similar plasma concentrations of the drug. Consequently, in chronic studies it may be a reasonable approach to attempt to establish the same plasma concentrations in the body of various species. To achieve this aim in animals that eliminate drugs more rapidly, it may be necessary to give more frequent and larger doses of a drug, than for those species which exhibit slower drug elimination. Estimations of reasonable correct multiple dosage regimens required to maintain the same concentrations of drug in different animal species can be readily calculated (Wagner et al., 1965; Goldstein et al., 1968). In this way a more rational basis for conducting toxicity studies in animals can be achieved than by arbitrarily giving the same dose per kilogram body weight or different doses to a variety of animals in a haphazard fashion.

Finally, a cautionary word with respect to dosage form effects on drug disposition. These can become quite marked especially in the case of relatively insoluble drugs which are often administered as suspensions. The suspension volume, nature of the vehicle and drug particle size are among the factors which can potentially modify absorption rate and hence drug kinetic patterns and perhaps effect the composition of drug metabolites.

E. Sampling of Body Fluids and Tissues

In the examination of drug disposition in the intact animal, the available sources for sampling body fluids and tissues are limited. Practical considerations restrict sampling to the blood and the more readily available excretory materials such as urine or the feces, unless the animal is subjected to surgical procedures. Analysis of expired air is limited to studies of volatile compounds or those drugs which are metabolized to gases capable of excretion via the lungs. Sampling via other excreted products such as salivary and mammary gland secretions, usually require specialized procedures for the collection of such material and for analysis of drug content which can be anticipated to be quite low. With few exceptions the sampling of body tissues, and in small animals this includes blood, can only be accomplished by sacrificing the animal.

In kinetic studies, to avoid individual variation it is generally preferable to carry out a complete concentration/time study in a single animal. This usually means resorting to the use of moderately large animal species, and in the case of plasma sampling, will involve catherization of a major blood vessel, such as the jugular vein, femoral vein, or the vena cava. Disposition events occur extremely rapidly following injection of an intravenous bolus and accordingly plasma sampling should be carried out frequently in the initial time period to avoid missing early phenomena. Concentration/time studies of plasma should not involve the sampling of more than 10 % of the blood volume of an animal during a complete study, to avoid the damage of hemorrhagic shock or causing hemodynamic changes which could give rise to spurious results. In carrying out such studies on a chronic basis, it is desirable that the animal be permitted to recover for at least one week before initiating a second experiment. In time studies of drug concentration in the tissues of small animals such as the mouse, it may not be possible to follow all the events in individual animals. One may be forced to use several animals at each time point in order to compensate for the variation in blood or tissue concentration that might occur.

Mass balance studies to determine the quantitative fate of the drug in the animal under investigation most often involve the collection of urinary and fecal materials. As with blood studies, urine should be sampled at frequent intervals to determine rate of excretion by this route. Measurement of a total 24-hour urine sample does not permit such analysis and indeed to sample urine adequately in a kinetic study it may be necessary to catheterize the animal. As a word of caution with regard to the interpretation of kinetic data, frequently the rate of urinary excretion of a drug may have little relevance to its blood concentration at any particular time. Urinary pH and flow rate may fluctuate with time, as may renal blood flow; and all these factors can alter urinary clearance of a drug, even if the level of the drug remains essentially constant in the blood.

The significance of differences in urinary pH between carnivores and herbivores with respect to renal excretion, has received comment previously. Hence, for precise estimation of urinary excretion of a drug, it is important to measure the pH of the sample immediately after it is collected. If analysis is to be delayed, samples should be stored frozen to prevent bacterial growth. The amounts of various metabolites present could be altered if the microorganisms are capable of metabolizing the drug. Decomposition of drugs by microorganisms may also occur in the gut. Moreover, analysis of fecal material may permit gross estimates only of the extent of absorption via the oral route due to complications of gastrointestinal metabolism and enterohepatic cycling. Estimation of the quantitative significance of biliary excretion with respect to pharmacokinetic studies can only be achieved by cannulation of the bile duct, a technique which has limitations, however, in studies which are not acute.

F. Conclusions

The foregoing considerations pertinent to *in vivo* studies on drug disposition introduce the new or prospective entrant into the field to certain of the preliminary decisions that he will be forced to make. The selection of species, dosage, route of administration and sampling techniques will depend on the objectives of his study. Perhaps it is not superfluous at this point to draw attention to the predictive value of knowledge concerning the physicochemical properties of the drug of interest. Similarly, the available information on the disposition of pharmacological agents of similar structure, which may be employed for quite different therapeutic purposes, warrants more than casual scrutiny. The less chemically oriented investigator is inclined to ignore such considerations, often to the detriment of his experimental design and occasionally, ipso facto, his ego.

III. SEPARATION OF DRUGS FROM BIOLOGICAL FLUIDS AND TISSUES

A. Introduction

The ability to separate drugs and their metabolites from biological samples is an essential requirement of almost all investigations of drug disposition. The extent and complexity of the separation procedures depends a great deal upon the nature of the investigation. A qualitative study designed to answer the question of whether a drug is metabolized and, if so, what is the identity of its metabolites, may involve complicated, inconvenient, and often costly separation methods. On the other hand, kinetic investigations in which drug concentrations may be estimated routinely, require separation techniques that are simple, convenient, and as inexpensive as possible without sacrificing reliability and accuracy. Independent of the final method of analysis, the most common methods of separation of drugs from biological materials involve extraction, adsorption, or precipitation. The major emphasis below is on practical considerations relating to sample preparation and solvent extraction. Further details of liquid extraction and chromatographic procedures are covered elsewhere in this volume.

B. Preparation of Biological Material for Extraction

The recovery of drugs from biological fluids or tissues by organic solvent extraction is occasionally lower than from aqueous solutions. Reduced recovery may be due to the influence of tissue constituents on the partition of the drug or to strong binding of the compound to tissue proteins or other macromolecules. Drug recoveries are usually higher and more uniform when, prior to solvent extraction, tissue samples are diluted 1–5 or 1–10 and homogenized using an electric powered blender or the conventional glass homogenizers. Diluted tissues suspensions usually result in lower "blank" values and often avoid troublesome emulsion formation.

When low recovery of a drug is due to high binding to tissue constituents, it becomes necessary to liberate the bound drug by employing protein denaturing or precipitating agents. The selection of the agent to be employed is generally determined by trial and error. Trichloroacetic acid in concentrations ranging from 1–20% has been found to be the most generally useful, although it sometimes may interfere with color reactions of certain phenol reagents. Sulfosalicylic acid, tungstic acid, are alternative protein precipitating agents, while freshly prepared magnesium hydroxide is useful for those materials which are unstable either in acidic media or subsequent to protein precipitation, are required to be extracted from an alkaline solution.

Occasionally, strong inorganic acids are used, usually to allow the extraction of acidic materials, and incidentally cause denaturation or precipitation of proteins. In this and the other cases, care should be taken to insure that drug molecules do not become trapped within or occluded on the precipitating protein. As recommended previously dilution of the tissue or fluid tends to reduce this problem, while if the precipitated material is not separated from the supernatant liquid prior to solvent extraction, then complete extraction of the drug can usually be insured by a more prolonged shaking of this suspension with the organic solvent. While not strictly solvent extraction, an equal volume of ethanol or acetone is frequently added to plasma to precipitate proteins and many electrolytes. The supernatant mixed solvent system is decanted off and by this method polar materials, e.g., para-aminobenzoic acid, which would otherwise be extremely difficult to extract with organic solvents, can be separated from plasma. The aqueous-organic phase can then be evaporated and reconstituted with a suitable organic solvent.

After precipitation of the protein and **centrifugation**, the drug may be largely present in the supernatant phase. If **good drug recovery** can be obtained from the supernate, this is advantageous **for handling**, since emulsion formation during extraction procedures may be **minimized**. Unfortunately, it is difficult to predict which substances will appear **solely in the** supernate. In the case of the narcotic analgesics, after precipitation of **tissue proteins** with trichloroacetic acid, morphine appears largely in the supernate **but with** the closely related surrogate, methadone, removal of the compound **by solvent** extraction can only be achieved by subjecting both the supernate and the **precipitated** fractions to organic solvent extraction (Way *et al.*, 1949). In the **case of certain** bases, such as amphetamine, lidocaine, etc., which are stable in **strong base**, tissues samples can be dissolved directly in 4 % sodium hydroxide solution **by slight** warming, and in this way avoid the problem of precipitation of **proteins**.

The following dilution procedures have **been** found suitable for many drugs:

urine: dilute 1:4 in water

plasma: dilute 1:5 with water, and, if **required**, with 5 % trichloroacetic acid

whole blood: dilute 1:5 with 5 % **trichloroacetic** acid

organs: following homogenization in **water to make** a 1:5 suspension, dilute to 1:10 with 10 % trichloroacetic acid

feces: soak in water, then shake and **dilute 1:50** with water or 5 % trichloroacetic acid

C. Influence of pH on Extraction

The pH at which solvent extraction **techniques** are applied to separate organic compounds on biological samples is of **some importance** and depending upon the drug, can be critical. Organic bases **are more readily** extracted by solvents from alkaline solution and as a general rule **this should** be effected at the lowest pH that permits quantitative recovery. **This can minimize** the extraction of naturally occurring basic substances and drug **metabolites** that might interfere with the analytical procedure. In certain cases **excessive alkalinity** is undesirable because the compound of interest may undergo **hydrolysis** or molecular rearrangement at high pH values.

The percentage of any drug that is **extracted** at a given pH will depend on the pKa of a compound and the partition **coefficient** of the unionized species between the two immiscible liquids. **Many drugs** have high partition coefficients and can often be extracted at several **pH units** below their pKa value. Thus, lidocaine (pKa 7.9) can readily be **extracted directly** from plasma (pH 7.4) into ether, without having to make the **sample basic**. On the other hand, their metabolites are usually less readily **extracted** and by a suitable use of pH, closely related drugs and metabolites **can be separated**.

Frequently, the problem arises of **interference** in the analytical method by naturally occurring materials in the **biological sample**. Should this occur, one effective way of eliminating these **contaminants is** to subject the solvent extract of the drug to a series of washes with **a buffer** solution which removes these contaminants but not the drug of **interest. The** selection of the appropriate buffers involves a somewhat empirical **approach**. However, it is important to recognize that buffer washes can **influence** extraction negatively, if, due to solubility in the solvent they change the **pH and hence** the partition of the drug.

In the case of acidic drugs, as with bases, a pH extraction profile of the drug can be established in a variety of buffer solutions with the organic solvents under study. The optimum pH is selected on the basis of quantitative extraction with concomitant low blank values. Again, such an optimum pH may be quite different from the pKa of the acid, for example, good partitioning of the barbiturates, with low "blank" values, can be effected at pH 7.4 despite extensive ionization. However, great care must be taken in the selection of the pH used in the extraction of labile acids. Thus, acetylsalicylic acid is best extracted into ether at pH 2.2. At this pH precipitation of proteins occurs, the stability of this drug is at an optimum, and effective recovery of this drug into the organic phase is achieved (Rowland and Riegelman, 1967).

Recovery of amphoteric compounds from biologic media is generally optimal at the isoelectric point, but there are exceptions to the rule. A striking example is morphine (pKa 9.85). The extraction of this narcotic from aqueous solution with organic solvents is generally performed between a pH of 8 to 10, but high recoveries of the drug from urine were also obtained by extraction after alkalinization with 16 N KOH. Moreover, the extraction procedure yielded much lower urine blanks in comparison with the conventional extraction procedure performed at about pH 9 (Fujimoto et al., 1954).

The purity of certain solvents may require consideration especially with regard to subsequent analysis of drugs by fluorometric or spectrophotometric techniques and this may necessitate alternate acid/base washings and sometimes redistillation should high "blanks" present a problem. In relation to the subsequent analytical method, it is pertinent to consider boiling point and water solubility. If solvent has to be removed from drug sample prior to analysis, boiling points less than 100°C are obviously desirable, and the most commonly used are ether, methylene chloride, hexane, chloroform and benzene. Similarly, when prior to analysis the drug must undergo an organic reaction under anhydrous conditions, the extent of water solubility in the solvent may condition one's choice.

The use of mixed solvent systems should also be considered under certain circumstances. For example, the extraction of certain drugs into ethylene dichloride may be excellent, but "blanks" are often high and the density of the solvent relative to water may pose inconveniences. Addition of a non-polar solvent (e.g., cyclohexane) may maintain extractability but decrease the "blank" value and even add a bonus to the investigator by changing solvent density to a value less than water. Finally, a word concerning the time and vigor of extractions which in the reported literature is often far longer than necessary and appears to coincide strongly with the gustatorial habits of a particular laboratory. Obviously the shortest time period giving favorable extractability should be determined, and excessively vigorous shaking is to be avoided since this favors emulsion formation.

D. Other Practical Considerations

Organic solvent extraction of aqueous tissue suspensions sometimes results in the formation of emulsions. A few simple precautions can frequently reduce this problem. The tube used in the extraction should not be significantly greater than the total volume of the aqueous-solvent system. Also, in general a slow tilt-action shaker is most suitable in minimizing emulsion formation. Should emulsions still occur, they can often be resolved by simple procedures of centrifugation or filtration. The addition of sodium chloride or small quantities of detergents (e.g., Triton X 100) are often effective, as is freezing the system in a mixture of dry ice and acetone. The investigator should be aware, however, that these latter procedures can affect the partition of a compound and a value for "tissue recovery" should be re-established when they are employed.

Finally, consideration should be given to the necessity of repetition of an extraction step in a given separation procedure. In many cases the use of multiple extractions to effect complete removal of a substance is quite unnecessary. Precisely how exhaustive such extractions need to be depends largely on the specificity and sensitivity of the analytical method as well as the partition behavior of the drug between two immiscible solvents. A single extraction step which may yield 80 or 90% recovery generally will provide data that can be reproduced consistently. The use of single extraction procedures is particularly advantageous for the routine estimation of large numbers of samples and for analytical procedures based on the relative recovery of the drug. The sacrifice in sensitivity due to aliquot sampling and extraction losses necessitated by single extraction procedures is generally well worth the time that is saved. The reduction in sensitivity is generally about 40 to 60%. For example, with an analytical procedure requiring two extraction steps, if the extraction loss for each step is 10% and the aliquot loss for each sampling is 20%, then the total percent recovery would be $90 \times 90 \times 80 \times 80$ or 51.84%.

IV. METHODS OF DRUG ANALYSIS IN BODY FLUIDS

A. Basic Considerations

In the development and application of separation and analytical techniques to the determination of drugs present in biological fluids or tissues, it is essential to know the potential and limitations of the technique selected. The validity of the methods depends on the assumption that a drug added to a tissue dispersion will behave identically with regard to separation as it would if present in the tissue of intact animals. The logical development of the methodology should therefore include:

1. Determination of the characteristics (linearity) of the instrumentation used for analysis of drug concentration by construction of an absolute concentration curve.

2. Determination of a calibration curve for the total procedure by application to aqueous drug solutions to obtain "aqueous recovery" values.

3. Calibration of the *total* procedure by application to biological samples to which known concentrations of the drug have been added, to obtain "tissue recovery" values.

4. Determination of the specificity of the procedure with respect to interference from both endogenous compounds (tissue blank) and drug metabolites. This usually involves application of techniques different from those used in the separation procedure to establish that the desired compound has been separated and is being solely estimated by the analytical procedure under application.

There is an unfortunate tendency on the part of the less objective investigator to equate the reliability, and even the quality of a research study, with the degree of sophistication of the analytical methods employed. Newer physical methods of analysis, while characterized in the main by their specificity and sensitivity, often require an almost unlimited budget for instrumentation and a high degree of technical expertise in their application. Moreover, even with such elegant equipment, it is usually necessary to expose the biological sample to "clean-up" procedures, before the measurements can be made.

Fortunately, a number of analytical techniques, which combine simplicity with economy, are available to the average investigator interested in drug disposition and the most widely used of these are spectroscopic methods. In such methods, the sample in a suitable solvent is irradiated with an electromagnetic wave of suitable wave-length. Depending upon the molecule under investigation, absorption of this radiation will occur at a particular wavelength, resulting in an excited molecule. Either absorption of this light is measured as in the case of photometric or ultraviolet analysis, or the emission of light at a different wavelength to the radiating light is measured (fluorometry). Each of these techniques is readily accomplished in even the most modest laboratory and in many cases they possess a high enough degree of sensitivity. The following discussion concerns the application of photometric, ultraviolet and fluorometric methods to drug analysis.

B. Colorimetric Analysis

Perhaps the most widely used of all procedures involves the measurement of the light absorbance of a compound in the visible region of the spectrum (360 to 700 mμ). The popularity is attributable to many factors including long history, reliability, precision and low cost of instrumentation. Very satisfactory colorimeters using optical filters can generally be purchased for a few hundred dollars. Spectrophotometers using a prism or grating as a monochromator designed essentially for routine colorimetry are somewhat more expensive but within the medium price range (Rao, 1967).

Quantitation in colorimetry (and ultraviolet spectrophotometry) is based on the combined Beer-Lambert law which relates optical density or absorbance to the concentration of absorbing species. A more detailed consideration of the principles involved is included in Chapter 21. The validity of the law should be tested for each system being quantitatively studied. This is usually carried out by measuring the absorbance of a series of known concentrations of the compound at a particular wavelength and plotting the values against concentration. Generally, linearity between absorbance and drug concentration in solution can be anticipated for the normal levels of the compound expected in biological samples. Certain acids, bases and salts in solution may deviate from the law since they become progressively less dissociated with increasing concentration.

The majority of drug molecules do not possess intrinsic absorption in the visible region and it is necessary, therefore, to subject such compounds to procedures which result in the formation of a molecular species which does have this property. This is generally effected by reacting the drug with another substance to produce a more conjugated derivative that is colored. The type of conjugated derivative to be formed is dependent upon the functional groups on the drug. For example, the presence of a primary amine as part of drug molecule invariably dictates the application of diazotization followed by dye coupling procedures to yield a colored derivative. N-(1-napthyl)ethylene diamine or p-nitroaniline are commonly used to couple with the diazotized product. The first procedure, known classically as the Bratton-Marshall method, has been widely used and will usually detect aromatic amines at concentrations as low as 1 μg/ml. Tissue blanks are relatively low but the presence of drug metabolites with the amine moiety intact would necessitate modification of the procedure to exclude them in the manner discussed below for phenols.

The phenolic group of a drug is often used as the marker for estimation and a wide variety of phenolic agents are available for forming colored derivatives of varying color intensity. A disadvantage of estimating a compound by phenolic procedures is the high tissue blanks that are often encountered. Unless the compounds are ingested in relatively high doses such as salicylates, it is advisable to use methods other than phenol estimation. In a mixture of phenols the problem becomes even more complicated. However, it sometimes still is possible to assay two closely related phenols individually even if they are not completely separated by extraction procedures. By determining the partition behavior of the two substances separately under certain fixed conditions, the relative amount of each compound in a mixture can be calculated after determining the phenol concentration under each set of conditions and solving simultaneous equations which define the partition behavior. The two phenolic metabolites of heroin, 6-monoacetylmorphine and morphine were estimated in this manner (Way, *et al.*, 1960). Alternatively, countercurrent distribution can be used to separate the two compounds before their estimation as phenols. This is a more precise but also more laborious procedure. As shown in Figure 18.1, a mixture of equal parts of 6-monoacetylmorphine and morphine added to brain homogenate was effectively separated and the amount of each substance present was determined nicely by countercurrent distribution (Way, Young and Kemp, 1965).

The most commonly employed method in the photometric analysis of drugs that are acids or bases involves dye complexation. Dye methods are discussed in detail by Axelrod (1960). Most of the dye procedures are concerned with the estimation of various organic bases of therapeutic interest. The usual procedure is to dissolve the dye in an aqueous solution and the compound of interest in an organic solvent. Upon shaking the two phases together, the complex if formed, remains soluble in the organic phase and can be readily separated from the large excess of dye in the aqueous phase. In practice the choice of solvent is limited to ethylene dichloride, chloroform and benzene, since drug-dye complexes are relatively insoluble in less polar solvents and more polar solvents usually extract considerable quantities of free dye. Benzene is the solvent to be preferred. Although many base-dye complexes are not sufficiently soluble in benzene, this can be circumvented usually by the addition of small quantities of isoamyl alcohol. The alcohol may also serve to reduce adsorption of the drug on glassware. Ethylene dichloride is often preferable to chloroform as a halogenated solvent, since the latter is known to react with bases producing compounds which are incapable of dye complexation.

The greater popularity for using dyes to estimate basic drugs over acidic ones is related to reasons we discussed earlier concerning the differences in distribution characteristics between acidic and basic drugs. The greater affinity of various tissues and organs for basic drugs impose limitations on the amounts of drug which can be administered therapeutically and dictates the application of more

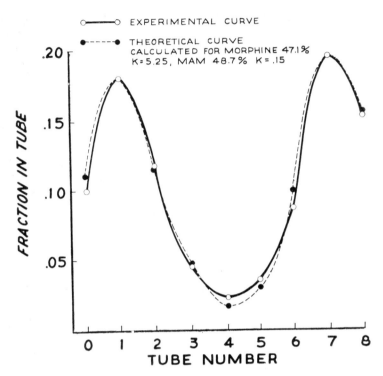

Fig. 18.1 Countercurrent distribution curve for extract of rat brain containing equal parts of added morphine and 6-monoacetylmorphine (MAM). (From Way, Young and Kemp, 1965.)

sensitive methods. The indicator dyes used generally have a high color index and as a consequence procedures involving dye methods often permit determinations of bases in concentrations as low as 0.1 to 0.5 μg drug per gm or ml of biologic material. The indicator dyes that have been used include bromthymol blue, bromocresol purple, bromocresol green and most widely of all, methyl orange (Brodie, Udenfriend and Dill, 1947). The methyl orange method has been successfully applied to a variety of therapeutic bases including several narcotic analgetics and antihistamines. Specific compounds and references are listed in a monograph (Way and Adler, 1962).

The chief disadvantage of the dye procedure is its lack of specificity. Since any amine which forms a solvent-soluble dye compound will be measured as the administered compound, the procedure must always be evaluated for its specificity and, if necessary, modified to exclude interfering contaminants. This can often be accomplished by washing the solvent extract of the base with a suitable buffer before reacting with the methyl orange. A high degree of specificity to the methyl orange procedure can also be conveyed by applying it in conjunction with countercurrent separation.

The development of countercurrent distribution procedures has greatly facilitated the separation and characterization of substances in biologic material. The principle and applications of the technique have already been discussed in detail in Chapter 20. The design in the fractionation process to correspond with the binomial expansion theorem, permitting rapid calculation of theoretical distribu-

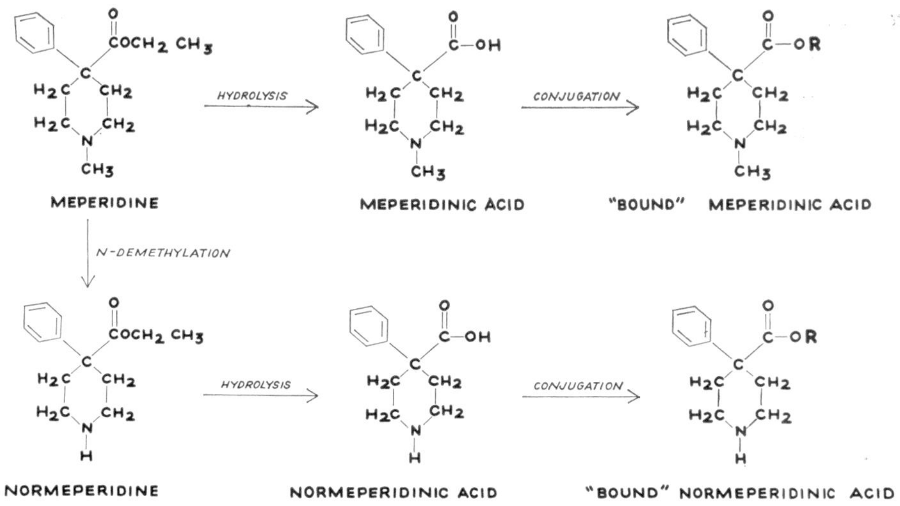

Fig. 18.2 Metabolic pathways of meperidine according to Plotnikoff, Way and Elliott, 1956.

tions (Way and Bennett, 1951) has greatly enhanced the application of non-specific procedures for estimating many compounds in body fluids.

An example of the applicability of combining the methyl orange method with countercurrent distribution can be illustrated by a study on the biotransformation of meperidine (Plotnikoff *et al.*, 1956). By combining a non-specific detection procedure with countercurrent distribution, meperidine and five of its biotransformation products were identified from urine of subjects receiving meperidine. As shown in Figure 18.2, meperidine, is hydrolyzed in the body to meperidinic acid which is then conjugated ("bound" meperidinic acid). In addition, meperidine is demethylated to normeperidine which is then hydrolyzed to normeperidinic acid and then partly conjugated ("bound" normeperidinic acid). The products were identified in the following manner. Meperidine and normeperidine were extracted from alkalinized urine with benzene and the solvent phase was subjected to countercurrent distribution. Using the methyl orange procedure to measure the fractionated organic bases, meperidine and normeperidine were identified by their partition ratios and the relative amounts of each present calculated from the areas of each curve (Fig. 18.3, M1 and N1). The amount of the corresponding acids of the two substances were identified by difference after noting that the amounts of meperidine and normeperidine present in the urine increased after esterification (Fig. 18.3, M2 and N2). An even greater recovery of meperidine and normeperidine resulted when the urinary consituents were subjected to acid hydrolysis before esterification, indicating conjugated or bound forms of meperidinic and normeperidinic acids (Fig. 18.3, M3 and N3).

C. Ultraviolet Analysis

For detection of drugs in body fluids, ultraviolet (uv) analysis is often tried first because of the simplicity of the procedure. This technique is applicable to a wide variety of compounds that are capable of absorption of energy from radiations in the wavelength 200 to 350 mμ. Absorption in this range is usually associ-

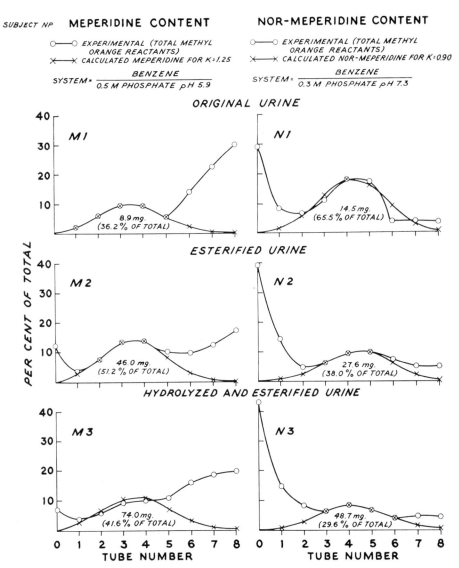

Fig. 18.3 Countercurrent distribution curves for free, hydrolyzed and conjugated metabolites of meperidine in urine estimated by the methyl orange dye procedure. From Plotnikoff, Way and Elliott, 1956.

ated with the displacement of outer electrons within the molecule giving rise to a new energy state. More detailed consideration of the principles of uv spectrometry is included in Chapter 21. From the practical standpoint the method is worth considering by virtue of its convenience since the most rudimentary spectrophotometer of the "black-box" variety is quite suitable for uv quantitation. A major drawback lies in lack of specificity since for most compounds absorption in the uv lies over a fairly wide range of wavelengths and there is generally very little fine structure in the spectrum. Nonetheless, the spectrum is usually characteristic for a given molecule and the extent of absorption at a given wavelength can be utilized for quantitative analysis.

The uv method is also of value in identification and estimation of purity of a compound. Both molar coefficient and wavelength at which maximum absorbance occurs are characteristic of the molecule. Comparison of these experimental values with those quoted in the literature may permit a check on purity. The method is relatively insensitive to temperature change and normally no special care is required to insure measurement at constant temperature from day to day. Although a wide variety of solvents are permissible, it is important to check that the solvent does not have absorption bands in the same region as that selected for measurement of the compound. It may be necessary to remove certain absorbing species from a particular solvent that would otherwise interfere with analysis. This is often accomplished by simple acid/base washing, passing the solvent through absorption columns or redistillation to remove aromatic substances.

It is essential that all solutions prepared for uv analysis be perfectly clear. Even slight turbidity or cloudiness can cause errors in the position of absorption maxima and in the degree of absorption, due to light scattering. Centrifugation of the sample or treatment with Celite is often effective in removing slight cloudiness, espcially if it occurs following a pH adjustment of the system.

Ultraviolet spectrometry is characterized by a high degree of precision and accuracy, but lacks sensitivity. A compound rarely has a sufficiently high molar extinction coefficient to permit quantitation at less than one μg per ml of solution. Improvement in sensitivity may be achieved in certain cases by the use of microcells following extraction and concentration of the molecular species of interest. The use of cells with a longer light path may be tried to enhance sensitivity but they are less convenient to handle in comparison with the widely used 1 cm cells and any advantage gained is often offset by increased blanks. Absorbance of a compound can be enhanced by converting it to a substance with a higher resonance. Paraldehyde, for example, can be estimated in plasma or brain by depolymerizing it to acetaldehyde which can then be separated and reacted with semicarbazide. The acetaldehyde semicarbazone thus formed can be determined at 224 mμ (Figot *et al.*, 1952).

The limited specificity of the method can be improved by a variety of techniques. One of these is to measure absorbance of the compound in a suitable solvent at various wavelengths. Since the ratio of absorbance between different wavelengths is characteristic for the compound, it is possible to calculate concentration in a biological sample containing interfering substances, by appropriate use of simultaneous equations. Another method involves utilization of the spectral shifts that occur with certain compounds when the pH of the medium is changed. Normally the spectrum is run at pH values at which the compound exists either as the acid or the base and a differential spectrum is obtained by using one of these solutions as the reference and the other as sample in the spectrophotometer. A calibration curve is then constructed at various concentrations of the drug. Frequently, interfering materials from biological samples exhibit little spectral shift with pH change and the procedure may significantly reduce tissue blank values. The specificity of uv analysis of barbiturates, chlorpromazine, salicylates, and morphine can be greatly improved by taking advantage of pH spectral shift (Feldstein, 1960). The utilization of bathochromic shift to enhance sensitivity and convey specificity to a uv procedure can be illustrated by the problems encountered with the alkylphosphate antagonist, pralidoxime.

The estimation of the alkylphosphate antagonist, pralidoxime (2-PAM), provides an interesting example in which uv analysis proved to be superior to colorimetric estimation. Chemical assay of the compound involved hydrolysis of the oxime to liberate hydroxylamine which can then be oxidized to nitrous acid. The latter is used to form a diazonium salt that is coupled with a dye for colorimetric estimation. However, the procedure, while applicable for estimation of 2-PAM in blood, proved to be unsuitable for estimating the compound in liver homogenates or subcellular fractions. A more convenient method was developed based on the enhanced molar absorptivity of 2-PAM in alkaline solution at 333 mμ (J. Way, 1962). In addition to this absorption peak in alkali, 2-PAM also exhibits a peak in acid solution at 292 mμ (Fig. 18.4). The measurement of increased molar absorption of 2-PAM in dilute alkaline solution offers a highly specific procedure for estimating 2-PAM, since any alteration of the auxochromic aldoximino functional group would also effect the bathochromic displacement of 2-PAM from 292 to 333 mμ. This was attributed to the existence of 2-PAM in

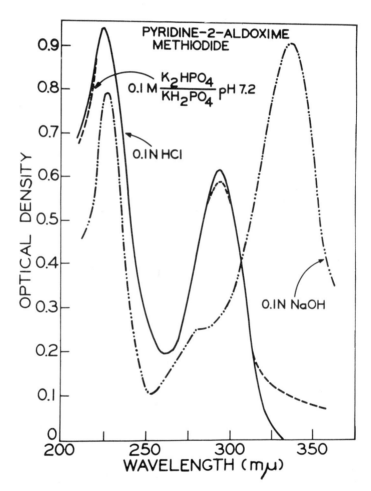

Fig. 18.4 Ultraviolet absorption spectra of 2-PAM (0.048 μmole/ml) in 0.1 N HCl ———; 0.5 M potassium phosphate buffer, pH 7.2 - - - - - and 0.1 N NaOH—··—. (From J. Way, 1962.)

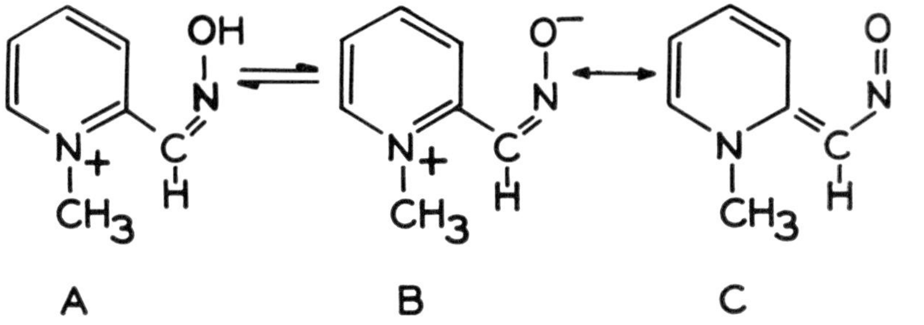

Fig. 18.5 The three forms of 2-PAM; the enolic form, A; the zwitterionic form, B in resonance with (C). (From J. Way, 1962.)

three chemical species (a) the enolic form; (b) the zwitterionic form; (c) and its resonance stabilized form (Fig. 18.5).

In our own experience we have usually found uv spectrophotometry to be less sensitive than colorimetry for estimating drugs in body fluids and we have also encountered more difficulty in eliminating tissue blanks. However, despite this generalization, there are many exceptions and in specific cases uv procedures can offer a high degree of specificity and sensitivity. In addition to 2-PAM, the estimation of the emetic agent, apomorphine may be used for illustrative purposes.

One of us was called upon to develop a procedure for apomorphine and study its physiologic disposition because it was suspected of being used illegally to stimulate race horses. Although several color reactions had been developed for the qualitative detection of apomorphine, none appeared suitable for its quantitative estimation. Apomorphine is a strong absorber of ultraviolet radiation but at its absorption peak high tissue blanks were noted, and, because of its labile nature, it was difficult to purify the compound without incurring appreciable loss. These problems were overcome by oxidizing the compound with mercuric chloride before extraction and determining the oxidized product.

Interestingly, the oxidation product exhibits different colors in different solvents. The color is green in water, blue in methanol, pink in benzene and violet in isoamylacetate. In isoamylacetate, the oxidation product exhibits 2 maxima at 540 mμ and 400 mμ in the visible region and a sharp peak of much greater absorptivity at 330 mμ (Fig. 18.6). Taking advantage of the greater absorbance in the ultraviolet region, a method was developed to estimate apomorphine quantitatively at 330 mμ with a high degree of specificity. As little as 0.1 μg/ml could be detected and zero blank absorbance was observed when various blank specimens were carried through the procedure (Kaul *et al.*, 1959).

D. Fluorescence Techniques

The most sensitive of the routine spectrometric methods available for drug analysis is that afforded by the use of fluorescence techniques. Indeed, fluorescence methods are often simpler, less hazardous and equally sensitive with regard to measurement as analytical methods involving radioisotopic techniques. Fluorescence results from specific electronic changes within a molecule following the absorption of light. Upon electromagnetic irradiation the molecule is excited to a higher energy state and subsequently returns to a lower energy level emitting a photon in the process. The difference between the energy of the initial and final states determines the energy of the emitted radiation or fluorescence.

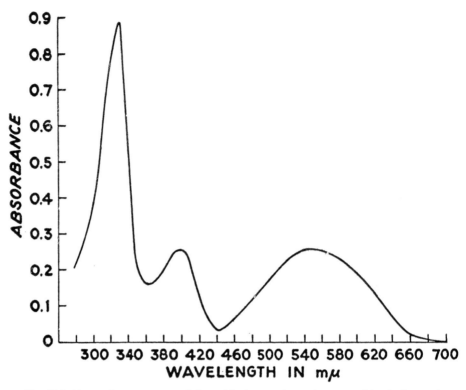

Fig. 18.6 Absorption spectrum of the oxidation product of apomorphine in isoamylacetate. (From Kaul *et al.*, 1959.)

In general, the emitted fluorescence has a greater wavelength than the absorbed light, implying an energy dissipation as heat in the overall process. Upon removal of the radiating source, usually light in the ultraviolet or low visible range, the lifetime of fluorescence is extremely short (10^{-4} to 10^{-10} secs.). Detection and measurement of fluorescence are limited primarily by the fluorescence efficiency of the molecule rather than sensitivity of instrumentation. High fluorescence efficiency is usually associated with molecules containing fairly large conjugated systems of rigid conformation such as phenols, aromatic amines and polycyclic compounds. However, it is possible to convert compounds of low fluorescence efficiency to more potent fluorphores by appropriate chemical reactions analogous to those used in colorimetry.

Fluorescence analysis differs from absorbance spectrometry in a number of significant ways. It is both more specific, since differences may exist even between cis-trans isomers, and more sensitive, enabling quantitation of concentration as low as 0.1 nanograms per ml in certain cases. In contrast to absorbance methods there are no absolute units for fluorescence measurement and quantitation is usually achieved by reference to standard solutions. In dilute solutions the relationship between concentration of a compound and fluorescence intensity can be derived from Beers law which reduces to

$$\text{Fluorescence Intensity} = 2.3 \times \text{Io} \times (\text{Ecl}) \times \text{quantum yield}$$

where Io = intensity of exciting light; E = molar extinction coefficient; c =

concentration; and l = pathlength. Quantum yield or efficiency (ϕ) is given by

$$(\phi) = \frac{\text{number of quanta emitted}}{\text{number of quanta absorbed}}$$

and can be estimated by comparison against a compound of known ϕ value (Udenfriend, 1962). It is apparent, therefore, that at low concentrations, when absorption of light is low, a linear relationship will exist between fluorescence intensity and concentration. At high concentrations quenching by the molecules themselves or other components of the system decreases true fluorescence efficiency and the relationship becomes non-linear. Quenching interactions have a certain degree of specificity, but as a general rule the most troublesome species are halide ions, oxygen, heavy metals and certain nitro compounds, which may have to be removed from the medium in which the drug is being measured. Fluorescence measurement is quite sensitive to temperature changes and it is prudent to carry out such assays at constant room/cell compartment temperature and it may be necessary to reread standards frequently. Since fluorescence intensity increases with decreasing temperature, it is possible to improve the sensitivity of certain fluorometric analyses by maintaining the sample at a temperature appreciably below that of room temperature.

Mention has been made previously of the problem of quenching by the molecules themselves or by other light absorbing species. When fluorescent techniques are employed near the limits of sensitivity, certain other practical difficulties may need to be overcome. These relate particularly to the cleaning of glassware, purification of solvents and the suitability of the extraction procedure. When using water as a solvent, triple distillation may be necessary for the fluorescence blank to be reduced to a low level. Similarly organic solvents should be of spectral grade, preferably "suitable for fluorescence assay," but in some cases will still require further purification. A common procedure is to expose the solvent to alternate acid/base water washes and then pass it over silica gel. However, careful redistillation may be required when highest sensitivity is needed.

Many common detergents contain fluorescent components and in the cleaning of glassware, particularly that used in the later stages of an analysis, it is good policy to rinse with hot concentrated nitric acid, followed by hot distilled water and finally copious volumes of cold distilled water. The nature of the extraction procedure used to isolate compounds can markedly influence the sensitivity of fluorescence analysis. The use of separating funnels lubricated with stopcock grease or rubber and cork stoppers are common sources of fluorescent contaminants. Trace impurities in filter paper are also capable of yielding high blank values. Traces of organic solvents which absorb in certain regions of the ultraviolet (e.g., benzene, acetone) may also survive the extraction procedure and interfere with fluorescence assay.

Regardless of such difficulties the use of fluorescent analysis is well established for the determination of a variety of compounds of interest to the pharmacologist, including vitamins, steroids, antimalarials, antibiotics, analgesics, sedatives, muscle relaxants and catecholamines. Sometimes the compound of interest possesses native fluorescence, but frequently it is necessary to convert a nonfluorescent species to a fluorophore by chemical means. For example, the interaction of penicillins with certain flavin amines results in the formation of fluorescent amides. The complexation of certain amines with the fluorescent dye eosin, has been employed to determine very low concentrations of these species. Condensation of catecholamines with ethylenediamine while relatively non-specific can be used for the determination of such compounds if adequate separative procedures are employed. Morphine is a weakly fluorescent compound. However, it can be rapidly and quantitatively oxidized to pseudomorphine (Fig 18.7) which is highly fluorescent. The emission and excitation spectra is shown in Fig. 18.8. By determining the emission at 440 mμ resulting from excitation at 250 mμ morphine levels as low as 25 nanograms could be measured (Kupferberg et al., 1964; Takemori, 1969). More recently dansyl chloride has been used to detect nanogram quantities of tetrahydrocannabinol, morphine, amphetamine and mescaline (Ho et al., 1971). Dansyl chloride forms highly fluorescent conjugates with primary and secondary amines and has been used as a sensitive end group reagent for peptide, phenols and protein analyses.

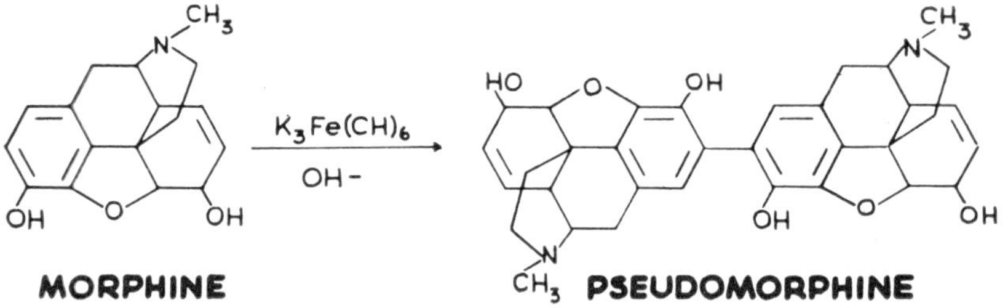

Fig. 18.7 Oxidation of morphine to pseudomorphine.

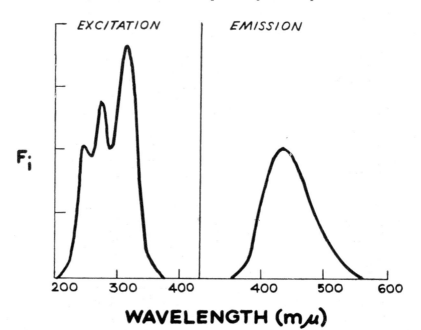

Fig. 18.8 Excitation (left) and emission (right) spectra of pseudomorphine obtained by oxidation of morphine by potassium ferricyanide. The excitation spectrum was obtained by setting the emission monochromator at 440 mμ. The emission spectrum was obtained by setting the excitation monochromator at 250 mμ. (From Kufperberg et al., 1964.)

The sensitivity of fluorometric techniques can sometimes be improved by taking advantage of changes in fluorescence which may accompany an alteration of the pH of the solvent. For example, salicylic acid does not fluoresce as the uncharged species, but is fluorescent as the anion. The measurement of extremely low concentrations of this drug in tissue samples may be facilitated by estimation of fluorescence intensity at pH values of 7 and 2. Frequently the fluorescence of endogenous components does not change with pH and it is possible to obtain a very accurate determination of blank value by this procedure. Variation of medium pH to improve quantitation is not restricted solely to acidic and basic molecules. Griseofulvin, a neutral molecule, is normally considered to be insensitive to pH changes in the environment. However, at a pH of less than 1, the fluorescence of this compound is completely abolished, due to protonation, while that of endogenous tissue contaminants is usually unchanged. Accurate blank values can be easily achieved by measuring the sample at pH 7 and again after addition of 6 M sulfuric acid, thus permitting the estimation of griseofulvin at concentrations below 0.1 microgram per ml of plasma (Rowland *et al.*, 1968).

One of the widest applications of fluorescence spectroscopy is the analysis of biogenic amines in various fluids and tissues. An example is the method of Ansell and Beeson (1968), for the simultaneous determination of norepinephrine, dopamine and serotonin in a single brain sample. This method is considered in some detail as it illustrates the use of various extraction, adsorption and fluorescent techniques in achieving a sensitive and specific assay procedure for these amines. Their procedure (Fig. 18.9) initially involves homogenization of the dissected brain sample with acid butanol. Although this simple step extracts the biogenic amines, it also removes other fluorescent materials. The latter are reduced by adding iso-octane to the butanol extract. This decreases the polarity of the organic phase allowing quantitative transfer of the amines into an aqueous phase, while leaving behind some of the polar fluorescent compounds. Further purification is achieved by adsorption of the catecholamines on alumina at pH greater than 7.0. The supernate above the alumina, containing the serotonin, is separated and both are treated separately. The separated serotonin is further cleaned by passing into butanol and reextraction into pH 7 phosphate buffer. Although serotonin possesses native fluorescence, the sensitivity of the assay is greatly increased by the formation of a fluorophor of this amine with ninhydrin, which is measured at $385/495$ mμ (excitation maximum/fluorescence maximum).

The catecholamines are eluted from the alumina with acid and then oxidized at pH 6.5 with an iodine, alkaline sulfite and acetic acid system added in a definite time sequence. The EDTA is added to stabilize the resultant fluorophors. The oxidized products exhibit a marked enhancement of the fluorescence. The fluorophor of norepinephrine is readily distinguished from that of dopamine by its rapid formation at $100°$ and subsequent destruction upon further heating at this temperature. The dopamine fluorophor is more stable but takes up to 24 hours for complete formation. Also, the difference in the excitation and fluorescent maxima of these two species reduces interference between them.

Before quantitation is achieved, it is necessary to run standards and blanks through all or various parts of the procedure. A tissue standard is carried through the entire assay by adding 250 ng of each amine to the initial homogenate and serves to estimate overall recoveries. An unextracted standard and reagent blank

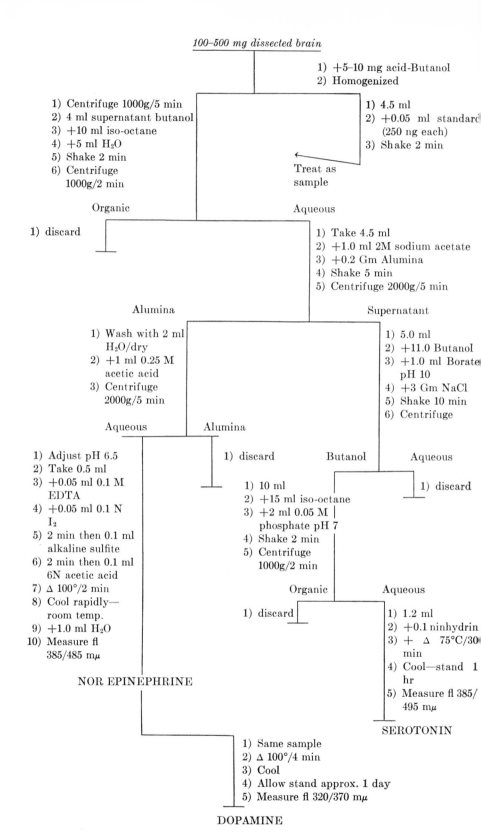

Fig. 18.9 Flow diagram of the assay procedure for the determination of norepinephrine, dopamine and serotonin from a single brain sample. (From Ansell and Beeson, 1968.)

are taken through the fluorophor formation steps to calibrate the fluorometer. Finally, a tissue blank is prepared by taking part of either the eluate from the alumina or phosphate pH 7 buffer, adding the premixed reagents used to make the fluorophor and measuring the fluorescence at the appropriate wavelength settings. In all cases the fluorescence value is the observed value less that of the reagent blank. The amine content of the sample is then given by

$$\frac{A - blank}{B - A} \times \frac{4}{4.5} \times 250 \text{ ng}$$

where A = Fluorescence of sample; B = fluorescence of sample plus 250 ng· standard; 4/4.5 = the 4 ml of butanol homogenate of the sample while 4.5 mls is volume of the homogenate to which the standard was added. Defining sensitivity as the amount of amine giving a reading twice that of the blank, these workers were able to detect 20 ng for norepinephrine, 30 ng for serotonin and 100 ng for dopamine.

For a comprehensive survey of the theoretical and practical aspects of fluorescence assay as well as the instrumentation, the reader is referred to the exellent monograph of Udenfriend (1962). References to established and recently introduced fluorescence methods of analysis, published monthly (*Traces*, G. K. Turner, Palo Alto, California) are available to interested investigators on request.

E. Assessment of Specificity

Since the reaction or property by which a drug is being measured may be shared by other substances with common functional groups, the specificity of the procedure for the compound in question needs always to be evaluated. The problem constantly arises concerning whether closely related metabolites of the parent compound or other ingested drugs are also being measured. Specificity of procedure is usually established by demonstrating that no substances are present that interfere with the quantification of the parent compound. This is not always easy to accomplish since the amount of drug present in biologic material is often extremely low and contaminated with other material. Even if the extraneous matter is not detected by the method of analysis, it renders difficult the isolation of the drug in the crystalline state for characterization by conventional methods (melting point, optical rotation, refractive index, etc.).

A rigid test for specificity which does not require the actual isolation of the pure compound can be accomplished by comparing the partition behavior of the recovered drug with that of the authentic substance between two immiscible solvent phases. Since the methods for estimating drugs in biologic media generally involves extraction techniques, the distribution of the drug between two phases can be conveniently followed with the same technique used to detect the drug in body fluids. Two procedures are generally employed to study distribution behavior; countercurrent distribution and comparative distribution ratios.

The distribution behavior of a drug between two immiscible solvent phases can be used to reveal the specificity of an analytical procedure, especially if the compound is acidic or basic. The distribution of such compounds between an organic solvent and water can then be altered by varying the pH of the aqueous phase with a series of buffers. In such systems, a comparison of the distribution ratios of the drug recovered from body fluids with those of the authentic compound should yield information concerning the identity or non-identity of the two substances. The probability for two dissimilar compounds to distribute in an identical manner between two phases at varying pH is indeed remote (Brodie and Udenfriend, 1945). Hence, if the two compounds being compared exhibit similar distribution ratios under such rigidly defined conditions, the likelihood is great that the two compounds are identical, and, therefore, it can be concluded that the analytical procedures measures the desired compound with a high degree of specificity.

A recent study on the fate of methotrimeprazine, a potent phenothiazine analgetic may be used to illustrate this procedure (Afifi and Way, 1968). After administering methotrimeprazine to rats and allowing a suitable interval for the drug to become at least partly metabolized, the livers and brains were homogenized, alkalinized and extracted with 1% n-butanol in cyclohexane. The method of analyzing the drug consisted of washing the solvent extract with a buffer of pH 6.4, back-extracting the drug from the solvent into acid and determining its absorbance at 250 mμ. To appraise for specificity of the procedure, therefore, four aliquots of the washed and unwashed organic solvent extract were equilibrated respectively with buffers of pH 4, 5, 6 and 7. The amount of methotrimeprazine remaining in the solvent was then determined by uv in the usual manner. The results were compared with those obtained from a similar treatment of authentic methotrimeprazine in aqueous solution or added to urine or liver homogenate.

As can be noted in Table 18.1, the respective fractions of the recovered drug from liver after equilibration of the solvent extract with buffers of various pH values were different from those for authentic methotrimeprazine. Moreover, the interfering material was more water soluble than the parent compound. After the organic solvent tissue extract was subjected to a single buffer wash, the distribution ratios of the recovered drug more nearly approached that of the authentic compound. After washing the solvent extract of liver three times with the buffer wash, the drug in the solvent phase now behaved similarly to methotrimeprazine. Thus, a comparative distribution ratio study not only revealed the non-selectivity of the original extraction procedure, but also conveyed the information on how to make it specific for the parent compound.

Another procedure for appraisal of specificity is countercurrent distribution.

TABLE 18.1

Distribution behavior of authentic and recovered methotrimeprazine in 1% n-butanol in cyclohexane and buffers of varying pH

The figures under each pH value denote the fraction of the compound remaining in the unwashed or washed organic solvent phase after equilibration with an equal volume of each buffer.

Methotrimeprazine	N*	Fractions Remaining at			
		pH 7	pH 6	pH 5	pH 4
Added to					
Water	0	0.98	0.93	0.73	0.35
Rat liver	0	1.01	0.94	0.73	0.34
Recovered from liver of injected rats	0	0.69	0.57	0.37	0.16
	1	0.87	0.71	0.47	0.25
	3	0.97	0.92	0.73	0.40

* Number of washings with 0.2 M phosphate buffer, pH 6.4. (From Afifi and Way, 1968.)

The principles and applications are discussed in detail in Chapter 20. An example will be provided here to illustrate its application in the assessment of the specificity of the procedure. The technique was utilized in a recent study on the metabolism of the antagonist analgetic pentazocine which was estimated by spectrofluorometry. In brief, the procedure is based on the extraction of pentazocine at pH 8–9 into benzene, washing the solvent extract twice with a phosphate buffer of pH 6.7, back-extracting the pentazocine into acid and assaying the fluorescence intensity of the acid extract (Berkowitz and Way, 1969).

To assess the specificity of the procedure, urine was collected from subjects receiving pentazocine and extracted with benzene. The benzene extract was subjected to an 8-plate countercurrent distribution and the experimental distribution curve was compared with authentic pentazocine similarly treated. Figure 18.10 depicts the experimental distribution curve obtained with (A) pentazocine added to water, (B) pentazocine added to urine, (C) 24 hours urine from a subject receiving pentazocine, and (D) the same urine after washing the benzene extract with buffer.

It is apparent that a fluorescent metabolite of pentazocine appears in urine, since a single substance curve was not obtained. However, after removal of the metabolite with the buffer wash, the remaining material behaved as a single

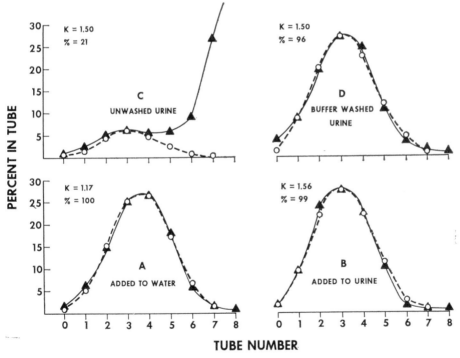

TUBE NUMBER

Fig. 18.10 Countercurrent distribution curves obtained on the benzene extracts of: A, pentazocine added to 5 ml of water, B, pentazocine added to 5 ml of urine; C, 5 ml of 0 to 24 hour urine after 50 mg of pentazocine orally; and D, 5 ml of same urine after washing the benzene phase twice with 10 ml of 0.2M phosphate buffer, pH 6.7, prior to countercurrent distribution. ——— = experimental; - - - - = theoretical. K value represents partition ratio, and percent value represents amount of fluorescence in sample that can be attributed to unaltered pentazocine. (System: benzene/0.2M phosphate buffer, pH 6.7). (From Berkowitz and Way, 1969.)

substance with a partition ratio similar to that of pentazocine added to urine. Hence, by washing the benzene extract of urine, a high degree of specificity was conveyed to the procedure. It may be noted that the partition ratio of pentazocine in water was different from that in urine. These shifts may occasionally be expected to occur when a compound is added to biological fluids.

In addition to the comparative distribution ratio and countercurrent distribution procedures, other techniques such as thin-layer or gas-liquid chromatography may be utilized to evaluate specificity of an assay procedure. The number of criteria to be applied is arbitrary and it is strictly up to the investigator to decide. Since it is not possible to establish absolute specificity for an analytical method, the more tests that are applied to check the specificity of the procedure, the greater is the assurance that contaminating products will not have been estimated.

REFERENCES

Abou-el-Makerem, M. M., Milburn, P., Smith, R. L., and Williams, R. T.: The biliary excretion of foreign compounds in different species. Biochem. J. *99:* 3p, 1966.

Adler, T. K.: Studies on morphine tolerance in mice. *In vivo* N-demethylation of morphine and N- and O-demethylation of codeine. J. Pharmacol. Exp. Ther. *156:* 585–590, 1967.

Afifi, A. and Way, E. Leong: Studies on the biologic disposition of methotrimeprazine. J. Pharmacol. Exp. Ther. *160:* 397–406, 1968.

Ansell, G. B. and Beeson, M. F.: A rapid and sensitive procedure for the combined assay of noradrenaline, dopamine, and serotonin in a single brain sample. Anal. Biochem. *23:* 196–206, 1968.

Anton, A. H.: The relations between binding of sulfonamides to albumin and their antibacterial activity. J. Pharmacol. Exp. Ther. *129:* 282–290, 1960.

Axelrod, J. The estimation of basic drugs by dye methods, pp. 714–730. In *Toxicology,* Vol. I, ed. by C. P. Stewart and A. Stolman, Academic Press, 1960.

Berkowitz, B. and Way, E. L.: Metabolism and excretion of pentazocine in man. Clin. Pharmacol. Ther. *10:* 681–689, 1969.

Boyes. R. N., Adams, H. J., and Duce, B. R.: Oral absorption and disposition kinetics of lidocaine hydrochloride in dogs. J. Pharmacol. Exp. Therap. *174,* 1–8 (1970).

Brodie, B. B. and Udenfriend, S.: The estimation of basic organic compounds and a technique for appraisal of specificity. J. Biol. Chem. *158:* 705–714, 1945.

Brodie, B. B., Udenfriend, S., and Dill, W.: estimation of basic organic compounds in biological material. V. Estimation by salt formation with methyl orange. J. Biol. Chem. *168:* 335–339, 1947.

Chiou, W., Riegelman, S., and Amberg, J.: Complications in using rabbits for the study of oral drug adsorption. Chem. Pharm. Bull. *17:* 2170 (1969).

Conney, A. H.: Pharmacological implications of microsomal enzyme induction. Pharmacol. Rev. *19:* 317, 1967.

Cserr, H. F.: Blood brain barrier in vertebrates. In *Proceedings of an International Symposium on Comparative Pharmacology,* p. 1024–1026, ed. by Cafruny, E. J., Cosmides, G. J., Rall, D. P., Schroeder, C. R., and Weiner, I. M. FASEB, Bethesda, Md., 1967.

Feldstein, H.: The use of ultraviolet spectra in toxicological analysis in toxicology: mechanisms and analytical methods. pp. 464–512. In *Toxicology,* Vol. I, ed. by Stewart, C. P. and Stolman, A., Academic Press, 1960.

Figot, P. P., Hine, C. H., and Way, E. Leong: The estimation and significance of paraldehyde levels in blood and brain. Acta Pharmacol. Toxicol. *8:* 290–304, 1952.

Freireich, E. J., Gehan, E. A., Rall, D. P., Schmidt, L. H., and Skipper, H. E.: Quantitative comparison of toxicity of anticancer agents in mouse, rat, hamster, dog, monkey and man. Cancer Chemotherap. Rep. *50:* 219–244, 1966.

Fujimoto, J. M., Way, E. Leong, and Hine, C. H.: A rapid method for the estimation of morphine. J. Lab. Clin. Med. *44:* 627–635, 1954.

Goldstein, A., Aronow, L., and Kalman, S. M.: *"Principles of Drug Action",* Hoeber, 1968.

Goldenthal, E. I.: Current views on safety evaluation of drugs. FDA Papers, May, 1968, pp. 13–18.

Ho, I. K., Loh, H. H., and Way, E. L.: Mini thin layer chromatography in the detection of narcotics in the urine. Proc. West. Pharmacol. Soc. *14:* 183–186, 1971.

Hogben, C. A., Schanker, L. S., Tocco, D. J., and Brodie, B. B.: Absorption of drugs from the stomach. II. Human, J. Pharmacol. Exp. Ther. *120:* 540, 1957.

Hume, D. S., Bush, M. T., Remick, J., and Douglas, B. H.: Comparison of gastric absorption of thiopental and pentobarbital in rat, dog and man. Arch. Int. Pharmacodyn. Ther. *171:* 122–127, 1968.

Kalow, W.: Pharmacogenetics and the predictability of drug responses. In *Drug Responses in Man*, A Ciba Foundation Volume, pp. 220–232, ed. by G. Wolstenholme and R. Porter, Little, Brown, Boston, 1967.

Kaul, P. N., Brochmann-Hanssen, E., and Way, E. Leong: A rapid and sensitive method of quantitative determination of apomorphine. J. Amer. Pharm. Assn. Scientific Ed. *48:* 638–641, 1959.

Kupferberg, H. J., Burkhalter, A., and Way, E. Leong: A sensitive fluorometric assay for morphine in plasma and brain. J. Pharmacol. Exp. Ther. *145:* 247–251, 1964.

Kupferberg, H. J., and Way, E. L.: Pharmacologic basis for the increased sensitivity of the newborn rat to morphine. J. Pharmacol. Exp. Ther. *141:* 105–112, 1963.

Lehman, A. J., Patterson, W. I., Daviddown, B., Hagah, E. C., Woodward, G., Laug, E. P., Frawley, J. P., Fitzhugh, O. G., Bourke, A. R., Draize, J. H., Nelson, A. A., and Vos, B. J.: Procedures for the appraisal of the toxicity of chemicals in food, drugs and cosmetics. Food, Drug, Cosmetic Law Journal, *10:* 679–748, 1955.

Lehman, A. J.: Appraisal of the safety of chemicals in food, drugs and cosmetics, pp. 60–67, 1959. Pub. Association of Food and Drug Officials of the U.S.A.

Levy, G.: Dose dependent effects in pharmacokinetics. In *Importance of Fundamental Principles in Drug Evaluation*, pp. 141–172, ed. by D. H. Tedeschi and R. E. Tedeschi, Raven Press, New York, 1968.

Parke, D. V.: *The Biochemistry of Foreign Compounds*, Pergamon Press, New York, 1968.

Plotnikoff, N. P., Way, E. Leong, and Elliott, H. W.: Biotransformation products of meperidine excreted in the urine of man. J. Pharmacol. Exp. Ther. *117:* 414–419, 1956.

Rall, D. P.: Role of pharmacological disposition in drug action. In *Importance of Fundamental Principles in Drug Evaluation*, pp. 173–182, ed. by D. H. Tedeschi and R. E. Tedeschi, Raven Press, New York (1968).

Rao, C. N. R.: *Ultraviolet Invisible Spectroscopy: Chemical Applications*, p. 8, Butterworth: London (1967).

Rolinson, G. and Sutherland, R.: The Binding of antibiotics to serum proteins. Brit. J. Pharmacol. Chemother. *25:* 638–650, 1965.

Rowland, M. and Riegelman, S.: Determination of acetylsalicylic acid and salicylic acid in plasma. J. Pharm. Sci. *56:* 717–720, 1967.

Rowland, M., Riegelman, S., and Epstein, W. L.: Absorption kinetics of griseofulvin in man. J. Pharm. Sci. *57:* 984–989, 1968.

Schanker, L. S., Shore, P. A., Brodie, B. B., and Hogben, C. A.: Absorption of drugs from the stomach. I. Rat. J. Pharmacol. Exp. Ther. *120:* 528, 1957.

Stowe, C. M. and Plaa, G. L.: Extrarenal excretion of drugs and chemicals. Ann. Rev. Pharmacol. *8:* 337–356, 1968.

Takemori, A. E.: An ultrasensitive method for the determination of morphine and its application in experiments *in vitro* and *in vivo*. Biochem. Pharmac. *17:* 1627–1635, 1968.

Udenfriend, S.: *Fluorescence Assay in Biology and Medicine*, Academic Press, New York (1962).

Wadell, W. J. and Butler, T. C.: The distribution and excretion of phenobarbital. J. Clin. Invest. *36:* 1217, 1957.

Wagner, J. A., Northam. J. I., Alway, C. D., and Carpenter, O. S.: Blood levels of drug at the equilibrium state after multiple dosing. Nature *207:* 1301, 1965.

Way, E. Leong: Metabolism of analgetics and antihistamines. *Symposium on Amine Metabolism*, Meet. Amer. Chem. Soc., Los Angeles, 1953.

Way, E. Leong: Distribution and metabolism of morphine and its surrogates. Chapter II in *The Addictive States*, A. Wikler, ed., Williams and Wilkins Co., Baltimore, 1968.

Way, E. Leong and Adler, T. K.: The Biologic disposition of morphine and its surrogates. World Health Organization, Geneva, 1962.

Way, E. Leong and Bennett, B. N.: Estimation of theoretical countercurrent distribution values. J. Biol. Chem. *192:* 335–338, 1951.

Way, E. Leong, Kemp, J. W., Young, J. M., and Grassetti, D. R.: The pharmacologic effects of heroin in relationship to its rate of biotransformation. J. Pharmacol. Exp. Ther. *129:* 144–154, 1960.

Way, E. Leong, Sung, C. Y., and McKelway, W. P.: The absorption, distribution and excretion of d,1 methadone. J. Pharmacol. Exp. Ther. *97:* 222–228, 1949.

Way, E. Leong, Young, J. M., and Kemp, J.: Metabolism of heroin and its pharmacologic implications. Bull. Narcotics *17:* 25–33, 1965.

Way, J. L.: The metabolism of C¹⁴ 2-PAM in the isolated perfused rat liver. J. Pharmacol. Exp. Ther. *138:* 258–263, 1962.

Williams, R. T.: Species comparative patterns of drug metabolism. Fed. Proc. *26:* 1029, 1967.

19

Techniques for Studying Drug Metabolism *In Vitro*

JAMES R. GILLETTE

I. INTRODUCTION

Studies of drug metabolism in living animals have made it possible to elucidate the pathways of drug metabolism and the factors which control the levels of drugs and their metabolites at receptor sites. Without corollary *in vitro* studies, however, the interpretation of many of these studies would be virtually impossible. Before the mechanisms of drug metabolism were extensively studied, for example, it was frequently assumed that the presence of a drug metabolite in a tissue indicated that the tissue contained an enzyme system which catalyzed the metabolism of the drug. Although this concept has occasionally led to an understanding of the metabolism and pharmacologic properties of a variety of drugs, including sympathomimetic amines, *in vitro* studies have usually revealed that the drugs are metabolized in liver or in organs other than those which concentrate the metabolite and that localization of metabolites in tissues is due to the presence of active transport systems or intracellular binding sites. Thus, much of our present-day knowledge on the mechanisms of drug action has been obtained by studying drug metabolism with isolated tissue preparations and correlating these findings with those observed in living animals.

Biochemical pharmacologists carry out *in vitro* studies for a number of reasons: 1) To determine in which tissues drug metabolism takes place. 2) To determine the steps involved in the formation of metabolites. 3) To discover the components of the enzyme systems that catalyze these various steps. 4) To identify the biochemical properties of the various components. 5) To determine the various mechanisms which control enzyme activity. To achieve these objectives, investigators may choose a variety of tissue preparations and techniques, each of which has its advantages and disadvantages.

II. ENZYME PREPARATIONS

A. Organ Perfusion

Perfusion of drugs through various organs may be carried out under conditions closely resembling those which occur in living animals. These studies may provide information on the rate and pathways of drug metabolism which occur in the organ being perfused. If the drug under study is metabolized slowly *in vivo*, this technique is virtually the only way to assess drug metabolism *in vitro*, for the activity of the preparations may be maintained for several hr. On the other hand, if the drug is rapidly metabolized, the rate may be limited by the blood flow rate through the organ, or by the diffusion of the drug from the blood to the intracellular enzyme system rather than by the activity of the enzyme system.

Although perfusion studies provide kinetic data which is relevant to drug metabolism *in vivo*, they provide little information on the various steps of drug metabolism which occur within the organ or the properties of the enzyme systems which catalyze these steps. The technique has failed to gain wide-spread popularity in the drug metabolism studies for a number of reasons. For the identification of the principal metabolities of drugs and thus the pathways of drug metabolism, it frequently offers no advantage over studies of urinary metabolites. It requires constant surveillance by experienced investigators and thus is rather inefficient in collecting data on kinetics of drug metabolism. It requires considerable amounts of blood from donor animals and rather complicated and expensive systems for maintaining oxygenated blood, proper blood flow and temperature control. Nevertheless, for evaluating organ function, organ perfusion has no peer and as the apparatus becomes more fully automated, its use should increase.

B. Tissue Slices

Tissue slices have been used as an alternative to organ perfusion in evaluating drug metabolism by various tissues. Since circulation of nutrients and oxygen through the capillaries is lost, however, the transfer of these substances from the medium to the innermost cells must depend on passive diffusion. It is therefore imperative that the slices be thin because the rate of diffusion is inversely related to the square of the distance the substances must traverse. Even with slices as thin as 0.5 mm, the concentrations of the nutrients and other substrates which are rapidly utilized by cells in the slice may not be identical throughout the slice. For this reason studies on the kinetics of drug metabolism obtained with tissue slices may not truly represent the kinetics of drug metabolism within the cell. Nevertheless, studies with tissue slices have provided valuable clues to the pathways of drug metabolism catalyzed by uncharacterized enzymes in cells and on the mechanisms of drug transport into tissues. The techniques are relatively simple and require little specialized equipment, although reproducibility of results requires experienced personnel.

C. Separated Cells

Since organs usually consist of several different kinds of cells, it sometimes is important to determine which cells contain the enzymes that catalyze metabolism of drugs. To this end, tissues are treated with enzymes such as collagenase and trypsin which hydrolyze the collagen that cements the cells together. The separated cells may then be isolated by differential centrifugation. With this technique Govier (1965) found that the acetylation of sulfanilamide occurs in reticular cells rather than in parenchymal cells of liver. Among the obvious advantages of this type of preparation is that the cells are constantly bathed by the medium, and thus diffusion barriers to oxygen, nutrients and substrates are minimized. Moreover it is the simplest preparation in which intracellular relationships remain intact. Practically, however, the technique has not gained widespread acceptance because yields of the cells are small and cross contamination is frequently great.

D. Tissue Cultures

The tissue culture technique provides a method for obtaining and maintaining cells having a common genetic background. With this technique it might be possible to maintain cell lines from patients having rare genetic defects in drug metabolism. With these cell lines, it might then be possible not only to elucidate the mechanism of the defect but also to screen drugs which would be dangerous in patients having similar genetic defects. Unfortunately, this technique has a number of disadvantages. The yield of cells is usually small and thus studies are restricted either to unusually active enzyme systems or to reactions which are followed with unusually sensitive analytical techniques. Moreover, it has not been possible to maintain cultures of liver parenchymal cells in which the drug metabolizing enzyme systems of the endoplasmic reticulum remain active through many generations. Although Nebert and Gelboin (1968a,b) have used tissue culture preparations from fetuses to evaluate the induction of 3,4-benzpyrene hydroxylase by polycyclic hydrocarbons, they have not been able to maintain active cell lines from these preparations indefinitely.

E. Tissue Homogenates

Homogenization of tissues represents a radical departure from the techniques discussed above. Once cell walls are broken the relationships among the various intracellular organelles are lost, steady-state levels of rapidly turning over substrates and cofactors differ from those which occur *in vivo*, and some intracellular components become damaged. Indeed, the liver endoplasmic reticulum which contains many of the enzymes that catalyze the metabolism of drugs breaks on homogenization to form microsomes. Without the homogenization technique, however, it would have been impossible to show that most lipid soluble drugs are metabolized by liver endoplasmic reticulum or that these enzymes require NADPH and oxygen. It would also have been impossible to demonstrate that liver microsomes convert some substances to intermediates which in turn are converted to other metabolites by enzymes in the soluble fraction.

Occasionally, the enzyme activity appears to be destroyed on homogenization of the tissues. Sometimes the medium used in homogenization causes the apparent inactivation, sometimes the homogenization damages intracellular components because the clearance of the homogenizer is insufficient or homogenization is too vigorous or prolonged. But inactivation of drug metabolism systems is most frequently caused by inactivation of cofactors required by the systems. For example, the metabolism of many drugs by liver microsomes frequently appears lower in homogenates than in tissue slices because pyrophosphatases in the nuclear and microsomal fractions hydrolyze cofactors which are required for the metabolism of many lipid soluble drugs and the formation of glucuronides. Moreover, ATPases in liver microsomes may impair the formation of ethereal sulfates and methylated derivatives by decreasing the formation of 3'-phosphoadenosine-5'-phosphosulfate (PAPS), and S-adenosylmethionine, which are required in these reactions.

F. Subcellular Fractions

Since many of the subcellular organelles contain enzymes that inactivate cofactors, it is generally advisable to study drug metabolism with isolated fractions of the enzyme rather than with whole homogenates. For gross separation of homogenates into nuclear, mitochondrial, microsomal and soluble fractions, the method of Schneider and Hogeboom (1950) is generally used. It should be kept in mind, however, that each of these fractions is highly heterogeneous; thus the nuclear fraction invariably contains whole cells as well as nuclei; the mitochondrial fraction contains lysosomes and peroxisomes as well as mitochondria; the microsomal fractions contain free ribosomes and both rough-surfaced and smooth-surfaced microsomes; and the soluble fraction contains enzymes which have leaked out of the subcellular organelles as well as those which are present in the cell sap. Moreover, organs usually consist of a number of tissues and thus the various fractions contain subcellular organelles from different kinds of cells.

Further purification of the various subcellular organelles is usually accomplished by centrifuging the fractions over continuous or discontinuous density gradients. The composition of the density medium used for the separation depends on the type of organelle to be isolated. For separating the various components in liver microsomes, the discontinuous gradient method of Dallner (1963) has gained widespread acceptance. In this method, the 9000 $\times$ g fraction rather than the microsomal fraction is subfractionated because isolated microsomes tend to clump and thus separation of the components is then virtually impossible. Owing to the poor yields of the various components, however, drug metabolism studies are rarely carried out with these subfractions. The recently developed zonal centrifugation techniques may improve the yield of the subcellular organelles, but this technique has thus far not been used to separate smooth and rough-surfaced microsomes.

Subcellular particles contain a host of enzyme systems which are important in drug metabolism. For example, liver microsomes contain systems that catalyze the oxidation of a wide variety of lipid-soluble drugs and steroids, the reduction of azo- and nitro compounds, and the formation of glucuronides. Mitochondria contain systems that catalyze the oxidation of monoamines and diamines, the formation of glycine and glutamine derivatives and the β-oxidation of long chain carboxylic acids.

G. Solubilization and Purification

In order to elucidate the mechanisms of these various systems, considerable effort has been made to solubilize and purify the enzymes. Among the techniques which have been used to solubilize the enzymes are: 1) alternate freezing and thawing of the suspension, 2) subjection of the suspension to hypotonic conditions, 3) subjection of the suspensions to high frequency sonic waves, 4) treatment of the suspension with organic solvents such as acetone and butanol, 5) treatment of the suspension with various detergents such as desoxycholate, cutscum and Lubrol, and 6) treatment of the suspension with lipolytic or proteolytic enzymes. The solubilization of a particular enzyme system, however, requires considerable knowledge of the stability of the enzyme system, hard work, patience and luck. Over the past 15 years many attempts have been made to solubilize the oxidative systems in liver microsomes, but it was only recently the Lu *et al.* (1969a,b) reported partial success in the solubilization of a system which catalyzes ω-oxidation of fatty acids and oxidation of drugs.

In carrying out studies with solubilized preparations, however, considerable caution should be used in interpreting results. During the solubilization process, enzymes that normally act in a lipid matrix are now exposed to an aqueous environment. The process of solubilization, particularly by treatment with enzymes, frequently causes drastic changes in the composition as well as the conformation of the enzyme. For example, cytochrome b_5 when solubilized by treatment with trypsin has fewer amino acid residues than it does when solubilized by treatment with detergents. Moreover, liver microsomal NADPH cytochrome *c* reductase when solubilized by steapsin does not catalyze the reduction of cytochrome P-450, which presumably is its normal electron acceptor.

The solubilization of enzyme systems from subcellular particles is seldom an end in itself, but is merely the requisite to the isolation and purification of the components of multiple enzyme systems. For this purpose a number of techniques have been employed, including selective precipitation of enzymes by salts such as NH_4Cl, organic solvents such as ethanol, selective inactivation by heat or organic solvents such as chloroform, and selective adsorption and desorption on various gels and ion exchange resins. In recent years, however, column chromatographic and electrophoretic methods have gained widespread popularity. The purification of most enzymes, however, still remains more of an art than a science, and hence the selection of a technique is based on purely pragmatic grounds.

Studies with purified enzymes have provided valuable information on the mechanisms of enzyme action. For example, the sequence of events in a multiple enzyme system may be confirmed with such preparations. Isolated enzymes also provide information on the number of enzymes in the organ which catalyze similar reactions. Purified enzymes have been used to produce antibodies, which in turn have been used to study the sequence of events in multiple enzyme systems. Allosteric changes of purified enzymes may be evaluated without possible misinterpretations by interfering substances. Isolation of enzymes has led to the discovery of similar enzymes having different amino acid sequences and of isozymes. The purification of enzymes has permitted evaluations of their rates of synthesis and catabolism in the body. The interpretation of kinetic studies is greatly simplified with purified preparations.

Nevertheless, the isolation and purification of enzymes is not the panacea many biochemists believe it to be. The relative concentrations of the various components of a multiple enzyme system and intracellular organelles may not be calculated since the recoveries of these components are usually not quantitative. Thus the rate limiting step in multiple enzyme systems may not be elucidated with purified enzymes alone. Moreover, the various components may undergo irreversible changes during the process of solubilization or isolation and thus the Michaelis constants (K_m) and maximum rates (V_m) obtained with purified enzymes may have little relevance to the effective K_m and V_m values in living animals.

It is also frequently a mistake to assume that a reaction catalyzed by a combination of purified enzymes has biological significance. Once the interrelations of a multiple enzyme system are destroyed by solubilization and purification even the sequence of events may be irreparably changed. Thus the assumption that studies of a reaction which occurs with enzymes purified from subcellular particles has a direct bearing on the mechanism of the reaction in living animals or even the subcellular particles is of questionable validity.

From these considerations, there obviously is no single enzyme preparation that adequately answers the needs of the biochemical pharmacologist. Indeed, some preparations have been frequently misused in attempting to show the relationships between enzyme activity and the metabolism of drugs *in vivo*. It is best to use a number of different kinds of preparations and to relate the findings obtained with one type of preparation to those obtained with another.

III. DERIVATION OF RATE EQUATIONS USED IN STUDYING THE KINETICS OF PSEUDOSINGLE SUBSTRATE ENZYME SYSTEMS

The rate of an enzyme-catalyzed reaction is not proportional to the concentration of the substrate, but reaches a limiting rate at high substrate concentrations. This property of enzyme-catalyzed reactions led Michaelis and Menten (1913) to assume that the substrate formed a complex with the enzyme and that the rate of the overall reaction depended on the rate of breakdown of the complex into the products of the reaction. To simplify the study of these events, Michaelis and Menten further assumed that the formation of the complex was much faster than the formation of the products; thus the concentration of the complex depended on the equilibrium between enzyme, substrate and complex. According to this view, the reaction sequence of an enzyme-catalyzed reaction is as follows:

$$(1) \qquad E + S \underset{\substack{k_2 \\ \text{fast}}}{\overset{\substack{\text{fast} \\ k_1}}{\rightleftharpoons}} ES \underset{\text{slow}}{\overset{k_3}{\longrightarrow}} P + E$$

where E represents the enzyme, S the substrate and P the products. The rate of reaction depends on the concentration of the complex (ES),

$$(2) \qquad v = [ES]k_3$$

where v is the rate, [ES] the concentration of the enzyme substrate complex and k_3 the rate constant. At any given substrate concentration a part of the total amount of enzyme is present as the complex and a part is free. Thus,

$$(3) \qquad [E_0] = [E] + [ES]$$

Dividing equation 2 by equation 3 gives the reaction rate per unit enzyme (Equation 4).

$$(4) \qquad \frac{v}{E_0} = \frac{[ES]k_3}{[E] + [ES]}$$

According to the assumption that equilibrium is established between the enzyme and the substrate, [ES] is given by the following relationships

(5) $$[E][S]k_1 = [ES]k_2$$

(6) $$[ES] = [E][S]/(k_2/k_1) = [E][S]/K_S$$

where $K_S = k_2/k_1$ and is the dissociation constant of the complex. Notice that the dimension of K_S is concentration. On substitution of equation (6) into equation (4),

(7) $$\frac{v}{E_0} = \frac{k_3[S]/K_S}{1 + [S]/K_S} = \frac{k_3[S]}{K_S + [S]}$$

At infinite substrate concentrations, however, all of the enzyme is present as ES and thus the maximum rate of the reaction (V_m) is

(8) $$V_m = k_3 E_0$$

On rearranging equation 7 and substitution of equation 8, the rate equation becomes:

(9) $$v = \frac{V_{max}[S]}{K_S + [S]}$$

Unfortunately, k_2 is not always much greater than k_3, as was assumed by Michaelis and Menten and thus the [ES] may not always reach the value predicted by the dissociation constant. Recognizing this, Briggs and Haldane (1925) developed a rate equation based on steady-state kinetics in which the rate of formation of the enzyme-substrate complex equals the rate of breakdown of the complex; i.e.,

$$[E][S] k_1 = [ES](k_2 + k_3)$$

Thus,

(11) $$[ES] = [E][S]/(k_2 + k_3)/k_1 = [E][S]/K_m$$

where $K_m = (k_2 + k_3)/k_1$. The general rate equation becomes

(12) $$v = \frac{V_m[S]}{[S] + K_m}$$

where K_m may be either equal to or greater than K_S, the dissociation constant of the enzyme-substrate complex. The common assumption that K_m is inversely proportional to the affinity of the enzyme for its substrate is thus not universally correct. Indeed, a more accurate definition of K_m is: that concentration of substrate which gives one-half the maximal rate of the reaction under the conditions of the assay.

IV. INHIBITION OF ENZYMES SYSTEMS

Inhibitors may block enzyme systems in a number of ways. Some may act by combining with cofactors or substrates, thereby lowering the effective concentrations of these substances. Others may act by combining either reversibly or irreversibly with the enzyme and thereby change the apparent affinity of the enzyme for the substrate, cofactor, or modified, or by altering the apparent

TABLE 19.1

Equations for various inhibition mechanisms

Mechanism	Partial	Complete
Competitive	$v = \dfrac{V_m}{1 + \dfrac{\alpha K_m[K_i + (I)]}{(S)[\alpha K_i + (I)]}}$	$v = \dfrac{V_m}{1 + \dfrac{K_m}{(S)}\left[1 + \dfrac{(I)}{K_i}\right]}$
Noncompetitive	$v = \dfrac{V_m}{\dfrac{K_i + (I)}{K_i + \beta(I)} + \dfrac{K_m[K_i + (I)]}{(S)[K_i + \beta(I)]}}$	$v = \dfrac{V_m}{\left(1 + \dfrac{(I)}{K_i}\right) + \dfrac{K_m}{(S)}\left(1 + \dfrac{(I)}{K_i}\right)}$
Mixed	$v = \dfrac{V_m}{\dfrac{\alpha K_i + (I)}{[\alpha K_i + \beta(I)]} + \dfrac{\alpha K_m[K_i + (I)]}{(S)[\alpha K_i + \beta(I)]}}$	$v = \dfrac{V_m}{\left(1 + \dfrac{(I)}{\alpha K_i}\right) + \dfrac{K_m}{(S)}\left(1 + \dfrac{(I)}{K_i}\right)}$
Uncompetitive	$v = \dfrac{V_m}{\left(\dfrac{K_i + (I)}{K_i + \beta(I)}\right) + \dfrac{K_m}{(S)}\left(\dfrac{K_i}{K_i + \beta(I)}\right)}$	$v = \dfrac{V_m}{\left(1 + \dfrac{(I)}{K_i}\right) + \dfrac{K_m}{(S)}}$

amount of active enzyme in the system. An inhibitor may thus cause changes in the apparent V_m, the apparent K_m or both. The mechanisms of inhibition have been classified according to how these parameters are affected (see Webb, 1963).

1. *Competitive inhibition.* At any given inhibitor concentration, the apparent K_m is increased, but the apparent V_m is unchanged. In completely competitive inhibition the enzymatic rate decreases to zero as the inhibitor concentration is increased. In partially competitive inhibition, however, the rate of the reaction approaches a limiting value (not zero) as the inhibitor is increased.

2. *Noncompetitive inhibition.* At any given inhibitor concentration the apparent K_m is not altered. In completely noncompetitive inhibition the apparent V_m decreases to zero as the inhibitor concentration increases, but in partially noncompetitive inhibition the V_m decreases to a limiting value (not zero) as the inhibitor concentration is increased.

3. *Mixed inhibition.* At any given concentration of inhibitor, the apparent V_m is decreased and the apparent K_m is increased. In completely mixed inhibition, the rate of the reaction decreases to zero as the inhibitor concentration is increased. In partially mixed inhibition, the rate of the reaction decreases to a limiting value as the inhibitor concentration is increased.

4. *Uncompetitive or coupled inhibition.* At any given inhibitor concentration, both the apparent K_m and the apparent V_m are decreased, but the ratio K_m/V_m remains unchanged.

The rate equations for each of these types of inhibition are given in Table 19.1.

V. PLOTTING TECHNIQUES

Equation 12 may be rearranged to form a number of linear equations, which may be used to evaluate the apparent K_m and the apparent V_m. The formula for the double reciprocal plot, commonly known as the Lineweaver-Burk plot

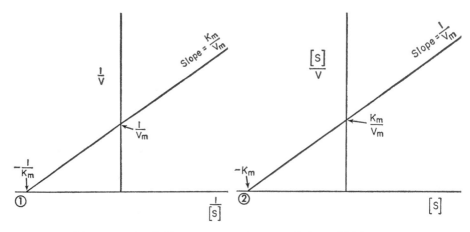

Fig. 19.1 Lineweaver-Burk Plot.   Fig. 19.2 [S]/v vs [S] Plot

(1934), is as follows:

$$\frac{1}{v} = \frac{1}{V_m} + \frac{K_m}{V_m}\cdot\frac{1}{[S]}$$

On plotting $1/v$ against $1/[S]$, the intercept on the y axis is $1/V_m$ and the slope of the line is K_m/V_m (Fig. 19.1). If the line is extrapolated to the x axis, the intercept is $-1/K_m$. Although this kind of plot has been widely used, it is probably the most inaccurate of the plotting techniques, because data obtained at low substrate concentrations are given more weight than data obtained at high substrate concentrations, even though data obtained at low substrate concentrations are usually less accurate. Moreover, the Lineweaver-Burk plot frequently fails to detect curvature of the line.

Because of the statistical inaccuracies of the double reciprocal plot, the [S]/v vs [S] plot, also suggested by Lineweaver and Burk (1934), has recently gained increasing popularity. The equation for this plot is:

$$[S]/v = (K_m/V_m) + ([S]/V_m)$$

On plotting $[S]/v$ against $[S]$, the intercept on the y axis is K_m/V_m and the slope of the line is $1/V_m$ (Fig. 19.2). When the line is extrapolated to the x axis the intercept is $-K_m$. Although this kind of plot weights the data obtained at low and high substrate concentrations about equally, it still frequently fails to detect curvature of the line.

The Hofstee plot (1956) is based on the following equation:

$$v = V_m - K_m\, v/[S]$$

On plotting v vs $v/[S]$ the intercept on the y axis is V_m, the slope is $-K_m$ and the intercept on the x axis is V_{max}/K_m (Fig. 19.3). Although K_m is not as easily determined by this plot as it is by the other plots, this plot weights the data obtained at low and high substrate concentrations about equally. Its principal virtue, however, is in its ability to detect curvature of the line. Indeed, the well-known Scatchard plot, based on an analogous equation, is widely used to detect the binding of substances to various kinds of sites on proteins.

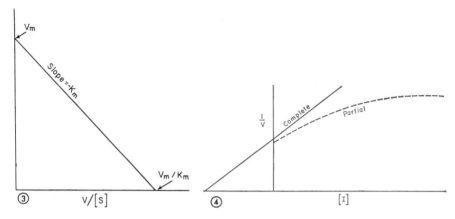

Fig. 19.3 Hofstee Plot.   Fig. 19.4 Dixon Plot.

The Dixon plot (1953) is used in the study of inhibitors. The formula on which it is based is similar to that used for the Lineweaver-Burk plot, but $1/v$ is plotted against $[I]$ (Fig. 19.4). Although this plotting technique may be useful in estimating K_i, it is principally used to differentiate between partial and complete inhibition. Indeed, of the commonly used plots it is the only one which is able to do this. For example, the formula for completely noncompetitive and partially noncompetitive inhibition are as follows:

$$\frac{1}{v} = \frac{1}{V_m}\left[1 + \frac{K_m}{[S]} + \left(1 + \frac{K_m}{[S]}\right)\frac{[I]}{K_i}\right] \quad \begin{array}{l}\text{completely}\\\text{noncompetitive}\end{array}$$

$$\frac{1}{v} = \frac{1}{V_m}\left[\frac{K_i([S] + K_m)}{[S](\beta[I] + K_i)} + \frac{([S] + K_m)[I]}{[S](\beta[I] + K_i)}\right] \quad \begin{array}{l}\text{partially}\\\text{noncompetitive}\end{array}$$

where β is a number between 0 and 1.

Inspection of these equations reveal that the Dixon plot of a completely noncompetitive inhibition gives a straight line with an intercept on the y axis at $1 + (K_m/[S])$ and a slope of $(1 + K_m/[S])/K_i$. If the line is extrapolated to the x axis the intercept is $-K_i$. In contrast, the Dixon plot of a partially noncompetitive inhibition gives a curved line which reaches an asymtope at $1/v = (1/V_m\beta)[1 + (K_m/[S])]$. Similarly, the Dixon plots of partially competitive and partially mixed inhibitions also give curved lines, but of course the asymtopes have different meanings.

VI. GENERAL CONSIDERATIONS IN THE STUDY OF ENZYME ACTIVITY

Before any of the plotting techniques described above may be used to evaluate enzyme activities, it is essential that two criteria be met: (1) the rate must be linear with time, (2) the activity must be proportional to enzyme concentration. By making sure that the enzyme activity is linear with time, one automatically makes sure that the enzyme is not inactivated, that the concentrations of the cofactors and the substrate remain relatively constant during the incubation, and that the accumulation of products from either the substrate or one of the cofactors does not affect the measurement of the initial rate. By making sure that the rate of reaction is proportional to enzyme concentration, one automatically ensures that the free concentrations of the substrates or the cofactors are not markedly decreased by being bound to nonspecific binding sites in components of the enzyme preparation, and that the cofactor generating systems such as NADPH generating systems, are adequate to maintain the cofactor in its fully active form.

Enzyme-activity and time-activity studies should be carried out at both the lowest and the highest concentrations of the substrate, if not at all substrate concentrations, to be used in the kinetic analysis. Some substrates, for example, stabilize the enzyme during incubation, whereas others may promote its inactivation. Moreover, some substrates and cofactors may be highly bound to saturable non-enzymic sites. Furthermore, inhibition by the product arising from the substrate would be more apparent at low substrate concentrations whereas inhibition by products arising from the cofactors would be more likely at high substrate concentrations.

Enzyme-activity studies are important in studying the possible presence of endogenous activators and inhibitors. For example, when a reversible endogenous inhibitor is present the specific activity of the enzyme will appear to decrease as the enzyme concentration is increased, whereas when an endogenous activator is present the specific activity will appear to increase. Time-activity studies reveal the presence of small amounts of endogenous substrates which compete with the substrate for the enzyme. When this occurs the activity appears to increase with time.

Both enzyme-activity and time-activity studies are useful in evaluating the effects of inhibitors. The activity of the enzyme decreases with time when the inhibitor acts by altering the enzyme irreversibly or when the inhibitor is metabolized to a more potent inhibitory metabolite. When an inhibitor is highly bound to either enzymic or nonenzymic sites in the enzyme preparation, however, the degree of inhibition decreases as the enzyme concentration is increased.

VII. INTERPRETATION OF KINETIC STUDIES

Although the kinetics of most enzyme reactions may be expressed in the general form of the Michaelis-Menten equation, it should be borne in mind that a number of assumptions have been made in the derivation of the equation. For example, it has been assumed that the total concentrations of the substrates, cofactors and inhibitors represent the free concentration of these substances in the immediate vicinity of the enzyme site; this implies that the amounts of these substances bound to the enzyme or to other components in the assay system are insignificant compared with their total concentrations and that there are no diffusion barriers between the medium and the enzyme site. It has been assumed that the products of the reaction are released rapidly from the enzyme and that the reaction is essentially pseudo irreversible during its initial phase. It has also been assumed that only one substrate molecule is bound to an enzyme site or that if the enzyme molecule possesses more than one site, the sites act independently.

In many biochemical pharmacology studies, the assumption is made that the free substrate concentration at enzymic sites is equal to the total substrate concentration. This is frequently invalid since many drugs are highly bound to tissue proteins, phospholipids or nucleic acids. In this situation, the rate equation for the metabolism of drugs becomes:

$$v = \frac{V_m(S_t - S_b)}{(S_t - S_b) + K_m}$$

where S_t is the total concentration of the substrate and S_b is the concentration of the bound substrate. The effect of nonenzymic binding in assay systems on the kinetics of the substrate metabolism will depend on the dissociation constant of the complex and the free concentration of the substrate. If at the highest total concentration used the free concentration of the substrate is still much lower than the dissociation constant, the rate equation becomes

b)
$$v = \frac{V_m(S_t)/(1 + B_t/K_b)}{K_m + (S_t)/(1 + B_t/K_b)}$$

where B_t is the concentration of the binding sites and K_b is the dissociation constant. Inspection of this equation reveals that the plots of the data will be linear, but the apparent K_m will be higher than the true K_m value, i.e. apparent $K_m = K_m[1 + (B_t/K_b)]$. On the other hand, if the free concentrations of the substrate are similar to the dissociation constant the equation is quadratic and the plots of the data will not be linear.

$$v = \frac{V_m S_t/[1 + B_t/(S + K_b)]}{K_m + S_t/[1 + B_t/(S + K_b)]}$$

In the metabolism of insoluble drugs, the rate of dissolution of the drugs may limit the rate of metabolism. Dissolution rates, however, depend on a number of factors and thus, the interpretation of studies in which the drug is present as a precipitate is virtually impossible. To overcome some of these difficulties, the drug is frequently added as a soluble complex with proteins. In these studies the total concentration of the protein as well as the total concentration of the substrate are frequently varied. When this is done, however, the plots will be linear only when the binding sites on the protein are virtually saturated, i.e. the free concentration of the drug is much greater than the dissociation constant of the drug-protein complex. Under these conditions the apparent K_m equals $K_m[1 + (B_t/S)]$.

With potent inhibitors, the enzyme concentration may approach and even exceed the inhibition constant. When this occurs, the free concentration of the inhibitor becomes much less than its total concentration. With noncompetitive inhibitors, apparent K_i values may be calculated but, of course, the values will depend on the enzyme concentration. Several approaches may be used to obtain the true K_i values: (1) The binding of I may be measured directly by using the equilibrium dialysis or ultrafiltration techniques described elsewhere in this book. (2) The degree of inhibition of the enzyme is determined at various enzyme concentrations by varying the (I). The apparent K_i values for each enzyme concentration are estimated by interpolation, not extrapolation, of the Dixon plots. These values are then plotted against the enzyme concentration. Extrapolation of a line connecting the points to the y axis give the true K_i value, whereas the slope of the line gives an estimate of the amount of inhibitor bound per mg protein when the free inhibitor concentration equals K_i. The basis for this plot is given by the following equation.

$$K_i(50) = K_i + \left[\frac{0.5(E)}{mg/ml} + \frac{(B)}{mg/ml}\right] mg/ml$$

where $K_i(50)$ is the apparent K_i, K_i is the true K_i, (E) is the amount of enzyme per mg protein, (B) is the concentration (amount per mg protein) of inhibitor bound to nonspecific sites in the enzyme preparation at the inhibitor concentration which blocks the enzyme 50 % and mg/ml is the protein concentration. Inspection of this equation reveals that when the inhibitor is bound solely to the enzyme, the slope of the line may be used to estimate the enzyme concentration in the preparation.

The effects of potent competitive inhibitors are more difficult to evaluate. When the K_i is much less than the enzyme concentration and the inhibitor is bound solely to the enzyme, the inhibition will appear to be noncompetitive at concentrations of substrate near the K_m value. But the Lineweaver-Burk and Dixon plots will be curved at very high substrate concentrations because the free concentration of inhibitor will rise as it is displaced from the enzyme by the substrate. On the other hand, if the inhibitor is bound to non-specific sites as well as enzyme sites in the enzyme preparation, the various plots may give straight lines at very high substrate concentrations, because the free concentration of the inhibitor may not rise appreciably as the inhibitor is displaced from the enzyme sites. This probably accounts for the finding that SKF-525A and Lilly 18947 may competitively block the metabolism of drugs by liver microsomes (Gillette, 1963), even though these inhibitors are highly bound to the enzyme preparation (Gillette, 1965).

Diffusion of polar substrates and cofactors across cell walls may limit the metabolism of drugs by intact cells, tissue slices or perfused liver. Indeed, the rate of diffusion may be so slow relative to the activity of the intracellular enzymes that the kinetics of metabolism are not related to the enzyme activity at all. In this case, both the K_m and the V_m will appear to be infinite. In most cases, however, the rate depends primarily on the enzyme reaction but the rate of diffusion is slow enough to exert a significant effect. In these cases, the plots will curve and will approach the values predicted by the Michaelis-Menten equation only at high substrate concentrations (*see* Lineweaver and Burk, 1934).

It is also possible that the active site of an enzyme is embedded in a lipid phase and that the rate depends only indirectly on the substrate concentration in the aqueous phase. If equilibrium is established between the substrate in the aqueous phase and that in the lipid phase, the various plots will be linear but the apparent K_m would equal the true K_m divided by the distribution ratio. Although it is conceivable that this process may play a role in the metabolism of lipid-soluble substrates by liver microsomes, no unequivocal evidence has appeared establishing the validity of this view.

In most studies on the effects of competitive inhibitors, it is generally assumed that the inhibitor is not metabolized by the enzyme. If the inhibitor is converted to products which do not interfere with the assay of substrate metabolism, the usual plotting techniques may be employed. If the inhibitor is metabolized by the same enzyme as the substrate these plotting techniques should show that the K_i value of the inhibitor is identical to its K_m value. Let S_1 be the substrate and S_2 be the inhibitor. Thus the rate equations will be:

$$v_1 = \frac{V_{m1}[S_1]/K_{m1}}{1 + [S_1]/K_{m1} + [S_2]/K_{m2}} = \frac{V_{m1}}{1 + \dfrac{K_{m1}}{[S_1]}\left(1 + \dfrac{(S_2)}{K_{m2}}\right)}$$

$$v_2 = \frac{V_{m2}[S_2]/K_{m2}}{1 + [S_1]/K_{m1} + [S_2]/K_{m2}} = \frac{V_{m2}}{1 + \dfrac{K_{m2}}{[S_2]}\left(1 + \dfrac{[S_1]}{K_{m1}}\right)}$$

where v_1, V_{m1}, and K_{m1} refer to the metabolism of the substrate and v_2, V_{m2}, and K_{m2} refer to the metabolism of the inhibitor.

When the inhibitor and the substrate are converted to the same product, however, the total rate of product formation becomes:

$$V_t = v_1 + v_2 = \frac{(V_{m1}[S_1]/K_{m1}) + (V_{m2}[S_2]/K_{m2})}{1 + ([S_1]/K_{m1}) + ([S_2]/K_{m2})}$$

If the concentration of the inhibitor, $[S_2]$, is held constant while the concentration of the substrate, $[S_1]$, is varied, the Lineweaver-Burk plot will be curved. It will reach an asymtope at $(K_{m2} + [S_2])/V_{m2}[S_2]$ and will insect the y axis at $1/V_{m1}$. If a Lineweaver-Burk plot of the metabolism of the substrate in the absence of the inhibitor is now superimposed on the plot the two lines will cross not only at the y axis but also at $1/S = (V_{m1} - V_{m2})/V_{m2}K_{m1}$ provided that the maximum rate of metabolism of the substrate, (V_{m1}), is greater than that of the inhibitor (V_{m2}). This relationship has been used by Sladek and Mannering (1969) to determine whether drugs are demethylated by the same enzyme in liver microsomes.

VIII. COSUBSTRATE ENZYME SYSTEMS

Although the kinetics of most enzyme reactions superficially resemble the form of the Michaelis-Menten model, virtually every enzymatic reaction is far more complex. For example, the model assumes that the product is released rapidly and that there are no complexes with cofactors or transitory intermediates, but for most enzyme systems these assumptions are not valid. Most drug metabolizing enzyme systems require cofactors such as acetyl-CoA, UDPGA, PAPS, S-adenosylmethionine, or one of the pyridine-adenine dinucleotides. These cofactors may participate in the various drug metabolizing systems through a variety of mechanisms; most of these mechanisms, however, may be related to four basic mechanisms that can be readily discerned from initial rate studies.

The cofactor (A) and substrate (S) may combine with the enzyme in a random order, as illustrated in the following model.

$$\begin{array}{ccc}
E & \underset{k_2}{\overset{k_1 S}{\rightleftharpoons}} & ES \\[2mm]
k_4 \big\Vert k_3 A & & k_6 \big\Vert k_5 A \\[2mm]
EA & \underset{k_8}{\overset{k_7 S}{\rightleftharpoons}} EAS & \xrightarrow{k_9} E + B + P
\end{array}$$

In this model it is generally assumed that k_9 is much smaller than the other rate constants and that equilibria are established among the various enzyme forms. It is also assumed that $k_3 = k_5$, $k_4 = k_6$, $k_1 = k_7$ and $k_2 = k_8$. When these assumptions are valid the rate equation is similar to the Michaelis-Menten equation:

$$v = \left(\frac{V_{max}(S)}{(S) + K_s}\right)\left(\frac{(A)}{(A) + K_a}\right)$$

where $K_s = k_2/k_1$ and $K_a = k_4/k_3$.

This equation may be rearranged to form linear equations as described for the Michaelis-Menten equation. Plotting of $1/v$ vs $1/S$ would reveal that varying the concentration of (A) changes the apparent V_{max} but does not change the K_s value. Similarly, plotting $1/v$ vs $1/(A)$ would give straight lines which would reveal that different concentrations of S change the apparent V_{max}, but do not alter K_a. Inhibitors which act on the same site as A would be competitive with respect to A but noncompetitive with respect to S.

If $k_3 \neq k_5$, $k_4 \neq k_5$, $k_1 \neq k_7$ and $k_2 \neq k_8$, plots of $1/v$ vs $1/S$ would show that varying the concentration of A changes both the apparent V_m and K_s and plots of $1/v$ vs $1/A$ would show that varying the concentration of S changes both the apparent V_m and K_a. Moreover, inhibitors that act on the same sites as A would be competitive with respect to A but either noncompetitive or mixed with respect to S.

By contrast, the steady-state equation derived according to the method of King and Altman (1956) is a binominal and thus will not be in the form of the Michaelis-Menten equation unless k_9 is much smaller than the other rate constants. When k_9 is large the various plots will be curved, and thus the K_m, V_{max} and the inhibitor relationships will not be readily evaluated. It follows, therefore, that when linear plots are obtained, it may be presumed that the system is virtually in equilibrium or is ordered (see below).

It is also noteworthy that the noncompetitive inhibition is illustrated by the same model except that (ES) rather than (EAS) is the active enzyme-substrate complex. When steady-state conditions rather than equilibrium conditions occur in the enzyme system the rate equation will not be of the Michaelis-Menten type. Lineweaver-Burk plots of noncompetitive inhibition under these conditions will thus not appear to be "noncompetitive" according to the usual criteria. It also follows, therefore, that when linear plots are obtained and noncompetitive inhibition is observed, it may be presumed that the enzyme system is in equilibrium or that E I cannot be converted to E I S directly.

In some mechanisms, the cofactor and the substrate may combine with the enzyme in a definite order. For example, the cofactor may react with the enzyme-substrate complex but not with the free enzyme and thus no enzyme-cofactor complex is formed. This kind of reaction may be illustrated by the following model.

$$E \underset{k_2}{\overset{Sk_1}{\rightleftharpoons}} ES \underset{k_4}{\overset{Ak_3}{\rightleftharpoons}} EAS \overset{k_5}{\longrightarrow} E + B + P$$

If equilibrium conditions are established among the various enzyme forms, the rate equation for this mechanism is:

$$v = \frac{V_m(S)(A)}{K_aK_s + (S)K_a + (S)(A)}$$

This equation may be rearranged to form linear equations which are analogous to those for the Michaelis-Menten equation. Plotting $1/v$ against $1/(S)$ reveals that varying the concentration of A changes both the apparent V_m and the apparent K_s. By contrast plotting $1/v$ against $1/(A)$ reveals that varying the concentration of S changes the apparent K_a but not the V_m. Inhibitors which react with the same site as A would be competitive with respect to A but uncompetitive with respect to S.

In the acetylation of drugs the enzyme is activated by acetyl CoA and the activated enzyme then reacts with the substrate (Weber and Cohen, 1967a,b). The mechanism may be visualized as follows:

$$E \underset{k_2}{\overset{k_1A}{\rightleftharpoons}} EA \underset{k_4}{\overset{k_3}{\rightleftharpoons}} EB \underset{k_6}{\overset{k_5}{\rightleftharpoons}} E' + B$$

$$E' \underset{k_8}{\overset{k_1S}{\rightleftharpoons}} E'S \underset{k_{10}}{\overset{k_9}{\rightleftharpoons}} EP \underset{k_{12}}{\overset{k_{11}}{\rightleftharpoons}} E + P$$

In this model there is no EAS complex and thus the rate requation equation is:

$$v = \frac{V_m(A)(S)}{(A)(S) + K_s(A) + K_a(S)}$$

Inversion of this equation reveals that on plotting $1/v$ vs $1/(S)$ the slope will be K_s/V_m, the intercept at the y axis will be $[1 + (K_a/(A))]/V_m$ and the intercept at the x axis will be $-[1 + (K_a/(A))]/K_s$. Thus, increasing concentrations of A will increase both the apparent V_{max} and the apparent K_s, but the ratio of K_s/V_{max} will be constant. Similarly, Lineweaver-Burk plots in which (A) is varied will have a slope of K_a/V_{max} but will intersect the y axis at $[1 + (K_s/(S))]/V_m$ and the x axis at $-[1 + (K_s/(S))]/K_a$. Thus increasing concentrations of A will increase both the apparent V_m and the apparent K_m, but the ratio of K_s/V_m will be constant. Inhibitors which interact with E but not E' will appear to be competitive with respect to A but uncompetitive with respect to S, whereas those which interact with E' but not E, will appear to be competitive with respect to S but uncompetitive with respect to A. In contrast inhibitors which react with both E and E' will appear to be noncompetitive with respect to both A and S. It seems probable that most instances of uncompetitive inhibition arise by selective interaction with different forms of an enzyme as illustrated in this mechanism.

In a fourth mechanism the cofactor and the substrate react simultaneously with the enzyme. This mechanism may be illustrated as follows:

$$E \underset{k_2}{\overset{(S)(A)k_1}{\rightleftharpoons}} EAS \overset{k_3}{\longrightarrow} E + B + P$$

Since, there are no binary complexes with either A or S in this mechanism, the rate equation is:

$$v = \frac{V_m[A][S]}{K_{as} + [A][S]}$$

where K_{as} is not the Michaelis constant in the usual sense, because its dimension is concentration[2]. On plotting $1/v$ vs $1/[S]$, the apparent K_m decreases with increasing concentrations of A_s but the V_{max} remains constant. Similarly on plotting $1/v$ vs $1/[A]$ the apparent K_a decreases with increasing concentrations of S, but again the V_m remains constant. One of the unique properties of this mechanism is that an inhibitor which acts competitively with respect to the cofactor will also act competitively with respect to the substrate.

Mechanisms that are more complex than these may occur, some of which may result in changes of the apparent K_m and V_m values that are not described here. Indeed many mechanisms may not be differentiated by studying the initial rates of product formation alone. When the reaction is reversible, however, many of the mechanisms may be differentiated by studying the inhibitory effects of various concentrations of the products as well as by studying the effects of various concentrations of the cofactor and substrate. In carrying out such studies, however, it should be remembered that the interpretations are based on the assumptions that the enzymes are pure and that the results are not obscured by side reactions, the presence of similar enzymes or the presence of endogenous inhibitors or activators.

IV. COUPLED ENZYME SYSTEMS

In order to maintain NADPH and NADH in their active form in an incubation system, other enzymes which catalyze the reduction of NADP and NAD are frequently added to the incubation system. It is not often realized, however, that regenerating systems which are adequate at high concentrations of the coenzyme may not be adequate at low coenzyme concentrations.

To illustrate this point, let us consider the kinetics of a coupled system in which an enzyme that utilizes NADPH has a low K_m with respect to NADPH and an enzyme that generates NADPH has a high K_m with respect to NADP. At infinite concentrations of the other substrates utilized in the coupled system, the rate equation for the NADPH generating system becomes:

$$v_1 = \frac{V_{m1}[NADP]}{K_{m1} + [NADP]}$$

while that of the NADPH utilizing enzyme is

$$v_2 = \frac{V_{m2}[NADPH]}{K_{m2} + [NADPH]}$$

In a coupled system, a steady-state between the oxidation of NADPH and the reduction of NADP is rapidly established and thus v_1 equals v_2. The rate therefore becomes:

$$\frac{V_{m1}[NADP]}{[NADP] + K_{m1}} = \frac{V_{m2}[NADPH]}{[NADPH] + K_{m2}} = v$$

This equation may be rearranged to the following linear equation:

$$\frac{[NADPH]}{[NADP]} = \frac{[NADPH](V_{m1} - V_{m2})}{K_{m1}V_{m2}} + \frac{V_{m1}K_{m2}}{K_{m1}V_{m2}}$$

On plotting $[NADPH]/[NADP]$ against $[NADPH]$, the slope is $(V_{m1} - V_{m2})/K_{m1}V_{m2}$ and the intercept is $V_{m1}K_{m2}/V_{m2}K_{m1}$.

TABLE 19.2

Let $V_{m1} = 10\ V_{m2}$ and $Km_1 = 100\ K_{m2}$

[NADPH]		[NADPH]/[NADP]	[NADP]	
100	K_{m2}	9.1	11	K_{m2}
10	K_{m2}	1.0	10	K_{m2}
1	K_{m2}	.19	5	K_{m2}

Let $V_{m1} = 10\ V_{m2}$ and $K_{m1} = 10\ K_{m2}$

100	K_{m2}	91	1.1	K_{m2}
10	K_{m2}	10	1.0	K_{m2}
1	K_{m2}	1.9	.5	K_{m2}
.1	K_{m2}	1.09	.09	K_{m2}

Table 19.2 shows the ratios of NADPH to NADP which would be expected to exist in a hypothetical system in which the maximum velocity of the NADPH generating enzyme was 10 times greater than that of NADPH oxidizing enzyme and the K_m value of the generating enzyme was 100 times that of the oxidizing enzyme. When the total concentration of coenzyme is well above the K_m of the oxidizing enzyme, ($111 \times K_{m2}$ = total conc.) about 91 % of the coenzyme would be in the reduced form, but when the total concentration of the coenzyme is about six times the K_m of the oxidizing enzyme, only about 17 % of it is in the reduced form. Thus this concentration of the NADPH generating enzyme would be adequate at the high coenzyme concentrations but would be useless in attempting to determine the K_m (NADPH) for the oxidizing enzyme. An even more complicated situation may occur with NADPH cytochrome c reductase, which is presumably a component of the drug oxidizing enzymes in liver microsomes. NADP competitively inhibits this enzyme with a K_i value which is similar to the K_m (NADPH). Although inhibition of the cytochrome c reductase by NADP would cause an apparent increase in the K_{m2}, it would also tend to increase the NADPH/NADP ratio.

From the constant term in the above equation it is possible to calculate the ratio of the enzyme activities needed to keep the NADPH/NADP ratio within acceptable limits at all concentrations of the cofactor. If a minimum NADPH/NADP ratio of 10 (91 % of the total in the reduced form) is acceptable, the V_{m1}/V_{m2} ratio should be 10 (K_{m1}/K_{m2}). Thus for a coupled system which consists of NADPH cytochrome c reductase (K_m(NADPH) of about 2×10^{-6} M) and glucose-6-phosphate dehydrogenase (K_m(NADP) of about 2×10^{-5} M) the V_{m1}/V_{m2} ratios should be about 100.

These considerations illustrate one of the difficulties in attempting to elucidate the "rate-limiting" step of a reaction in intact cells, tissues and organs. An enzyme which generates a cofactor may limit the metabolism of a drug in living animals and in the cellular preparation even though assays of tissue homogenates indicate it to be in excess of the cofactor utilizing enzyme. For example, in perfused liver the generation of NADPH may limit the demethylation of aminopyrine under certain conditions (Thurman and Scholz, 1969). Moreover, formation of the ethereal sulfate conjugate of salicylamide in man may be limited by the availability of inorganic sulfate and hence by 3'-phosphoadenosine-5'-phosphosulfate (PAPS), the cofactor required for ethereal sulfate formation.

It seems apparent that some of the discrepancies between *in vitro* and *in vivo* studies of drug metabolism may be explained by difference between the steady-state levels of cofactors in cells and their levels in the *in vitro* systems.

REFERENCES

Briggs, G. E. and Haldane, J. B. S.: A role on the kinetics of enzyme action. Biochem. J. *19:* 338–339, 1925.

Dallner, G.: Studies on the structural and enzymic organization of the membranous elements of liver microsomes. Acta Path. Microbiol. Scand. (Suppl.) 166–193, 1963.

Gillette, J. R.: Metabolism of drugs and other foreign compounds by enzymatic mechanisms. Progress in Drug Research *6:* 11–73, 1963.

Gillette, J. R.: Reversible Binding as a Complication in Relating the *in vitro* Effects of Drugs to Their *in vivo* Activity, pp. 9–22. In *Drugs and Enzymes*, Proceedings of the 2nd International Pharmacological Meeting. Pergamon, Oxford, 1965.

Govier, W. C.: Reticuloendothelial cells as the site of sulfanilamide acetylation in the rabbit. J. Pharmacol. Exp. Ther. *150:* 305–308, 1965.

Hofstee, B. H. J.: Graphical analysis of single enzyme systems. Enzymologia *17:* 273–278, 1956.

King, E. L. and Altman, C.: A schematic method of deriving the rate laws for enzyme-catalyzed reactions. J. Phys. Chem. *60:* 1375–1378, 1956.

Lineweaver, H. and Burk, D.: The determination of enzyme dissociation constants. J. Am. Chem. Soc. *56:* 658–666, 1934.

Lu, A. Y. H., Junk, K. W., and Coon, M. J.: Resolution of the cytochrome P-450 containing a hydroxylation system of liver microsomes into three components. J. Biol. Chem. *244:* 3714–3721, 1969a.

Lu, A. Y. H., Strobel, H. W., and Coon, M. J.: Hydroxylation of benzphetamine and other drugs by a solubilized form of cytochrome P-450 from liver microsomes: lipid requirement for drug demethylation. Biochem. Biophys. Res. Commun. *36:* 545–551, 1969b.

Michaelis, L. and Menten, M. L.: Die Kinetik der Invertinwirkung. Biochem. Z. *49:* 333–369, 1913.

Nebert, D. W. and Gelboin, H. V.: Substrate-inducible microsomal aryl hydroxylase in mammalian cell culture: 1. Assay and properties of induced enzyme. J. Biol. Chem. *243:* 6242–6249, 1968a.

Nebert, D. W. and Gelboin, H. V.: Substrate-inducible microsomal aryl hydroxylase in mammalian cell culture. II. Cellular responses during enzyme induction. J. Biol. Chem. *243:* 6250–6251, 1968b.

Schneider, W. C. and Hogeboom, G. H.: Intracellular distribution of enzymes. V. Further studies on distribution of cytochrome *c* in rat liver homogenates. J. Biol. Chem. *183:* 123–128, 1950.

Thurman, R. G. and Scholz, R.: Control of mixed function oxygenases in perfused rat liver. The Pharmacologist *11:* 260, 1969.

Webb, J. L.: *Enzyme and Metabolic Inhibitors*, Vol. *1*, 1963. Academic Press, New York and London.

Weber, W. W. and Cohen, S. N.: N-acetylation of drugs: Isolation and properties of an N-acetyltransferase from rabbit liver. Mol. Pharm. *3:* 266–273, 1967a.

Weber, W. W. and Cohen, S. N.: The mechanism of isoniazid acetylation by human N-acetyltransferase. Biochim. Biophys. Acta *151:* 276–278, 1967b.

20

Isolation Procedures—Liquid Extraction and Isolation Techniques

ELWOOD O. TITUS

I. INTRODUCTION

The enormous growth of interest in the metabolism and distribution of chemical substances in the body has brought with it a flood of methods for the determination of drugs and their metabolites in biological material. Analytical procedures usually include some preliminary purification of the desired component. Since the methods by which this is achieved are generally similar to those for the fractionation of metabolites, no distinction will be made between analytical and preparatory methods of separation. Almost all separatory procedures make use of repeated partitions of a substance between two phases. The latter may be pairs of immiscible liquids as in countercurrent distribution and partition chromatography, a liquid and a solid surface as in chromatography, a liquid and a vapor phase in gas chromatography, etc. A useful guide to the suitability of various methods for different types of molecules has been published by Pfleiderer (1965). The extraction techniques with which this chapter is particularly concerned have been exhaustively reviewed by Craig and Craig (1956).

II. THEORY OF EXTRACTION

The theory that underlies all extraction procedures states that a solute will distribute between two immiscible liquids such as water and a hydrocarbon so that the ratio of concentration in the organic phase to the concentration in the aqueous phase always equals k, the Nernst partition constant. To the extent that there is dimerization or other concentration dependent change in the molecular species of solute in either phase, there will be concentration-dependent changes in the ratio, k, so that its true value will be measurable only in very dilute solutions. This is often the case for drugs that contain free carboxylic groups, which tend to dimerize, or long aliphatic side chains, which can associate appreciably at low concentrations.

Since in most cases the ionized forms of acidic or basic drugs remain entirely in the aqueous layer of a liquid pair the distribution of these substances between organic solvents and aqueous solutions is very sensitive to pH. If, for example, the solute in question is an organic amine and if the pH of the aqueous phase is sufficiently acidic so that salt formation with organic base is appreciable, then at least two equilibrium conditions, which must both be satisfied in the final partitition, will contribute to the distribution of amine. The relative concentrations of free base in solvent and water must satisfy the Nernst partition constant. At the same time free base entering the aqueous phase will have been protonated until the concentration of the resultant cation comes into equilibrium with the hydrogen ion and free base in the aqueous phase. If the aqueous half of a liquid-liquid pair is strongly buffered so that the concentration of hydrogen is not altered by small amounts of the amine to be distributed, the pH can be the most important determinant of the final distribution of drug.

In actual extractions the number of molecular or ionic species involved is of little concern. The important information is the relative amount of solute in each component of the solvent pair. If k represents the ratio of the concentration of a drug in an organic phase to the concentration in the aqueous phase, and V_0 and V_a represent the volumes of the two phases, a constant, K, equal to k $\times$ V_0/V_a will equal the ratio of the absolute amount of drug in the organic phase to the absolute amount in the aqueous phase. This "effective distribution constant" is a convenient form for the expression of distribution data since the fraction of the total solute in the organic phase at equilibrium is then simply $K/(K + 1)$. K of course is a valid constant only when the relative volumes of the two solvents and other conditions such as pH, temperature, salt content of the phases, etc. are specified.

III. SIMPLE EXTRACTION PROCEDURES

A. General Considerations

Many drugs and their metabolites are rather lipophilic acids or bases that are extractable into organic solvents in the non-ionized form. Extraction into solvents from aqueous tissue extracts that have been adjusted to appropriate pH will sometimes separate small amounts of drugs and their metabolites from other tissue components to an extent which permits further fractionation by micro methods such as gas chromatography or thin-layer chromatography. If a drug has ultraviolet absorption or fluorescent properties that adequately identify it, or if other determinative procedures of adequate specificity are available, a few simple extraction steps will often provide sufficient purification to permit its analytical determination in the extracts.

The removal of protein from the aqueous phase is usually imperative if emulsification is not to hinder these extractions. Tissues are therefore frequently homogenized in 0.1 N HCl to extract basic drugs. Water extracts may be treated with 5% trichloroacetic acid or 0.4 N perchloric acid to precipitate proteins. Two extractions of the protein-free filtrate with cold peroxide-free ether will frequently suffice to remove remaining trichloracetic acid without significant loss of basic drugs. Perchloric acid may be largely removed by titration with K_2CO_3 to give insoluble $KClO_4$.

Once the protein has been removed from a tissue extract and the pH adjusted to minimize ionization of the drug or metabolite to be extracted, there remains the question of the most suitable solvent. The partition coefficient, k, will depend on the relative ability of the solute to associate with water or solvent. A few simple generalizations may be useful in relating the choice of solvent to the structure of the solute to be extracted. Lipophilic structures pass from water nto hydrocarbon solvents because the CH_2 moieties of the drug associate with those of the solvent, with concomitant exclusion of the water between them. It is energetically less expensive to maintain a water envelope about a pair of CH_2 groups than to maintain separate envelopes about two such moieties. The aliphatic hydrocarbons, however, provide essentially no opportunity for dipole-dipole interaction and none for hydrogen bonding. Solutes with polar or polarizable groups will therefore tend to have partition coefficients more favorable to water.

In general, addition of groups such as NH_2 or OH increase the solubility of drugs in more polar liquids, the effect being most often due to hydrogen bonding between solute and solvent. Consideration of the possibility of hydrogen bonding may help in predicting effects of changes in solvent or of alterations in the structure of the solvent. Ethers, amines, aldehydes and ketones will act as proton acceptors in the formation of such bonds. The hydroxyl groups of water and alcohols can serve both as donors and acceptors. Alcohols such as butanol and its homologues, which have sufficiently large non-polar groups so that they form a second phase with water, are thus excellent solvents for the extraction of more polar drugs.

The utility of relatively simple extraction procedures was pointed out by Brodie et al. (1947a) in their discussion of general methods for the determination of organic bases in biological material. These authors recommended the use of the least polar solvent that would adequately remove the drug from aqueous tissue homogenates made alkaline with NaOH. Since most metabolic alterations increase the polarity of the drug, this precaution minimizes the extraction of metabolites. Such of the latter as are taken into the organic phase may frequently be removed by shaking the solvent with alkaline aqueous solutions. The organic solvent may then be washed by shaking with water and the desired base can be concentrated by a final extraction from the organic solvent into a small volume of strong acid such as 0.1 N HCl or H_2SO_4. Hexane, cyclohexane, benzene and ethylene dichloride have been used extensively in such procedures. Since the concentration of drug or metabolite in these extracts is usually of the order of micro- or nanograms per ml, adsorption on the glass walls of the containers is sometimes appreciable. Inclusion of 1.5% isoamyl alcohol in the extracting solvent is a routine precaution that will usually prevent this.

Not infrequently drugs are metabolized to derivatives so similar in polarity to the parent substance that both metabolite and drug are extensively extracted by the same solvent. Partition of the extracted material between solvent and a buffer of appropriate pH will sometimes separate the individual components sufficiently to permit analytical determination. Chlorpromazine and its metabolite, chlorpromazine sulfoxide, are both extracted from alkalinized biological material into heptane containing 1.5% isoamyl alcohol in the analytical procedure of Salzman and Brodie (1956). The sulfoxide, however, may be separated from the chlorpromazine by extraction into 0.1 M acetate buffer, pH 5.6. In another example (Dingell et al., 1964) imipramine and its metabolite desmethylimipramine (DMI) are similarly extracted into heptane. When the extract is shaken with 0.2 M phosphate, pH 5.9, about 80% of the DMI but only 10% of the imipramine is removed into the aqueous phase.

The dependence of partition coefficients on the pH of the aqueous phase is, of course, particularly marked at pH values near the pKa of the drug, since there the degree of ionization is changing most rapidly. A plot of partition coefficient versus pH in a series of buffered liquid pairs will thus distinguish between otherwise closely related substances that differ slightly in pK. Such plots have proved useful as tests for the specificity of analytical procedures. Thus if material recovered from tissue by the analytical procedure displays the physical properties of the desired drug or metabolite and also has the same partition coefficient as authentic substance at several pH values, the analytical procedure may be considered trustworthy (Brodie et al., 1947a).

B. The Use of Solvents of Varying Polarity

In some simple extraction procedures it may be advantageous to vary the polarity of the extracting solvent. In the experiments of Titus and Weiss (1952), for example, it was desirable to recover as many as possible of the excreted metabolites of pentobarbital-C^{14} for analysis by chromatography and countercurrent distribution. Extraction of dog urine with butanol yielded ten metabolites. With such polar solvents as this, extraction of inorganic substances from biological material is appreciable and substances recovered by evaporation of butanol extracts must often be separated from salts by repeated trituration with methanol or by electrolytic desalting before further fractionation.

The extraction of drugs or their metabolites from body fluids into solvents of relatively high polarity and their subsequent displacement into an aqueous phase by the addition of non-polar solvent is sometimes an effective means for partial purification. In the procedure of Shore (1959) for the determination of norepinephrine, tissue extracts are made alkaline and saturated with salt, then shaken with butanol. The addition of heptane to the washed butanol extract greatly enhances the recovery of norepinephrine when the latter is back extracted into aqueous acid. In this instance the procedure was dictated by the polar nature of the catecholamine which, even as the free base, is only slightly extractable into the solvents generally used for amine determinations. A procedure similar in principle has been used by Goldbaum and Domanski (1966) to isolate the neutral drugs Carbromal, Bromural, Valmid, Noludar, Meprobamate, Doriden and Soma. These were recovered by the evaporation of ether extracts of tissue or urine after organic bases and acids had been washed out with acid and alkali. After the residues were dissolved in ethanol:hexane (4:10) and one part of water was added, a lower phase containing the desired drugs separated from a heptane phase containing most of the tissue lipids. Microgram quantities of the drugs were thus recovered in sufficient purity to permit their final resolution by gas chromatography. A very similar procedure has been used to recover progesterone from biological specimens for thin layer chromatography (Watson et al., 1967).

The necessity to recover metabolites from biological material dictates that water will be one of the two liquids phases in most extraction experiments. Non-aqueous liquid pairs, however, are occasionally useful for the further fractionating by countercurrent distribution of material already partially purified. The partition coefficient in such a system may also be used as an identifying physical constant. The latter device is particularly useful when drugs or metabolites are recovered in amounts too small for identification by the usual criteria. A potentially very useful application has been described by Beroza and Bowman (1965a, 1965b) (Bowman and Beroza, 1965, 1966) who have separated trace amounts of pesticides by gas chromatography. In cases where different materials gave identical retention times or where further identification was necessary, fractions were dissolved in the upper phase of an immiscible solvent pair and shaken with the lower phase. The concentration of solute in the upper phase was determined by quantitative gas chromatography before and after extraction. For the chlorinated hydrocarbons, which could be determined by electron affinity methods, distribution data could be obtained with nanogram amounts. Constants for 131 pesticides have been tabulated (Bowman and Beroza, 1965). Solvent systems used in this work were hexane with either acetonitrile or 90% dimethyl sulfoxide, isooctane with dimethyl formamide or 80% octane and heptane/90% ethanol.

Other immiscible systems are, of course, possible. Craig and Craig (1956) adopted the very useful device of listing common solvents in the order of increasing dielectric constant as below:

Pentane	Benzene	o-Dichlorobenzene
Isopentane	Toluene	Carbon disulfide
Hexane	Ethylene dichloride	The higher ethers
Heptane	Tetrachloroethylene	Diisopropyl ether
2,2,4-Trimethylpentane	Methylene chloride	Diethyl ether
Cyclohexane	Carbon tetrachloride	Furan
Cyclopentane	Chloroform	Furfural
Thiophene	Pentanol	Pyridine homologs
Methyl ethyl ketone	Tertiary pentanol	Pyridine
Methylcyclohexanone	Butanol	Morpholine
Acetone	Secondary butanol	Aniline
Dioxane	Propanol	Phenol
Amyl acetate	Ethanol	Acetic acid
Isopropyl acetate	Methanol	Formamide
Ethyl acetate	Acetonitrile	Water
Methyl acetate	Nitromethane	Hydrochloric acid
Nitrobenzene	Nitroethane	Sulfuric acid
Cyclohexanol	Methoxyethylene glycol	Salt solutions

In general, solvents are miscible with others listed nearby but immiscible with those far removed. The list is useful in devising liquid pairs for extraction studies such as those just described or for countercurrent distribution. For those solvents which are insoluble in water the list also indicates the order of increasing ability to remove more polar solutes from aqueous solution.

C. The Extraction of Ion Pairs

Favorable distribution coefficients may be obtained by means other than variation of the solvents. The extraction of pharmaceutical amines and quaternary ammonium compounds as ion pairs with anionic dye molecules has been long known. These extractions provide some specificity since they are carried out in acidic solutions. Ionized organic bases are therefore removed only if they can form ion pairs soluble in the extracting solvent. The well-known dye extraction methods (Brodie et al., 1947b; Ballard et al., 1954; Axelrod, 1960; Schill, 1965, 1965a) for the estimation of organic bases in biological material use this principle.

Biles has investigated the extraction of quaternary amines (Divatia and Biles, 1961; Hull and Biles, 1964).

Some very useful theoretical studies of ion pair extraction have appeared recently. Higuchi and Michaelis (1968) (Higuchi et al., 1967) have observed that the extraction of dextromethorphan from aqueous solutions of low pH into mixtures of cyclohexane and chloroform or pentanol depends on the presence of bromide ions. Extractability is ascribed to the formation of complexes between the ion pair and the polar solvent that is dissolved in cyclohexane. The data indicate that complexes containing three to five molecules of solvent per ion pair can be expected. The extraction of codeine, lidocaine, promazine and strychnine as ion pairs with a number of inorganic anions has been studied by Schill et al. (1965). Iodide and thiocyanate in chloroform-water systems gave useful coefficients which permitted the separation of these amines when the solvents were used in partition chromatography. Similar pairs with methadone, papaverine, emetine, meclizine and pyrilamine are extractable (Persson and Schill, 1966). This and other publications from the same group (Gustavii and Schill, 1966a, 1966b) will be of interest to those concerned with analytical applications of association complexes and the computation of conditions for their use in separations.

Ion pair extractions of pharmaceutical amines with more lipid soluble anions such as p-toluene sulfonate have been studied by Doyle and Levine (1967) to devise systems appropriate for partition chromatography. At pH values low enough for significant protonation of amino acids these substances will form complexes with tetraphenyl borate that partition between ether and water with k values in the range of 5 to 50 (Beyermann, 1965). The formation of extractable tri-n-butyl ammonium salts of transfer ribonucleic acids has made possible the use of countercurrent distribution for the separation of RNA's specific for individual amino acids (Karau and Zachau, 1964).

D. Enhancement of Extractability by Enzymatic Reactions

Since many drugs and metabolites are excreted as glucuronides or sulfuric acid esters which are essentially not extractable into organic solvents, it is often necessary to hydrolyze these derivatives. Incubations with β-glucuronidase and sulfatase have long been used as a means of achieving this without the potentially harmful effects of chemical hydrolysis on the parent compound. Beyer (1965) has recently determined the optimal conditions for the application of these enzymatic procedures to a variety of drug metabolites.

The methylation of phenolic hydroxyls by S-adenosyl methionine and specific methylating enzymes has been used to convert catecholamines (Axelrod and Tomchick, 1958) and 5-hydroxytryptamine (Axelrod and Weissbach, 1961) to readily extractable derivatives.

IV. COUNTERCURRENT DISTRIBUTION

A. General Principles

Despite the variety of methods for obtaining favorable distribution coefficients, simple extraction procedures will seldom recover drugs or metabolites from biological material in sufficient purity for chemical characterization. Various systems for separation by multiple extraction were reviewed some years ago by Craig and Craig (1956). By far the most satisfactory of these is countercurrent distribution. This procedure is applicable both on the preparative scale and at trace levels of solute. The fractionated material can usually be totally accounted for by evaporation of the solvents. Since the pattern of distribution of a substance is predictable from its partition coefficient, the procedure is useful analytically. Small amounts of impurities are measurable by means of discrepancies between observed and theoretical distribution patterns.

Countercurrent distribution in a series of separatory funnels is possible but prohibitively time consuming for more than about ten transfers. An all glass distribution train has been described by Craig et al. (1951a) (Craig and Craig, 1956; Titus, 1960) and commercial models are available. In essence, countercurrent distribution is a series of single extractions. Ideally each solute obeys the Nernst distribution law so that K remains independent of concentration or of the presence of other solutes. As noted earlier $K = p/q$ where p represents the fraction of a component in the upper phase and q the fraction in the lower phase and $p + q = 1$. In practice the apparatus provides a series of tubes numbered 0, 1, 2- - -r and each of these contains the same fixed volume of the lower layer. These lower layers may be designated as L_0, L_1, L_2- - -L_r as in Figure 20.1. To begin the process a unit quantity of solute is dissolved in L_0. An equal volume of upper layer, U_0, is added, the tube is shaken and allowed to settle. If K is assumed as one for illustrative purposes, one-half the material is now in each phase, the total in tube 0 is 1 and no transfer has taken place. The upper phase U_0 is now moved over L_1, a new upper phase, U_1, is introduced over L_0 and the phases are again equilibrated. One transfer has been accomplished and one-half the total material is in each of tubes 0 and 1.

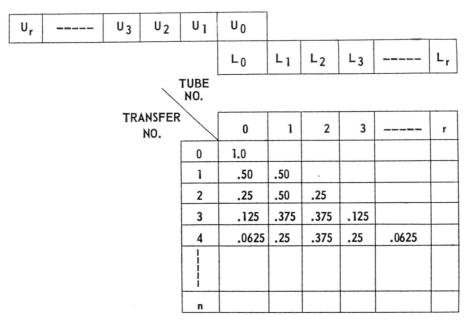

Fig. 20.1 The fraction of total solute (K = 1) in individual tubes during successive transfers in the countercurrent distribution apparatus.

Since the contents of each tube are equally distributed between the two phases, the next transfer will carry one-fourth of the total from tube 1 into tube 2 as U_0 moves over L_2. All of the upper layers are moved forward simultaneously in the Craig apparatus so that in the same transfer U_1 will bring one-fourth over L_1 and one-fourth will remain in L_0. Introduction of a fresh upper layer, U_2, over L_0, equilibration and transfer will continue the process. It can be seen by construction of diagrams like Figure 20.1 that as the process continues the solute becomes distributed through the apparatus as a gradually broadening band. For $K = 1$ the tube or tubes of maximum concentration will always occur in the center of the band and will be in the center of the apparatus upon completion of the run. For substances of K greater than one, the fraction, $K/(K + 1)$, carried forward by the upper layer at each transfer will be more than one-half and the band will be displaced toward the higher numbered tubes. With a sufficient number of transfers the bands containing substances of different K can be separated completely.

Distribution data are customarily plotted with the total amount of solute in both layers as ordinate against tube number as abscissa. The tubes are numbered from 0 and the numbers increase in the direction in which the upper layer moves. It is important to remember that countercurrent distribution is really a series of discontinuous steps and only the points at whole number values for tube number have physical significance.

Detailed descriptions of the physical manipulations in countercurrent distribution are available (Craig *et al.*, 1951a; Craig and Craig, 1956; Hecker, 1955; Titus, 1960). In the basic procedure, a fixed volume of the lower layer from a previously equilibrated pair of immiscible solvents is placed in each tube. These lower layers remain in place throughout subsequent operations. The sample is dissolved in tube 0 and a fixed volume of upper layer is added. After equilibration, which is achieved by rocking the whole train of tubes, the phases are allowed to settle and the apparatus is gradually tilted so that the upper phase drains off through a side port into an adjacent reservoir tube. The latter delivers the upper layer into the next equilibration tube when the apparatus is tilted back. At each step fresh upper layer must be added to tube 0 and after each sequence of rocking and tilting each upper layer moves forward one position. All of these operations are mechanized in modern apparatus and trains of several hundred tubes are entirely practical.

The process is complete when the foremost of the advancing upper layers has reached the last tube. This first sample of upper layer to pass through the apparatus may lose volume as it travels because of adhesion of droplets to glass surfaces, etc. For this reason it is sometimes desirable to wet all surfaces adequately by letting one or two volumes of blank upper layer precede the sample to be fractionated. The extra upper layers can be allowed to pass out of the apparatus. When the upper layer which was first equilibrated with solute has reached the last tube samples are withdrawn for analysis. Since the total amount of solute in each tube is to be plotted, time may often be saved by concentrating the solute in one of the two phases before analysis. When that solute is an organic acid or base, alkali or acid may be added to each tube and the whole apparatus rocked until the solute concentrates in the organic solvent. If systems containing water and a higher alcohol are used, the addition of a few ml of methanol may give a homogeneous phase.

The conventional operation described above is most commonly used and the easiest to describe mathematically. If further transfers are applied, each additional step will result in emergence of one volume of upper layer from the last unit in the train and the bands will eventually emerge from the apparatus in a manner analogous to the elution of fractions from a chromatographic column. This "single withdrawal technique" has been mechanized by the addition of a fraction collector at the end of the distribution train (Craig and Craig, 1956) and is sometimes advantageous. If, for example, the composition of the lower layer interferes with the analytical determination of the separated components, the distribution may be continued by the single withdrawal procedure until all of the desired fractions have appeared in the emergent upper layers. Enhanced resolution of slow moving bands may sometimes be obtained if faster moving material is allowed to pass out of the apparatus while many more transfers are applied to the fractions remaining within.

In graphical presentations of data obtained by the single withdrawal procedure the first sample to emerge is usually plotted furthest to the right and subsequently emerging fractions are plotted from right to left until this curve meets that representing the contents of the machine, which is plotted as usual. By this procedure the peaks representing individual components are arranged in order of increasing K.

A double withdrawal procedure (Craig and Craig, 1956) has also been described and discontinuous extraction trains permitting the transfer of either phase have been described by Jantzen (1948), Tschesche and Könige (1950) and Verzele (1953).

B. Mathematical Treatment

The ease with which the distribution patterns of individual solutes can be predicted from partition coefficients is one of the attractive features of countercurrent distribution. The mathematical treatment may be visualized with aid of diagrams like Figure 20.1 (Williamson and Craig, 1947; Stene, 1944). When a substance is first equilibrated between two solvents in tube 0, a fraction, p, of the total material passes into the upper layer. This fraction is moved forward to the next tube at the first transfer and the fraction, q, remaining in the lower layer, is left behind. At the second equilibration, the quantity p in tube 1 will distribute according to the equilibrium constant $K = p/q$ so that a fraction, p^2, of the total is now in the upper layer ready to be transferred. A fraction, pq, remains in the lower layer, L_1. In tube 0 the fraction q will have similarly equilibrated so that U_1 now contains pq and q^2 remains in L_0. After the second transfer a quantity p^2 has moved into tube 2, 2 pq is in tube 1 and q^2 remains in tube 0. It can readily be seen that after n transfers the fraction of the total solute in any tube, r, will be given by the rth term of the binomial expansion $(q + p)^n = 1$.

Since $p = K/(K + 1)$ and $q = 1 - p = 1/(K + 1)$ the binomial expansion becomes

(1)
$$\left(\frac{1}{1 + K} + \frac{K}{K + 1}\right)^n = 1$$

Theoretical curves may be plotted from the following expression which gives $T_{n,r}$ the fraction of a solute present in the rth tube after n transfers (Rietz, 1927).

$$(2) \qquad T_{n,r} = \frac{n!}{r!(n-r)!}\left(\frac{1}{K+1}\right)^{n} K^{r}$$

Way and Bennett (1951) have pointed out that solutions of this expression have been tabulated (National Bureau of Standards, 1950). In the standard table $T_{n,r}$ is treated as a function of p and q, these letters having the same significance as above, i.e., $K/(K+1)$ and $1/(K+1)$ respectively. Theoretical distribution curves may then be constructed from tabulated values once p and q have been calculated from K. A useful table of p and q values as a function of K has been included in the paper of Way and Bennett (1951).

It is often convenient to use the relationship between successive terms of a binomial expansion (Williamson and Craig, 1947).

$$(3) \qquad \frac{Tr}{Tr-1} = K\frac{(n+1-r)}{r}$$

If the value of any point on the curve is known, all the other points can be calculated, providing K is known. Even when experimental values for partition coefficients are at hand, it is often advantageous to use a K determined from the distribution data. It is not always certain that conditions within the apparatus exactly duplicate those for the determination of standard values and not infrequently the chemical identity of a metabolite may be unknown. Since the tubes near the peak of a distribution curve are most likely to contain pure solute, values from two adjacent points in this region are used to calculate K according to equation 3. The K thus obtained is then used to construct a theoretical curve by calculation of values for the terms preceding and following the initially chosen points.

The distribution curves generated in stepwise fashion by the binomial expansion of Figure 20.1 assume the form of the normal curve of error as the number of transfers approaches infinity. At values of n of about 25 or more, however, discrepancies between the curves plotted by the two methods are usually less than the uncertainty in the analytical determinations. The treatment of counter current distribution curves by statistical methods has therefore provided a number of useful mathematical tools. Values for K, for example, may be calculated from the position N, of the maximum in a distribution curve by the expression

$$(4) \qquad N = n\left(\frac{K}{K+1}\right)$$

The assumption that the distribution curve is continuous is inherent in the derivation of this expression (Bock, 1950) from statistical considerations and the formula is exact only when n becomes infinite. It may be used without appreciable error, however, for distributions of more than 20 transfers when $K/(K+1)$ has values between 0.1 and 0.9 (Craig, 1944).

Equation 5, essentially the formula for the normal curve of error, may be used to plot distribution curves for values of K between 0.2 and 5 when 20 or more transfers are used.

$$(5) \qquad y = \frac{1}{\sqrt{2\pi\ nK/(K+1)^2}}\ e^{-(x^2/2nK/(K+1)^2)}$$

Here y is the fraction of substance in a given tube, x is the distance from the maximum, y_0, and the theoretical curve is constructed by plotting points on either side of the maximum. The procedure is simple. With the aid of equation 4 K is calculated from the position of the maximum concentration in the experimental curve and the value of the recurrent expression, $2\ nk/(K+1)^2$, is computed. For each of the two fractions which are on opposite sides of the peak and x units removed, the concentration can be obtained by dividing the concentration at the peak by the antilog of $x^2 \times 0.434/2nK/(K+1)2$. If it is desirable to have the ordinates of the theoretical curve in terms of the fraction of the total rather than in concentration, the value of the peak height should be taken as y_0 which is, of course, simply

$$\frac{1}{\sqrt{2\pi\ nK/(K+1)^2}}$$

It may happen that the best plot of an experimental distribution curve will give a maximum at a fractional tube number. Although fractional tube numbers are without physical significance in the actual experiment, the position of the maximum may still be used to calculate a best value for K.

The calculations considered to this point apply only to the conventional procedure in which no component leaves the apparatus. A plot of the concentrations in the emergent fractions when the single withdrawal procedure is used must be treated somewhat differently. In a 100 tube apparatus, for example, the first fraction to emerge will be the 100th tube of a 100 transfer distribution. The second will be the 100th tube of a 101 transfer distribution, etc. It has been shown by Stene (1944) that the contents of the emergent fractions correspond to the terms of a Pascal distribution. Ghosh et al. (1965) have published a procedure for constructing theoretical curves from tables of probability distribution. Theoretical curves may be conveniently calculated with the expression (Craig and Craig, 1956)

$$y = \frac{1}{\sqrt{2n/K}}\ e^{(-2x^2/2n/K)}$$

Here n is the average number of transfers in the band, i.e., the tube numbers of the maximum of the emergent curve, and the calculations are performed as with equation 5. This expression is an approximation which gives good results with distribution of about 100 transfers or more.

C. Use of Computers

In analytical applications of counter current distribution, a theoretical curve which coincides with the largest possible number of experimental points in one band is calculated. The difference between observed concentrations and those predicted by theory may then be plotted as a function of tube number to give the distribution of impurities. If the second pattern indicates the presence of several compounds, the process may be repeated until a curve for the distribution of each impurity has been obtained. The process must of course terminate whenever the differences to be plotted become statistically insignificant because of uncertainties in the experimental values.

This procedure is extremely useful in such applications as assessing the radiochemical purity of isotopically labeled drugs, but it can be time consuming. It is therefore fortunate that computerized analysis of distribution curves is now being undertaken (Pohl, 1965). Priore and Kirdani (1968) have examined in detail the problems in designing a program to carry out the steps outlined above. In their program, a staged least squares procedure is employed in fitting a mixed binomial model. One binomial distribution at a time is added until the limit of statistical significance is reached. The program has been tested in a study of the fractionation of estriol metabolites (Kirdani and Priore, 1968).

D. Predicting Separability

The extent to which two components of distribution constant K_A and K_B are separable is predictable and depends primarily on the ratio of these constants, often referred to as the separation factor, β. Thus at a β of 10, relatively few transfers will separate a mixture; whereas, at a β of 1, the mixture is inseparable under any circumstances. It is important to note that the separation of two substances is optimal when the geometric mean of K_A and $K_B = 1$ (Hecker, 1953; Craig and Craig, 1956). In this case the distribution curves of A and B after n transfers will lie symmetrically on either side of the middle tube of the apparatus, $r = n/2$. An equivalent statement by Hecker (1953) is that a volume fraction, α, must be 1 for the most efficient separation

$$\alpha = K_A \times k_B = k_A \times k_B \times V^2$$

Here V is the ratio of the volume of upper and lower phases. Countercurrent distributions are usually carried out with equal volumes of the two phases, but if may occasionally be advantageous to vary the ratio of volumes. If the Nernst distribution constants k_A and k_B are known, the ratio, V, may be adjusted so that $V = 1/\sqrt{k_B \times k_A}$ in order to set α equal to 1.

Hecker (1953) has published a detailed analysis of the conditions required for separation. With the aid of tables and curves from this publication, the planning of countercurrent distribution separations is relatively rapid. Table 1 lists a series of values for n, the number of transfers required, for various degrees of purification of two component mixtures. These are taken from the data of Hecker (1953) and apply to the special case $\alpha = 1$.

As the number of components in a mixture increases, larger numbers of transfers are required. Although the bands widen as more transfers are applied, the fraction of total tubes occupied by a particular component lessens. The width of a band containing 99% of a solute is approximated by the expression $6\sqrt{nK/(k+1)^2}$ (Craig and Craig, 1956).

In general, partial resolution of a mixture of four components ranging in K from 0.1 to 10 can be achieved with about 25 transfers and complete separation would require about 100 transfers. In undertaking the countercurrent distribution of an unknown mixture, it is common practice to select a solvent pair in which the total solutes distribute equally, since such a system is most likely to give effective resolution. When the resolution of two closely related substances is a problem, it may be worthwhile to try a number of solvent systems, since a

TABLE 20.1

Number of transfers required for separation of two components by countercurrent distribution

β	% of pure component recoverable				
	99.73	95	80	60	50
11.0	22				
10.0	24				
9.0	27				
8.0	30				
7.0	35	21			
6.0	42	25			
5.0	53	32	22		
4.5	61	36	25		
4.0	72	43	29	21	
3.5	89	53	36	26	22
3.0	116	70	48	34	29
2.7	143	86	59	42	36
2.4	185	111	76	55	46
2.2	229	137	94	67	57
2.0	292	175	120	86	72
1.9	346	208	142	102	87
1.8	413	248	169	121	103
1.7	508	305	208	149	127
1.6	649	389	266	191	162
1.5	872	523	357	256	218

relatively small increase in the ratio, β, of their distribution constants can greatly lessen the transfers required for separation (Table 20.1). Analytical methods used with countercurrent distribution depend, of course, on the nature of the solute. In analytical applications where it is important to determine whether impurities of unknown properties are present, weight determination may be the most satisfactory procedure. This can be practical, even when very small weights are to be determined, if aliquots are evaporated under nitrogen in tared hemispherical dishes of very thin platinum or glass (Craig *et al.*, 1951a, 1951b).

E. Choice of Solvent Systems

The choice of a system of two liquid phases between which the solute to be examined distributes approximately evenly is important to the success of counter-current distribution. A few practical considerations should be kept in mind: (1) Since the phases must separate quickly, systems prone to emulsification should be avoided. (2) High boiling solvents or salt solutions may be undesirable if it is necessary to recover the solute. (3) The distribution constant should be independent of concentration. Since solutes are rapidly diluted during distribution, deviations from a linear partition isotherm cause skewing of the distribution curves less frequently than might be expected. Self-association of solute molecules in the less polar phase, a potential source of deviation, can often be suppressed by appropriate choice of solvent. Inclusion of acetic acid in the solvent mixture is sometimes effective, especially with solutes containing COOH moieties (Ahrens and Craig, 1952).

In general the greatest difference between partition coefficients of chemically similar solutes will be observed with solvents that differ most in polarity or the ability to form hydrogen bonds, *i.e.*, solvents most widely separated in the list cited earlier.

Solvent combinations that have been used for a great variety of substrates have been tabulated by von Metzch (1953, 1956). The extensive review by Craig and Craig (1956) is a useful guide to the choice of solvent mixtures. Systems for phospholipids (Cole *et al.*, 1953; Olley and Lovern, 1953; Olley, 1956) and fatty acids (Ahrens and Craig, 1952) have been published. A brief summary of representative systems useful for various drugs and natural products has appeared (Titus, 1960). Some general conclusions from the above studies can be briefly summarized.

As might be expected (and illustrated by specific examples in Chapter 18), organic solvents and aqueous buffers are generally useful for alkaloids and basic drugs. Chloroform or sometimes ethylene dichloride is widely used for alkaloids, quinoline antimalarials, etc. Benzene or cyclohexane is appropriate for less polar substances such as substituted anilines. Phosphate, which does not tend to form extractable ion pairs, is perhaps the most widely used buffer. Methanol-water mixtures have also been used as a second phase with chloroform but at the sacrifice of the selectivity offered by the control of pH. The latter system and occasionally water-benzene systems can be used for neutral molecules of intermediate polarity.

For substances of increasing polarity, butanol may often be substituted for chloroform. For basic polar substrates, butanol systems with slightly acidic buffers are often useful, but butanol systems tend to emulsify at higher pH.

Sugars, glycosides and other highly hydroxylated compounds can be distributed in systems prepared from water and ethanol-chloroform or ethanol-chloroform-glycol monoether mixtures. Aqueous solutions, often containing dilute acetic acid or ammonia, may be used with butanols for the distribution of peptides and have been used for some cardiac glycosides.

For extremely lipoidal substances, the choice of solvent pairs is somewhat limited since these compounds are insoluble in water, often cause emulsification and may associate in nonpolar solvents. Successful systems for these usually include petroleum ether or hexane and a mixture of organic solvents just polar enough to separate as a second phase. Methanol or ethanol containing a little water, nitromethane, nitroethane, acetonitrile and methylcellosolve, have been used in various combinations as the second phase.

Ion pair formation has found use in countercurrent systems as well as simple extractions. *p*-Toluene sulfonic acid in butanol-water and buffered sodium stearate in amyl alcohol-water systems have been used for the very water soluble antibiotic, streptomycin. The isolation of transfer-RNA in a system containing tri-n-butyl amine is a dramatic example of the use of ion pairs to achieve a useful distribution constant.

The formation of complexes other than ion pairs seems to have had little use as a means of controlling K. Scholfield *et al.* (1963), however, have taken advantage of the preferential formation of silver complexes by the cis isomer of monoenoic methyl esters to separate cis and trans isomers in a hexane-90% methanol system containing 0.2 M $AgNO_3$. A mixture of methyl trienoates was also partially separated into six fractions. As might be expected, the most rapidly moving of these was all-trans and that most retarded by its preferential solubility in the aqueous phase was all-cis (Scholfield *et al.*, 1966).

In applying countercurrent distribution to studies of drug metabolism, it may be advantageous to devise distribution systems for both the administered drug and the expected products. Not infrequently the metabolites are more polar than the parent substances, so that a convenient rule of thumb is to select a solvent pair in which the ingested drug has a K of approximately 5 in favor of the organic solvent. The partition coefficients of the metabolites are then more likely to fall within the desired range. The magnitude of some of these changes can be illustrated with a few examples: In a butanol-0.25 M pyrophosphate system at pH 9.4, pentobarbital has a K of 12. The alcoholic and acidic metabolites, 5-ethyl-5-(3-hydroxy-1-methylbutyl) barbituric acid and 5-ethyl-5-(1-methyl-3-carboxypropyl) barbituric acid have coefficients of 0.67 and 0.15, respectively. Metabolic removal of an N-ethyl group from the antimalarial 4-(3-diethyl amino-2-hydroxypropylamino)-7-chloroquinoline increased K from 1.1 to 17 in a $CHCl_3$-phosphate buffer system. Changes of about the same magnitude result from the oxidation of chlorpromazine to the sulfoxide. Metabolism of some of the phosphorodithioate insecticides causes especially dramatic changes (Knaak and O'Brien, 1960). Metabolic deamidation of 0,0-dimethyl-S-(N-methyl carbamoylmethyl) phosphorothiate, which has a K of 41.5 in chloroform-pH 7 buffer, gives a product with a K of approximately 3×10^{-3} (Uchida *et al.*, 1964).

Whether countercurrent distribution or some other method of fractionation is best suited for a particular situation depends on several factors. If all the components of a reaction mixture must be quantitatively accounted for, distribution avoids the possibility of irreversible adsorption or chemical reactions on an active surface that are sometimes encountered in adsorption chromatography.

Distribution may be a useful adjunct to micro methods. The separation from tissue extracts of very small amounts of drugs in sufficient purity to permit gas chromatographic fractionation may become an important application as increasingly effective drugs are studied at ever smaller doses.

When less water-soluble neutral substances, such as steroids, differ appreciably in three dimensional structure but not in solubility properties, adsorption on a solid surface may be more selective than partition between solvents, so that adsorption chromatography becomes the method of choice.

The distribution of some molecules so strongly favors water that multicomponent mixtures such as ethanol-water-chloroform are required to get reasonable quantities into both phases. The selectivity of this type of system is lower because the composition of the two phases is not widely different. A great many transfers must be applied for effective separations, and automatic equipment is necessary. For such substances, partition chromatography may offer a means of achieving the effect of many transfers in equipment less demanding of space. In this procedure, the less polar component of a solvent pair is passed through a column in which the other solvent is suspended on a more or less inert agent, such as silicic acid or diatomaceous earth. The procedure is analogous to countercurrent distribution in that separation depends largely on differences in partition coefficient, but adsorption of the solute by the suspending agent undoubtedly plays a role in many systems. In the more effective applications, good resolution has often been obtained by slow elution with solvents in which the solutes are but slightly soluble. The manner in which the aqueous phase is suspended on the column is usually critical and care is required. The space saving advantages of partition chromatography on a preparative scale may thus be achieved at the cost of considerable time and solvent.

For the separation of organic acids and bases, countercurrent distribution will often be the method of choice. The systems of organic solvents and aqueous buffers used for the distribution of such substances are highly selective (Craig *et al.*, 1945) and require relatively few transfers for good separations. When precise determination of the composition of a mixture is necessary, distribution is often also advantageous, since even with systems requiring many transfers, the use of automatic equipment and computer programs for analysis of the results provide data quickly and conveniently.

REFERENCES

Ahrens, E. H., Jr. and Craig, L. C.: The extraction and separation of bile acids. J. Biol. Chem. *195:* 763–778, 1952.

Axelrod, J.: The estimation of basic drugs by dye methods. In *Toxicology, Mechanisms and Analytical Methods*, Vol. I, ed. by C. P. Stewart and A. Stolman, pp. 714–729, Academic Press, New York, 1960.

Axelrod, J. and Tomchick, R.: Enzymatic O-methylation of epinephrine and other catechols. J. Biol. Chem. *233:* 702–705, 1958.

Axelrod, J. and Weissbach, H.: Purification and properties of hydroxy-indole O-methyl transferase. J. Biol. Chem. *236:* 211–273, 1961.

Ballard, C. W., Isaacs, J., and Scott, D. G. W.: The photometric determination of quaternary ammonium salts and of certain amines by compound formation with indicators. J. Pharm. Pharmacol. *6:* 971–985, 1954.

Beroza, M. and Bowman, M. C.: Extraction of insecticides for clean up and identification. J. Ass. Offic. Agr. Chem. *48:* 358–370, 1965a.

Beroza, M. and Bowman, M. C.: Identification of pesticides at nanogram level by extraction p-values. Anal. Chem. *37:* 291–292, 1965b.

Beyer, K. H.: Zur fermentativen Aufarbeitung toxikologischen Untersuchungsmaterials. 6. Mitteilung zur Chemie und Analytik der Schlafmittel. Z. anal. Chem. *212:* 139–145, 1965.

Beyermann, K.: Distribution of tetraphenyl borates of amino acids and oligo peptides between aqueous solutions and organic solvents. Z. anal. Chem. *212:* 199–211, 1965.

Bock, R. M.: A derivation of the concentration distribution equation for the Craig countercurrent apparatus. J. Amer. Chem. Soc. *72:* 4269–4270, 1950.

Bowman, M. C. and Beroza, M.: Extraction p-values of pesticides and related compounds in six binary solvent systems. J. Ass. Office Agr. Chem. *48:* 943–952, 1965.

Bowman, M. C. and Beroza, M.: Device and method for determining extraction p-values with unequilibrated solvents or unequal phase volumes. Anal. Chem. *38:* 1427–1428, 1966.

Brodie, B. B., Udenfriend, S., and Baer, J. E.: The estimation of basic organic compounds in biological material. I. General principles. J. Biol. Chem. *168:* 299–309, 1947a.

Brodie, B. B., Udenfriend, S., and Dill, W. The estimation of basic organic compounds in biological material. V. Estimation by salt formation with methyl orange. J. Biol. Chem. *168:* 335–339, 1947b.

Cole, P. G., Lathe, G. H., and Ruthven, C. R. J.: Application of counter-current methods to the fractionation of lipid material from human placenta. Biochem. J. *55:* 17–23, 1953.

Craig, L. C.: Identification of small amounts of organic compounds by distribution studies. II. Separation by countercurrent distribution. J. Biol. Chem. *155:* 519–534, 1944.

Craig, L. C. and Craig, D.: Extraction and distribution. In *Technique of Organic Chemistry*, ed. by A. Weissberger, Vol. 3, 2nd ed., pp. 172–311, Interscience, New York, 1956.

Craig, L. C., Golumbic, C., Mighton, H., and Titus, E.: Identification of small amounts of organic compounds by distribution studies. III. Use of buffers in countercurrent distribution. J. Biol. Chem. *161:* 321–332, 1945.

Craig, L. C., Hausmann, W., Ahrens, P., and Harfenist, E. J.: Automatic countercurrent distribution equipment. Anal. Chem. *23:* 1236–1244, 1951a.

Craig, L. C., Hausmann, W., Ahrens, P., and Harfenist, E. J.: Determination of weight curves in column processes. Anal. Chem. *23:* 1326–1327, 1951b.

Dingell, J. V., Sulser, F., and Gillette, J. R.: Species differences in the metabolism of imipramine and desmethylimipramine. J. Pharmacol. Exp. Ther. *143:* 14–22, 1964.

Divatia, G. J. and Biles, J. A.: Physical chemical study of the distribution of some amino salts between immiscible solvents. J. Pharm. Sci. *50:* 916–922, 1961.

Doyle, T. D. and Levine, J.: Application of ion-pair extraction to partition chromatographic separation of pharmaceutical amines. Anal. Chem. *39:* 1282–1287, 1967.

Ghosh, S. B., Schaad, L. J., and Bush, M. T.: Binomial probability distribution tables for the calculation of withdrawn series of counter-current distribution. Anal. Chem. *37:* 1122–1123, 1965.

Goldbaum, L. R. and Domanski, T. J.: Detection and identification of micrograms of neutral drugs in biological samples. J. Forensic. Sci. *11:* 233–242, 1966.

Gustavii, K. and Schill, G.: Determination of amines and quaternary ammonium ions as complexes with picrate. I. Constants needed in the calculation of extraction conditions. Acta Pharm. Suec. *3:* 241–258, 1966a.

Gustavii, K. and Schill, G.: Determination of amines and quaternary ammonium ions as picrate complexes. II. Interference by foreign anions. Acta Pharm. Suec. *3:* 259–268, 1966b.

Hecker, E.: A simple separation function for countercurrent distribution and its importance in practice. Z. Naturforsch. *8b:* 77–86, 1953.

Hecker, E.: Verteilungsverfahren im Laboratorium. Verlag Chemie, 1955.

Higuchi, T. and Michaelis, A. F.: Mechanism and kinetics of ion pair extraction. Rate of extraction of dextromethophanium ion. Anal. Chem. *40:* 1925–1931, 1968.

Higuchi, T., Michaelis, A., Tan, T., and Hurwitz, A.: Ion pair extraction of pharmaceutical amines. Role of dipolar solvating agents in extraction of dextromorphan. Anal. Chem. *39:* 974–979, 1967.

Hull, R. L. and Biles, J. A.: Physical chemical study of the distribution of some amine salts between immiscible solvents. II. Complexation in the organic phase. J. Pharm. Sci. *53:* 869–872, 1964.

Jantzen, E.: Das fractionierte Destillieren und das fractionierte Verteilen, Dechema, Monographic, Vol. V, No. 48, Verlag Chemie, Berlin, 1948.

Karau, W. and Zachau, H. G.: Isolierung von serinspezifischen Transfer ribonuclein säurefraktionen. Biochim. Biophys. Acta *91:* 549–558, 1964.

Kirdani, R. Y. and Priore, R. L.: Statistical analysis of data from countercurrent distribution. II. Some applications and limitations of the method. Anal. Biochem. *24:* 377–392, 1968.

Knaak, J. B. and O'Brien, R. D.: Effect of EPN on *in vivo* metabolism of malathion by rat and dog. J. Agr. Food Chem. *8:* 198–203, 1960.

National Bureau of Standards: Tables of the binomial probability distribution. Applied Mathematics Series, Vol. 6, Washington, D. C., 1960.

Olley, J.: Application of countercurrent distribution to phospholipid chemistry. Chem. In. (London) pp. 1120–1130, 1956.

Olley, J. and Lovern, J. A.: The lipids of fish. III. Acetone-insoluble fraction of an acetone extract of the flesh of the haddock. Biochem. J. *54:* 559–569, 1953.

Persson, B. A. and Schill, G.: Extraction of amines as complexes with inorganic ions. Part 2. Determination of constants when the amine is extracted as complex and base. Acta Pharm. Suec. *3:* 281–302, 1966.

Pfleiderer, G.: Möglickeiten und Grenzen in der Anwendung moderner biochemischer Analysenverfahren. Z. anal. Chem. *212:* 64–77, 1965.

Pohl, F. A.: Comprehension and evaluation of chemical data. Z. anal. Chem. *209:* 19–35, 1965.

Priore, R. L. and Kirdani, R. Y.: Statistical analysis of data from counter-current distribution. I. Method for estimation of quantity and partition coefficient of each compound in the distribution. Anal. Biochem. *24:* 360–376, 1968.

Rietz, H. L.: In *Mathematical Statistics*, Open Court, La Salle, Illinois, 1927.

Salzman, N. P. and Brodie, B. B.: Physiological disposition and fate of chlorpromazine and a method for its estimation in biological material. J. Pharmacol. Exp. Ther. *118:* 46–54, 1956.

Schill, G.: Photometric determination of amines and quaternary ammonium compounds with bromothymol blue. Part 4. Extraction constants and calculation of extraction conditions. Acta Pharm. Suec. *2:* 13–43, 1965a.

Schill, G.: Photometric determination of amines and quaternary ammonium compounds with bromthymol blue. Part 5. Determination of dissociation constants of amines. Acta Pharm. Suec. *2:* 99–108, 1965b.

Schill, G., Modin, R., and Persson, B. A.: Extraction of amines as complexes with inorganic anions. Acta Pharm. Suec. *2:* 119–136, 1965.

Scholfield, C. R., Butterfield, R. O., and Dutton, H. J.: Fractionation of geometric isomers of methyl linolenate by argentation countercurrent distribution. Anal. Chem. *38:* 1694–1697, 1966.

Scholfield, C. R., Jones, E. P., Butterfield, R. O., and Dutton, H. J.: Argentation in countercurrent distribution to separate isologues and geometric isomers of fatty acid esters. Anal. Chem. *35:* 1588–1591, 1963.

Shore, P. A.: A simple technique involving solvent extraction for estimation of nor-adrenaline and adrenaline in tissues. Pharmacol. Rev. *11:* 276–277, 1959.

Stene, S.: Theory of systematic extraction and related convection problems. Ark. Kemi, Mineral. Geol. A18, No. 18, 1944.

Titus, E. O.: Countercurrent distribution. In *Toxicology, Mechanisms and Analytical Methods*, ed. by C. P. Stewart and A. Stolman, Vol. I, pp. 392–419, Academic Press, New York, 1960.

Titus, E. and Weiss, H.: The use of biologically prepared radioactive indicators in metabolic studies: Metabolism of pentobarbital. J. Biol. Chem. *214:* 807–820, 1955.

Tschesche, R. and Konige, H. B.: Apparatus for countercurrent distribution for preparative purposes. Chem. Ing. Tech. *22:* 214–215, 1950.

Uchida, T., Dauterman, W. C., and O'Brien, R. D.: The metabolism of dimethoate by vertebrate tissues. J. Agr. Food Chem. *12:* 48–52, 1964.

Verzele, M.: A new method of separation on a preparative scale based on countercurrent distribution. Bull. Soc. Chim. Belges *62:* 619–639, 1953.

Von Metzsch, F. A.: The choice of solvents for the distribution between two liquid phases. Angew. Chem. *65:* 586–598, 1953.

Von Metzsch, F. A.: Anwendungsbeispiele multiplikativer Verteilungen. Angew. Chem. *68:* 323–334, 1956.

Watson, D. J., Romanoff, E. B., Kato, J., and Bartosik, D. B.: A method for the determination of progesterone in biological specimens. Anal. Biochem. *20:* 233–245, 1967.

Way, E. L. and Bennett, B. M.: Rapid estimation of counter-current distribution values. J. Biol. Chem. *192:* 335–338, 1951.

Williamson, B. and Craig, L. C.: Identification of small amounts of organic compounds by distribution studies. V. Calculation of theoretical curves. J. Biol. Chem. *168:* 687–697, 1947.

21

Isolation and Identification Procedures— Spectral Methods

HENRY M. FALES

I. INTRODUCTION

As little as ten years ago any pharmacologist would have been gratified to elucidate the structure of even one metabolite of a new drug. Structural methods were neither powerful nor sensitive enough to deal with the small quantities usually encountered. This picture is changing rapidly, thanks to the advent of modern physical methods such as gas chromatography and mass spectrometry. With this change, the requirements of industry, governmental drug control agencies and, most importantly, of biochemistry itself have been upgraded correspondingly. This trend will doubtless continue as metabolites continue to shed light on the processes of drug action.

Ideally, the pharmacologist desires to know the fate of every carbon atom within the drug. This necessitates the preparation of drugs labeled with ^{14}C in as many positions as possible—no mean task. During metabolism of the drug, account is first taken of any radioactivity exhaled as carbon dioxide or lost in urine and fecal matter; the pharmacologist then turns his attention to the very small amounts of radioactive material which may be isolated from bile, urine, or blood. The isolation and concentration processes themselves usually supply some information on the polarity and general structural class of an unknown metabolite and it is at this stage that physical methods may be first invoked. While the pharmacologist often refers to such a concentrate as "highly purified" because it contains much of the original radioactivity and exhibits only one spot on paper or thin layer chromatography, it is seldom really suitable for the classical physical tools. The sample usually contains many biological substances which may not be apparent from the colorimetric or chromatographic techniques used during its isolation. There is also inclined to be large amounts of material arising from solvent residues, paper or thin layer chromatographic throw and ubiquitous stopcock grease. In fact, it has been our experience that the matrix, or main component of such an extract, will bear little relation to the metabolite under investigation. The pharmacologist purifying a metabolite must therefore continually bear in mind the relation of mass to radioactivity. Obviously, it will usually be impossible to obtain an accurate measure of mass *via* a microbalance but if the mass of the sample is *ten times* more than expected on the basis of its radioactivity, a re-evaluation is obviously necessary.

It is probably for these reasons that gas chromatography-mass spectrometry has recently attracted so much attention. In this technique extensive prior purification can often be eliminated because the molecular weight and consequently the volatility (expressed in terms of retention time) of the initial drug are known, and hence its metabolites may be correspondingly approximated. Once the molecular weight of the unknown metabolite is established, it is often a relatively simple problem to make an intelligent guess at its structure. Simple chemical reactions (acetylation, reduction, etc.) can be performed on the unknown and their success or failure confirmed by a second gas chromatographic-mass spectrometric analysis. Where it is possible to obtain as much as 0.25–1 mg of pure metabolite, one can now employ the very powerful method of nuclear magnetic resonance which uses the proton arrangement around the core of the molecule as a structural probe. In fact, mass spectrometry and nuclear magnetic resonance supply highly complementary data, for the latter method may leave ambiguous the exact number of protons in the molecule, particularly in a sample that is somewhat impure. In mass spectrometry, such a decision is a very simple matter.

In the following chapter the older and now classical methods of infrared and ultra-violet spectroscopy will be briefly discussed, especially from the pharmacologist's viewpoint, although their utility today is very limited. The much more powerful methods of nuclear magnetic resonance and gas chromatography-mass spectrometry will then be discussed at greater length. As an example of each of the methods, I have chosen a minor metabolite (II) obtained recently in a study of the metabolism of probenecid (I) (Guarino et al., 1969).

$$\text{HOOC} - \underset{\text{I}}{\bigcirc} - \text{SO}_2\text{N} \underset{\text{CH}_2\text{CH}_2\text{CH}_3}{\overset{\text{CH}_2\text{CH}_2\text{CH}_3}{<}} \qquad \text{HOOC} - \underset{\text{II}}{\bigcirc} - \text{SO}_2\text{N} \underset{\text{H}}{\overset{\text{CH}_2\text{CH}_2\text{CH}_3}{<}}$$

II. INFRARED SPECTROMETRY

A. Theory, Use and Correlations

This method furnishes a chart showing peaks resulting from all combinations of stretching and bending vibrations of various parts of a molecule; because of the interactions of these modes complete analysis is extraordinarily difficult even in such a simple case as methane. On the other hand, this very complexity leads to a spectrum which is often entirely unique for the molecule in question and the region below 1600 cm^{-1} supplies an excellent molecular "fingerprint." The region above 1600 cm^{-1} contains relatively few bands and reflects comparatively high energy vibrations which are most easily interpreted since they are relatively unaffected by the rest of the molecule. This higher frequency region has three zones of principal interest. One, 2800–3600 cm^{-1}, reflects the ROH, RNH, RCH, or generally X—H stretching vibrations. The next region, 2000–2800 cm^{-1} reflects triple bond stretching vibrations as found in nitriles, acetylenes, diazo groups, etc. Finally, the region between 1500 cm^{-1} and 2000 cm^{-1} often supplies valuable data on the double bond stretching mode as found in ketones, olefins, benzene rings, esters, acids, imines, etc. Because this region has been so extensively studied it is often possible to discover a subtle change in structure such as that brought about by ring contraction by observing a small shift in carbonyl frequency. The difference between saturated and unsaturated ketones, aldehydes and esters, acids and their sodium salts, imines and immonium salts, and conjugated and unconjugated double bonds is easily observed. Unfortunately, similar correlations for OH and NH groups in the 3200–3600 cm⁻¹ region are obscured due to intermolecular hydrogen bonding and a distinction between these functions cannot usually be made unless sufficient sample is available for measurements to be made at high dilution in inert solvents.

The infrared method has particular advantage as a means of identification and analysis of isotopically labeled compounds, since complex molecules differing only by substitution of a single deuterium will usually exhibit quite different spectra.

B. Quantitative Analysis

It is somewhat surprising that infrared has been used so little for the quantitative analysis of drugs and apparently many pharmacologists are not aware of its potential in this regard. Perhaps this is due to the fact that early instruments often used somewhat poorly designed comb and pulley systems to indicate absorption. Also, early spectral charts were calibrated in terms of transmission rather than absorbance so that the linear relationship between peak height and concentration was obscured. Calibration of absorbance with known mixtures is a simple process however, and the method is without peer for certain analyses, e.g., D_2O in H_2O, etc. Also, this is one of the few methods applicable to insoluble solids. An unknown may be intimately mixed in a KBr matrix with an internal standard such as KCNS and pressed into a clear disc for analysis. In fact, of all methods, infrared is perhaps the most generally applicable since samples can be prepared as above or simply ground into a nujol or fluorolube paste and smeared on a KBr sampling plate. This is fortunate indeed because many solvents one might ordinarily use, such as H_2O, dimethylsulfoxide (DMSO), dimethylformamide (DMF), absorb too strongly in the infrared and tend to dissolve the sodium chloride cells usually employed. Calcium fluoride, KRS-5 and other insoluble materials may be used for selected regions of the spectrum when such solvents must be utilized.

C. Sampling Methods

We have found attenuated total reflectance (ATR) (Wilks Scientific Corporation, South Norwalk, Conn. 06854) devices to be very useful for sampling very small quantities of valuable material. In this method the sample is dissolved in a small amount of easily evaporated solvent such as chloroform and spread on an orange-colored KRS-5 (thallium bromide iodide) plate. The beam enters the side of the crystal and exits many reflections later. Besides high sensitivity, an important feature of this technique is that the material can be easily recovered by simply rinsing the plate with the same solvent.

Ultramicromethods employing very small KBr disks have been described and it is comparatively easy to obtain good spectra on 10–100 μg of pure material. With highly sophisticated microscope arrangements, spectra can be obtained down to about 1 μg. A usable spectrum can also be obtained by placing the sample directly on the thermocouple window, but the complex spectrum of air will necessarily be superimposed since cancellation of a reference beam is not possible.

Solution spectra are more easily interpreted, and carbon disulfide, carbon tetrachloride, and chloroform are favorite solvents. Unfortunately, handling micro solution cells is rather difficult and alignment within the beam is criticas Also problems arise in transferring small volumes of volatile liquid such a chloroform.

While more difficult to interpret, spectra on crystalline substances often disclose subtle differences in crystalline form and polymorphs may be easily distinguished from one another. For this reason the conclusion that two sub-stances are not identical should be made only on the basis of solution or melt spectra.

D. Newer Developments

Excellent instrumentation requiring minimum maintenance is available today in the $3,000 to $10,000 range and no special skill is required to run a spectrum. The main disadvantage of IR spectrometry from the pharmacolo-gist's viewpoint is the extremely limited amount of structural information which is discernible due to the complexity of interacting vibrations. It does not seem that this problem will be resolved in the near future, even with the most sophisti-cated computers that may become available. In a very recent development (Lamb and Jaklevic, 1968) it has been shown that a pair of dissimilar metals containing a small amount of organic matter sandwiched between their faces exhibit a voltage-current relationship analogous to an infrared spectrum. The amount of material present on the metallic crystal faces may be, (in fact *must* be) only about one molecule thick so that sensitivity is greatly enhanced. The resolution obtained at present is less than that of conventional methods.

E. Application to a Metabolite

Figure 21.1 shows an infrared spectrum of the N-dealkylated probenecid (II) found as a metabolite of I. In general, it would be difficult to ascertain the pres-ence of the NH group in the presence of the carboxylic OH group, but the sharp band at 3300 cm^{-1} (3.1 μ) is probably due to this group. The carboxyl is easily observed by presence of the broad envelope extending from 3400 cm^{-1} (2.9 μ) to 2300 cm^{-1} (4.3 μ) and the sharp band at 1695 cm^{-1} (5.9 μ). The two sharp peaks at 2900 cm^{-1} (3.4 μ) on the bottom of the COOH envelope are mainly

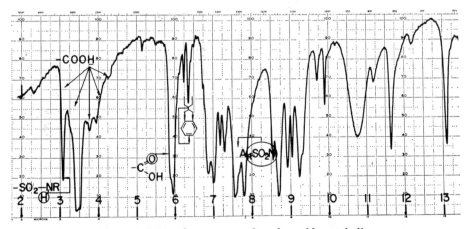

Fig. 21.1 Infrared spectrum of probenecid metabolite.

due to aliphatic C—H groups of the N-propyl side chains. Aromatic C=C vibrations are seen at 1560 and 1600 cm^{-1} (6.35 and 6.25 μ) and the broad intense band at 1330 cm^{-1} (7.55 μ) may be due to the sulfonamide group.

Although correlations are often made in regions below 1430 cm^{-1} (7 μ), they are most usually valid only within a given set of closely related compounds.

III. ULTRAVIOLET AND VISIBLE SPECTROMETRY

A. Advantages, Requirements and Correlations

Spectroscopy in the ultraviolet (uv) and visible region of the spectrum is undoubtedly familiar to all pharmacologists and is a favorite method for bio-chemical and drug analysis. It is useful wherever there is enough conjugation in a molecule to provide absorption or when a compound may be converted to an absorbing species by a relatively simple chemical reaction. Ultraviolet methods are particularly useful in drug metabolism studies since synthetic organic drugs are quite often aromatic compounds. Nature often assists by oxidizing sites activated by aromatic rings or carbonyl groups; the resulting increase in con-jugation changes the ultraviolet or visible spectrum. The accessible region of the spectrum today extends below 200 mμ, well into the region of the isolated C=C and C=O and CN absorptions. Unfortunately this region has received relatively little attention probably because of lack of solvents transparent in this region. Practically, the minimum structural feature required for the use of ultraviolet is either a double bond conjugated with a carbonyl or C=N group, or an aromatic ring. In a few cases (anesthesia gases, etc.) end absorption due to halogen atoms may be utilized.

When applicable, ultraviolet analysis is probably the first physical method that will be applied because any change in conjugation is seen with such ease. The data are valuable even in a negative sense to show that no structural change has occurred. The absorption coefficient of the original material provides a good approximation of the amount of mass present. Interpretation is fairly simple since even extensive aliphatic changes in the aliphatic portion of the molecule will result in relatively small changes in the uv of the basic unsaturated system. Thus a steroid containing an aromatic A-ring will have a spectrum nearly super-imposable with that of benzene (or more correctly o-xylene) itself. Occasionally, relatively small changes in structure will shift the position of a peak by small amounts, but in highly characteristic fashion. Thus, a complete set of rules is available for delineating the substitution pattern of an $\alpha\beta$-unsaturated ketone. Even the small difference in wavelength of a peak brought about by a change in substitution pattern on an aromatic ring from *ortho* to *para* may be highly char-acteristic, although it must be obtained at fairly high resolution with an instru-ment in good condition.

B. Solvents and Quantitation

Nearly any solvent of any degree of polarity (water, ethanol, hexane, DMF, DMSO, etc.) may be employed as long as it does not contain groups which absorb in the uv. The method is highly quantitative since a ratio recording system is usually employed and frequent calibration is not required. Since the uv-visible spectrophotometer is used so often for quantitative analysis, I feel that it is important to obtain an instrument of the highest possible quality, perhaps economizing on the infrared spectrometer if necessary. Such an instrument usually costs between $15,000 and $20,000.

C. Spectrum Modification

There are many operations which can be performed on a sample in the ultraviolet cell itself after the original spectrum has been obtained. Shifts on acidification and basification often dramatically disclose the presence of an aromatic amine or acid or phenol group. If one wishes to distinguish an aniline from a pyridine or other tertiary aromatic amine, a simple expedient is to add a small amount of acetic anhydride to the aqueous solution of the amine. Provided the amine contains an unsubstituted NH group, it will undergo smooth acetylation, and the resulting acetamide will now show no shift on acidification. Sodium borohydride may also be used for reaction *in situ*. This reagent will reduce most conjugated (and unconjugated) carbonyl groups causing a diminution of absorption and a hypochromic shift of the absorption band. Sodium borohydride is usually used in a neutral or basic medium but it may be employed even with weakly acidic solutions provided an excess of reagent is added.

Hydrogenations can be performed by simply adding a small amount of platinum catalyst to the uv cell and bubbling in hydrogen through a small capillary tube. Chelation with iron salts or boric acid often causes dramatic shifts in the absorption of enols, phenols, and catechols or amino phenols.

D. Measurement of Molecular Weight

The molecular weight of an unknown metabolite can often be obtained with considerable accuracy by forming a derivative with a molecule which contains an intensely absorbing chromophore which absorbs in a region of the spectrum not occupied by chromophores of the unknown molecule. This method has been applied to the determination of the molecular weights of aliphatic amines by converting them to their picrates or styphnates, etc. These derivatives undergo complete dissociation at the concentrations employed in uv analysis, and since the absorption coefficient of picric acid is known along with the weight of amine picrate, the molecular weight of the nonabsorbing aliphatic amine may be easily calculated.

E. Artifacts and Experimental Precautions

When a spectrum suggests that a molecule contains *two* superimposed chromophores, one chromophore may be conveniently isolated by adding a model compound containing the other chromophore to the reference cell, adjusting its concentration by trial and error to reveal the spectrum of the other moiety. This method is considerably easier than graphical subtraction of a complex curve, but in this and other double beam spectrophotometric methods there is a constant danger that one will enter a region of the spectrum where the reference cell absorbs beyond the limits of detection by the phototube. When this occurs the pen will simply drift up or down according to the "dark current" electronic balance of the amplifier. This is easily misinterpreted as a true absorption band. Indication of insufficient energy may be observed on some instruments by noting that the slit has opened to its limit. Alternatively, the reference solution may be run in the sample beam against an air blank.

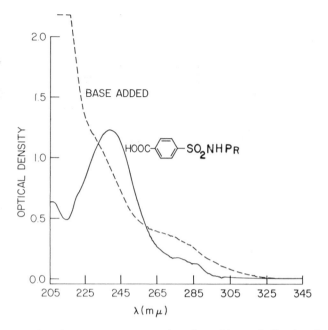

Fig. 21.2 Ultraviolet absorption spectrum of probenecid metabolite in ethanol ———;
with sodium hydroxide added — — —.

F. Application to a Metabolite

Figure 21.2 shows the ultraviolet spectrum of metabolite II in alcohol at a
concentration of .0148 g/l. Since:

$$\epsilon = \frac{\text{O.D.}}{C \times 1} = \frac{1.23}{6.08 \times 10^{-5} \times 1 \text{ cm}} = 20{,}300$$

where: ϵ = extinction coefficient
    O.D. = optical density
      C = molarity = g/l/m.wt. = .0148 g/l/243 = 6.08×10^{-5}
      1 = cell length in cm

The peak at 242 mμ (ϵ 20,300) is mainly due to resonance interaction of the
carboxyl group with the benzene ring (A). Addition of base creates

    A   B   C

the anion whose resonance form B does not give rise to absorption in this region.
The resonance form C analogous to A requires juxtaposition of two negative
charges and so does not contribute importantly at this wavelength. As a result,
a shift toward lower wavelengths (higher light energy) occurs, as required to
bring forms such as C into consideration. The very high absorption below 225
mμ is partly due to the sodium ion.

IV. NUCLEAR MAGNETIC RESONANCE

A. Advantages, Theory, "Acidity Concept"

The methods of nuclear magnetic resonance spectrometry provide a more complete structural description of a complex molecule than any other technique short of x-ray crystallography. The apparatus is complex and expensive, costing between \$20,000 and \$90,000 depending on complexity. The less expensive instruments are relatively easy to run, even for a novice, while the more expensive instruments require the full time and attention of a skilled technician. It is also true that a professional nmr spectroscopist can obtain a much greater amount of useful data from a limited amount of material.

Nmr spectra consist of a series of peaks whose area is proportional to the number of protons they represent, distributed along a horizontal scale corresponding to a magnetic field. The position of a band along this scale is a reflection of the degree to which protons are shielded by their bonds to other atoms. In effect, this is a kind of "acidity" scale and it is not surprising that compounds such as methane are found at one end ($\delta = 0.00$) while carboxylic acid protons are at the other limit ($\delta = 12$). Unlike other spectral methods, there are no extinction coefficients; and since area is directly proportional to the number of protons, a complete analysis of the spectra is theoretically possible. In fact, the main features of a spectrum are nearly always easily interpretable. At low resolution a series of broad overlapping peaks would be seen, each peak representing the protons in a given environment within the molecule. At higher resolution these broad peaks are observed to contain considerable fine structure. These narrow peaks are due to the interaction between the hydrogen nuclei within four bond lengths from each other. The resulting complexity often requires extreme analysis, but where it can be deciphered, information can be obtained concerning the spatial relationships between the protons.

Many synthetic aromatic drugs are ideal molecules for analysis by nmr methods since they often contain hydrogen atoms on a complex carbon skeleton insulated from each other by relatively long distances. The method is considerably less useful with molecules such as lipids where the overlap of hydrogen interactions extends from one end of the molecule to the other. Even in these cases quantitative statements may often be made concerning the number of double bonds present, the methyl-to-methylene group ratio, etc.

The method of decoupling may be used to disentangle interactions of protons from one another and locate precisely the position of the center of a complex band on the magnetic field scale. Although decoupling experiments are tedious, a very complete analysis of the spectrum may result.

B. Time Scale, Hydrogen Bonding and Inductive Effects

Nmr spectrometry is fundamentally different from most other types of spectrometry because the time scale for the response of the hydrogen nuclei to changes in the magnetic field is in the range of milliseconds. One therefore observes millisecond averages of any structural changes which may be occurring in the molecule. By contrast infrared and ultraviolet spectrometry furnish an instantaneous view of molecular phenomena. Rather than being a handicap, this averaging results in a simplification of the spectrum and can be employed with great success to

Table 21.1 Approximate Chemical Shifts of Typical Proton Functions Relative to Tetramethylsilane ($\delta = 0.00$).

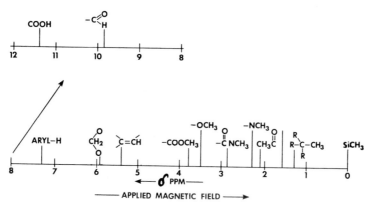

study phenomena such as hydrogen bonding, enolization, and even rotational and conformational isomerism of molecules. Still, some unusual complexities may result. Thus, hydroxyl groups will often show up as rather broad bands appearing anywhere within the spectrum, due to hydrogen bonding. A free hydroxyl group unperturbed by its neighbors is found at very high fields in spite of its "acidity" because the unshared electrons of the oxygen atom are effective in shielding the hydrogen nucleus from the effect of the magnetic field, so a higher *applied* field is necessary to overcome their effect. If hydrogen bonding to another OH group is occurring however, the proton will be spending more time remote from the shielding electrons of either oxygen. The result is that a hydroxyl group will appear at high field when at low concentrations where it is relatively free from neighbors. As the concentration is increased it will move progressively to lower fields due to hydrogen bonding. Intramolecularly hydrogen bonded enols are found at low fields independent of concentration. The *width* of the band is a function of its *rate* of exchange, and it is often advantageous to add a trace of hydrogen chloride or trichloracetic acid to an unknown alcohol in order to sharpen such a peak and make it more easily visible.

Certain structural groups containing protons in well defined symmetrical entities may be particularly easily observed in nmr spectrometry since they give rise to single sharp peaks (Table 21.1). The shift to lower fields is easily seen when the protons are attached to a carbon which is itself attached to an electronegative atom such as nitrogen or oxygen. In other words, the inductive effect of oxygen, nitrogen or halogen withdraws electrons rendering the protons more "acid."

C. Solvents and Peak Shifts Due to Chemical Changes

The nmr method is suitable for very polar, water soluble compounds such as sugars and amine salts, and it is fortunate that a wide variety of solvents suitable for magnetic resonance spectrometry are available in deuterated form otherwise absorption from the solvent would obscure the spectrum. Deuteriochloroform, carbon tetrachloride, deuteriodimethylsulfoxide, deuteriomethanol and D_2O are among the most useful solvents. Often, useful data may be revealed by the addition of small amounts of non-protonic acids such as deuteriotrifluoroacetic and deuterioacetic acids. Unfortunately, most bases are not available in deuterated form and combinations must be chosen which do not absorb in the region of interest. If acid is added to an amine, a downfield shift (toward higher δ values) of approximately 1 part per million will occur because the protons attached to the carbon bearing the nitrogen will be rendered more acidic by the presence of the positive charge upon the nitrogen. Quaternization will have the same effect. On the other hand, basification of a carboxylic acid with sodium hydroxide or other base will result in an upfield shift (toward lower δ values) of the protons alpha to the carboxyl group by about the same amount. Phenols will often show a similar upfield shift of the ring protons on basification telling whether the proton is *ortho* or *para* to the adjacent oxygen (Highet and Highet, 1965).

If exchangeable hydrogens are present (OH, NH, COOH, etc.), addition of a small amount of D_2O to the sample tube will remove the peak at that chemical shift. Under more forcing conditions, deuterioacetic acid or NaOD may be employed to exchange protons alpha to ketones or carboxylic acids. In some cases protons adjacent to an aromatic or heterocyclic ring will also exchange.

It is always advisable to run an unknown in several solvents, at least one of which is aromatic, preferably benzene. The dimagnetic shift (towards higher field, lower δ values) brought about by electrons circulating within the benzene ring may bring about dramatic shifts of peaks due to certain functional groups while not affecting others.

D. Newer Developments

The main disadvantage of nuclear magnetic resonance spectrometry for studies of drug metabolism is that it requires fairly large amounts (1–3 mg) of material in an advanced state of purity. On the other hand if the spectral impurities are known and do not occupy too much of the spectral region of the metabolite, the spectrum may still be usable. More expensive instruments have higher signal-to-noise ratios by virtue of their higher radio frequencies (100 megacycles) and useful spectra can often be obtained by a skilled operator on quantities as small as 50–100 μg. Even smaller amounts can be studied by the use of repetitive scan methods (CAT) which average out instrumental noise. Unfortunately, when this method is used, impurities in the solvents often become the limiting factor since their signal is also enhanced. A promising method employing a computer and other components (Fourier transform analysis) speeds up the accumulation of signals by providing more spectra in a given period of time, although a computer must be used to convert the spectra to the usual form.

It is clear that if enough sample were at hand nmr would be the method of choice, and extensive efforts are being made to enhance the sensitivity of the technique. A particularly fascinating proposal has been put forward recently by Shirley (1969) wherein nmr is coupled to radioactivity. The method, radiative detection of nmr (nmr/RD), depends on analysis of the angular dependence of counting rate of a radioactive nucleus placed in a magnetic field. For many nuclei alignment is possible and the counting rate is non-uniform. When a given radio frequency (the nmr Larmor frequency) is superimposed on the sample the nuclei are misaligned and the counting rate in a given direction changes. The method is still in its infancy and suffers from the fact that not all nuclei may be

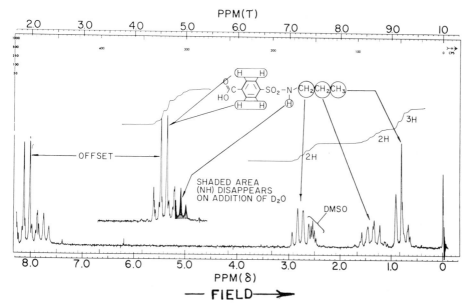

Fig. 21.3 Nuclear magnetic resonance spectrum at 60 megahertz in deuteriochloroform solution with tetramethylsilane as an internal reference ($\delta = 0.00$).

studied at present, but since only 10^{-7} mole is necessary to give a good statistical result, it is clear that the method merits extensive study.

E. Application to Metabolite

Figure 21.3 shows the nmr spectrum of the probenecid metabolite run in deuteriodimethylsulfoxide at 60 mc. Note that the reference point of the magnetic field $\delta = 0$ contains a sharp peak. This is tetramethylsilane used as an internal reference added to the sample. It contains perhaps the least "acidic" protons known and is used as a reference point for this reason. The terminal methyl of the propyl group is a triplet due to splitting by the adjacent methylene protons. The general rule for first order analysis of protons is that a band will be split into a multiplet containing one more band than the number of adjacent protons ($n + 1$ rule). For the same reason the H on the nitrogen at $\delta = 7.7$ (shaded area in offset spectrum) is a triplet. That it is indeed due to an exchangeable NH proton is proved by its disappearance on addition of D_2O. The other 2 CH_2 groups at $\delta 1.3$ and $\delta 2.8$ are more complex since they are split by 5 and 3 protons respectively. Note that the latter is a quadruplet as expected although it is obscured by the non-deuterated methyls of the incompletely deuterated dimethylsulfoxide. This group is also at higher δ value (more "acidic") because of the inductive effect of the sulfonamido nitrogen. All 3 groups contain the correct number of protons as measured by the integrator scan at the top of the spectrum.

Finally, the aromatic (and thus more "acidic") protons are seen as a pair of doublets at $\delta 8.1$, one doublet for the hydrogens *ortho* to the carboxyl and the other *ortho* to the sulfonamido substituent. The protons on either side of the substituents absorb at identical values because of symmetry and cannot be distinguished.

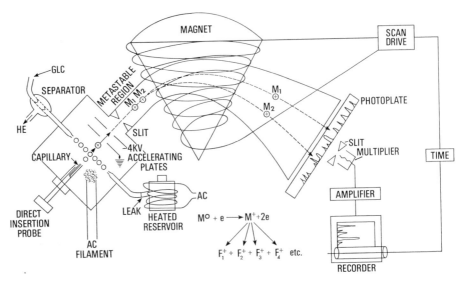

Fig. 21.4 Outline of a typical magnetic sector-single focussing mass spectrometer.

V. MASS SPECTROMETRY

A. Basic Considerations

The basic requirement of mass spectrometry is that the sample must have a finite, though small, vapor pressure at accessible temperatures. While this seemingly strict limitation appears to be disadvantageous, surprisingly, it is met by the vast majority of non-polymeric organic compounds, especially those encountered in most studies of drug metabolism. Upon vaporization, within a chamber maintained at 10^{-6} (Fig. 21.4), an electron current is run through the sample vapor, forming radical ions some of which undergo fragmentation to other ions. These ions are then accelerated according to their mass and charge by an electric field (4KV). After passing through a defining slit, the ions enter an evacuated free-flight region and finally are bent by a magnetic field in indirect proportion to their mass and in direct proportion to their charge. The ions are then either collected on a photographic plate placed in the path of the beams or, more commonly, detected as they strike an ion photomultiplier tube.

In this method the magnetic field is varied causing one mass after another to pass across the exit slit and into the photomultiplier tube. Output is in the form of a bar graph (actually quite narrow peaks) of detector response versus mass. In an ideal case the molecular ion is the last peak observed in the spectrum (except for satellites due to the normal abundance (1 %) of ^{13}C) and quite easily discerned. Often this is not the largest peak in the spectrum by any means. This "molecular ion" supplies the molecular weight of the unknown and can be measured using a double-focussing mass spectrometer with sufficient accuracy to yield the elemental formula based on the fact that the mass of CH_4 equals 16.0313 while that of oxygen equals 15.9949 (C = 12.000000). Thus the formula $C_{11}H_{12}N_2O_2$ (204.0899) differs from $C_{10}H_8N_2O_3$ (204.0535) by a difference in mass of 0.0364 units. Using this type of spectrometer, fragment ions can also be determined as to formula and the process of structural elucidation may consist simply of assembling the pieces. In many cases, reassembly is almost trivial; in other cases almost prohibitively complex.

B. Fragmentation Rules, Isotope Ratios, and Formula Calculations

A few rules follow:

1. Cleavage occurs on the carbon adjacent to heteroatoms:

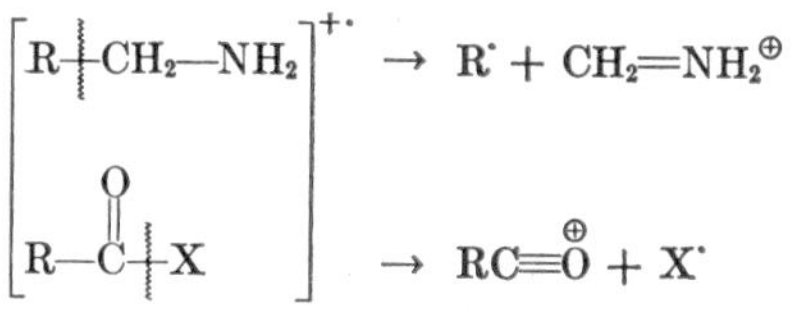

$$\left[R \!-\!\! CH_2\!-\!NH_2 \right]^{+\cdot} \rightarrow R\cdot + CH_2\!=\!NH_2^{\oplus}$$

$$\left[\underset{\substack{\parallel \\ O}}{R\!-\!C}\!-\!X \right] \rightarrow RC\!\equiv\!\overset{\oplus}{O} + X\cdot$$

2. Cleavage occurs preferentially next to benzylic, allylic, quaternary, tertiary, secondary and primary carbon atoms in that order:

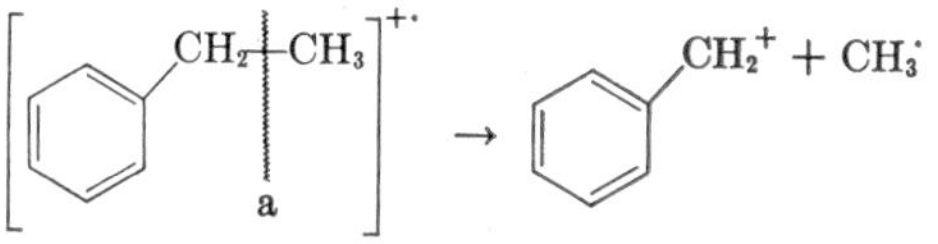

benzylic

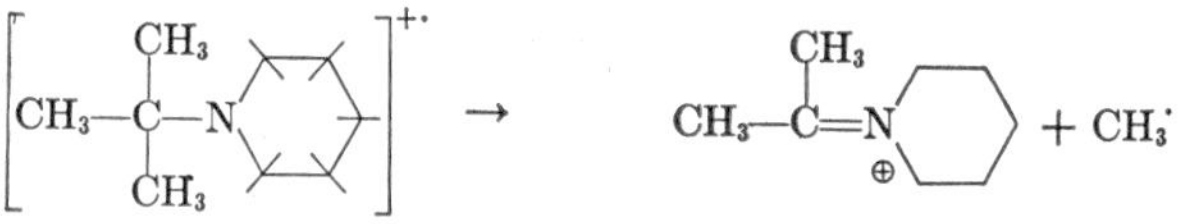

quaternary *and* adjacent to nitrogen

3. When C=X(X = O, N C, etc.) is present, along with a γ-hydrogen, rearrangement of this proton may occur with cleavage of the α,β-bond:

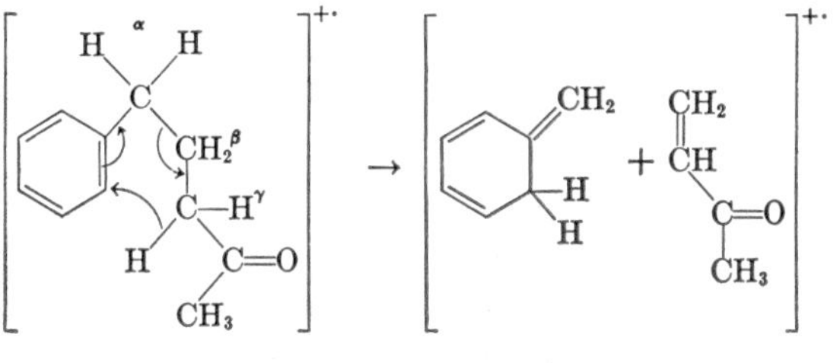

or

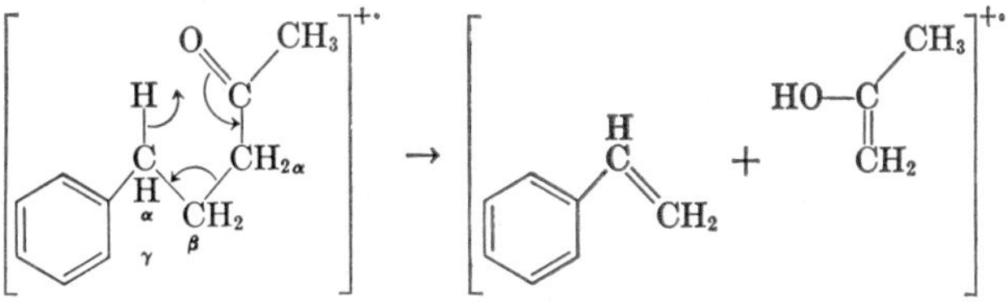

The charge may reside with either fragment

4. Loss of small molecules such as CO, H_2O, CO_2, H_2, HCN, etc., occurs easily, even where mechanistically unusual:

5. Double bonds in rings trigger retro-Diels-Alder type cleavage:

6. Ring formation, aromaticity, conjugation, and heteroatoms, particularly sulfur, iodine or other electron rich atoms, stabilize the molecular ion peak.

7. Certain atoms commonly found on synthetic drugs such as Cl, Br, I, S, etc. are found as natural isotopic mixtures, facilitating interpretation of a spectrum. The number of such atoms is often ascertained by mere inspection of the pattern. Compare the molecular ion region of a monobromide with that of a dibromide:

monobromide   bromide

8. The molecular ion is at odd mass if it contains an odd number of nitrogen atoms and at an even mass if it contains either no nitrogen atoms or an even number of nitrogen atoms. Addition of one or more heteroatoms such as chlorine, bromine, or iodine, etc. does not alter this fact.

9. The ratio of peak heights corresponding to (molecular ion + 1)/molecular ion × 100 gives an approximation of the number of carbon atoms in a molecule since there is about 1 % ^{13}C in nature.

C. Dynamic Range

The great value of mass spectrometry lies in its extreme sensitivity (even a few ions may give a definable peak) and dynamic range. Thus a 6 pen galvanometer is often used for recording spectra since it may cover the range of sensitivity from 1 to 300. The utility of this extreme sensitivity is sometimes overstated, however. If one considers that it is necessary to volatilize a finite amount of material within an ion chamber in such a condition that an electron beam can furnish ions for approximately 10 seconds during a scan, it is apparent that considerable skill may be necessary to obtain a useful spectrum from an unknown metabolite. Furthermore, the method is destructive; the sample cannot be recovered once volatilized.

Even in favorable cases it is difficult to estimate the correct temperature as well as the rate of heating required to volatilize optimally a sample so that it may be scanned within a few seconds. Nor is slow careful heating always an answer. Tyrosine, for example, undergoes polymerization at temperatures lower than that required to obtain a useful spectrum. The only practical method in such cases is to apply a rather rapid burst of heat for a short period of time. The "ion monitor," an electrode inserted within the ion beam prior to mass discrimination of the ions, has been used routinely to indicate the presence of measurable amounts of ions within the beam. While this device is indeed useful for samples of the order of .01 to 10 μg it is too insensitive, as currently designed, to be useful with some of the very small samples encountered in drug metabolite studies.

Instead of attempting to scan a spectrum for a period of a few seconds while the ions are present in the ion chamber, one can use a photoplate to integrate simultaneously all of the ion beams thus obviating the need for scanning. Unfortunately the photoplate is considerably less sensitive than an ion multiplier and the two factors tend to cancel each other.

D. Sampling Conditions and Use of Gas Chromatography

Sample handling can be difficult since the sample must be placed within a small area of the direct insertion probe for maximum sensitivity. This requirement often means that one must concentrate relatively large volumes of solution down to a few microliters, finally evaporating the solvent completely from the residue after placing it within the capillary. Reservoir methods, wherein a sample is placed in a heated chamber exterior to the ion chamber and admitted as a vapor through a small leak, are of almost no use in drug metabolism studies since they require quantities of the order of $\frac{1}{4}$–1 mg in order to supply sufficient vapor to fill the exterior chamber. Almost all metabolites are today admitted by the direct insertion probe system where a probe is admitted directly to the ion chamber and the sample volatilized directly into the electron beam over a path length of a few mm.

From the foregoing considerations it is obvious that gas chromatography is an excellent technique for admitting a sample and can be used more often than not. A surprisingly large number of compounds, originally not thought to be susceptible to gas chromatography, have been found to be perfectly stable at the relatively high temperatures involved. Still, the combination of gas chromatography with mass spectrometry is not without some drawbacks. The apparatus is complex, costly and sometimes destructive toward the sample. Since most mass spectrometers require a high vacuum in the ion chamber, it is essential to remove most of the carrier gas before admission. This is usually carried out by taking advantage of the higher rate of diffusion of the helium used as a carrier gas, relative to other compounds.

Separators in use today depend either upon diffusion of the helium through a fritted glass or preferential diffusion of helium from a molecular beam system. All separator devices are required to be at temperatures somewhat higher than that of the column itself and this is undoubtedly largely responsible for the sample decomposition which is often observed. Furthermore, neither glass nor metal, no matter how carefully protected are without some catalytic action. In order to insure complete scavenging of the sample and carrier gas from both separator and ion chamber it is necessary to insure that both are at considerably higher temperatures than required for direct insertion probe methods. In spite of these difficulties, the use of combined gas chromatography-mass spectrometry has obvious advantages, since the sample is entering the ion chamber at a smooth rate as indicated by the total ionization monitor which doubles as a gas chromatograph detector. In cases where extremely high sensitivity is required, spectra can be repeatedly scanned during the period when the sample is *expected* to be eluted from the column. This of course assumes that the retention time is known.

Spectra can often be obtained in this manner on samples that are too small to give definable peaks on the total ion monitor.

E. Quantitative Methods

Repeated spectra of a single component are generally fairly reproducible but quantitative analysis is not easy because of the difficulty of controlling sample admission to the source. Of course, when fractional milligram quantities of very stable samples are available the mixture may be admitted via the heated reservoir-leak system previously described. Under these conditions good quantitative results can be obtained. The intensity of each fragment peak in the spectrum is a quantitative value so that high reliability is available through cross-checking if time is taken to measure several peaks throughout the spectrum.

One way around the difficulties involved above consists of using an isotopically labeled derivative of the material in question. The unknown sample is mixed with a known amount of derivative and the total admitted to the ion chamber via the direct insertion probe. The ratio of the labeled internal standard to unknown provides a direct answer.

The high dynamic range of the mass spectrometer makes this method very appealing and it is somewhat surprising that it has not been used more often. Using this approach, one could either scan the complete spectrum which might provide many analytical points (provided the labeled group was not lost easily as a fragment) lending great confidence to the result. Using gas chromatography, accuracy could be increased by stopping the magnetic scan so that only one peak, the best from an analytical point of view (most intense, least obscured, etc.) is placed on the multiplier. The mass spectrometer is then a specific detector for the gas chromatographic system responding only to the molecular weight of the compound in question and the G.C. peak area is a measure of quantity of sample. Maximum sensitivity is obtained since time is not lost in the scanning process and because the detector may be operated at its maximum gain with the slits opened wide enough to encompass only one mass unit.

A compromise method is available wherein an electronic device switches the accelerating voltage between two or more values (Hammar, Holmstedt and Ryhage, 1968). This automatically places two peaks whose mass is inversely proportional to the accelerating voltage in front of the detector at alternate times. Since two peaks in the mass spectrum of any given compound will always bear fixed relationships to each other in terms of intensity, this ratio constitutes a very specific detector for a given compound, and only a very short time is lost in the switching operation. Obviously, this system could be employed either in the internal standard method outlined above for a single compound or as a G.C. detector specific only for one compound.

Ideally, one might place a separate detector at the position each mass occupies as it is dispersed by the magnet. So-called double collector methods are in fact used for very accurate analysis of isotope ratios at low mass. They do not appear to have been applied to the field of high molecular weight compounds probably because locating such detectors along the ion paths is difficult.

F. Structural Analysis

In terms of structural analysis, it is obvious that it is most important to assign correctly the molecular ion peak corresponding to the molecular weight of the compound. This can be an extremely difficult task. Experimentally it is often useful to operate at the lowest possible temperature to minimize thermal and electron-induced fragmentation. Lowering the ionizing voltage to just above onset of ionization and increasing the gain often permits clear identification of the molecular ion, for it is the last peak in the mass spectrum to disappear as the ionizing voltage is lowered.

Increasing the sample size, and consequently pressure, is a very useful expedient with most drugs since they often contain one or more nitrogen or other heteroatoms. Under such conditions a proton is often transferred from one molecule of sample to another and an ion is seen at a mass corresponding to molecular weight $+ 1$.

A modern version of this same method is the use of a chemical ionization source (Field, 1968; Fales *et al.*, 1969) where an external gas such as methane or isobutane is added along with the unknown at relatively high pressures ($\sim$1 mm). Ions of the matrix gas supply the proton (in the case of CH_4 *via*, the Bronstead acid CH_5^+) to the unknown and fragmentation is diminished since the energies involved are lower than in electron impact spectrometry at 70 electron volts. The ion $M + 1$ is not a free radical as in the case of electron impact spectrometry and for this reason also is more stable. We feel that this method holds much promise for the future, particularly in the field of gas chromatography-mass spectrometry as applied to metabolites. Because of the high pressure allowed in such a source the gas chromatograph eluate may be admitted directly to the ion chamber without prior separation of the carrier gas.

After all experimental methods have been exhausted, the spectrum itself may be used to assist in the identification of the molecular weight peak. This is done on a logical basis. Thus, it is obvious that except for hydrogen the smallest loss that can occur is CH_3 (loss of CH, C, O, N, are almost never encountered) and so a peak at $M^+ - 14, 13, 12$, etc. is evidence for the fact that the molecular ion is not as assigned or that the sample is impure. Large fragment ions should be logically derived from the assigned parent or molecular ion. Thus a peak at $M - 16$ would not be likely to be encountered in a molecule containing only CH and O since it would correspond to unlikely loss of CH_4 or O but if the compound contains $CONH_2$, loss of NH_2 is not unusual.

Metastable ions (m*) formed by decompositions occurring outside the ion chamber (Fig. 21.4) are observed as broad peaks in the spectrum extending over several mass units and the relationship $m/e^* = (m/e^2$ daughter ion$)/(m/e$ parent ion) holds not only for the molecular ion itself, but for all the fragment ions in the spectrum which give rise to a metastable ion. Metastable ions may also be used to identify the molecular ion where mixtures or impure samples are encountered. These ions are often found in heterocyclic polyfunctional materials and are very useful in a full interpretation of the spectrum.

One must always consider the possibility that the highest mass ion is actually the result of the loss of H_2O, CO_2, CH_3OH, C_2H_5OH, etc., occurring either thermally or under electron impact, and it is most useful to maintain a flexible attitude

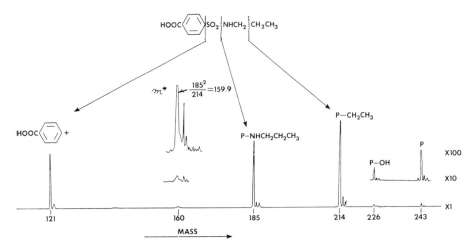

Fig. 21.5 Mass spectrum at 70 electron volts of probenecid metabolite.

towards an apparent molecular ion in considering the spectrum of an unknown metabolite. This is particularly true since many metabolites are alcohols, acids and other oxidation products prone to lose small molecules thermally.

G. Application to Metabolite

Figure 21.5 shows an actual scan of the 70 electron volt mass spectrum of the metabolite II. Notice that the molecular ion at m/e 243 is very small but easily discernible. Loss of OH is common in aromatic acids since the acyl ion is stable (Rule 1). Loss of ethyl to m/e 214 is typical for a n-propylamine (Rule 1) and this cleavage is followed by loss of NHCH$_2$ (m/e 185) as the sulfonyl group mimics its carboxyl counterpart (Rule 1). The broad band at m/e 159.9 proves that the process can take place in two steps as indicated (P $\rightarrow$ P-CH$_2$CH$_3$ $\rightarrow$ (P-CH$_2$CH$_3$)-NHCH$_2$) since the mass of the metastable ion corresponds to $185^2/214$. Finally, a cleavage of the whole sulfonamido side chain (m/e 121) occurs for similar reasons (sulfonyl group cleavage and phenyl radical stability). The peaks at m/e 245 (P + 2), 216, 187 are due to the 5% ^{34}S in nature and disclose its presence in the ions. Naturally it is absent in the benzoic acid ion at m/e 121. Using isobutane as a reactant gas supplying t-butyl ions, the same compound exhibited only m/e 121 (5%) and a quasi-molecular ion at m/e 244 corresponding to M + 1 and its ^{13}C and ^{33}S and ^{34}S satellites. Some recent papers using mass spectrometry and combined gas chromatography-mass spectrometry in studies of drug metabolism (and for investigations where the problems encountered are likely to be typical in such studies) are included under Pertinent Reading.

H. Computer Approaches

Reassembling fragments from cleavages based on the aforementioned rules may appear difficult but since it is largely a "numbers game" even those relatively unschooled in organic chemical principles or carbonium ion chemistry often find the process not only straightforward but intellectually stimulating. Today rapid advances are being made in the application of computers to such analysis. On one hand, a computer may attempt to reassemble all fragments following a set of simple rules, rapidly running through all the possibilities until the correct structure is uncovered. Alternatively, the computer may be given the spectra of a series of compounds of known formulae containing combinations of CHN and O in a "learning machine" approach (Jurs *et al.*, 1969). The spectrum of an unknown substance, is then compared and a reasonable formula deduced based on the rules "learned."

Computer systems should be considered in using any of the above methods. It is a comparatively simple matter to digitize any analog signal and store the resulting spectrum either in a computer disc file or on paper or magnetic tape. The value of such stored data is in direct proportion to the number of samples run. For a drug metabolism study, one might place in such a file the spectrum of every known derivative of the drug, perhaps even synthesizing simple derivatives just for this purpose. The object would not be to try to match an unknown metabolite exactly with one of the synthetic analogs, but to seek spectra-structure correlations which shed light on the structure of the metabolite.

Beyond such sophisticated use, the computer can also be programmed to assist in routine tasks and elegant graphs are easily prepared using a computer run plotter. This type of output is useful not only from an esthetic point of view, but the information content of the spectrum is often much easier to grasp after extraneous detail has been removed by the computer. Unfortunately, programs to accomplish all of these ends are not yet standardized and these sophisticated output devices are likely to be found today only in the laboratories of experts in the field who perhaps require them least.

VI. SUMMARY

In spite of the fact that great advances have been made in the sensitivity of physical methods it is clear that most physical techniques are still not at the stage of development where the pharmacologist can use them for investigation of a solution containing submicrogram quantities of radioactive materials in solutions containing a great deal of other matter. For the present, the pharmacologist will continue to rely heavily on deductive methods, depending upon chemical reactions to bring about changes in the solubility character and chromatographic characteristics of a radioactive component.

Although further advances may be made in the sensitivity of physical methods, more attention should be paid to design of methods to isolate and concentrate trace quantities on a micro scale, eliminating the introduction of impurities from work-up procedures. For example, in most of the methods mentioned above an N-methyl impurity in a drug containing an NH group can be easily discovered. On the other hand, a large quantity of plasticizer, such as butyl phthalate, commonly found in Tygon tubing, might cause major confusion. In the final stages of purification a nearly surgical cleanliness may be required.

A new class of purified solvents is needed which contain no residual impurities; thin layer and paper chromatographic substrates are needed containing far less organic matter so that a spot may be reliably eluted free from annoying impurities. The only alternative to such techniques is to extend physical methods to the nuclear level (Shirley, 1969) itself obviating entirely the need for such extensive purification procedures and while some years away, this is probably the ultimate answer to drug metabolism studies.

REFERENCES

Fales, H. M., Milne, G. W. A., and Vestal, M.: J. Amer. Chem. Soc. *91:* 3682, 1969.

Field, F. H.: Accounts Chem. Research *1:* 42, 1968.

Guarino, A., Conway, W. D., and Fales, H. M.: Eur. J. Pharmacol. *8:* 244,1969.

Hammar, C. G.: Combined GC-MS for identification of chlorpromazine and its metabolites. Agresslogie *9:* 109, 1968.

Hammar, C. G., Holmstedt, B., and Ryhage, R.: Mass fragmentography, identification of chlorpromazine and its metabolites in human blood by a new method. Anal. Biochem. *25:* 532–548, 1968.

Highet, R. J. and Highet, P. F.: J. Org. Chem. *30:* 902, 1965.

Jurs, P. C., Kowalski, B. R., and Isenhour, T. L.: Anal. Chem. *41:* 21, 1969.

Kapadia, G. J. and Fales, H. M.: Krebs cycle conjugates of mescaline. Identification of fourteen new peyote alkaloid amides. Chem. Commun. *24:* 1688-1689, 1968.

Lambe, J. and Jaklevic, R. C.: Physical Rev. *165:* 816, 1968.

Luukkainen, T. and Adlercreutz, H.: Mass spectrometric studies in the specificity of estriol determination in urine by GLC. Ann. Med. Exp. Biol. Fenn. *45:* 264, 1967.

Mize, C., Avigan, J., Steinberg, D., Pittman, R. C., Fales, H. M., and Milne, G. W. A.: A major pathway for the mammalian oxidative degradation of phytanic acid. Biochem. Biophys. Acta *176:* 720-739, 1969.

Nair, P. P. and Zenaida, L.: Identification of α-tocopherol from tissues by GC-MS, etc. Arch. Biochem. Biophys. *127:* 413-418, 1968.

Polito, A. J., Akita, T., and Sweeley, C. C.: Gas chromatography and mass spectrometry of sphingolipid bases. Characterization of sphinga-4,14-dienine from plasma sphingomyelin. Biochemistry *7:* 2609-2614, 1968.

Schwartz, M. A., Bommer, P., and Vane, F. M.: Diazepam metabolites in the rat: characterization by high-resolution mass spectrometry and nuclear magnetic resonance. Arch. Biochem. Biophys. *121:* 508, 1967.

Shirley, D. A.: Anal. Chem. *41:* 69A, 1969.

Sjovall, J. and Vikko, R.: Analysis of solvolyzable steroids in human plasma by GC-MS. Acta Endocrinol. *57:* 247, 1968.

Smith, D. L. and Grostic, M. F.: Mass spectrometric identification of the metabolites of methyl N-(o-aminophenyl)-N-(3-dimethyl aminopropyl) anthranilate. J. Med. Chem. *10:* 375-379, 1967.

PERTINENT READING

Infrared

Bellamy, L.: *The Infra-red Spectra of Complex Molecules,* John Wiley & Sons, Inc., New York, N. Y., 1958.

Rao, C. N. R.: *Chemical Applications of Infrared Spectroscopy,* Academic Press, New York, 1963.

Martin, A. E.: *Infrared Instrumentation and Techniques,* Elsevier Publishing Co., New York, 1966.

Nakanishi, K.: *Infrared Absorption Spectroscopy, Practical,* Holden-Day, San Francisco, Calif., 1962.

Szymanski, H. A., and Alpert, N. L.: *IR, Theory and Practice of Infrared Spectroscopy,* Plenum Press, New York, 1964.

Ultraviolet

Hershenson, H. M.: *Ultraviolet and Visible Absorption Spectra—A Literature Index* 1930–1963, Academic Press, New York 1956.

Gillam, A. E. and Stern, E. S.: *An Introduction to Electronic Absorption Spectroscopy in Organic Chemistry,* Edward Arnold Publishers, London, 1954.

Nuclear Magnetic Resonance

Bible, R. H.: *Interpretation of NMR Spectra; an Empirical Approach,* Plenum Press, New York, 1967.

Bhacca, N. S. and Williams, D. H.: *Applications of NMR Spectroscopy in Organic Chemistry; Illustrations from the Steroid Field,* Holden-Day, San Francisco, Calif. 1964.

Jackman, L. M.: *Applications of Nuclear Magnetic Resonance Spectroscopy in Organic Chemistry,* Pergamon Press, New York, 1959.

Mass Spectrometry

Biemann, K.: *Mass Spectrometry—Organic Chemical Applications,* McGraw-Hill, New York, 1962.

Beynon, J. H.: *Mass Spectrometry and its*

Application to Organic Chemistry, Elsevier Publishing Co., New York, 1960.

Budziekiewicz, H., Djerassi, C., and Williams, D. H.: *Mass Spectrometry of Organic Compounds*, Holden-Day, Inc., San Francisco, Calif., 1967.

McLafferty, F. W.: *Interpretation of Mass Spectra*, W. A. Benjamin, Inc., New York, **1966.**

General

Silverstein, R. M. and Bassler, G. C.: *Spectrometric Identification of Organic Compounds*, John Wiley & Sons, Inc., New York, 1967.

Fleming, I. and Williams, D. H.: *Spectroscopic Methods in Organic Chemistry*, McGraw-Hill, New York, 1966.

22

Qualitative and Quantitative Applications of Thin-Layer, Gas-Liquid, and Column Chromatography

GRANT R. WILKINSON

I. INTRODUCTION

Chromatographic techniques, because of their simplicity, speed, efficiency, sensitivity, versatility and economy, play a significant and vital role in isolating, identifying and quantifying a drug and/or metabolite. These procedures gen erally require a small volume of a relatively concentrated solution of the materials of interest and, consequently, they are most frequently applied to suitable organic solvent extracts of the biological media to be analyzed. A certain degree of specificity and concentration may be incorporated into this extraction procedure, and the material of this chapter is based on the assumption that such extracts are available.

Chromatography is a physical method of separation in which the components to be separated are distributed between two phases, one a stationary bed of large surface area and the other a fluid that penetrates through or along the stationary bed. Either a liquid or gas may serve as the mobile phase while liquids or solids function as the stationary phase. The mechanism of solute retardation is by adsorption, partition, ion exchange or molecular sieving. Although one mechanism is usually made to predominate, frequently all four mechanisms are present during a chromatographic separation. One classification of chromatography is made according to the physical states involved, i.e., gas-liquid, gas-solid, liquid-liquid, liquid-solid. Another classification depends upon the mechanism by which separation occurs. Also common, however, is reference to the different techniques according to the design of the instrumental apparatus rather than the more fundamental characteristics, i.e., thin-layer, column and gas chromatography.

No attempt will be made to list the innumerable applications of chromatographic procedures in drug metabolism studies. Information of this nature may be found through the texts listed in the bibliography. Instead, this chapter describes some of the basic principles underlying the various techniques with particular emphasis upon techniques which permit direct identification and subsequent quantification of a particular compound after separation from related metabolites and tissue constituents, etc. Purely separatory and preparative aspects will not be mentioned, for this only involves in general a scaling modification of the basic procedure. Consequently, emphasis will be placed upon thin-layer and gas-liquid chromatography, the most widely used procedures. In

458

view of the revived interest in analytical column chromatography, this subject will be briefly mentioned. Coverage of these topics does not imply that other techniques such as paper chromatography, electrophoresis, gel permeation, etc. do not have a place in the analytical armamentarium. In certain circumstances and applications these methods are invaluable, but in general they currently do not contribute heavily to the "drug metabolism" work load.

II. THIN-LAYER CHROMATOGRAPHY

Thin-layer chromatography (TLC) has replaced to a large extent paper chromatography in the majority of applications involving separation of drugs and metabolites. The advantages of TLC are a much shortened development time (an hour or less is normally required), detection methods which are increased from 10 to 100 times when applied to thin-layer chromatograms, a reproducibility which is fair providing the coating procedures are controlled, individual spots which are more discrete and less diffuse, and the use of a greater variety of detection techniques.

A. Basic Principles and Techniques

The standard procedure in TLC is preparation of the plate by spreading a slurry consisting of a specific sorbent powder and suitable liquid, usually water, on a glass plate. After the thin-layer of sorbent has dried, it is activated, if necessary, and then the sample mixture is applied to one end of the plate, either as a spot or a line. The plate is developed by placing it vertically in a suitable chamber, the bottom of which is filled with the solvent system. Solvent is drawn through the layer by capillary action and, because of differences in solute/ system interactions, the components of the mixture are separated into individual spots. Subsequently the spots can be suitably visualized and, if required, quantified.

1. Adsorbents. The choice of sorbent depends primarily upon such properties of the sample components as solubility (hydrophilic or hydrophobic) and chemical characteristics (acidic, basic, amphoteric or neutral, and lability towards chemical reaction with the sorbent or solvent). Table 22.1 lists some of the major types of sorbents with details of their principles of use, and types of sample and solvents suitable for use with them.

Although the various adsorbents may be used in pure form, normally other substances are present. Binders such as calcined calcium sulfate are frequently added, 10–20% w/w, to make the adsorbent adhere more firmly to the plate. Additives may also be incorporated to modify the physical and chemical properties of the adsorbents and also to aid visualization of the completed chromatogram. The layer of adsorbent should be of uniform thickness, and for analytical separations a thickness of 250 μ is routinely used. A uniform powder particle size distribution (5–80 μ) is essential for producing the minimum spreading or tailing of spots and also for structural strength and increased speed of development. Details concerning the method of preparing the plates are usually provided with the adsorbent and it is advisable that a good commercial applicator is employed to coat the glass plates.

Silica gel is probably the most popular adsorbent, and it produces a highly active acidic chromatoplate mainly used to separate acidic and neutral com-

TABLE 22.1

Selectivity of various TLC techniques

Technique	Separation Due To Differences In	Sample	Sorbents	Solvents
Adsorption Chromatography	Polarity due to functional groups	Neutral/acidic non-polar $\updownarrow$ to polar Neutral/basic non-polar $\updownarrow$ to polar	Silica-gel Kieselguhr Alumina	Non-aqueous
Partition Chromatography A. Normal	Solubility due to: 1. Number and polarity of constituents 2. Molecular size and shape	Polar to medium polar	Silica-gel Cellulose Kieselguhr	Aqueous-nonaqueous mixture Non-aqueous moves
B. Reversed phase	3. Chain length, etc.	Non-polar to medium polar	Silica-gel impregnated with nonpolar oils	As above, but aqueous moves
Ion exchange	pH-depending on charge; size and shape of molecule	Forms ions	Anion or cation exchangers	Aqueous
Thin-layer electrophoresis	Charge and size of molecule	Forms ions	Silica-gel Cellulose	Aqueous buffers
Polyamide	Hydrogen bridge bonding, aromatic —OH, —NO$_2$ and quinones	Strongly polar	Polyamide and acetylated polyamide	Aqueous

pounds which are not too hydrophilic. However, by use of buffers and appropriate solvents it can be used for basic or hydrophilic substances. Commercially it is possible to obtain silica gel with hydrated silicon dioxide as a binder, an agent superior to anhydrous calcium sulfate generally employed with other sorbents. Alumina is also popular and preferred for non-polar and weakly polar basic and neutral substances. Alumina is much more chemically reactive than silica gel and it may cause artifacts with chemically sensitive compounds, e.g., ester hydrolysis, isomerization of double bonds, and other reactions (Bobbitt, 1963). Kieselguhr is a neutral adsorbent of low activity which is used primarily for partition chromatography of strongly hydrophilic and amphoteric compounds. Powdered cellulose has also been used as the support phase for partition chromatography. Of more specialized application are such adsorbents as ion-exchange resins for separating of ionic and non-ionic compounds. Polyamide powder has been used to separate very strongly polar substances such as phenols.

Activation, a term used to describe the ability of a sorbent to attract other compounds electrostatically, is of importance in adsorption chromatography. Water occupying the adsorptive sites reduces the activity and separating power of a given adsorbent considerably. Consequently, it is necessary to control the activity mainly by controlling the time and temperature of drying and subsequent activation of the layers. Various grades of activity of both silica gel and alumina are obtainable. Although it is not usually necessary to know the precise activity of the adsorbent layer, so long as desirable separations are achieved, a simple routine procedure may be used to obtain such information (Stolman, 1965). For many drug applications, activation by heating the coated plate at 110°C for 30 to 90 minutes is usually satisfactory. After activation the plate is protected against moisture by storing in a suitable desiccator. Should the plate become deactivated by the adsorption of atmospheric moisture, one can reactivate by re-heating.

If a separation of a drug and its metabolites is unsatisfactory, a different adsorbent may be substituted. Rather than different adsorbents, however, the use of different solvent systems is more expedient and economical.

2. Sample application. Samples to be separated are applied to the prepared plate as spots with a suitable capillary tube, micropipette or microsyringe. The solvent used for application preferably should boil between 50° and 100°C so that it does not evaporate too rapidly but nevertheless may be easily removed. Furthermore, it should be non-polar to a point where the sample is concentrated at the center of the spot and not around the edge. If large samples are to be applied, application of the solution in stages is preferable. Also, the spot is dried with a current of warm air after each application. For analytical chromatography, samples from 5 to 100 μg are usually applied; too large a sample will overload the plate and cause tailing of the spots, and high Rf values. Plastic templates are often used to simplify placing the spots on a line 15 to 25 mm from the lower end of the plate and from 10 to 20 mm apart. It is preferable to apply the samples at the end of the plate opposite to the direction of film application or the end of the plate which was coated last. This eliminates any portion of the layer which may not be uniform as a result of the applicator adjusting to each plate.

3. Solvent systems. Much of the flexibility of TLC is derived from the wide variety of solvent systems which may be successfully used with the technique. Selection of a suitable solvent is empirically based upon the separation desired. Solvents can be arranged according to their eluting effect in an "eluotropic series," and several series have been suggested (Stahl, 1969; Bobbitt, 1963; Haer, 1968). There is a close relationship between polarity and elution effects and, in general, the more polar a solvent the greater the elution. When separating a mixture for the first time, it is best to choose a very low polar solvent and, if the sample doesn't migrate from the origin, then to try a solvent of higher polarity. If the sample moves with the solvent front, a solvent of less polarity should be utilized. In selecting a suitable solvent, the radial technique is particularly useful. In this procedure, after application of the test spots, trial solvents are applied to each of them by means of a capillary tube. The spots are allowed to migrate radially. That solvent which moves the sample about halfway between the point of origin and the solvent front and resolves it into several rings, is the one to use. Most common solvent systems are mixtures composed of high and low polarity components. To obtain an optional elution, therefore, the only modification required is to increase or decrease the proportion of the polar solvent.

Reagent grade solvents should preferably be used and the mixed systems should be accurately and frequently prepared. Many investigators feel that better separations and reproducibility are obtained when mixtures are kept as simple as possible (Bobbitt, 1963). Some caution is required with multi-component systems, for they may separate and demix during chromatography, producing secondary solvent fronts.

Chromatography of acids and bases sometimes produces "tailing" of the spots because more than one ionic species of the substance(s) is present. Small amounts of acidic (acetic acid) or basic (ammonia, diethylamine) solvents may be added to the developing system to buffer and keep the components exclusively in the un-ionized form. Sharper separations are frequently obtained with this technique compared to pretreating and buffering the sorbent material.

4. Development. Ascending development of the spotted-plate is generally employed for routine separations. The plate is placed vertically into a chamber or tank of suitable size and with sufficient solvent to cover the bottom of the plate by about 1 cm. Rapid equilibration of the atmosphere of the chamber with the solvent vapors is achieved by lining the side of the chamber with a sheet or strip of filter-paper dipping into the solvent. The chamber is then firmly sealed and the plate developed over a sufficient time until the solvent front has migrated about 10 cm. Depending upon the solvent system, this migration may take from 10 minutes to several hours.

For better resolution of complex mixtures of components of similar structure, the use of uni-directional, multi-developmental techniques with the same or different solvent systems of decreasing polarity may be of value. Similarly, two-dimensional development, frequently at right angles and with two different solvent systems, can be successfully applied.

5. Detection methods. Visualization of the chromatogram is carried out as a separate and distinct operation after the plate has been developed and dried (c.f., GLC). In general the chemical nature of the separated compounds and the nature of the adsorbent determine the method of detection.

For colored substances no problem is encountered in detection. Many organic substances fluoresce and as such may be located as fluorescent spots on a dark background by irradiating the plate with ultra-violet light. Advantage has been taken of the reverse situation where a fluorescent agent such as fluorescein is incorporated into the adsorbent layer. With this technique, the isolated substances appear as dark spots on an intensely yellow-green fluorescent background.

Chromatograms of radioactive compounds can be visualized by making x-ray prints of the plate. Depending upon the activity of the spot, exposure times may vary from a few hours to weeks. Location of radioactive materials may also be made by scanning the plate with a suitable counting device.

The inorganic nature of most adsorbent layers permits location of spots by a wide variety of chemical reagents, often very corrosive, applied as a spray. A number of universal spray reagents have been developed based primarily upon converting organic compounds to carbon by either dehydration or oxidation. For example, concentrated and 50% sulfuric acid and chromic/sulfuric acid are applied to the plate and heated to between 100° and 200°C until the charred spots appear. Iodine, either as a vapor or spray, is an exceptionally effective universal reagent which produces a brown spot with most organic substances and, furthermore, is reversible. A certain degree of specificity may be obtained in detection by using spray reagents which only react with certain types of compounds. Bobbitt (1963), Kirchner (1967) and Stahl (1969) have listed a wide variety of the more frequently used specific reagents with details of their preparation, color reactions, and specificity.

The detection limit for visualization of a compound depends predominantly upon the technique used for detection. With highly fluorescent substances and intensely colored spots, as little as 5 to 10 nanograms may be detected; however, this limit must be decreased for less chromatophoric substances. The detection of radioactive substances is obviously dependent upon the specific activity of the labelled compound.

For every chromatogram the position, size, color, and color intensity of each spot should be recorded. For permanent documentation of the separation, a number of methods are available. Most commonly the chromatograms is either copied upon transparent paper or reproduced by photography or other means, such as "Xeroxing." It is possible to preserve the layer intact by spraying it with a plastic material which after setting may be peeled off along with the adhered sorbent.

B. Qualitative Techniques

Because of the wide separatory power of TLC, unequivocal identification of the separated individual spots based solely upon their chromatographic behavior is difficult. Some often valuable information may be obtained by the use of specific visualization procedures but generally, when using TLC alone, one must compare the behavior of the unknown with a reference compound(s). The power of TLC in the identification of drugs and their metabolites is well illustrated by its application to the elucidation of the metabolism of the phenothiazines where large numbers of biotransformation products are formed (Green and Forrest, 1966). The combined use of a differential solvent extraction and TLC with a number of different systems permits the identification of many of these metabolites (Afifi and Way, 1968; Forrest et al., 1968). However, even with the availability of reference compounds some difficulties and incorrect identifications may arise as exemplified by the recent controversy concerning the "pink spot" observed on both paper and thin-layer chromatograms after developing urine extracts from patients with Parkinson's disease and from some schizophrenics (Boulton et al., 1967). As a consequence of this difficulty, and also when reference compounds are not available, further evidence of identification must frequently be obtained by more structure-revealing techniques (Section II, B, 2).

1. R_f values. As in paper chromatography the ratio of the migration distance of the substance spot to the distance of the solvent front from the point of application is known as the R_f value of the substance. Ideally, in any given system this should be constant and characteristic for a particular substance.

In practice, however, many variables affect the reproducibility of R_f values and the latter should therefore be used with caution.

Variations in the adsorbent, such as uniformity of layer thickness on the same and different plates, activation of the layer and intra-batch differences, may affect R_f values. The degree of saturation of the developing chamber with solvent vapor and the solvent running distance, particularly with multi-component systems, influences migration. The R_f values are also found to be affected by the presence of impurities and the nature of the solvent in which the substance is applied. Overloading the plate causes tailing, and furthermore, R_f values vary with the quantity of substance applied to the plate, most noticeably with very small and very large quantities. It is advisable, however, to apply the unknown in various amounts. With short development times, variations due to temperature fluctuations are often insignificant but increasingly important as the running time increases.

The possible existence of a number of charged moieties or complexes and the existence of an equilibrium between two or more species may cause a single pure substance to appear as a mixture because of the "multiple-spot phenomenon" (Keller and Giddings, 1961). Such artifacts can lead to erroneous interpretation concerning new "metabolites" of a compound, e.g., pralidoxime (Way and Way, 1968). The appearance of multiple-spot phenomena can be greatly minimized by the conversion of all ionized compounds to a single common anion (Way et al., 1966). Chemical reaction on the plate prior to or during development may also give rise to the multi-spot phenomenon, a point to be considered when selecting a particular adsorbent/solvent system. These variations in absolute R_f values from one plate to another has led to the use of relative R_f values which are analogous to relative retention times in gas chromatography (Section III, B, 1). That is, the R_f value of the unknown is expressed as a ratio relative to a reference spot.

The difficulties in obtaining reproducible R_f values necessitates strict standardization of all the procedures involved in the separation—varied only when absolutely necessary. Furthermore, qualitative analysis on TLC is never positive unless authentic standards are run on the same plate and under identical conditions. For unequivocal identification of a spot relative to its reference, it is advisable to chromatograph the substance both uni- and bi-directionally in a number of adsorbent/solvent systems with different elution properties. Table 22.2 illustrates the usefulness of R_f values in identifying a number of closely structurally related sympathomimetic amines and the changes induced in these values by using different adsorbents and/or solvent systems.

2. Ancillary techniques. Unless pure reference compounds are available, a particular unknown spot is impossible to positively identify by TLC. It is then necessary to apply more rigorous structure elucidating techniques to the isolated substance. The adsorbent containing the desired component may be simply scraped off the plate and eluted from the inorganic support with a suitable solvent. The pure substance may then be isolated by evaporating the solvent, although it is advisable to re-extract with a less polar solvent to remove any adsorbent that might be initially extracted. Such techniques as infra-red, nuclear magnetic resonance and mass spectrometry may then be applied to the residue (Chapter 21).

TABLE 22.2

R_f Values of some "amphetamines" and "ephedrines" [a]

Support	Solvent	R_f Values $\times 10^2$				
		Amphetamine	Methylamphetamine	Norephedrine	Ephedrine	Methylephedrine
Alumina	CHCl₃-MeOH (50:50)	57	81	13	69	84
Silica gel	CHCl₃-MeOH (50:50)	29	20	19	23	30
Silica gel	CHCl₃-diethylamine (9:1)	74	79	23	35	64
Silica gel	CHCl₃-acetonediethylamine (5:4:1)	84	70	83	33	69
Silica gel	n-butanol-acetic acid-water (5:4:1)	60	49	55	50	41
Silica gel	MeOH-acetone (50:50)	59	24	67	30	36
Silica gel	MeOH-acetone NH₃ (35%) (47.5:47.5:5)	85	56	92	78	67
Silica gel	MeOH-acetone triethanolamine (1:1:0.03)	63	27	71	28	42
Silica gel	Isopropanol-NH₃ (5%) (10:1)	46	32	44	29	39
	Dimethylformamide-ethylacetate/+ 3 drops n-octanol (1:9)	21	16	18	20	38

[a] Reproduced with permission from Beckett *et al.* (1967).

C. Quantitative Techniques

Like visualization, the quantitation of a TLC plate is a separate procedure from the actual development. Consequently, it is frequently a more complicated and less convenient technique of estimation than is GLC, which uses real-time detection. Quantitative analysis of thin-layer chromatograms may be divided into two general categories; the separated components may be measured on the plate or they can be determined after elution from the adsorbent. Rigid standardization of all of the procedures is mandatory, and in such cases the precision of the various methods is from 3 to 10 %, depending upon the exact method of estimation and the type of compound being measured. Bobbitt (1963), Stahl (1969), Malins and Mangold (1966) and Shellard (1968) present excellent discussions of quantitative techniques and their limitations.

1. Analysis on the plate. The simplicity of these techniques probably makes them the most desirable. The size of a spot is mainly determined by the amount of substance applied to the plate; consequently, the precise measurement of spot areas or size may be used for quantification. Spot area does not increase linearly with the amount of substance applied; therefore it is advisable to prepare calibration curves for each plate. In many cases the square root of the spot area is linearly related to the logarithm of the weight of substance present, but the linear range for this relationship must be determined for each compound. Quantification via reproductions is often more precise than analysis of the fractions upon the plate itself.

A number of commercial photo-densitometers are available for scanning TLC plates either manually or automatically, and many are equipped with mechanical or electrical integrators. The curves recorded by this photometric method are dependent not only upon the color intensity of the spot but also upon its area and shape. When spray reagents are used to develop the color of the spot, caution must be taken that the color-formation occurs at a uniform and reproducible rate.

Soft β-emitters such as tritium and carbon-14 labelled compounds may be quantified directly upon the plate by several types of automatic radioscanners. The recorder deflection is directly proportional to the quantity of radioactive substance under the scanning counter and thus simplifies calibration. An alternative, but more tedious method for labelled compounds, is to evaluate densitometrically the x-ray films developed from the radioactive chromatogram.

2. Analysis of eluted fractions. Substances separated on a chromatogram may be scraped off the plate, eluted with a suitable solvent and then quantified by a number of techniques: gravimetric, spectrophotometric, colorimetric, fluorometric, gas-liquid chromatographic, biological and radiometric procedures, all have been successfully applied. The problems with this approach are that complete recovery of the substance is difficult and erratic, and frequently, the adsorbent produces a significant reading which must be corrected. Radioactively labelled substances may be directly counted in a liquid scintillation counter without subsequent elution from the adsorbent. This and the direct radioactive scanning method with the better scanners are considered by many investigators to be the best all-round quantitative procedures with respect to accuracy and precision.

D. Recent Innovations

1. Pre-coated plates. In recent years considerable effort has been directed towards simplification of the TLC technique by introducing pre-coated, ready-to-use layers. Advantages of such layers include convenience, time and labor savings, ease of storage and improved quality. The pre-coated glass plates which are commercially available offer better uniformity, homogeneity and physical stability than do home-made plates. They suffer, however, the same disadvantages of the latter, being fragile and unsuitable for direct record purposes. The introduction of layers pre-coated upon thin, inert, flexible plastic sheets has overcome these disadvantages. These sheets may be cut to any desired size and filed for permanent record. Other advantages over conventional plates include greater flexibility, simplicity of handling and minimum storage requirement. Being foils, they resemble paper chromatograms, but they retain the resolution, sensitivity and separating speed of conventional TLC. A variety of adsorbents with or without additives are commercially available, and it is possible with many to use even the most rigorous activation and visualization techniques. The overall convenience and performance of these pre-coated sheets recommend them not only to investigators requiring only occasional usage, but also, the more regular user.

2. Impregnated glass fiber TLC. An increasingly popular flexible TLC sheet is that in which silica gel adsorbent is impregnated into a uniform glass fiber matrix. The entire physically stable sheet is consequently sorbent and the need for binders and other possible organic contaminants is removed. In general, separations require from 50 to 75 % less developmental time than conventional plates, and the other advantages of these layers are similar to those of pre-coated sheets. An excellent text includes this new technique (Haer, 1968).

III. GAS CHROMATOGRAPHY

Since its inception in 1952, gas chromatography has developed into a major analytical tool of widespread application in a variety of scientific disciplines. The speed, separatory power, sensitivity, accuracy, specificity and simplicity of the technique has made it particularly applicable to both the qualitative and quantitative study of drugs and poisons. A number of excellent reviews and texts are available (see the bibliography).

A. Basic Principles and Techniques

In gas chromatography the components to be separated are carried through a column by an inert gas termed the carrier gas. The mixture is distributed between the carrier gas and a stationary phase which selectively retards the sample components according to their partition coefficients and/or adsorption characteristics. This results in the formation of separate component bands in the carrier gas which are swept out of the column and suitably detected. The resulting chromatogram consists of a recording of the detector response against the time after introduction of the mixture into the system (Fig. 22.1).

The stationary phase within the chromatographic column may be an active solid such as molecular sieve, silica gel or charcoal, in which case the procedure is referred to as gas-solid chromatography (GSC). This technique is generally used for the separation of permanent gases and as such has little application in drug metabolism studies. On the other hand, the use of a non-volatile liquid as the stationary phase (gas-liquid chromatography (GLC)) offers a wide versatility in identifying and determining any material having an appreciable vapor pressure (1 to 1000 mm Hg) at column operating conditions ($-70°$ to $400°C$).

1. Carrier gas. The most commonly used carrier gases are nitrogen, helium, hydrogen, and argon, all supplied from a high pressure cylinder with a suitable regulator to ensure a constant rate of flow. The choice of gas and the degree of purity are largely determined by the type of detector being used. In order to maintain stability, prevent contamination and save reconditioning time, the carrier gas should continually flow through the column.

2. Sample introduction. The sample to be analyzed is introduced into the

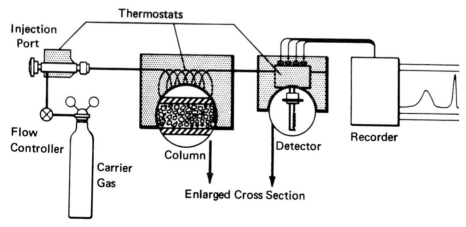

Fig. 22.1 Schematic diagram of a typical gas chromatographic system (reproduced with permission from McNair and Bonelli, 1967).

carrier gas stream at the injection port. The techniques and procedures for sample introduction vary according to the apparatus design and the physical state of the sample, whether liquid, gas or solid. Frequently, the drugs and metabolites being studied are dissolved in an organic solvent, in which case the standard technique for injection is by use of a micro-syringe inserted through a self-sealing septum. The sample should be introduced into the column as instantaneously as possible, i.e., as a "plug"; poor injection procedures may result in peak-tailing and a significant loss of column efficiency.

The temperature of the injection port is extremely important—hot enough to vaporize the sample almost instantaneously so that no loss in efficiency results. On the other hand the temperature must be low enough so that thermal decomposition and rearrangement does not occur. A practical test is to raise the temperature of the injection port. If the column efficiency or peak shape improves, the temperature was too low; if the peaks emerge sooner and give odd shapes, the temperature may be too high. Usually the injection port is maintained at 50° to 100°C higher than the column temperature.

3. Chromatographic column. The column of the gas chromatograph is frequently called the heart of the system, for it is here that separation of components occurs. Consequently, the success or failure of a particular separation depends to a large extent on the choice of column.

The most widely used type is the packed column where the liquid stationary phase is coated as a thin film upon an inert support material of large surface area. The coated support is then packed into suitable columns usually from 0.0625 to 0.25 inch external diameter and up to 50 feet in length.

Another type is the capillary column (Golay column, wall-coated open tubular (WCOT) column), in which the tubing wall of the column functions as a support for the liquid phase. These columns are long, and open tubes of small diameter ranging from 0.01 to 0.03 inches internal diameter and from 100 to 500 feet in length. Column efficiencies of several 100,000's theoretical plates are common thereby increasing the separation and resolution of compounds (packed columns exhibit from 1000–10,000 plates). The sample size permitted, however, with such columns is small.

Also commercially available are support-coated (SCOT) columns which are open tubes, the walls of which are coated with liquid phase which is itself coated upon an inert support material. They are intermediate in structure and performance between packed and capillary columns.

a. *Liquid phase.* The versatility and selectivity of GLC is due to the wide choice of stationary phases available. Hundreds of different phases have been described and although many do offer unique separations, in studies involving drugs and their metabolites, most analyses may be performed on a relatively few liquid phases.

Unfortunately, there is no accurate theoretical guide to the choice of a liquid phase. The literature may yield information on similar separations but beyond this only empirical trial and error approaches will lead to a suitable choice. The classification of phases according to their polarity is a useful concept in that a selection may often be aided by application of the rule that "like dissolves like." Hence, non-polar phases are best for non-polar samples and conversely, polar phases are best for polar samples.

A general purpose liquid phase which has found wide applicability in the past is the methyl siloxane polymer SE-30. This non-selective phase provides a separation based mainly upon molecular weight and volatility, and it exhibits very little column bleed at temperatures as high as 300°C. Recently, other extremely thermo-stable stationary phases, known as the OV-silicones, have become commercially available. Besides allowing columns to be successfully operated for long periods at temperatures up to 275–350°C, they have the added advantage of offering a range of polarities from non-polar (OV-1, OV-101) through to intermediate polar (OV-17, OV-25, OV-225). These few phases may be capable of achieving the necessary separation for the vast majority of bio-medical applications.

b. *Support phase.* A large number of different materials have been used in the search for an ideal support upon which to coat the liquid stationary phase as a thin film with large surface area. Ottenstein (1963) has reviewed the properties of many, such as glass beads, Teflon, sand, Tide and the more commonly used types of diatomaceous earth. A compromise must be made between chemical inertness and column efficiency.

Generally, the smaller the particle size of the support material, the more efficient the column. It is far more important, however, that the particle size range should be narrow, commonly 60/80, 80/100, and 100/120 mesh.

The amount of liquid phase applied to the support should be sufficient to coat the particles with a thin uniform layer. Since retention time is proportional to the amount of liquid phase, too much liquid phase increases analysis time, and also decreases column efficiency. The present day trend is towards lightly loaded columns, i.e., from 1 to 10 % liquid phase.

Techniques for coating the liquid phase onto the support either by the filtration process (Horning et al., 1959) or the slurry procedure (Purnell, 1962) are well described in basic GLC texts. Some controversy exists as to the advantages of each method but many investigators feel that for low loaded columns the filtration technique produces more reproducible and efficient columns.

Although the support material should be completely inert, this ideal has yet to be achieved in practice. As a consequence, solute may be adsorbed during chromatography resulting in complete loss of the solute, or peak-tailing and non-linear response curves. This problem is particularly troublesome when analyzing sub-microgram quantities of drugs, especially those compounds containing polar hydroxyl, carbonyl, carboxyl and amino groups. A variety of methods have been designed to overcome this problem (Ottenstein, 1963). One procedure is to acid-wash the support material and, although the precise mechanism of this inactivation is not known, it frequently renders the material less adsorptive.

Since the adsorptive character of the support is often due to the presence of silanol (Si-OH) groups, inactivation is frequently directed towards masking of this group. Generally this is accomplished by forming silyl ethers of the silanol functions by treating the support with either hexamethyldisilazane or dimethylchlorosilane.

Attempts have been made to saturate the adsorptive sites with a polar phase prior to coating the support with the final stationary phase. Precoating of the support with inert plastics like Teflon and PVP has also been reported.

For the basic nitrogen containing solutes, pre-coating the support with a stable alkali such as potassium hydroxide is possible. For acidic solutes, phosphoric acid, stearic acid or terephthallic acid are used to treat and pre-coat the support phase. Caution should be taken with such "inert" supports in that the inactivation treatment may not be reproducible, and the modifications can possibly affect the partitioning characteristics of the stationary phase and also may catalyze and cause chemical decomposition or prevent elution of certain solutes.

The recent introduction of (a) "textured" and porous glass beads (Filbert and Hair, 1968, 1969; MacDonell, 1968) which provide columns with efficiencies comparable to diatomaceous earths but without the latter's adsorptive characteristics, and (b) "brush border" support phases (Halasz, 1969; Little *et al.*, 1970) in which the stationary phases are permanently bonded to the support, should provide interesting improvements in the "art" of chromatography.

c. *Column tubing material.* Techniques for packing the dry, coated support into a column is well described in most basic texts. For many applications stainless steel tubing is satisfactory. However, for drugs which undergo metal-catalyzed degradation (e.g., steroids and pesticides), it is necessary to use glass columns. Many workers consider that an all-glass chromatographic system from injection septum to detector base is necessary for many biomedical studies, particularly those involving sub-microgram quantities of drugs.

d. *Column conditioning.* The primary purpose of conditioning the chromatographic column is to elute volatile impurities which are present and which otherwise would either appear as distant peaks, a "noisy" unstable recorder baseline, or as a high and slowly decreasing background signal. A common conditioning procedure is to operate the column, preferably disconnected from the detector, about 50°C above the probable working temperature with normal carrier gas flow rates. From 3 to 24 hours of conditioning should be sufficient for most systems.

With lightly loaded columns this procedure may be modified by allowing the column to stand for several hours at its maximum recommended temperature without the carrier gas flowing. This allows redistribution of the liquid phase and coating of the support and column tubing. Normal conditioning procedures with carrier gas flowing are then followed. Street (1968) recommends a relatively sophisticated conditioning technique including pre-treatment of the column tubing, and certainly the improved performance of his columns appears to outweigh the extensive work involved.

A procedure frequently carried out after conditioning, and at periodic intervals during the life of the column, is *in situ* silanization. By making a number of injections of a silylating reagent, the total chromatographic system is deactivated and, as a consequence, adsorption is often significantly reduced.

e. *Column temperature and flow rate.* For any particular column the speed, efficiency and resolution of analysis are controlled by the interaction of carrier gas flow rate and column temperature. To obtain the optimal chromatogram for the required purpose, these two parameters must be adjusted after consideration of the temperature limitations of the stationary phase and the characteristics of the detector.

With packed columns the carrier gas flow rate is usually set at between 20 and 60 ml/min. Unless operating close to the stationary phase temperature limit, it is more convenient to adjust the column temperature to obtain the desired separation. Too low a temperature will result in broad peaks and possibly the solute may not even be eluted. If the temperature is too high, the solute will come off the column rapidly; the peak will be sharp but resolution will be lost. A compromise must be made between resolution and speed of analysis. When a mixture contains components with greatly differing boiling points, then either temperature or flow programming may be necessary to achieve the desired separation in a reasonable time.

4. Detectors. The operating principles and characteristics of the large number of detectors used to monitor the column effluent vary considerably. A number of articles compare the various types with respect to such parameters as sensitivity, response time, linear range, response and noise level (Ettre and Zlatkis, 1967; Gill and Hartmann, 1967; McNair and Bonelli, 1967). Development in the past has been towards a universal detector responding to all compounds (e.g., thermal conductivity, argon and flame ionization detectors), but more recently the major emphasis has been towards more specific systems (e.g., electron capture detector) (also see Section III E, 4).

Historically, the most widely used detector has been that based upon thermal conductivity, primarily because of its response to all compounds, excellent linearity, simplicity of use and non-destructive characteristics. However, its relatively low sensitivity precludes its widespread use in metabolism studies where often only small quantities of drug are available.

The flame ionization detector is at the present time the most popular universal detector in use. This detector is rugged, easy to operate, requires little maintenance, has a wide dynamic range and a practical sensitivity limit for most compounds in the nanogram range. Furthermore, the detector is not sensitive to water, although this statement should be interpreted with caution (Anders and Mannering, 1967).

For compounds with a high electron affinity, e.g., alkyl halides, conjugated carbonyls, nitriles, nitrates and organometals, the electron capture detector exhibits excellent specificity and ultra-sensitivity. Whereas the use of tritium foil as the source of standing current limits the application to temperatures below 225°C, the recent commercial availability of nickel-63 foil has expanded the application to 350°C.

B. Qualitative Techniques

With GLC a problem similar to that found in TLC exists; its extraordinary ability to separate complex mixtures into their various component parts and the intrinsic sensitivity of the technique produce a significant problem in the identification of the chromatographic peaks. The various approaches to solution have recently been reviewed by Leathard and Shurlock (1968). Like all separatory methods, GLC when used alone to identify a compound requires the availability of a reference sample of that compound to which the behavior of the unknown can be compared.

1. *Retention time.* Defined as the time from the start of the analysis to the peak of the compound under consideration, retention time is a complex function of many variables. However, for a particular instrument and chromatographic system, the retention time for a given compound is a constant, independent of the presence of other compounds within the sample, and consequently, can be used to identify a compound. Practically, it is desirable to express this time

TABLE 22.3

Retention time data of some "amphetamines" and "ephedrines" [a]

Compound	Column I 2 m glass ¼″ o.d. 2.5% SE 30 120°C		Column II 1 m S.S. ⅛″ o.d. 2% PEG 20M 5% KOH 140°C		Derivatives, Column II		
					140°C Acetone RT (min)	180°C	
	RT (min)	RRT	RT (min)	RRT		N-acetyl RT (min)	N-propionyl RT (min)
Amphetamine	2.4	1.00	0.85	1.00	in solvent peak	4.0	4.1
Norephedrine	6.9	2.87	8.6	10.12	2.8	28.6	30.0
Norpseudo-ephedrine	6.9	2.87	8.4	9.88	3.0	29.5	30.8
Ephedrine	8.4	3.50	6.3	7.50	2.7	17.8	19.2
Pseudoephedrine	8.4	3.50	6.3	7.50	2.5	16.0	16.0
Methylephedrine	9.5	3.95	4.7	5.53	tertiary amine		
Ethylephedrine	13.0	5.42	6.5	7.65	tertiary amine		

[a] Reproduced with permission from Beckett et al. (1967).

relative to a standard component, i.e., relative retention time, for this approach has the advantage of being dependent only upon the column temperature and type of liquid phase.

Table 22.3 illustrates the value and limitations of retention times in identifying a series of closely related sympathomimetic amines. Such small structural differences as the addition of methyl, ethyl or hydroxy groups cause sufficient changes in partitioning behavior where all drugs may be easily identified, even on an SE-30 column. The problem of positive unequivocal identification using a single column is shown by the behavior of the epimers of ephedrine and norephedrine, respectively; it is impossible to differentiate these epimers using the SE-30 column. By using a more polar column, polyethylene glycol 20M, more solute/solvent interaction occurs as evidenced by the increased column temperature, the increase in retention times, and almost complete inversion of elution order. Under these conditions norpseudoephedrine is separated from norephedrine. Pseudoephedrine and ephedrine are still not separated under the experimental conditions but no doubt this could have been achieved either by increasing their retention times or using a different column. For unequivocal identification it is therefore mandatory that retention data from a number of columns, preferably of widely different polarities, be used.

An alternative and often superior approach to multi-column identification is to form suitable derivatives of the unknown; the probability of two different compounds with the same retention times producing the same derivative is small, and the more derivatives formed, the smaller this possibility becomes. Derivative formation is dealt with more fully in Section III, D, but Table 22.3 shows the ease with which all of the "ephedrines," including the epimers, are easily separated and identified by forming the respective acetone, N-acetyl and N-propionyl derivatives. Such approaches have proven extremely valuable in elucidating the biotransformation kinetics of these drugs in man (Rowland and Beckett, 1966; Beckett and Wilkinson, 1965; Wilkinson and Beckett, 1968).

Some caution should be taken in assuming that a compound's retention time is constant and reproducible. This is usually true for symmetrical peaks. If the peak is asymmetric, however, the retention time is dependent upon the amount of compound injected. As the amount is decreased, the peak becomes flatter and retention time increases. Consequently, unknown and reference samples should be injected in about equal amounts.

2. *Ancillary techniques.* One of the most useful and valuable contributions of GLC to drug and metabolite identification has been indirect rather than direct. The outstanding separatory powers of the GLC has been utilized to obtain a pure sample of the unknown which can subsequently be examined by more powerful and revealing structure elucidating techniques such as infra-red, nuclear magnetic resonance and mass spectrometry (Ettre and Zlatkis, 1967). The sample size required by these procedures is relatively small (0.5–200 μg), and an analytical chromatograph can be used to separate and collect the required component. A variety of simple to sophisticated methods have been devised to trap and collect the unknown peak as it elutes from the column (Anders and Mannering, 1967; Burchfield and Storrs, 1962). Most problems arise from the small sample size, the necessity to collect the sample in a small compact area, difficulties in premature condensation or complete failure to condense the sample.

An alternative to the above approach has been to introduce the column effluent directly into the ancillary instrument which automatically scans the field as frequently as every 1 to 10 seconds, i.e., "time of flight" methods. Gas-liquid chromatography-mass spectrometry (GLC-MS) is a particularly powerful and successful combination, the application of which should expand prodigiously over the next years. Figure 22.2 illustrates the potential of GLC-MS in that it is possible to identify and distinguish between the mass spectra of methylamphetamine and amphetamine extracted from urine containing levels of drugs that exist after administration of therapeutic doses of these drugs (Beckett *et al.*, 1967). Larger sample sizes are required for combined GLC-infra-red but the technique has been successfully utilized.

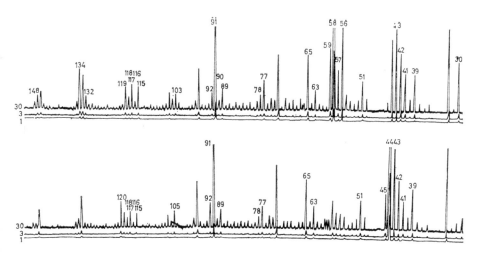

Fig. 22.2. Time of flight mass spectra of amphetamine (*bottom*) and methylamphetamine (*top*) obtained by GLC-MS of extracts of 5 ml urine containing 4 μg drug base/ml (reproduced with permission from Beckett *et al.*, 1967).

C. Quantitative Techniques

The prime use of GLC in biotransformation studies is quantitative analysis of the various drugs and metabolites separated. Not only is the technique one of the most sensitive available (10^{-9} to 10^{-12} g range), it is also extremely precise and accurate—providing the proper techniques are used. Good chromatographic performance is the key to accurate quantification.

Assuming that both the detector and recorder yield linear signals, quantitative analysis can be achieved by peak height or peak area measurement methods. Both methods have their advantages and disadvantages. Although peak height measurement is rapid and easy, it is readily influenced by any factor affecting retention time, such as changes in column temperature and flow rate. Furthermore, plots of peak height versus sample size have a more limited linear range than the corresponding plots for peak area. Fundamentally, peak area is directly related to the amount of sample component producing the response and it is much less affected by slight changes in chromatographic parameters. Several methods are available for its measurement (in order of their increasing precision): planimetry, triangulation, multiplication of the peak height by the corresponding width at half peak height, cutting out the peaks and weighing, mechanical disc integration, and finally electronic digital integration. Excellent reviews of comparisons have been published (Johnson, 1968; Gill and Hapgood, 1967).

Conversion of peak height or area to the amount injected into the chromatograph, or more importantly to the amount present in the extracted biological sample, requires calibration of the system and the extraction procedures.

Calibration curves can be prepared directly by injecting exactly known amounts of drug into the chromatograph. However, the precision of this method is poor, the method is tedious, and one must assume that detector sensitivity is constant from day to day. A more recommendable approach is the internal standard method, consisting of adding a constant amount of internal standard to known but varying amounts of drug. Peak height or area ratios of drug to internal standard are used to construct a calibration curve. Using this technique, the quantities injected need not be accurately measured nor need the detector response be known or remain constant, for any changes will not affect the height/area ratio. The choice of internal standard is important; the chosen compound should be well resolved from all other peaks but it should elute close to the peak(s) of interest and give a response not too different from the component being measured. Some investigators prefer to use compounds structurally similar to the drug. A further characteristic frequently sought is a similarity of physico-chemical properties between the drug and internal standard. In this case the internal standard is used not only for quantifying the chromatographic part of the procedure but also, by adding marker to the biological sample prior to extraction, errors introduced by losses of material during extraction and clean-up can be obviated.

D. Derivatives for GLC

A field of GLC, the importance of which will undoubtedly increase in the future, is the formation of suitable derivatives of drugs and metabolites. The purposes for which this procedure may prove useful include increased stability during chromatography, increased volatility for analysis, reduced adsorption, more positive identification, improved separation and specificity over inter-ference or background, and increased sensitivity of detector response.

Often a labile compound exposed to chromatography will undergo thermal and/or catalytic decomposition, e.g., steroids. Such behavior manifests itself as distorted peaks, extraneous peaks and non-linear response. Reduction of the column temperature and an all-glass system may obviate some of the problem but often not too successfully. By forming a suitable derivative, the stability of the compound will possibly be increased and frequently the derivatization increases volatility allowing analysis at a lower temperature. This latter approach may also be applied to compounds which, because of molecular weight and vapor pressure considerations, cannot be chromatographed *per se* under reasonable conditions.

Despite the recent advances in technology of column support and coating techniques, it is not always possible to eradicate completely solute/system adsorption interactions. By forming a suitable derivative in which the "polar" interacting groups are masked by "non-polar" moieties, this problem may be overcome. For example, with morphine and related narcotics, difficulties arise in quantification, particularly in the sub-microgram area. The reason is that the chromatographic peak tails badly and the response is dependent upon the prior history of the column in addition to the amount of drug injected (Fig. 22.3). These typical manifestations of adsorption may be overcome by forming the trimethylsilyl ether derivative: a good symmetrical peak is obtained and the response is not only linear but at any level it is greater for the derivative than the free base (Fig. 22.3). This solution to adsorption has permitted the determination of nanogram amounts of morphine in biologic fluids (Wilkinson and Way, 1969).

The rationale behind derivative formation in drug and metabolite identification was referred to and exemplified in Section III, B, 1. Such an approach may also be usefully employed where difficulties exist with biological "blank" interference and background. Forming a derivative which requires different chromatographic conditions may remove the interference.

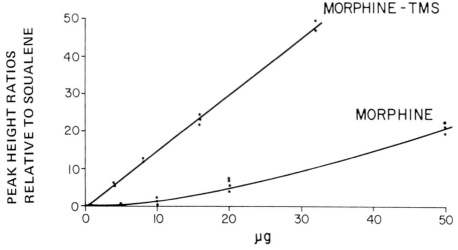

Fig. 22.3. Absolute FID response curves for morphine and its trimethylsilyl (TMS) derivative. (Wilkinson, unpublished data.)

TABLE 22.4

Comparison of detector responses to various derivatives of β-phenylethylamine

Derivative	FID Response coulombs/mole	H³-EC Response coulombs/mole	EC/FID
Trifluoroacetate	1.06	3	3
Pentafluoropropionate	1.15	401	350
Heptafluorobutyrate	1.14	1,778	1,565
Pentadecanefluorooctanoate	1.14	5,474	4,822
Pentafluorobenzoyl	0.96	79,685	83,021

The potential in quantitative analysis of forming derivatives in order to enhance the detector response and therefore lower the limit of sensitivity is only slowly being recognized in the biomedical area. In the past, emphasis has been directed towards the formation of derivatives with high electron capturing properties allowing picogram amounts of drug to be detected by the electron capture detector (Clarke et al., 1968). Often the increase in sensitivity may be several thousand fold compared to the parent compound, illustrated in Table 22.4 by the formation of various fluorinated derivatives of the model compound, β-phenylethylamine. The extreme sensitivity of the pentafluorobenzoyl derivative readily permits plasma levels of structurally related drugs and metabolites after their therapeutic administration (Wilkinson, G. R., 1970). Similar approaches will undoubtedly be used with the other sensitive specific detectors, e.g., the formation of nitrogen containing derivatives for use with the sodium thermionic detector (Section III, E, 4).

The types of derivatives that may be prepared depends upon the reactive functional groups incorporated into the parent molecule. A fairly comprehensive listing of common derivatives is tabulated in Table 22.5, where derivatization includes degradative as well as synthetic reactions; e.g., the determination of acetylcholine by degradation to dimethylaminoethyl acetate (Jenden et al., 1968).

Derivatives are most frequently formed separately and prior to chromatography by semi-micro, organic synthetic techniques, in which cases a number of factors need to be considered. The conversion process should be quantitative, preferably in high yield; it should be rapid and simple to perform but also reproducible and not subject to gross changes due to manipulations. Finally the derivative should be sufficiently stable to any manipulations performed before and after the chromatographic injection.

In qualitative analysis it is often possible to form the derivative in the injection port or on the chromatographic column by following the injection of the parent compound with an injection of the derivatizing agent. Anders et al. (1966) found this "peak-shift" technique useful in the rapid and unequivocal identification of the primary metabolite of the potent inhibitor of drug metabolism, SKF 525-A. The technique has also been applied to the study of alkaloids, steroids, amines and barbiturates (Anders and Mannering, 1967).

Much valuable information upon the synthesis and GLC of derivatives is contained in the reviews by Anders and Mannering (1967), Gudzinowicz (1967), Hammarstrand and Bonelli (1968), and Pierce (1968).

TABLE 22.5
Derivatives of organic compounds suitable for GLC[a]

Functional Group	Derivative
—OH, or poly—OH	Acetate, ether, trimethylsilyl ether, trifluoroacetate, etc.
—CHO,—CO—	Oxime, hydrogenate to —OH, oxidize to —COOH
—COOH	Methyl ester to *n*-butyl ester, trifluoroethanol ester, etc.
—NH₂, —NH—, —N— (with vertical bond above N)	Acetyl, TMS-derivative, benzoyl, trifluoroacetyl, etc.
—N=N—	Reduction to diamine
—NO₂, —NO, —NO₃, etc.	Reduction to amine, with LiAlH₄ and direct or derivative GLC
—SH	Acetate, ether, trimethylsilyl ether, trifluoroacetate, etc.
—S— or —S—S—	Either direct GLC or split to —SH and form derivative (above)
—SO—, SO₂, —SO₃, SO₄	Reduction to —SH as above
—O—	Direct or split with HI and analyze halides
—Cl, —F, —Br, —I	Direct or hydrolyze off halide and examine as alcohols or glycols
—ClO₃, —ClO₄, —IO₃, —IO₄, —BrO₃	Reduction to halide
—COOR	Hydrolyze and analyze alcohol and/or acid as above
R—CH₃	Direct or oxidize to alcohol, aldehyde, ketone, or acid
R=CH₂	Reduce to saturated hydrocarbon or oxidize at double bond to acid or add halogens
R≡CH	Reduce to saturated hydrocarbon, or oxidize, or add halogens
—CN	Hydrolyze to acid or reduce to amine

[a] Reproduced with permission from Crippen and Smith (1965).

E. Recent Innovations and Future Trends

1. Pyrolysis-GLC. In the fields of polymer-chemistry, pathology and bacteriology the technique of combined pyrolysis-GLC has proven extremely useful in the identification of compounds. In this procedure the sample is exposed to a sufficiently high temperature to cause thermal degradation, and the pyrolysis products so formed are swept into the chromatographic column for separation. The chromatogram or pyrolysis pattern under standard conditions is a characteristic "fingerprint" of the compound pyrolyzed. The potential of the technique is exemplified by Figure 22.4 where the qualitative and quantitative differences in the pyrolysis patterns allows unequivocal characterization of sodium secobarbital and sodium phenobarbital.

Unfortunately little research has been undertaken in the biomedical field, particularly with respect to drugs recovered from biological systems, and the degree of purity required (Kirk, 1968; Perry, 1968). As an identification tool the pyrolysis-GLC shows great promise but, until much more investigation is carried out, the actual potentialities and limitations will remain obscure.

2. Resolution of optically active isomers. Many drugs are optically active and are administered either as the racemic mixture or the most pharmacologically

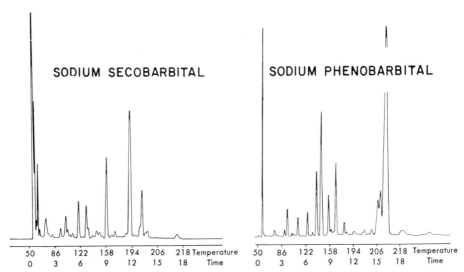

Fig. 22.4. Pyrolysis "fingerprint" patterns of sodium seconal and sodium phenobarbital (reproduced with permission from Barber Colman Company).

active isomer. The question often arises as to whether drug distribution, metabolism, excretion or receptor interactions are stereospecific. The inability to resolve small amounts of drug necessitated the separate administration of the two isomers. It is now possible, however, to resolve certain enantiomers directly by GLC.

By forming a derivative with an optically active agent, separation of the diastereoisomers is possible on ordinary chromatographic columns (Gil-Av *et al.*, 1965; Halpern and Westley, 1965, 1966). Most of the reported investigations have been concerned with amino-acids; but Gunne and Gallad (1967) and Gunne (1967), using the method of Gordis (1966), have recently reported studies with amphetamine. Using N-trifluoroacetyl-1-prolyl chloride as the resolving agent, complete resolution of racemic amphetamine was obtained, and the peak areas were in the ratio 1:1 (Fig. 22.5). Collection and analysis of urine showed that more (−)-amphetamine was excreted in man than (+)-amphetamine and this trend increased with time after administration. From these findings it was concluded that the metabolism of amphetamine in man is stereospecific, the (+)-isomer being more rapidly and extensively metabolized than the (−)-isomer. Similar findings were obtained for racemic methylamphetamine (Gunne, 1967).

A more recent approach to the resolution of enantiomers is that of direct resolution of the racemate by using an optically active stationary phase either in a capillary column (Gil-Av *et al.*, 1966; Feibush and Gil-Av, 1967) or in a packed column (Gil-Av and Feibush, 1967).

Whether either of these techniques can be applied to other classes of drugs than the amines remains to be seen but certainly the potential is exciting.

3. Analysis of glucuronides. Many drugs are metabolized to and excreted as their glucuronic acid conjugates (*cf.* Chapter 10). Classical methods of analysis are based upon determination of the aglycone level before and after hydrolysis with either acid or enzyme preparations. A number of recent reports have indicated the feasibility of determining glucuronides directly by GLC (Tamura and Imanari, 1964; Knaak *et al.*, 1967; Horning *et al.*, 1967; Horning, 1968). In order

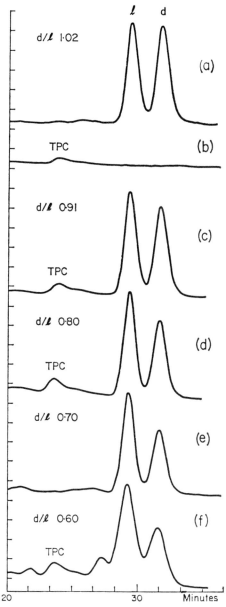

Fig. 22.5. Chromatograms showing the separation of the diastereoisomers formed by reaction of trifluoroacetyl-1-prolyl chloride and d- and l-amphetamine: (a) 5 μg racemic amphetamine; (b) urine extract before administration of amphetamine; (c) urine extract 0–12 hr after administration of 10 mg dl-amphetamine; (d) urine extract 12–24 hr after; (e) urine extract 24–36 hr after; (f) urine extract 36–48 hr after. The portions of the chromatograms recorded during the first 20 min have been omitted. (Reproduced with permission from Gunne, 1967).

to obtain sufficiently volatile compounds, it is necessary to form a derivative, e.g., methylation of the acid function and then silylating or acetylating the alcoholic groups of the carbohydrate residue. Studies have been limited mostly to compounds of fairly small molecular weight; however, Horning *et al.* (1967) and Horning (1968) reported the separation of glucuronides of various steroids.

4. Detectors. Increasing emphasis is being placed upon the development of detectors highly specific for a chemical atom or chemical group within a molecule. The electron capture detector is a prime example. Another example is the micro-coulometric detector, which, depending upon the electrodes and electrolyte solution, may be highly selective to halogen, sulfur or phosphorus. This detector has been successfully used to study chlorpromazine and its metabolites in urine (Burchfield *et al.*, 1965; Johnson *et al.*, 1965).

The alkali flame detector, which is a conventional flame ionization detector modified by fusing the sulfate salt of either sodium, rubidium, cesium onto the electrode, is specific to organophosphorus, organohalides and organonitro compounds, depending upon the configuration of the electrodes. Not only is this detector very specific but it is often from ten to a thousand-fold more sensitive than the flame ionization detector for these compounds (Aue *et al.*, 1967; Hartman, 1969).

Nitrogen may also be specifically determined by the electrolytic conductivity detector; however, its relative insensitivity will probably preclude its widespread use in drug metabolism studies (Coulson, 1966).

A recent and exciting approach to detection has been described by Hammar *et al.* (1968). Termed "mass fragmentography," the technique uses a linked GLC-MS with an accelerating voltage alternator (AVA). This unit allows the mass spectrometer to be set to continuously monitor any three mass numbers of the compounds emerging from the chromatograph. Only those compounds which fragment to give the chosen ions will be detected. Besides the extremely and variable high specificity of the instrument, it is also capable of being more sensitive than most ordinary detectors used in GLC. Using this technique, it was possible for the first time to unequivocally identify chlorpromazine and a number of its metabolites which were present in extremely small concentrations in the plasma of patients undergoing chronic therapy. As a tool for characterization, mass fragmentography has much to offer, but whether it may be usefully used as a quantitative detector remains to be investigated.

The increased specificity of the above detectors is advantageous in that elimination of interference from the solvent peak, column bleed and normal body constituents present in extracts of biological materials are much reduced. The sensitivity limits and specificity of the detectors may be increased in the future by the formation of suitable derivatives.

5. Automation. The present trend in all routine, repetitive, tedious, time consuming operations is towards automation, and considerable progress has already been achieved in this area with respect to GLC. A number of commercially available analytical chromatographs are designed for automatic injection whereby as many as 72 samples may be pre-loaded and automatically injected according to a programmed cycle. Peak attenuation and area integration may also be automatically performed, and in the more sophisticated instruments the electronic integrator is linked to a small digital computer into the memory of which can be placed the necessary information for obtaining all the desired qualitative and quantitative data. "The system automatically collects, attenuates and monitors all input signals, measures peak areas and retention times, allocates overlapping peak areas, identifies peaks, applies response factors, calculates component concentrations and types a complete analytical report in a form ready for distribution" (Electronic Associates, Inc., 1967).

In toto these computerized GLC systems are probably too expensive and complex for investigational work and small organizations. However, each of the component parts deserves consideration for the increased work load, precision and accuracy that it affords.

IV. COLUMN CHROMATOGRAPHY

Column chromatography (CC) is the oldest chromatographic technique. Its development as an analytical tool, however, has been retarded compared to TLC and GLC. This is particularly true with respect to its application in drug metabolism studies where, because of high capacity, its primary use has been as a gross separatory technique for "clean-up" and/or isolation of drugs and metabolites. The major reasons for the lack of interest in the past have been that the technique utilizing conventional apparatus is lengthy and tends to be accompanied by low resolution. Also, the design of a suitable liquid detector system has lagged behind the related area involving gases. Both mechanistically and practically, CC closely resembles TLC and this too has led to its demise in qualitative and quantitative analysis.

Perhaps the most popular use of CC is with an ion-exchange sorbent which permits separation of ionic species, e.g., proteins, enzymes, peptides, amino acids and nucleic acids.

A. Column Preparation

The conventional column is generally a glass tube, although metal and plastic tubes are in use. It is tapered at the bottom, equipped with a stopcock, and the bottom of the tube is frequently plugged with cotton or glass-wool padding just above the taper, or more preferably a glass frit or teflon filter disc is used to prevent loss of sorbent. The top of the column is often constructed with a reservoir for the mobile phase, or alternatively a constant speed pump may be used.

The sorbents used are the same as those utilized in TLC for adsorption, partition, ion-exchange chromatography, etc. Generally they are poured gently as a slurry into the tube and, after allowing setting by gravity or pressure from the top of the tube, the sorbent is rinsed with the mobile phase before use. Alternatively, the sorbent may be poured as a dry powder into the tube and packed down by tamping. Prior to use, the column is rinsed to remove any entrapped air within the packing which otherwise might deleteriously affect column performance. Wet packing, in general, is more popular than dry packing because it is more convenient and gives more homogeneous columns. The particle size and distribution of the sorbents is important for maintaining constant flow and elution patterns. Small sized particles allow a larger surface area of contact for the 2 phases, thus permitting a closer approach to equilibrium. On the other hand, small particles tend to pack tighter and hinder flow.

B. Solvents Systems and Development

The guide lines outlined in Section III, A, 3 for solvent selection in TLC also apply to CC. When transferring procedures from TLC to CC, one rule is generally valid: solvents used for a column separation should be less polar than solvent systems which produced the best results with TLC. Modification to reduce the R_f value to 0.2 or less is frequently successful.

The sample, dissolved in a liquid less polar than the one used for development, is evenly applied to the top of the column in as concentrated solution as possible (to reduce band spreading), and care must be taken not to disturb the top surface of the packing, which must always be covered with liquid. Three choices of development are then possible: frontal, displacement, elution (Heftmann, 1961). Elution analysis is the most popular method and this consists simply of allowing solvent to continuously flow through the column "washing out" the separated component bands. A number of different eluants may be successively applied or alternatively gradient elution may be used.

C. Detection and Determination

The procedure of detecting compounds directly on the column has to a large extent been replaced by methods directed towards analyzing the effluent as it leaves the column, or after collection of fractions isolated dependent upon volume or time. Spectrophotometry, refractive index, flame ionization, polarography and many other methods have been used to monitor the column effluent. In general, until recently the apparatus for continuous analysis of the eluate were complicated and of questionable accuracy and reproducibility. This led to the employment of eluate fraction collection and subsequent analysis by standard techniques. Although tedious and time-consuming, this is probably still the most common detection method. By the use of retention volumes, qualitative analysis may be achieved; but the often low resolution of the column does not encourage unequivocality of the identification, and frequently TLC or GLC may be used as supplementary proof of fraction purity.

D. Recent Innovations

In recent years there has been a revived interest in CC, also termed liquid chromatography, as an analytical technique. This in part has been due to the realization that long columns of narrow bore can achieve performance efficiencies approaching GLC. In order to achieve rapid analysis, the liquid chromatograph requires operation at high pressures (<3000 psi) (Huber and Hulsman, 1967). Highly efficient column packing materials have been developed which provide columns with about 1000 plates/meter (Horvath and Lipsky, 1969; Kirkland, 1969). Coupled with this development has been the evolution of reliable, sensitive on-line detectors.

High pressure liquid chromatographs (HPLC) are now becoming commercially available with these characteristics. In usage they are analogous to a gas chromatograph. However, HPLC offers advantages over GLC including (a) the ability to analyze materials of very low vapor pressure without preparation of derivatives, (b) analyses of thermally unstable materials, (c) the ability to select another operating parameter since the solvent liquid used as carrier may have a distinct influence on separation.

Application of this new technique is as yet limited. Horvath *et al.* (1967), however, have produced some very elegant separations of nucleotides using capillary columns packed with ion-exchange resin coated glass beads; and Kirkland (1969), using a synthetic mixture of some substituted urea herbicides, was able to separate these by partition chromatography within 6 minutes at room temperature and at nanogram levels (Fig. 22.6). The potentialities of HPLC appear to be extremely attractive for the separation, identification and determination of drugs and their metabolites but only time and much effort will determine whether it may be applied with the sensitivity, simplicity and facility that are desirable.

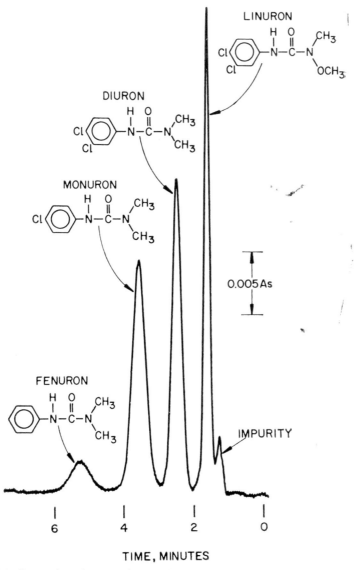

Fig. 22.6. Separation of some substituted urea herbicides by high pressure chromatography; sample 1 μl of 67 μg/ml each in dibutyl ether (reproduced with permission from Kirkland, 1969).

V. LITERATURE SOURCES

This section is designed to provide the reader with access to more authoritative material on the various described techniques and to indicate source material upon past, current and future innovations.

A number of texts have been published concerned with the general area of chromatography (Cassidy, 1957; Heftmann, 1961; Lederer and Lederer, 1957; Stock and Rice, 1967; and Wilson *et al.*, 1968). The biennial Fundamental Review section of *Analytical Chemistry* devotes a number of articles to the general and more specific areas of chromatography, listing the significant experimental papers, pertinent reviews and textbooks published during the review period. Other review material may be found in the various editions of *Advances in Analytical Chemistry and Instrumentation, Chromatographic Reviews* and *Advances in Chromatography*. Current research papers primarily of fundamental rather than biomedical interest are generally to be found in *Journal of Chromatography, Journal of Chromatographic Science* (formerly *Journal of Gas Chromatography*), *Chromatographia, Analytical Chemistry, Separation Science*, and other journals devoted to analytical methodology. Details of the application of the techniques to drugs and metabolism of drugs are frequently to be found buried as incidentals to the major purpose of the publication devoted to pharmacology, toxicology, forensic science and clinical science. Each issue of *Journal of Chromatography* contains a short review abstract of published papers applied to various classes of compound by different chromatographic procedures, and this can be a useful source-entry for literature searching.

In the short time that TLC has been in use, a large number of articles have been published. Textbooks by Bobbitt (1963), Stahl (1969), and Kirchner (1967) provide excellent introduction to the fundamental principles and also present details of a large number of applications. Shorter reviews have been written by Maier and Mangold (1964), Malins and Mangold (1966) and Mangold *et al.* (1964). Recent reviews by Stolman (1965) and Kirk (1968) have covered the application of TLC to drugs and other compounds of toxicological interest. Many of the manufacturers of TLC chemicals and apparatus maintain reasonably current bibliographies on the various application areas.

As an introduction to GLC, McNair and Bonelli (1967) provide excellent coverage with particular emphasis on practical considerations. More extensive treatment of the subject is to be found in textbooks by Dal Nogare and Juvet (1962), Ettre and Zlatkis (1967), Pecsok (1961), Purnell (1962), and Schupp (1968). An early publication upon the biomedical application of GLC is that of Burchfield and Storrs (1964), and other similar applications have been treated by Goldbaum *et al.* (1963), Lipsett (1965), Szymanski (1964, 1968) Wotiz and Clark (1966), and Kroman and Bender (1968). Anders and Mannerings' review (1967) provides excellent coverage of recent advances in technology and GLC analytical procedures for important toxicological compounds. But by far the most comprehensive and up-to-date text devoted to drugs is the extremely valuable book by Gudzinowicz (1967), which should become a standard reference book for all workers involved in this area.

The fundamentals of conventional column chromatography are well covered by Huber (1968) and the general chromatography texts cited previously. Many of the innovative papers covering HPLC have appeared in the *Journal of Chromatographic Science.*

VI. SUMMARY

A chromatographic system should separate all of the desired components and provide easy access to the analytical information thus obtained. Ideally, the system should allow repetitive separations, real-time detection, high resolution and speed of separation, high precision of both retention and quantitative data, high sensitivity, on line combination with other methods, and finally it should be suitable for automation. From the economic standpoint, cost, ease of operation and flexibility are important.

Of the described techniques, GLC fits these criteria more closely than TLC or CC. The fact that the sample must be volatile is the major disadvantage of the procedure. Other negative features include cost, the necessity of reference samples, fairly extensive supervision, particularly in developmental investigations, and capability of only being able to analyze one sample at any one time.

TLC is more limited than GLC with respect to the reproducibility, but its overall flexibility permits separation by a number of mechanisms and different systems. Furthermore, a number of samples may be separated simultaneously. Also, the technique is simple, cheap and no components are overlooked since the sample is detected on the chromatographic system.

The range of applicability of CC in the form of HPLC, i.e., compounds of molecular weight between 100 and 10,000, includes the majority of drugs. Thermal stability does not need to be considered, and, like TLC, a variety of separating mechanisms and systems are possible. Instrumental design includes many of the characteristics of GLC. The high instrumental cost and limited sensitivity of the available detectors towards certain types of compounds appear to be the only disadvantages of the technique. It is to be expected that HPLC will play an increasingly important and exciting role in the future of separation, identification and determination of drugs and their metabolites.

REFERENCES

Afifi, A. H. M. and Way, E. L.: Studies on the biologic disposition of methotrimeprazine. J. Pharmacol. Exp. Ther. *160:* 397–406, 1968.

Anders, M. A., Alvares, A. P., and Mannering, G. J.: Inhibition of drug metabolism. II. Metabolism of 2-diethylaminoethyl 2,2-diphenylvalerate HCl (SKF 525-A). Mol. Pharmacol. *2:* 328–334, 1966.

Anders, M. A. and Mannering, G. J., Application of gas chromatography to toxicology. In *Progress in Chemical Toxicology*, Vol. 3, ed. by Stolman, A. Academic Press, New York, 1967.

Aue, W. A., Gehrke, C. W., Tindle, R. C., Stalling, D. L., and Ruyle, C. D.: Application of the alkali flame detector to nitrogen containing compounds. J. Gas Chrom. *5:* 381–382, 1967.

Beckett, A. H., Tucker, G. T., and Moffatt, A. C.: Routine detection and identification in urine of stimulants and other drugs which may be used to modify performance in sport. J. Pharm. Pharmacol. *19:* 273–294, 1967.

Beckett, A. H. and Wilkinson, G. R.: Urinary excretion of (−)-norephedrine, (−)-ephedrine and (−)-methylephedrine in man. J. Pharm. Pharmacol. *17:* 107S–108S, 1965.

Bobbitt, J. M.: *Thin-layer Chromatography.* Reinhold, New York, 1963.

Boulton, A. A., Pollitt, R. J., and Maer, J. R.: Identity of a urinary "pink spot" in schizophrenia and Parkinson's disease. Nature *215:* 132–134, 1967.

Burchfield, H. P., Johnson, H. P., Rhoades, J. W., and Wheeler, R. J.: Selective detection of phosphorus, sulfur, and halogen compounds in the gas chromatography of drugs and pesticides. J. Gas Chrom. *3:* 28–36, 1965.

Burchfield, H. P. and Storrs, E. E.: *Biochemical Applications of Gas Chromatography*. Academic Press, New York, 1962.

Cassidy, H. G.: *Fundamentals of Chromatography*, Vol. X of *Technique of Organic Chemistry*, ed. by Weissberger, A. Interscience, New York, 1957.

Clarke, D. D., Wilk, S., and Gitlow, S. E.: Gas chromatographic determination of dopamine and related compounds. In *Biomedical Applications of Gas Chromatography*, Vol. 2, ed. by Szymanski, H. A. Plenum Press, New York, 1968.

Coulson, D. M.: Electrolytic conductivity detector in gas chromatography. In *Advances in Chromatography*, Vol. 3, ed. by Giddings, J. C. and Keller, R. A. Dekker, New York, 1966.

Crippen, R. C. and Smith, C. E.: Procedures for the systematic identification of peaks in gas-liquid chromatographic analysis. J. Gas Chrom. *3:* 37–42, 1965.

Dal Nogare, S. and Juvet, R. S.: *Gas Chromatography—Theory and Practice*. Interscience, New York, 1962.

Ettre, L. S. and Zlatkis, A.: *The Practice of Gas Chromatography*. Interscience, New York, 1967.

Feibush, B. and Gil-Av, E.: Gas chromatography with optically active stationary phases. Resolution of primary amines. J. Gas Chrom. *5:* 257–260, 1967.

Filbert, A. M. and Hair, M. L.: Glass beads as a chromatographic support material. II. Etched glass beads. J. Gas Chrom. *6:* 218–223, 1968.

Filbert, A. M. and Hair, M. L.: Pore-size effects on column performance in gas-liquid chromatography. J. Chrom. Sci. *7:* 72–78, 1969.

Forrest, I. S., Bolt, A. G., and Serra, M. T.: Distribution of chlorpromazine metabolites in selected organs of psychiatric patients chronically dosed up to the time of death. Biochem. Pharmacol. *17:* 2061–2070, 1968.

Gil-Av, E., Feibush, B., and Sigler, R. C.: Resolution of amino acids by gas chromatography. J. Chrom. *17:* 408–410, 1965.

Gil-Av, E., Feibush, B., and Sigler, R. C., Separation of enantiomers by gas-liquid chromatography with an optically active stationary phase. Tetrahedron Letters, (10), 1009–1015, 1966.

Gil-Av, E. and Feibush, B., Resolution of enantiomers by gas-liquid chromatography with optically active stationary phases. Separation on packed columns. Tetrahedron Letters, (35), 3345–3347, 1967.

Gill, J. M. and Habgood, H. W., Symposium on quantitative gas chromatography—fundamentals to automation (various authors). J. Gas Chrom. *5:* 595–646, 1967.

Gill, J. M. and Hartmann, C. H., Characteristics of ionization detectors and gas chromatography electrometers. In symposium on quantitative gas chromatography—fundamentals to automation. J. Gas Chrom. *5:* 595–646, 1967.

Goldbaum, L. R., Schoegel, E. L., and Dominguez, A. M.: Application of gas chromatography to toxicology, In *Progress in Chemical Toxicology*, Vol. 1, ed. by Stolman, A. Academic Press, New York, 1963.

Gordis, E.: Gas chromatographic resolution of optical isomers in microgram samples of amphetamine. Biochem. Pharmacol. *15:* 2124–2126, 1966.

Green, D. E. and Forrest, I. S.: *In vivo* metabolism of chlorpromazine. Can. Psychiat. Ass. J. *11:* 299–302, 1966.

Gudzinowicz, B. J.: *Gas Chromatographic Analysis of Drugs and Pesticides*. Dekker, New York, 1967.

Gunne, L. M.: The urinary output of d- and l-amphetamine in man. Biochem. Pharmacol. *16:* 863–869, 1967.

Gunne, L. M. and Galland, L.: Stereoselective metabolism of amphetamine. Biochem. Pharmacol. *16:* 1374–1377, 1967.

Haer, F. C.: *Introduction to Chromatography on Impregnated Glass Fiber*. Ann Arbor Science, Ann Arbor, 1968.

Halasz, I. and Sebastion, I.: New stationary phase for chromatography. Angew. Chem. Internat. Edit. *8:* 453–454, 1969.

Halpern, B. and Westley, J. W.: Optical resolution of D, L amino acids by gas chromatography and mass spectrometry. Biochem. Biophys. Res. Comm. *20:* 710–714, 1965.

Halpern, B. and Westley, J. W.: High-sensitivity optical resolution of amines by gas chromatography. Chem. Comm. 34–35, 1966.

Hammar, C. G., Holmstedt, B., and Ryhage, R.: Mass fragmentography-identification of chlorpromazine and its metabolites in human blood by a new method. Anal. Biochem. *25:* 532–548, 1968.

Hammarstrand, K. and Bonelli, E. J.: *Derivative Formation in Gas Chromatography*. Varian Aerograph, Walnut Creek, 1968.

Hartmann, C. H.: Alkali flame detector for organic nitrogen compounds. J. Chrom. Sci. *7:* 163–171, 1969.

Heftmann, E., *Chromatography*. Reinhold, New York, 1961.

Horning, E. C., Horning, M. C., Ikekawa, N., Chambaz, E. M., Jaakonmaki, P. I., and Brooks, C. J. W.: Studies on analytical separations of human steroids and steroid glucuronides, J. Gas Chrom. *5:* 283–289, 1967.

Horning, E. C., Moscatelli, E. A., and

Sweeley, C. C.: Polyester liquid phases in gas-liquid chromatography. Chem. and Ind. 751–752, 1959.

Horning, M. G.: Gas phase analytical methods for the study of urinary acids. In *Biochemical Applications of Gas Chromatography*, Vol. 2, ed. by Szymanski, H. A. Plenum Press, New York, 1968.

Horvath, C. G. and Lipsky, S. R.: Column design in high pressure liquid chromatography. J. Chrom. Sci. *7:* 109–116, 1969.

Horvath, C. G., Preiss, B. A., and Lipsky, S. R.: Fast liquid chromatography: an investigation of operating parameters and the separation of nucleotides on pellicular ion exchangers. Anal. Chem. *39:* 1422–1428, 1967.

Huber, J. F. K.: Liquid chromatography in columns. In *Comprehensive Analytical Chemistry*, Vol. 2B, *Physical Separation Methods*, ed. by Wilson, C. L., Wilson, P. W. and Strouts, C. R. N. Elsevier, New York, 1968.

Huber, J. F. K. and Hulsman, J. A. R.: A study of liquid chromatography in columns. The time of separation. Anal. Chim. Acta *38:* 305–313, 1967.

Jenden, D. J., Hanin, I., and Lamb, S. I.: Gas chromatographic microestimation of acetylcholine and related compounds. Anal. Chem. *40:* 125–128, 1968.

Johnson, H. W.: The quantitative interpretation of gas chromatographic data. In *Advances in Chromatography*, Vol. 5, ed. by Giddings, J. C. and Keller, R. A. Dekker, New York, 1968.

Johnson, D. E., Rodriguez, C. F., and Burchfield, H. P.: Determination by microcoulometric gas chromatography of chlorpromazine metabolites in human urine. Biochem. Pharmacol. *14:* 1453–1469, 1965.

Keller, R. A. and Giddings, J. C.: Multiple zones and spots in chromatography. In *Chromatographic Reviews*, Vol. 3, ed. by Lederer, M. Elsevier, New York, 1961.

Kirchner, J. G.: Thin-layer Chromatography. Vol. XII of *Techniques of Organic Chemistry*, ed. by Weissberger, A. Interscience, New York, 1967.

Kirk, P. L.: Chromatographic advances in chromatography. In *Advances in Chromatography*, Vol. 5, ed. by Giddings, J. C. and Keller, R. A. Dekker, New York, 1968.

Kirkland, J. J.: High speed liquid chromatography with controlled surface porosity supports. J. Chrom. Sci. *7:* 7–12, 1969.

Knaak, J. B., Eldridge, J. M., and Sullivan, L. J.: Systematic approach to preparation and identification of glucuronic acid conjugates. J. Agri. Food Chem. *15:* 605–609, 1967.

Kroman, H. S. and Bender, S. K.: *Theory and Applications of Gas Chromatography in Industry and Medicine*. Grune and Stratton, New York, 1968.

Leathard, D. A. and Shurlock, B. C.: Gas chromatographic identification. In *Advances in Analytical Chemistry and Instrumentation*, Vol. 6, *Progress in Gas Chromatography*, ed. by Purnell, J. H. Interscience, New York, 1968.

Lederer, E. and Lederer, M.: *Chromatography—A Review of Principles and Applications*. Elsevier, New York, 1957.

Lipsett, M. B.: *Gas Chromatography of Steroids in Biological Fluids*. Plenum Press, New York, 1965.

Little, J. N., Dark, W. A., Farlinger, P. W., and Bornbaugh, K. J.: GC packings with chemically-bonded stationary phases. J. Chrom. Sci. *8:* 647–652, 1970.

MacDonell, H. L.: Very lightly loaded textured glass beads for gas-liquid partition chromatography. Anal. Chem. *40:* 221–224, 1968.

Maier, R. and Mangold, H. K.: Thin-layer chromatography. In *Advances in Analytical Chemistry and Instrumentation*, Vol. 3, ed. by Reilley, C. N. Interscience, New York, 1964.

Malins, D. C. and Mangold, H. K.: Thin-layer chromatography. In *Standard Methods of Chemical Analysis*, Vol. 3, Pt. A, ed. by Welcher, F. J. Van Nostrand, Princeton, 1966.

Mangold, H. K., Schmid, H. H. O., and Stahl, E.: Thin-layer chromatography (TLC). In *Methods of Biochemical Analysis*, Vol. 12, ed. by Glick, D. Interscience, New York, 1964.

McNair, H. M. and Bonelli, E. J.: *Basic Gas Chromatography*. Varian Aerograph, Walnut Creek, 1967.

Ottenstein, D. M.: Column and support materials for use in gas chromatography. J. Gas Chrom. *1:* 11–23, 1963.

Pecsok, R. L.: *Principles and Practice of Gas Chromatography*, Wiley, New York, 1961.

Perry, S. G.: Pyrolysis gas chromatography of involatile substances. In *Advances in Chromatography*, Vol. 7, ed. by Giddings, J. C. and Keller, R. A. Dekker, New York, 1968.

Pierce, A. E.: *Silylation of Organic Compounds*. Pierce Chemical Co., Rockford, 1968.

Purnell, H.: *Gas Chromatography*. Wiley, New York, 1962.

Rowland, M. and Beckett, A. H.: The "amphetamines." Clinical and pharmacokinetic implications of recent studies on an assay procedure and urinary excretion in man. Arzneimittel-Forsch. *16:* 1369–1373, 1966.

Schupp, O. E.: Gas chromatography, Vol. XIII of *Techniques of Organic Chemistry*, ed. by Weisberger, A. Interscience, New York, 1968.

Shellard, E. J.: *Quantitative Paper and Thin-layer Chromatography*. Academic Press, London, 1968.

Stahl, E.: *Thin-layer Chromatography—A Laboratory Handbook*, 2nd Ed., Springer Verlag, New York, 1969.

Stock, R. and Rice, C. B. F.: *Chromatographic Methods*. Chapman Hall, London, 1967.

Stolman, A.: Thin-layer chromatography application in toxicology. In *Progress in Chemical Toxicology*, Vol. 2, Academic Press, New York, 1965.

Street, H. V.: Forensic problems in the gas chromatography of amines and alkaloids. J. Chrom. *37:* 162–171, 1968.

Szymanski, H. A.: *Biomedical Applications of Gas Chromatography*, Vol. 1. Plenum Press, New York 1964.

Szymanski, H. A.; *Biomedical Applications of Gas Chromatography*, Vol. 2, Plenum Press, New York, 1968.

Tamura, Z. and Imanari, T.: Gas chromatography of O-glucuronides. Chem. Pharm. Bull. *12:* 1386–1388, 1964.

Way, J. L. and Way, E. L.; The metabolism of the alkylphosphate antagonists and its pharmacologic implications. Ann. Rev. Pharmacol. *8:* 187–212, 1968.

Way, J. L., Brady, W. T., and Tong. H. S.: Multiple spot phenomena of 2-PAM and metabolite on paper chromatograms. J. Chromatog. *21:* 280–285, 1966.

Wilkinson, G. R.: The GLC separation of amphetamine and ephedrines as pentafluorobenzamide derivatives and their determination by electron capture detection. Anal. Letters, *3:* 289–298, 1970.

Wilkinson, G. R. and Beckett, A. H.: Absorption, metabolism and excretion of the ephedrines in man. I. The influence of urinary pH and urine volume output. J. Pharmacol. Exp. Ther. *162:* 139–147, 1968.

Wilkinson, G. R. and Way, E. L.: Submicrogram estimation of morphine in biological fluids by gas-liquid chromatography, Biochem. Pharmacol., *18:* 1435–1439 1969.

Wilson, C. L., Wilson, D. W., and Strouts, C. R. N.: *Comprehensive Analytical Chemistry*, Vol. 2B, *Physical Separation Methods*. Elsevier Co., New York, 1968.

Wotiz, H. H. and Clark, S. J.: *Gas Chromatography in the Analysis of Steroid Hormones*. Plenum Press, New York, 1966

23

Applications of Tracer Techniques in Drug Metabolism Studies

RONALD KUNTZMAN

I. STUDIES WITH RADIOACTIVE DRUGS

During the last 20 years the use of compounds containing a radioactive atom has facilitated progress in drug metabolism. In these studies the most frequently used isotopes have been carbon-14 and hydrogen-3 (tritium). The use of a radioactive compound simply provides a nonspecific detection method which is independent of the chemical and physical properties of the molecule. The fact that the detection method is nonspecific has many advantages and some disadvantages. Whereas other detection methods (discussed elsewhere in this book) can supply information about the nature of the compound under investigation; radioactivity, *per se*, cannot. For example, while it is possible that a drug, but not its major metabolite, may fluoresce, both the parent drug and its metabolites will be radioactive if the radioactive atom was put in a stable part of the molecule. Since a lack of specificity is inherent in radioactive techniques, other methods of separation, such as solvent extraction or chromatography, must be used to obtain the required specificity. This chapter will not describe principles and methods of quantifying radioactivity but will present examples of the many ways that radioactive compounds can aid in the study of drug metabolism and some examples of pitfalls will be given. For a general background in tracer techniques, the reader should consult references listed in the appendix.

A. Sources of Error Due to the Nonspecificity of the Detection Method

Before discussing the advantages of using radioactivity to study drug metabolism, some possible sources of error will first be described.

1. Design of the labeled compounds. The isotope of choice for drug metabolism studies is carbon-14. Although labeling with tritium has been used successfully in drug metabolism studies, it has many pitfalls inherently. While carbon-14 is usually introduced into a specific part of the molecule, tritium is often incorporated into an already synthesized compound by various isotope exchange procedures using either tritium gas or tritiated solvent and a hydrogen-transfer catalyst. These procedures lead to the exchange of hydrogen by tritium and the radioactive compound thus produced is randomly labeled. Compounds containing "labile" hydrogen positions, i.e., hydrogen atoms attached to oxygen, nitrogen or sulfur atoms, will contain much of the incorporated tritium in these positions

489

and this labile tritium must first be removed before the compound is used. Following the removal of 'labile' tritium, purification of the crude tritiated compound must be achieved. This is often accomplished by a combination of techniques which include preparative paper, thin layer, column or gas chromatography, sublimation, solvent extraction and crystallization.

After purification the compound should be subjected to critical analysis in as many different ways as possible. This will usually involve chromatography in several systems (different from those used to purify the compound), coupled with reverse isotope dilution analysis. Compounds containing carbon-14 must also be purified, but experience has taught most investigators that the purification of compounds specifically labeled with C^{14} is much easier to accomplish than is the purification of compounds randomly labeled with tritium.

When using a compound labeled with carbon-14, the isotope should be incorporated into the molecule at a position where it is likely to appear in the major metabolites. This can usually be accomplished by synthesizing the parent compound with the label located either at a benzyl carbon or a carbon in an aromatic ring. These positions would be preferable to carbon-14 in a methyl group attached to an oxygen or a nitrogen, since both of these carbons are likely to be enzymatically removed by demethylation reactions leaving the major part of the molecule no longer labeled. However, if information only on N or O demethylation is required, then a radioactive methyl carbon atom could be justified as the label of choice to form labeled formaldehyde or carbon dioxide for quantification. For example, Adler et al. (1955, 1967) were able to demonstrate that morphine and norcodeine are biotransformation products of codeine by using a $C^{14}H_3$ label on either the 3-hydroxyl or the ring nitrogen and the amount of $C^{14}O_2$ evolved was used as a measure of the degree of demethylation.

2. Use of Tritium Labeled Compounds. In some studies tritium is specifically, rather than randomly, introduced into the molecule; but even when this is done, a problem associated only with tritium labeling may occur. To illustrate this and some other pitfalls of tracer analysis, the results of an experiment with progesterone is presented. Progesterone, labeled with tritium in the 7α- position, was administered to rats. Because necessary caution was not heeded, several problems were encountered. In this study only the total radioactivity in each tissue was measured and no attempt was made to incorporate specificity into the study. The nature of the radioactivity was not determined, i.e., the question of whether the radioactivity was associated with progesterone or progesterone metabolites was not investigated; and, therefore, the results have a diminished value.

As can be seen in Table 23.1, the changes in tissue distribution of the radioactivity with time did not appear to reflect the decay of a single substance. One hour after the administration of 50 microcuries of tritium labeled progesterone, the liver and kidney contained considerably more radioactivity than did the brain or blood. However, as the level of radioactivity decreased in all tissues, by 24 hours the uneven distribution of the radioactivity was no longer evident. After 24 hours the radioactivity that was measured no longer had anything at all to do with either progesterone or its metabolites. The tritium from the progesterone had been transferred to body water and 24 hours following progesterone administration, water was the only labeled compound in the various

TABLE 23.1

Decrease in tissue radioactivity with time after the administration of 50 μc of 7α-H³-progesterone intraperitoneally

	dpm/gm				
Time (Hr)	Blood	Liver	Brain	Kidney	Lung
1	1,438,560	4,144,452	584,226	3,592,776	1,012,119
5	603,840	864,621	523,311	708,753	490,947
24	388,960	333,591	335,637	314,154	293,260
48	312,080	223,200	253,611	250,077	234,260
72	120,160	106,206	112,344	115,227	90,768
168	37,520	41,943	40,083	37,944	28,272
336	2,880	4,929	3,441	2,976	2,139

TABLE 23.2

Distribution of radioactivity and triprolidine in guinea pig tissues one hr after 40 mg/kg of C¹⁴ triprolidine intramuscularly

Tissue	Radioactivity[a] μg/gm or ml	Triprolidine[b] μg/gm or ml
Muscle	13.5	13.8
Heart	23.6	23.0
Lung	146.7	130.1
Brain	27.9	24.5
Spleen	51.6	39.6
Plasma	8.7	5.1
Kidney	77.0	52.6
Liver	48.6	8.9
Urine	240.0	7.2

[a] The radioactivity was converted to μg/gm by dividing the dpm obtained in each tissue by the specific activity of the administered triprolidine (150 dpm/μg).

[b] Determined using the methyl orange method.

tissues. This was indicated by the fact that when tissue homogenates were freeze-dried, all the tissue radioactivity was found in the water and no radioactivity remained in the tissue residue.

B. Use of Radioactive Techniques to Determine the Distribution, Excretion and Metabolism of a Drug

1. Determination of parent drug and metabolites in tissue and urine. An example, using triprolidine as a typical drug, of how radioactivity can be used to determine the tissue distribution of both the parent compound and its metabolites is presented in Table 23.2. To make this determination, a radioactive drug and a specific method for the drug's measurement are needed. Triprolidine was synthesized with a carbon-14 in the molecule, and a modification of the methyl orange procedure of Burns *et al.* (1955) provided a specific method for the measurement of triprolidine. The specificity of the method for triprolidine was proven by thin layer chromatography which indicated that under the extraction conditions for methyl orange analysis, the only radioactive compound extractable into benzene from tissue homogenates and urine after C^{14} triprolidine administration was unchanged triprolidine.

The total radioactivity in the various tissues and urine was determined either by adding an aliquot of a tissue homogenate or urine to Bray's scintillation mixture (Bray, 1960), or by dissolving the tissue in NCS reagent (obtained from Nuclear Chicago) before the addition of scintillation mix. Triprolidine C^{14} (40 mg/kg, 150,000 dpm/mg) was administered to guinea pigs and the animals were killed one hour later. The amount of radioactivity and the amount of triprolidine was determined in the various tissues. The results in Table 23.2 show that in the muscle, heart, lung and brain, about 90–100 % of the radioactivity represented triprolidine as indicated by the similarity between the level of drug measured by the radioactive and the methyl orange procedures. In the plasma, kidney, liver and especially the urine, however, much of the radioactivity was not present as triprolidine, but instead as unidentified metabolites. The large discrepancy between the amount of triprolidine and radioactivity in the urine indicated that triprolidine is extensively metabolized *in vivo*.

2. Determination of the route of drug and metabolite excretion. Radioactive techniques can be used to account for the excretion of all of an administered drug whether it is present, unchanged or as metabolites. Triprolidine C^{14} (40 mg/kg) was administered to two guinea pigs, and urine and feces were collected for the next several days. The radioactivity in the urine was determined by adding 0.5 ml of urine to Bray's scintillation mixture. The radioactivity in the feces was determined by extracting 20 mg of dried ground-up feces 4 times with 5 ml of a 50 % methanol:water solution and then counting an aliquot of the extract. More than 50 % of the radioactivity in the feces was extracted by the first extraction and no significant radioactivity was found in the fourth extraction. Alternatively, when the radioactivity cannot be extracted, C^{14} or H^3 in feces can be determined by combustion techniques (Kelly *et al.*, 1961) in which the feces and any radioactive compounds in them are burned to CO_2 and H_2O, and the radioactivity of the CO_2 or tritiated H_2O is quantified. Regardless of the method of quantification, the counts per minute obtained are converted to decompositions per minute, taking into account the counting efficiency of the isotope in each sample. Following the administration of triprolidine C^{14} to guinea pigs, all of the administered radioactivity could be accounted for in the urine and feces within 48 hours (Table 23.3).

3. Identification of drug metabolites. When the urine obtained in the above study was extracted with benzene and the extract chromatographed, it was found that less than 5 % of the urinary radioactivity was unchanged triprolidine. In further studies the metabolites of triprolidine C^{14} have been identified using techniques which illustrate how a radioactive label can help in the isolation procedures subsequent to structure determination by mass spectroscopy (Kuntzman *et al.*, 1968). Schwartz *et al.* (1967) have originally used a radioactive drug and mass spectroscopy for the determination of the metabolites of diazepam.

C. Determination of Metabolite Patterns

1. Species differences. An extremely important use for a radioactive drug is its value in determining the pattern of drug metabolism. This determination allows the selection of an animal species which metabolizes the drug most like

TABLE 23.3

The excretion of radioactivity in the urine and feces of guinea pigs administered 40 mg/kg of C¹⁴ triprolidine intramuscularly

		Guinea pig 1 dpm	Guinea pig 2 dpm
Day 1	Urine	985,000	576,000
	Feces	1,262,000	612,000
Day 2	Urine	53,000	51,600
	Feces	378,000	1,653,000
Total	Urine	1,038,000	627,600
	Feces	1,640,000	2,265,000
		2,678,000	2,892,600

Guinea pigs 1 and 2 were given 2,620,000 and 2,535,000 dpm of triprolidine respectively.

man for chronic toxicity studies. To do this, the nonspecificity of radioactivity is used to maximum advantage. The drug is administered to various animal species, and their urine is collected. A small aliquot of the urine may then be chromatographed directly or the urine may first be extracted with various organic solvents at various pH's, and then the extracts chromatographed. An excellent solvent which we have developed to extract very polar metabolites is a mixture of dichloromethane:isopropanol:water (75:25:2). This solvent has the polarity of butanol but can easily be evaporated to dryness at room temperature under a stream of nitrogen. Without identifying any or all of the metabolites of the drug, the characteristics (Rf, solvent partition, etc.) of the various radioactive metabolites will be known. Following the first administration of labeled drug to man, the characteristics of the drug metabolites obtained from human urine are compared to that previously obtained in various animal species, and the animal that metabolizes the drug most like man is selected as one of the species for chronic toxicity studies.

In addition to determining the characteristics of the metabolites in urine, the nature of the metabolites obtained by incubating the drug *in vitro* with the liver microsomal enzyme system will also point out species differences in the metabolism of drugs. Progesterone C¹⁴ was incubated with liver microsomes from various animal species in the presence of a TPNH generating system. An aliquot of the incubation mixture was extracted with dichloromethane, which was then evaporated to dryness under nitrogen and the residue was dissolved in methanol. An aliquot of the methanol extract was then chromatographed in a system consisting of decalin-nitromethane-methanol (100:50:50) for 6 days. Under these conditions, progesterone ran off the end of the paper and only the polar metabolites remained on the chromatogram. Each chromatogram was cut into 2 cm sections and each section was added to Bray's scintillation mix and quantified in a liquid scintillation spectrometer.

As can be seen in Table 23.4, no two species metabolized progesterone in an identical manner. For example, microsomes from the female rat formed a major metabolite which moved 5 cm from the origin of the chromatogram, while microsomes from the females of all the other species failed to form this metabolite.

TABLE 23.4

Species differences in the metabolism of progesterone by liver microsomal enzymes

Cm. from origin	Female guinea pigs	Female rabbits	Female mice	Male rats	Female rats
2 (16α-OH)	±	++	++	+++++	0
5	0	0	0	0	++
7 (6β-OH)	++	+	+++	+++	0
13	++	±	+	±	0
23	+	0	0	+++++	0
30	+	±	0	0	0

Liver microsomes were incubated with progesterone-4-C^{14} and were extracted and chromatographed. Pluses indicate the relative amount of each radioactive peak. The metabolites found at 2 and 7 cm from the origin which have 2 or more pluses have been identified as 16α- and 6β-hydroxyprogesterone.

In addition, one can also see marked differences in metabolites formed by liver microsomes from the male and female rat. If data of this type were available from studies with urine obtained from various species, a determination of which species metabolized the drug most like man could then be made even without knowing the identity of the metabolites. In the example just cited in Table 23.4, only 2 of the metabolites of progesterone have been identified. These are 6β-hydroxyprogesterone and 16α-hydroxyprogesterone and the chromatographic mobilities of these are indicated in Table 23.4.

2. Effect of substrate concentration on the pattern of metabolites. Not only can one obtain different patterns of metabolites when several species are studied, but a change in the substrate concentration may also lead to differences in the pattern of metabolites formed by liver microsomal enzymes. Since the use of a radioactive substrate may allow the measurement of smaller amounts of products than could normally be measured by other techniques, smaller substrate concentrations are often used when the substrate is labeled than when it is not. The metabolites obtained with the different amounts of substrate will often be different, not only quantitatively but also qualitatively. When testosterone is incubated with the liver microsomal enzyme system of the male rat, 6β, 7α- and 16α-hydroxy-testosterone are formed. These hydroxylated products in turn can be further metabolized by the same enzyme system and the amount of further metabolism is dependent on the concentration of substrate (testosterone), as can be seen in Table 23.5. Various amounts of radioactive testosterone were incubated with liver microsomes. The 6β-, 7α- and 16α-hydroxytestosterone and the metabolites of these hydroxytestosterones which were formed were separated and quantified as previously described (Jacobson *et al.*, 1969).

The results shown in Table 23.5 indicate that the pattern of metabolite formation depends on the substrate concentration. When 16 mμmoles of testosterone were used as substrate, metabolites of 6β, 7α and 16α-hydroxytestosterone were found after the incubation, while metabolites of these 3 hydroxytestosterones were not found when 164 mμmoles of testosterone were used as substrate. This change in the pattern of testosterone metabolism has been shown to result from the competitive inhibition by testosterone of the metabolism of the 6β,- 7α- and 16α-hydroxytestosterone formed during the incubation. Therefore, in the presence

TABLE 23.5
Profile of metabolites formed during the incubation of high and low concentrations of testosterone

Testosterone per incubation (mμmoles)	6β-, 7α- and 16α-hydroxytestosterone formed (mμmoles)	Metabolites of 6β-, 7α- and 16α-hydroxytestosterone formed (mμmoles)
16	6.06	1.47
33	11.06	1.58
67	16.21	0.94
164	23.78	0.00

Various amounts of testosterone-4-C^{14} were incubated with liver microsomes obtained from 100 mg of liver for 15 min at 25° in the presence of an NADPH-generating system. Each incubation flask contained the same amount of radioactivity (.05 μc). The amount of 6β-, 7α- and 16α-hydroxytestosterone formed and the amount of metabolites of 6β-, 7α- and 16α-hydroxytestosterone formed were determined as previously described (Jacobson et al., (1969)).

of a high testosterone concentration the hydroxylated testosterones are not further metabolized.

The ability of a substrate to inhibit the further metabolism of its metabolites is a general concept, and several examples can be cited. Aminopyrine, which is metabolized to monomethyl-4-aminoantipyrine by rat liver microsomes, inhibits the conversion of the latter compound to 4-aminoantipyrine, i.e., the tertiary amine inhibits the conversion of the secondary amine to the primary amine (Dingell and D'Encarnacao, 1966). Similarly, Levin and Conney (1967), in studying the hepatic metabolism of 7,12-dimethylbenz(α)anthracene to monohydroxymethyl compounds, demonstrated a similar type of inhibition of the further metabolism of these hydroxylated compounds. Thus, it is apparent from these studies and those presented here on testosterone that when a low concentration of substrate is used in an incubation, a different pattern of microsomal metabolism may be obtained than when a high concentration of substrate is used.

D. Use of a Radioactive Precursor to Label Endogenous Compounds

In addition to the use of a labeled drug to study drug disposition, radioactive compounds can be used to study the mechanism of drug metabolism. A microsomal hemoprotein, which when reduced binds carbon monoxide, has been implicated as the terminal oxidase for microsomal drug and steroid metabolism (Kuntzman, 1969). To study the turnover of this hemoprotein, labeled δ-aminolevulinic acid can be administered to rats. This compound is converted to heme which then becomes part of the hemoprotein of liver microsomes. This was demonstrated by experiments which showed that the labeled component found in the microsomes after δ-ALA administration had the solubility characteristics of a hemoprotein. Addition of cold trichloroacetic acid (TCA) to the microsomes obtained from rats 2 to 72 hours after δ-ALA administration resulted in the precipitation of the protein and 99% of the radioactivity, indicating that the radioactivity was associated with protein.

Similarly, as would be expected if the label was in a protein or hemoprotein, all the radioactivity precipitated when the microsomes were suspended in acetone:water. When the microsomes were suspended in cold acid:acetone, which precipitates protein but solubilizes the heme moiety of a hemoprotein, over 99 % of the radioactivity was solubilized indicating that the radioactivity was in the heme moiety. Methylethylketone has also been used to split and extract the heme from a hemoprotein, and extraction of the microsomes with this solvent resulted in the extraction of over 93 % of the radioactivity into the methylethyl-ketone, (Levin and Kuntzman, 1969).

The CO-binding hemoprotein and cytochrome b_5 are the only hemoproteins that occur in liver microsomes. Cytochrome b_5 can be easily removed from the microsomes leaving only the CO-binding hemoprotein in the CO-binding par-ticles (microsomes minus cytochrome b_5). The radioactivity which is incorporated into the hemoprotein of the CO-binding particles disappears biphasically (Fig. 23.1); and since cytochrome b_5 has already been removed from these particles, the results suggest the presence of two CO-binding hemoproteins in the CO-binding particles (Levin and Kuntzman, 1969). In this way radioactivity can be used to study the turnover of endogenous substances which are important in drug metabolism. Radioactive precursors have been used to study the turnover and storage of many endogenous compounds not associated with drug metabolism; and this technique, therefore, has importance in all areas of pharmacology and biochemistry.

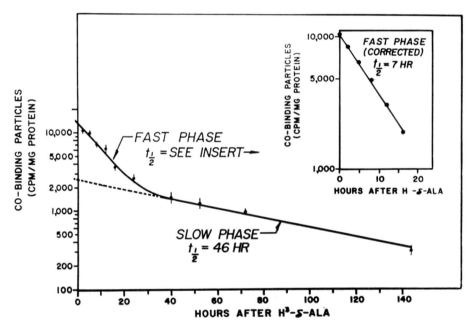

Fig. 23.1. Disappearance of labeled hemoprotein from the CO-binding particles obtained from control rats. Rats were injected i.v. with ^{3}H-δ-ALA (0.234 mg/kg) and killed at various times. Each value represents the mean ±S.E. for 4 rats. Values used for the determination of the corrected half-life of the fast phase (insert) were obtained by extrapolation of the slow phase to zero time and subtracting the cpm/mg protein of the slow phase from the uncorrected fast phase portion of the curve. The ratio of the fast phase hemoprotein to the slow phase hemoprotein was obtained by extrapolation of the curves for the 2 phases to zero time and subtracting the cpm/mg protein at zero time for the slow phase intercept from the cpm/mg protein at zero time for the fast phase intercept and dividing by the cpm/mg protein at zero time for the slow phase intercept.

II. ANALYSIS OF DRUGS IN BIOLOGICAL MATERIALS BY THE FORMATION OF A RADIOACTIVE DERIVATIVE

Since the rate of metabolism of a drug may vary as much as ten-fold in different individuals, methods are needed to determine the concentration of drug in human plasma so that the amount of drug administered can be varied to reflect differences in the rate of metabolism. The amount of drug in human plasma is often small because of tissue localization and/or the low dosage usually administered. To satisfactorily measure nanogram amounts of drugs in plasma, the technique of making a radioactive derivative has been recently applied to the field of drug metabolism. In procedures of this type, a non-radioactive drug is administered to man, plasma samples are obtained, the drug is extracted from the plasma and then reacted with a radioactive compound to form a derivative which can be separated from the excess radioactive reagent and quantified in a liquid scintillation spectrometer. Many types of derivatives are theoretically possible and will undoubtably be useful in future studies. Here, I will give several examples which have already been utilized for the study of drug metabolism in man.

A. Determination of Secondary Amines by Reaction with Acetic Anhydride H[3]

The reaction of primary and secondary amines with tritiated acetic anhydride has been used to measure the small amounts of desmethylimipramine (Hammer and Brodie, 1967), norchlorcyclizine (Kuntzman et al., 1967) and phenmetrazine (Quinn et al., 1967) in human plasma. The reaction scheme is shown in Figure 23.2. The sensitivity of the method depends on the high specific activity of the acetic anhydride which is used. Desmethylimipramine (DMI) and norchlorcyclizine are extracted from plasma with hexane and reacted with H[3]-acetic anhydride in this solvent as described by Hammer and Brodie (1967).

When the plasma concentrations of more polar drugs are to be determined, a solvent more polar than hexane can be used for the extraction and acetylation. We have recently applied this method to the determination of pseudoephedrine,

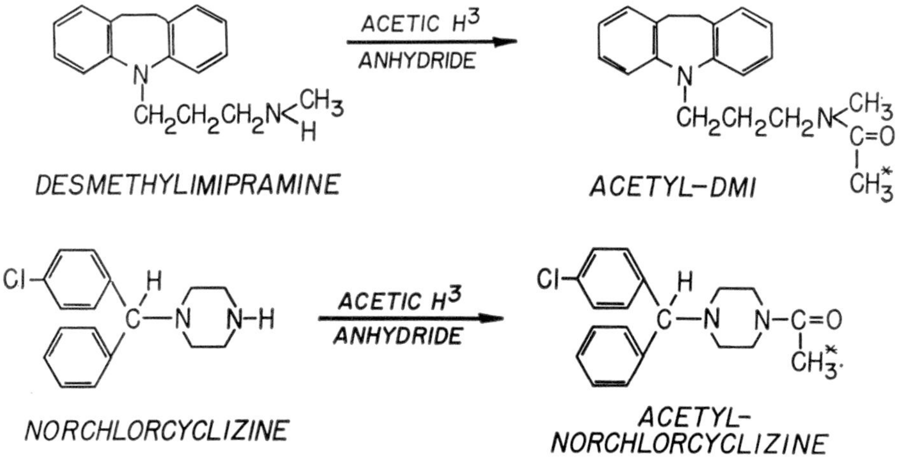

Fig. 23.2. Reaction scheme for the acetylation of desmethylimipramine and norchlorcyclizine with radioactive acetic anhydride.

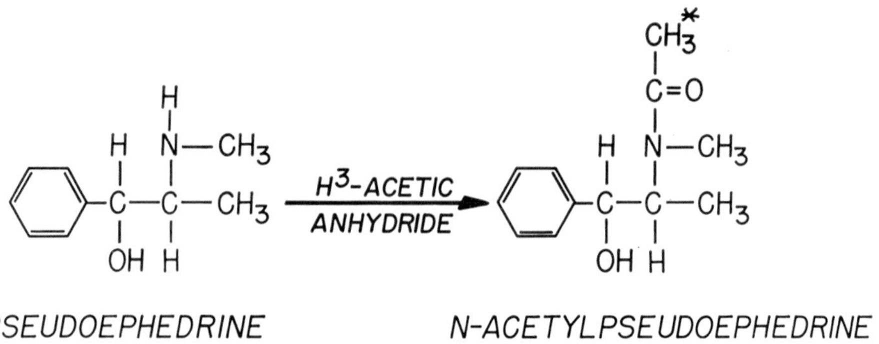

Fig. 23.3. Reaction scheme for the acetylation of pseudoephedrine with radioactive acetic anhydride.

which cannot be extracted from plasma into hexane. This drug was extracted into chloroform and acetylated in this solvent (Fig. 23.3). Following acetylation, the radioactive acetylated amine must be separated from the large excess of unreacted H^3-acetic anhydride. The extent to which this can be achieved will ultimately determine the blank and the sensitivity of the procedure.

Hammer and Brodie (1967) have indicated that the lower limit of sensitivity for desmethylimipramine using the separation procedure which they describe is 5 mμg/ml of plasma. Better sensitivity is obtained when the method is modified for the determination of norchlorcyclizine. Acetylnorchlorcyclizine, which retains an ionizable nitrogen, can be extracted from hexane into acid and then can be re-extracted into heptane after the addition of excess base to the aqueous phase as previously described (Kuntzman et al., 1967). In the method developed for pseudoephedrine, still another procedure has been used to separate the acetylated derivative from the blank. Following acetylation in chloroform, the solvent containing the acetylated amine is washed twice with 0.1 N NaOH, and the radioactivity in the chloroform (after evaporation) is determined directly in the scintillation mixture of Bray (1960). This procedure allows a lower limit of sensitivity of 0.2 μg of pseudoephedrine per ml of plasma.

When greater sensitivity (0.01 μg/ml) is needed, 100 μg of cold acetyl pseudoephedrine is added to an aliquot of the chloroform phase which is then evaporated to dryness. The residue is dissolved in a few drops of methanol and chromatographed on aluminum oxide GF using the lower phase of a solvent system containing chloroform, methanol, water and acetic acid in the proportions 20:7.5:-20:1, respectively. After chromatography the alumina in the ultraviolet absorbing area corresponding to the R_f for acetylated pseudoephedrine is scraped into vials and the radioactivity is quantified in the scintillation mixture described by Bray (1960). To correct for the recovery of the tritiated derivative on the chromatogram, a known amount of a C^{14} acetylated pseudoephedrine can be added to the 100 μg of cold acetylated pseudoephedrine after the reaction of pseudoephedrine with the tritiated acetic anhydride. The recovery of the C^{14} acetylated pseudoephedrine is determined and a correction is then made for the amount of tritiated derivative lost during the purification.

B. Determination of Tertiary Amines

Although the above methods for measuring small amounts of primary and secondary amines are extremely useful in studies of drug action, many drugs are tertiary amines and do not react with acetic anhydride. Two radioactive derivative procedures have been recently described which allow the determination of tertiary amines.

1. Enzymatic demethylation. By using lyophilized rat liver microsomes as a reagent for enzymatic demethylation, some tertiary amines can be converted to secondary amines, and the acetic anhydride procedure can then be used to assay the secondary amines as shown in Figure 23.4 (Kuntzman et al., 1967). For example, the antihistaminic, chlorcyclizine, can be demethylated by adding lyophilized microsomes (equivalent to 30 mg of liver) and an NADPH generating system directly to plasma which contains chlorcyclizine. Following the incubation of this plasma mixture for 5 minutes at 37°C, the norchlorcyclizine that is formed is assyed as described above by acetylation with H^3-acetic anhydride (Table 23.6).

The deficiency of this procedure, which has previously been discussed by Kuntzman et al. (1969), is that it cannot be used to assay all tertiary amines. The method can be used only when the rate of demethylation of the tertiary amine to the secondary amine in the presence of lyophilized microsomes is faster than the rate of metabolism of the secondary amine which is thus formed. The demethylation of chlorcyclizine meets these criteria (Kuntzman et al., 1969) and this method has been used for the determination of the plasma concentration of chlorcyclizine and norchlorcyclizine in man following the administration of chlorcyclizine.

The results in Table 23.7 show the plasma level of both chlorcyclizine and its metabolite, norchlorcyclizine, at various times after the administration of 2.0 mg/kg of chlorcyclizine to 4 human subjects. As can be seen, the metabolite norchlorcyclizine remained in man for more than 30 days, whereas chlorcyclizine

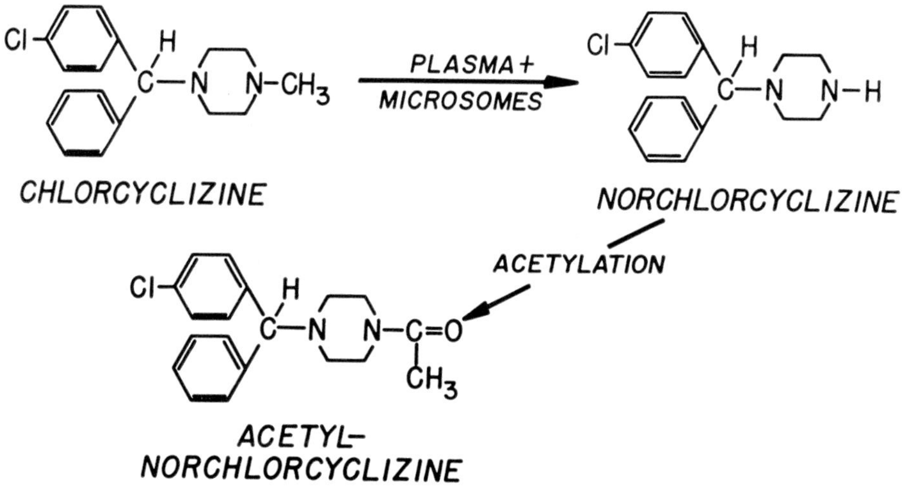

Fig. 23.4. Reaction scheme for the enzymatic demethylation of chlorcyclizine in plasma and subsequent reaction of norchlorcyclizine with radioactive acetic anhydride.

TABLE 23.6

Analysis of chlorcyclizine in plasma by enzymatic N-demethylation and reaction with H^3-acetic anhydride

Amount of chlorcyclizine added to plasma μg/ml	Incubated with enzyme (lyophilized microsomes)	cpm	cpm minus blank
0.00	yes	627	0
0.50	no[a]	619	0
0.50	yes	26,120	25,493
0.01	no[a]	620	0
0.01	yes	1,148	528

[a] Enzyme and cofactors were incubated with plasma and chlorcyclizine was added after the incubation at zero time. In the other samples (yes) chlorcyclizine was incubated with enzyme and cofactors as described in the text.

TABLE 23.7

Plasma level of chlorcyclizine and norchlorcyclizine in man following the administration of 2 mg/kg of chlorcyclizine

Time	Chlorcyclizine μg/ml ± S.D.	Norchlorcyclizine μg/ml ± S.D.
1 hour	0.018 ± 0.025	0.032 ± 0.022
5 hours	0.051 ± 0.007	0.034 ± 0.012
24 hours	0.020 ± 0.012	0.032 ± 0.009
2 days	0.004 ± 0.007	0.031 ± 0.013
3 days	0.000	0.031 ± 0.009
6 days	0.000	0.023 ± 0.004
10 days	0.000	0.018 ± 0.002
14 days	0.000	0.013 ± 0.002
30 days	0.000	0.004 ± 0.001

The above averages represent the data obtained from 4 humans given chlorcyclizine.

disappeared much more rapidly. The finding that norchlorcyclizine is retained for such a protracted period has been related to the extensive binding of this compound to tissue and plasma protein (Kuntzman *et al.*, 1967).

2. Reaction with C^{14} methyl iodide. An alternate method for the determination of tertiary amines has recently been developed by Harris *et al.* (1968). In this procedure the tertiary amine is reacted with C^{14} methyl iodide and converted into a quaternary amine which can be quantified after the removal of the excess methyliodide. Harris *et al.* (1968) have used this method to measure the concentration of imipramine in dog plasma, and simultaneously have used the acetylation procedure to measure desmethylimipramine, the major metabolite of imipramine. The method has also been used to measure chlorpromazine and may have more widespread applicability for the determination of tertiary amines than does the enzymatic method.

Needless to say, other radioactive derivative methods not already described may be applicable to the study of drug metabolism. The criteria to be used in the development of such a procedure are that the radioactive compound quantitatively reacts with the drug to be measured and that the radioactive derivative which is formed can be separated from the excess radioactive reagent. The ultimate sensitivity of a radioactive derivative method will depend on how well this second criteria is met, since as with most drug assay methods, the extent of the blank limits the overall sensitivity of the method.

C. Determination of Drug Levels by Chelation with Radioactive Metal

Another use for radioactivity should be suggested which, although not used in the past, may have applicability in the future. Many compounds can form chelates with metals such as copper, and one of these is shown in Figure 23.5. When copper is added to plasma containing this drug, the chelate is formed and the chelated copper can be extracted into ether; while in the absence of the drug, copper would not extract. The determination of drug level was, therefore, accomplished by measuring the amount of ether extractable copper. This colorimetric method lacked sensitivity but provided the basis for a more sensitive procedure.

B.W. 356C61 (Fig. 23.5) will also form a complex with nickel, which, like the copper complex, can be extracted into ether. In this procedure, Ni^{63} is added to

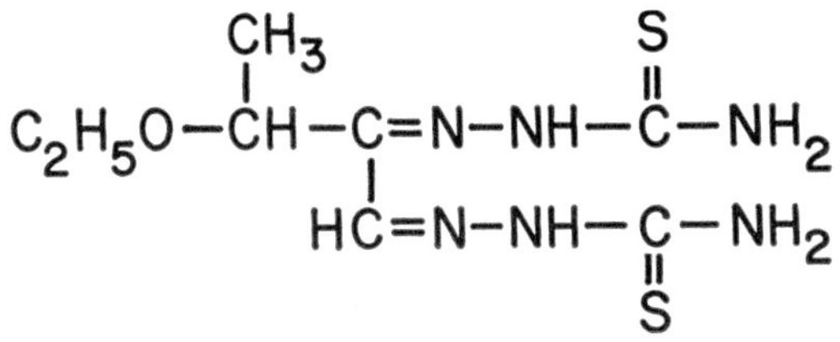

$$C_2H_5O-\underset{\underset{HC=N-NH-\underset{\underset{S}{\|}}{C}-NH_2}{|}}{\overset{\overset{CH_3}{|}}{CH}}-C=N-NH-\overset{\overset{S}{\|}}{C}-NH_2$$

Fig. 23.5. Structure of BW 356C61.

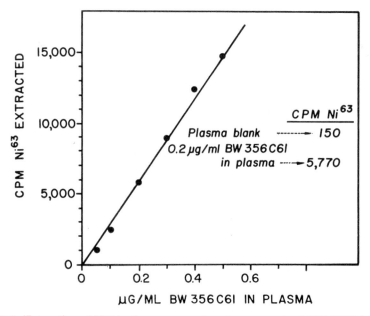

Fig. 23.6. Extraction of Ni^{63} in the presence of various amounts of BW 356C61. Ni^{63} (10 $\mu c/30\ \mu g$) was added to plasma containing BW 356C61. The plasma was extracted with 5 volumes of ether and the extractable radioactivity was quantified.

plasma containing the drug, and the plasma is extracted with ether; and the extractable radioactivity is determined as a measure of the amount of drug present (Fig. 23.6).

When B.W. 356C61 was not present in plasma, the radioactivity which extracted was equivalent to 150 cpm; however, in the presence of 0.2 μg/ml of B.W. 356C61, the extracted radioactivity amounted to 5,770 cpm. The linearity of Ni^{63} extraction at various concentrations of B.W. 356C61 can also be seen in Figure 23.6. Since many compounds form metal chelates, this method may have widespread applicability and may be more fully exploited in the future. For example, fatty acids can be assayed by reaction with copper; therefore the possibility exists that a method for the determination of fatty acids based on the formation of the above type of radioactive derivative can be developed.

III. CONCLUDING REMARKS

The use of radioactivity in drug metabolism studies has been discussed from two main points of emphasis. In the first, a radioactive drug is administered to animals or incubated *in vitro*, and the radioactivity is used as a non-specific detection method. This approach is most useful in studies to determine the metabolism of the drug in animals and in very early human studies with a very limited number of subjects. In the second approach, nonradioactive drug is administered and a radioactive derivative is made after the extraction of the drug from the plasma. This approach is most useful where sensitive procedures are needed for the measurement of nonradioactive drugs in blood and other biological materials. The latter approach may result in a more sensitive assay procedure, since the specific activity of the reacting reagent can be much greater than the specific activity of a drug administered to man.

Acknowledgments

I would like to thank M. Jacobson, W. Levin, I. Tsai, E. Sernatinger and S. Haber for their collaboration on the studies presented in this chapter.

REFERENCES

Adler, T. K., Fujimoto, J. M., Way, E. Leong, and Baker, E. M.: The metabolic fate of codeine in man. J. Pharmacol. Exp. Ther. *114:* 251–262, 1955.

Adler, T. K.: Studies on morphine tolerance in mice. I. In vivo N-demethylation of morphine and N- and O-demethylation of codeine. J. Pharmacol. Exp. Ther. *56:* 585–590, 1967.

Bray, G. A.: A simple efficient liquid scintillator for counting aqueous solutions in a liquid scintillation counter. Anal. Biochem. *1:* 279–285, 1960.

Burns, J. J., Berger, B. L., Lief, P. A., Wollack, A., Papper, E. M., and Brodie, B. B.: The physiological disposition and fate of meperidine (Demerol) in man and a method for its estimation in plasma. J. Pharmacol. Exp. Ther. *114:* 289–298, 1955.

Dingell, J. V. and D'Encarnecao, P. W.: Studies on the demethylation of second-

ary and tertiary amines. Pharmacologist *8:* 181, 1966.

Hammer, W. and Brodie, B. B.: Application of isotope derivative technique to assay of secondary amines: estimation of desipramine by acetylation with H^3-acetic anhydride. J. Pharmacol. Exp. Ther. *157:* 503–508, 1967.

Harris, S. R., Efron, D., and Gaudette, L.: Radioactive derivative formation for the simultaneous estimation of plasma imipramine and desimipramine. Pharmacologist *10:* 166, 1968.

Jacobson, M., Levin, W., and Kuntzman, R.: Testosterone inhibition of 6β, 7α and 16α-hydroxytestosterone metabolism by rat liver microsomes. Biochem. Pharmacol. *18:* 2253–2262, 1969.

Kelly, R. G., Peets, E. A., Gordon, S., and Buyske, D. A.: Determination of C^{14} and H^3 in biological samples by Schöniger combustion and liquid scintillation techniques. Anal. Biochem. *2:* 267–273, 1961.

Kuntzman, R., Tsai, I., and Burns, J. J.: Importance of tissue and plasma binding in determining the retention of norchlorcyclizine and norcyclizine in man, dog and rat. J. Pharmacol. Exp. Ther. *158:* 332–339, 1967.

Kuntzman, R. and Tsai, I.: A sensitive radiochemical method for the assay of some tertiary amines. Pharmacologist *9:* 240, 1967.

Kuntzman, R., Sernatinger, E., Tsai, I. and Klutch, A.: New methodology for studies of drug metabolism. In *Importance of Fundamental Principles in Drug Evaluation*, ed. by D. H. Tedeschi and R. E. Tedeschi, pp. 87–103, Raven Press, New York, 1968.

Kuntzman, R.: Drugs and enzyme induction. Ann. Rev. Pharmacol. *9:* 21–36, 1969.

Levin, W. and Conney, A. H.: Stimulatory effect of polycyclic hydrocarbons and aromatic azo derivatives on the metabolism of 7,12-dimethylbenz(α)anthracene. Cancer Res. *27:* 1931–1938, 1967.

Levin, W. and Kuntzman, R.: Biphasic decrease of radioactive hemoprotein from liver microsomal CO-binding particles: effect of 3-methylcholanthrene. J. Biol. Chem. *244:* 3671–3676, 1969.

Quinn, G. P., Cohn, M. M., Reid, M. B., Greengard, P., and Weiner, M.: The effect of formulation of phenmetrazine plasma levels in man studied by a sensitive analytic method. Clin. Pharmacol. Ther. *8:* 369–373, 1967.

Schwartz, M. A., Bommer, P., and Vane, F. M.: Diazepam metabolites in the rat: characterization by high resolution mass spectrometry and nuclear magnetic resonance. Arch. Biochem. Biophys. *121:* 508–516, 1967.

References needed to acquire a working background in tracer methodology

Chase, G. D. and Rabinowitz, J. L.: *Principles of Radioisotope Methodology.* Burgess Publishing Co., Minneapolis, Minn., 1962.

The Radiochemical Manual. Edited by B. J. Wilson, The Radiochemical Centre, Amersham, 1966.

Aronoff, S.: *Techniques of Radiochemistry*, Iowa State College Press, 1956.

Selected references utilizing tracer methodology to study drug metabolism

Adamson, R. H., Ague, S. L., Hess, S. M., and Davidson, J. D.: The distribution, excretion and metabolism of hydroxyurea-14C. J. Pharm. Exp. Ther. *150:* 322–327, 1965.

Angelucci, R., Artini, D., Cresseri, A.,

Giraldi, P. N., Logemann, W., Nannini, G., and Valzelli, G.: Some aspects of the metabolism of triazine derivatives active in experimentally induced virus infections. Brit. J. Pharmac. *24:* 274–281, 1965.

Birtley, R. D. N., Roberts, J. B., Thomas, B. H., and Wilson, A.: Excretion and metabolism of 14C-pyridostigmine. Brit. J. Pharmac. *26:* 393–402, 1966.

Charalampous, K. D. and Tansey, L. W.: Metabolic fate of B-(3,4-dimethoxyphenyl)-ethylamine in man. J. Pharm. Exp. Ther. *155:* 318–329, 1967.

Cresseri, A., Giraldi, P. N., Logemann, W., Tosolini, G., and Valzelli, G.: Some aspects of the metabolism of triazine derivatives active in experimentally induced virus infections. Brit. J. Pharmac. Chemother. *27:* 486–490, 1966.

Dacre, J. C. and Williams, R. T. : The role role of the tissues and gut micro-organisms in the metabolism of 14C-protocatechuic acid in the rat. Aromatic dehydroxylation. J. Pharm. Pharmac. *20:* 610–618, 1968

Dacre, J. C., Scheline, R. R., and Williams, R. T.: The role of the tissues and gut flora in the metabolism of 14C-homoprotocatechuic acid in the rat and rabbit. J. Pharm. Pharmac. *20:* 619–625, 1968.

Davison, C. and Williams, R. T.: The metabolism of 5,5¹-methylene-disalicylic acid in various species. J. Pharm. Pharmac. *20:* 12–18, 1968.

DiCarlo, F. J., Hartigan, J. M., Jr., Coutinho, C. B., and Phillips, G. E.: Absorption, distribution and excretion of pentaerythritol and pentaerythritol tetranitrate by mice. Proc. Soc. Exp. Biol. Med. *118:* 311–315, 1965.

DiCarlo, F. J., Crew, M. C., Melgar, M. D., and Haynes, L. J.: Prazepam metabolism by dogs. J. Pharmaceut. Sci. *58:* 960–962, 1969.

Dreyfuss, J., Swoap, J. R., Chinn, C., and Hess, S. M.: Excretion and distribution of thiazesim-14C with its biotransformation *in vivo* and *in vitro*. J. Pharmaceut. Sci. *57:* 1497–1505, 1968a.

Dreyfuss, J. A., Cohen, I., and Hess, S. M.: Metabolism of thiazesim, 5-(2-dimethylaminoethyl)-2,3-dihydro-2-phenyl-1,5-benzothiazepin-4 (5H)-one, in the rat. *In vivo* and *in vitro*. J. Pharmaceut. Sci. *57:* 1505–1511, 1968a.

Elliott, T. H., Parke, D. V., and Williams, R. T.: The metabolism of cyclo-14C-hexane and its derivatives. Biochem. J. *72:* 193–200, 1959.

Ellison, T., Gutzait, L., and Van Loon, E. J.,: The comparative metabolism of d-amphetamine-14C in the rat, dog and monkey. J. Pharm. Exp. Ther. *152:* 383–387, 1966.

Emmerson, J. L., Welles, J. S., and Anderson, R. C.: Studies of the tissue distribution of d-propoxyphene. Toxicol. Appl. Pharmacol. *11:* 484–488, 1967.

Furst, C. J.: Studies on the distribution and excretion of a metabolite of guanethidine in the rat. Brit. J. Pharmac. Chemother. *32:* 57–64, 1968.

Hague, D. E., Fabro, S., and Smith, R. L.: The fate of ¹⁴C-thalidomide in the pregnant hamster. J. Pharm. Pharmac. *19:* 603–607, 1967.

Hucker, H. B., Ahmad, P. M., and Miller, E. A., Absorption distribution and metabolism of dimethylsulfoxide in the rat, rabbit and guinea pig. J. Pharm. Exp. Ther. *154:* 176–184, 1966.

Hucker, H. B., Zacchei, A. G., Cox, S. V., Brodie, D. A., and Cantwell, N. H. R.: Studies on the absorption, distribution and excretion of indomethacin in various species. J. Pharm. Exp. Ther. *153:* 237–249, 1966.

Hug, C. C., Jr. and Mellett, L. B.: Tritium-labeled dihydromorphine: Its metabolic fate and excretion in the rat. J. Pharm. Exp. Ther. *149:* 446–453, 1965.

Husain, M. A., Roberts, J. B., Thomas, B. H., and Wilson, A.: Metabolism and excretion of 3-hydroxyphenyltrimethylammonium and neostigmine. Brit. J. Pharmac. *35:* 344–350, 1969.

Kamm, J. J., Taddeo, A. B., and Van Loon, E. J., Metabolism and excretion of tritiated dextromethorphan by the rat. J. Pharm. Exp. Ther. *158:* 437–444, 1967.

Kaighen, M. and Williams, R. T.: The metabolism of 3-¹⁴C-coumarin. J. Med. Pharm. Chem. *3:* 25–43, 1961.

Koechlin, B. A., Schwartz, M. A., Krol, G., and Oberhansli, W.: The metabolic fate of ¹⁴C-labeled chlordiazepoxide in man, in the dog and in the rat. J. Pharmacol. Exp. Ther. *148:* 399–411, 1965.

McMahon, R. E., Culp, H. W. and Marshall, F. J.: The metabolism of a-dl-acetylmethadol in the rat: the identification of the probable active metabolite. J. Pharm. Exp. Ther. *149:* 436–445, 1965.

McMahon, R. E. Marshall, F. J., and Culp, H. W.: The nature of the metabolites of acetohexamide in the rat and in the human. J. Pharm. Exp. Ther. *149:* 272–279, 1965.

Misra, A. L., Jacoby, H. I., and Woods, L. A.: The preparation of tritium nuclear-labeled morphine and evidence for its *in vivo* biotransformation to normorphine in the rat. J. Pharmacol. Exp. Ther. *132:* 317–322, 1961.

Mule, S. J., Clements, T. H., and Gorodet-zky, C. W.: The metabolic fate of ³H-cyclazocine in dogs. J. Pharm. Exp. Ther. *160:* 387–396, 1968.

Murphy, P. J. and Wick, A. N.: Metabolism of β-phenethylbiguanide. J. Pharmaceut. Sci. *57:* 1125–1127, 1968.

Parke, D. V.: The metabolism of ¹⁴C-nitrobenzene in the rabbit and guinea pig. Biochem. J. *62:* 339–346, 1956.

Parke, D. V.: The metabolism of ¹⁴C-aniline in the rabbit and other animals. Biochem. J. *77:* 493–503, 1960.

Parke, D. V.: The metabolism of m-dinitro-¹⁴C-benzene in the rabbit. Biochem. J. *78:* 262–271, 1961.

Parke, C. V. and Williams, R. T.: The metabolism of benzene containing ¹⁴C-1-benzene. Biochem. J. *54:* 231–238, 1953.

Parke, D. V. and Williams, R. T.: The metabolism of benzene. (a) The formation of phenylglucuronide and phenylsulphuric acid from ¹⁴C-benzene. (b) The metabolism of ¹⁴C-phenol. Biochem. J. *55:* 337–340, 1953.

Roberts, J. B., Thomas, B. H., Wilson, A.: Metabolism of ¹⁴C-neostigmine in the rat. Brit. J. Pharm. *25:* 763–770, 1965.

Roberts, J. B., Thomas, B. H., and Wilson, A.: Distribution and excretion of ¹⁴C-neostigmine in the rat and hen. Brit. J. Pharmac. *25:* 234–242, 1966.

Schreiber, E. C., Min, B. H., Zeiger, A. V., and Lang, J. F.: Metabolism of diethylpropion-1-¹⁴C hydrochloride by the human. J. Pharmacol. Exp. Ther. *159:* 372–378, 1968.

Schwartz, M. A., Koechlin, B. A., Postma, E., Palmer, S., and Krol, G.: Metabolism of diazepam in rat, dog and man. J. Pharm. Exp. Ther. *149:* 423–435, 1965.

Smith, D. L., Forist, A. A., and Gerritsen, G. C.: Metabolism of 3,5-dimethyl-pyrazole-¹⁴C in the rat. J. Pharm. Exp. Ther. *150:* 316–321, 1965.

Smith, D. L., Wagner, J. G., and Gerritsen, G. C.: Absorption, metabolism and excretion of 5-methyl-pyrazole-3-carboxylic acid in the rat, dog and human. J. Pharmaceut. Sci. *56:* 1150–1157 1967.

Titus, E. O. and Weiss, H.: The use of biologically prepared radioactive indicators in metabolic studies: Metabolism of pentobarbital. J. Biol. Chem. *214:* 807–820, 1955.

Tocco, D. J., Egerton, J. R., Bowers, W., Christensen, V. W., and Rosenblum, C.: Absorption, metabolism and elimination of thiabendazole in farm animals and a method for its estimation in biological materials. J. Pharm. Exp. Ther. *149:* 263–271, 1965.

24

Autoradiography in Drug Disposition Studies

WILLIAM J. WADDELL

I. INTRODUCTION

Autoradiography is the production of an image in a photographic emulsion by the emission from a radioactive element. The term autoradiography is preferred to that of radioautography. Prefixes are added to words to further classify the concept. Therefore, the process is "auto-" radiography for a "self-" radiograph and not a "radio-" autograph or one's transmitted signature.

A. Selection of Isotope

Radioactive elements may be selected to study the disposition of specific atoms or ions. The isotopes of iodine (^{125}I and ^{131}I) have been widely used as sodium iodide. Other elements used as inorganic salts include ^{45}Ca, ^{85}Sr, ^{90}Sr, ^{22}Na, ^{18}F, ^{36}Cl, ^{82}Br, ^{80m}Br, ^{203}Hg, ^{65}Zn, ^{109}Cd, ^{75}Se, ^{233}U, ^{204}Tl, ^{137}Cs, ^{160}Tb, ^{166}Ho, ^{169}Yb, ^{144}Ce, ^{147}Pm, and ^{103}Ru. However, where biological interest pertains to organic molecules, the choice of isotopes is limited. The only useful isotopes of organic compounds containing carbon and hydrogen are ^{14}C and ^{3}H. Fortunately, ^{14}C is almost ideal for all applications in autoradiography except those requiring high resolution. In the latter case the very weak emission from ^{3}H is highly suitable. Radioisotopes of oxygen or nitrogen do not have half-lives long enough for autoradiography. For molecules containing sulfur or chlorine, ^{35}S and ^{36}Cl are appropriate labels. Because the energy of the beta particles from ^{35}S and ^{14}C are virtually the same, similar resolution may be obtained. Peptides containing tyrosine may be iodinated with ^{125}I or ^{131}I for autoradiography and retain most of their original biological specificity.

The monoenergetic radiation from ^{125}I is much more useful in autoradiography than the gamma radiation from ^{131}I because the quantized energy from ^{125}I allows the selection of radiant energy levels for different applications. For example, ordinary x-ray film may be used with ^{125}I for resolution comparable to that of ^{14}C; however, thin emulsions may be used to absorb energy only from the electrons of 3 kev and thus allow resolution similar to that of ^{3}H.

The difference in the half-life of ^{45}Ca and that of ^{18}F has enabled a comparison of the distribution of the two isotopes in the same animal (Appelgren, et al., 1961). To detect ^{18}F, autoradiograms were prepared from sections of the animal soon after injection. After allowing a 2-day time interval for decay of the ^{18}F, another set of autoradiograms was prepared from the same sections to detect the ^{45}Ca.

B. Processing of Tissue

The biological material containing the radioactive element must be in close contact with the photographic emulsion. This usually involves a thin section of the tissue. For most isotopes the autoradiographic resolution is better as the section becomes thinner, but this necessitates a longer exposure time. Beta particles from ^3H penetrate only about 1 μ of tissue; thicknesses greater than 1 μ do not shorten the exposure time.

Ordinary histological procedures may be used only for autoradiography where isotopes are incorporated into molecules that are not soluble in alcohol, formalin, etc. Classical examples are nucleosides and amino acids labeled with ^{14}C or ^3H and incorporated into nucleic acids and proteins. The latter are fixed in the tissue by the treatment and consequently the histological solutions do not remove or translocate the compounds.

The situation is entirely different for most drugs, for they are not incorporated into large molecules. Placing tissue in fixing solutions of formalin or osmium, dehydrating in ethanol, and embedding in paraffin or plastic, all involve the risk of translocating soluble compounds to a position other than that which existed *in vivo*. Examination of the fixing or processing solutions for evidence of removal into the solutions of only a small percentage of the isotope offers no assurance that translocation within the tissue has not occurred. The only technique suitable for studying the distribution of drugs is that of freezing the living tissue; sectioning and processing of the frozen tissue must be performed without allowing thawing or the use of any solvents.

C. Application of Photographic Emulsion

The tissue section may be placed in contact with the photographic emulsion by one of several techniques. However, for autoradiography of drugs in tissues, it is absolutely essential that contact of the tissue with any solutions be avoided. Therefore, the technique of floating stripping film on a water bath and dipping the specimen under the film cannot be used. Similarly, coating the specimen with liquid emulsion by brushing, dipping, or from a film within a wire loop, each allows possible translocation of the drug in the specimen.

Apposition of the freeze-dried tissue to x-ray film or a nuclear tract plate is the only alternative for soluble compounds. Separation of the tissue from the photographic plate after exposure simplifies development of the photographic emulsion and staining of the tissue. The drawback is that correlation of the autoradiographic image with the specimen is difficult at higher resolution.

Attachment of the specimen to a dry emulsion such as a nuclear tract plate has been accomplished with limited success. The use of minimal amounts of solvent to facilitate adhesion (Hammarström, *et al.*, 1965) or of solvents that do not dissolve the labeled compound (Masuoka and Placidi, 1968) are the best available compromise for localization at the cellular and subcellular level.

II. TECHNIQUES

A. Whole-Body

The most comprehensive technique currently available for the initial survey of the distribution of a drug is that of whole-body autoradiography. Tissues or fluids which ordinarily would not be sampled can be assessed readily by this method. Furthermore, gradients of concentration within a tissue can be detected; a high concentration in a few cells of a tissue may be obscured by homogenization and analysis of the entire tissue.

The technique of whole-body autoradiography for soluble compounds was developed by Ullberg (1954, 1961, 1965), who has done extensive studies on a wide variety of compounds. An illustrated description of the basic principles has been presented (Waddell and Brinkhous, 1967). The animal receives the labeled drug, is frozen alive and is processed without allowing thawing and without the use of any solvents.

The species of animals used include mice, rats, fish, birds, monkeys, cats, dogs, and human embryos. The most widely used animal has been the mouse, which has the advantages of requiring less isotope and being easier to section.

The animals are anesthetized and then frozen by immersion at various times after administration of the labeled compound in hexane or acetone cooled with dry ice. Since the freezing in the interior of the animals occurs slowly, large ice crystals form within these tissues. Hence, subcellular localization of compounds is not possible.

The selection of times for freezing an animal after injection of a drug must be based on the information available on the rate of elimination of the compound from the animal by metabolism and excretion. In general, a geometric increase in time intervals is most useful. In order to have time intervals for comparison, we routinely have employed freezing times which are approximately multiples of 3, namely 2 minutes, 6.5 minutes, 20 minutes, 1 hour, 3 hours, 9 hours, and 24 hours. In certain cases, rapid elimination of the drug by the kidneys must be circumvented by ligation of the renal pedicles to avoid apparent localization from failure of the agent to reach equilibrium. An example of this is given in Section IV, A for urea-^{14}C in pregnant mice.

The frozen animal is frozen into a block of carboxymethylcellulose ice on the microtome stage. Although the Jung, type K, microtome has been used, the Leitz, model 1300, sledge microtome is more suitable, for its smaller size allows it to be mounted in an ordinary commercial freezer instead of a walk-in freeze room (Waddell and Marlowe, 1969). The microtome stage must be designed for mounting in the vice by the front end of the stage.

Sections from 5 μ to approximately 80 μ thick are taken onto $\times$ 800 Scotch tape (Minnesota Mining & Mfg. Co.). Before removal from the freezer, the sections must be allowed to dry thoroughly so that no ice remains which can melt and allow movement of the isotope. After drying, if covered to prevent condensation of moisture on the sections, the sections may be transferred from the freezer to room temperature.

X-ray films which produce the most satisfactory autoradiograms are Kodak industrial type AA and Gevaert Structurix D-7. Both are fine grain films which have been demonstrated not to produce chemical artifacts. Approximately six times faster, Kodak No Screen and Kodirex may be used for rapid screening and timing of autoradiograms. However, they occasionally produce artifacts and should not be relied on for interpretation. Some investigators have used photographic emulsions such as Ilford G-5, 10 μ thick, pre-applied to glass plates. The increased cost and likelihood of breakage, however, hardly justify the small improvement in resolution for whole-body sections.

Exposure of the photographic emulsion by the radioactivity of the tissue section should be at freezer temperatures to prevent autolysis of the tissue. After exposure of the x-ray film, sections with isotopes which have a long half-life may be placed against fresh x-ray film for additional sets of autoradiograms with either a longer or a shorter exposure time. This procedure is useful for revealing relative concentrations of radioactivity for areas that have either very high or very low concentrations after the first exposure. When no further autoradiograms are needed, the section can be stained with histological dyes to verify localizations of radioactivity.

Compounds that fluoresce under ultraviolet light can be visualized in the tissue sections and their locations recorded with color film. The fluorography and autoradiography of tetracycline compounds have been compared by Blomquist and Hanngren (1968). Whole-body tissue sections can be used for histochemical localizations (Appelgren, 1967) for comparison with the autoradiograms. Furthermore, the areas can be removed, extracted, and the extract chromatographed to identify the chemical nature of the radioactivity revealed by the autoradiogram.

B. Cellular and Subcellular

Although the whole-body technique will allow localization of an increased concentration of an isotope in a tissue or occasionally a cell type, other techniques must be used for single cells and subcellular localization. The method presented by Hammarström et al. (1965) uses ⚹ 688 Scotch tape for collecting the sections. A nuclear tract plate is prepared by dipping the plate in a 12% solution of glycerine in absolute ethyl alcohol and allowing it to drain for 10 minutes in a vertical position before approximating the section on tape. After the emulsion is exposed, soaking in xylene removes the tape but leaves the section attached to the nuclear tract plate. The Ilford G-5 nuclear tract plates with 10 μ emulsions are most satisfactory. The increased resolution gained by the finer grained Ilford K and L emulsions is warranted only for tissues that are well preserved and relatively free of ice crystal artifacts. Kodak NTB emulsions seem to produce more pressure artifacts than the Ilford plates.

Comparison of various techniques of autoradiography for diffusible compounds by Stumpf and Roth (1966) clearly demonstrates that no solutions can be used in processing the tissue. These investigators have dried thin sections of liver and uterus at temperatures below $-60°C$. These freeze-dried sections were dry mounted on microscope slides which had been precoated with either Kodak NTB-3 or NTB-10 emulsion. Other techniques which thawed the frozen section, embedded the tissue in paraffin or dipped the section in liquid emulsion were demonstrated to translocate diffusible compounds. Many other similar attempts have been and are currently being made to localize diffusible compounds by autoradiography at the electron microscope level. For a summary, the proceedings of a recent conference may be consulted (Roth, 1969).

III. FUNCTIONAL LOCALIZATIONS

A. Water Compartments

The water compartments classically defined as extracellular water and total tissue water may be visualized in whole-body, sagittal sections of mice injected

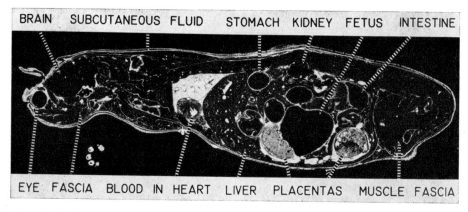

BRAIN   SUBCUTANEOUS FLUID   STOMACH KIDNEY FETUS   INTESTINE

EYE FASCIA BLOOD IN HEART   LIVER   PLACENTAS   MUSCLE FASCIA

Fig. 24.1. An autoradiogram of a whole-body, 20 μ section of a pregnant mouse that received inulin-carboxyl-^{14}C intravenously 1 hour prior to freezing. The renal pedicles had been ligated prior to injection. White areas correspond to radioactivity.

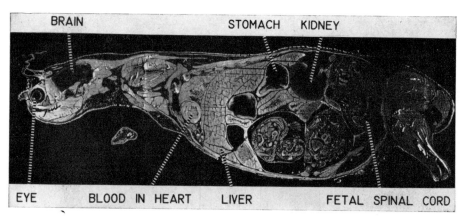

BRAIN   STOMACH   KIDNEY

EYE   BLOOD IN HEART   LIVER   FETAL SPINAL CORD

Fig. 24.2. An autoradiogram of a whole-body, 20 μ section of a pregnant mouse that received urea-^{14}C intravenously 1 hr prior to freezing. The renal pedicles had been ligated prior to injection. White areas correspond to radioactivity.

with inulin-carboxyl-^{14}C or urea-^{14}C. Figure 24.1 is an autoradiogram of a pregnant mouse whose kidneys were ligated before the intravenous injection of inulin-carboxyl-^{14}C. The animal was frozen 1 hour after the injection. The kidneys were ligated to prevent renal elimination and thus allow for equilibrium of the compound in the extracellular water. Note that inulin of any detectable amount did not cross the placenta into the fetus during this time. The thin, fine lines along the fascial planes in the muscle are visual indication of the inhomogeneity of the extracellular water in muscle tissue. The line beneath the skin corresponds to the subcutaneous layer of water around the body. Figure 24.2 is a whole-body autoradiogram of a section from a mouse whose kidneys had been ligated prior to the intravenous injection of urea-^{14}C. The animal was frozen 1 hour after injection. Radioactivity clearly appears in the fetus and is relatively uniform throughout the body. Notice, however, the limited penetration into the brain and spinal cord of mother and fetus.

Another compound that has been used for the estimation of total body water

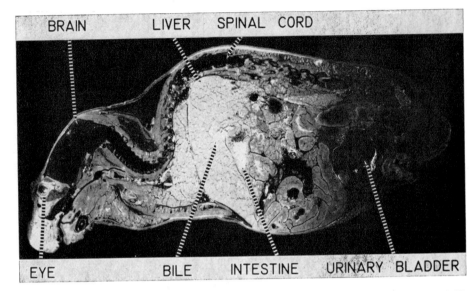

Fig. 24.3. An autoradiogram of a whole-body, 20 μ section of a mouse that received N-(acetyl-^{14}C)-4-aminoantipyrine intravenously 1 hr prior to freezing. The renal pedicles had been ligated prior to injection. White areas correspond to radioactivity.

is N-acetyl-4-aminoantipyrine. Figure 24.3 is a whole-body autoradiogram of a mouse that received N-(acetyl-^{14}C)-4-aminoantipyrine intravenously 1 hour prior to freezing. The kidneys had been ligated prior to injection to prevent renal elimination of the compound. The high concentration of the compound in the bile and upper intestine reveals biliary secretion which had not been heretofore suspected. The small percentage eliminated by this route apparently does not invalidate it as an indicator of total body water. The limited penetration into the central nervous system is quite similar to that of urea.

B. pH Gradients

The increased localization of compounds in tissues and areas can be due to pH gradients which exist between these areas or tissues when the drug of interest is a weak acid or a weak base. An example of this is the weak acid, 5,5-dimethyl-2,4-oxazolidinedione (DMO), which is not metabolized and which has been demonstrated to distribute according to pH gradients (Waddell and Butler, 1959). Figure 24.4 is a whole-body autoradiogram of a mouse that was given DMO-^{14}C intravenously 1 hour prior to freezing. The animal's kidneys were ligated prior to administration of the compound. Readily seen is a higher concentration of the compound in the fetuses than in the tissues of the mother. Also, the periphery of the lens of the eye and the retina have a higher concentration of the compound than other tissues. Comparison of the distribution of DMO in the eye with the distribution of urea in the eye suggests that more DMO is present than can be accounted for by the water content. This may be due either to an increased alkalinity of the retina and the lens or an increased alkalinity of the vitreous humor. A high concentration of a compound in a fluid filled cavity sometimes results in migration of the compound to the lining of the cavity during the freeze-drying process. This possibly could have occurred, causing

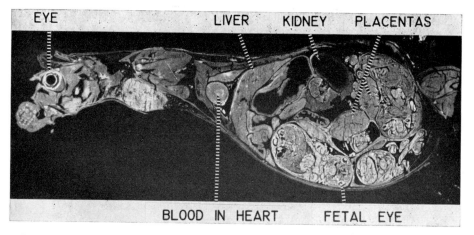

Fig. 24.4. An autoradiogram of a whole-body, 80 μ section of a pregnant mouse that received 5,5-dimethyl-2,4-oxazolidinedione-2-¹⁴C 1 hr prior to freezing. The renal pedicles had been ligated prior to injection. White areas correspond to radioactivity.

DMO to migrate to the periphery of the lens and retina from the vitreous humor of the eye. The distribution of the bases nicotine (Andersson *et al.*, 1965), mepivacaine (Kristerson *et al.*, 1965), and atropine (Albanus *et al.*, 1968) to pH gradients has been demonstrated. These bases accumulate in a high concentration in the urine and stomach.

C. Fat Solubility

The very high solubility of some compounds in body fat is clearly seen in whole-body autoradiograms of mice that had received DDT-¹⁴C and dieldrin-¹⁴C (Bäckström, *et al.*, 1965) and thiopental-¹⁴C (Cassano, *et al.*, 1967).

D. Specific Affinities

The remarkable, selective localization of vitamin A in the retina of the eye (Ullberg, 1965) and of dihydroxyphenylalanine in the adrenal medulla (Ullberg, 1961) are striking examples of a technique that may provide leads to biochemical mechanisms.

E. Metabolism

Most compounds that have been investigated by whole-body autoradiography have been found to exhibit radioactivity in the liver. Metabolic conversion of the administered compound and accumulation of the products in the liver undoubtedly account for this activity. Occasionally, secretion by the liver of the parent compound or its metabolic product is so efficient that, instead of a high activity in the liver, only an increased concentration in the bile may be seen. Figure 24.5 is an example of how the technique may be used to reveal secretion of a compound by the liver into the bile of a fetus in utero. This is an autoradiogram of a pregnant mouse at 17.5 days of gestation that received phenobarbital-¹⁴C 24 hours before freezing. The secretion of radioactivity into the bile and small intestine of the fetus is clearly apparent.

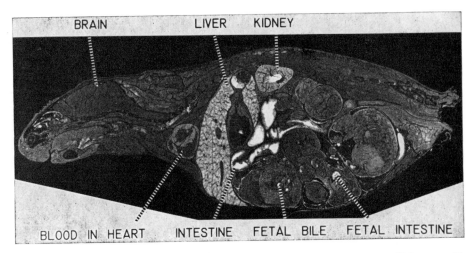

Fig. 24.5. An autoradiogram of a whole-body, 40 μ section of a pregnant C57 mouse 24 hr after intravenous injection of phenobarbital-^{14}C. White areas correspond to radioactivity.

IV. DECEPTIVE LOCALIZATIONS

A. Equilibrium Kinetics

If the concentration of a compound in the blood is changing rapidly because of renal excretion, metabolism, elimination by the lungs, or rapid accumulation in some compartment, there is no opportunity for the agent to equilibrate with tissues whose rate of exchange with blood is slow. In such tissues early after injection, the concentration in the blood is higher than that in the tissue. Later, the relative concentrations are reversed. What the concentration ratio for such tissues would be between the tissue and blood at equilibrium is not known. It cannot be assumed that the concentration ratio would have been unity. The time course of distribution of urea-^{14}C in pregnant mice is an example of such distribution behavior (Waddell, 1968). At early times after injection there is very little or no radioactivity in the brain, eye, spinal cord, and fetus of the mouse. At later times the concentration is approximately equal to that in other tissues, and at even later times after injection the concentration is much higher than that in other tissues. The rapid elimination of urea by the kidney together with slow equilibrium with the fetus, brain, and spinal cord results in information that may lead to erroneous conclusions.

B. Transfer of Label

Figure 24.6 is an autoradiogram of a rat that was hypophysectomized when 20 days old and that received insulin-^{125}I every 12 hours for 4 injections. The last injection was 12 hours prior to freezing. Virtually the only radioactivity in the entire animal is seen in the thyroid gland, concentrated there after removal from the insulin.

Figure 24.7 is an autoradiogram of a rat that was hypophysectomized when 20 days old and that received an injection of human growth hormone labeled with ^{125}I every 12 hours for 4 injections. The final injection was given 12 hours

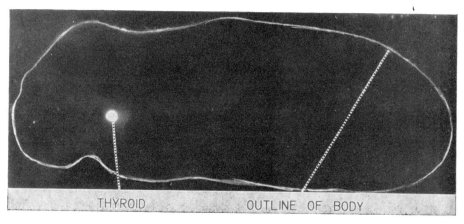

THYROID   OUTLINE OF BODY

Fig. 24.6. An autoradiogram of a whole-body, 20 μ section of a rat that was hypophysec-tomized when 20 days old and that was frozen 12 hr after the last of 4 injections of insulin-^{125}I at 12 hr intervals. Except for the outline of the body, white areas correspond to radio-activity. The approximate position of the body was outlined with ink.

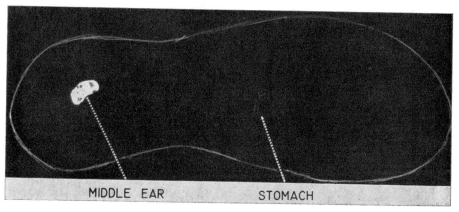

MIDDLE EAR   STOMACH

Fig. 24.7. An autoradiogram of a whole-body, 20 μ section of a rat that was hypophysec-tomized when 20 days old and that was frozen 12 hr after the last of 4 injections of human growth hormone-^{125}I at 12 hr intervals. Except for the outline of the body, white areas cor-respond to radioactivity. The approximate position of the body was outlined with ink.

prior to freezing. Aside from a minimal amount in the stomach, the only radio-activity in the body was in a discrete area within the head, which was finally identified as the middle ear. Further investigation of the tissue revealed a middle ear infection with *Pseudomonas* apparently resulting from the hypophysectomy. The logical conclusion to make is that the ^{125}I was being removed from the human growth hormone at a rate or in a manner different from its removal from insulin.

Metabolism of compounds containing ^{14}C to $^{14}CO_2$ results in release of most of the radioactive CO_2 into the atmosphere. A small percentage of the radioactivity is retained in the animal primarily in bone, liver, pancreas, intes-tine, kidney, salivary gland, retina and sclera of the animal. (Waddell *et al.*, 1969).

Acknowledgments

The assistance of Miss Carolyn Marlowe is gratefully acknowledged.
Supported in part by National Institutes of Health Grants CA-5323, CA-07056
and DE-02668.

REFERENCES

Albanus, L., Hammarström, L., Sundwall, A., Ullberg, S., and Vangbo, B.: Distribution and metabolism of H³-atropine in mice. Acta physiol. Scand. *73:* 447–456, 1968.

Andersson, G., Hansson, E., and Schmiterlöw, C. G.: Gastric excretion of C¹⁴-nicotine. Experientia *21:* 211–217, 1965.

Appelgren, L.-E.: Sites of steroid hormone formation; autoradiographic studies using labelled precursors. Acta physiol. Scand. Suppl. *301:* 1–108, 1967.

Appelgren, L.-E., Ericsson, Y., and Ullberg, S.: A comparison of the distribution of radioactive fluorine and calcium by use of double-isotope autoradiography. Acta physiol. Scand. *53:* 339–347, 1961.

Bäckström, J., Hansson, E., and Ullberg, S.: Distribution of C¹⁴-DDT and C¹⁴-dieldrin in pregnant mice determined by whole-body autoradiography. Toxicol. Appl. Pharmacol. *7:* 90–96, 1965.

Blomquist, L. and Hanngren, Å.: Whole-body autoradiography and fluorography of two tetracycline compounds in tumor-bearing mice. Acta Med. Scand. *184:* 1–11, 1968.

Cassano, G. B., Ghetti, B., Gliozzi, E., and Hansson, E.: Autoradiographic distribution study of "short acting" and "long acting" barbiturates: ³⁵S - thiopentone and ¹⁴C-phenobarbitone. Brit. J. Anaesth. *39:* 11–20, 1967.

Hammarström, L., Appelgren, L.-E., and Ullberg, S.: Improved method for light microscopy autoradiography with isotopes in water-soluble form. Exp. Cell Res. *37:* 608–613, 1965.

Kristerson, L., Hoffman, P., and Hansson, E.: Fate of mepivacaine in the body: 1. Whole-body autoradiographic studies of the distribution of ¹⁴C-labelled mepivacaine in mice. Acta Pharmacol. Toxicol. *22:* 205–212, 1965.

Masuoka, D. and Placidi, G.-F.: A combined procedure for the histochemical fluorescence demonstration of monoamines and microautoradiography of water-soluble drugs. J. Histochem. Cytochem. *16:* 659–662, 1968.

Roth, L. J., and Stumpf, W. E., editors: *International Conference on High Resolution Autoradiography of Diffusible Substances.* Academic Press, New York, 1969.

Stumpf, W. E. and Roth, L. J.: High resolution autoradiography with dry mounted, freeze-dried frozen sections; comparative study of six methods using two diffusible compounds ³H-estradiol and ³H-mesobilirubinogen. J. Histochem. Cytochem. *14:* 274–287, 1966.

Ullberg, S.: Studies on the distribution and fate of S³⁵-labelled benzylpenicillin in the body. Acta Radiol. (Stockholm), Suppl. *118:* 1–110, 1954.

Ullberg, S.: Autoradiographic localization in the tissues of drugs and metabolites. In *Proceedings of the First Pharmacological Meeting*, Vol. 5, p. 29, Pergamon Press, Oxford, 1961.

Ullberg, S.: Specific localization of labelled hormones and vitamins; whole-body autoradiographic observations. In *Isotopes in Experimental Pharmacology*, Chap. 6, p. 63, Univ. of Chicago Press, Chicago, 1965.

Waddell, W. J.: Distribution of urea-¹⁴C in pregnant mice studied by whole-body autoradiography. J. Appl. Physiol. *24:* 828–831, 1968.

Waddell, W. J. and Brinkhous, W. K.: The Ullberg technique of whole body autoradiography. J. Biol. Photographic Assoc. *35:* 147–154, 1967.

Waddell, W. J. and Butler, T. C.: Calculation of intracellular pH from the distribution of 5,5-dimethyl-2,4-oxazolidinedione (DMO). Application to skeletal muscle of the dog. J. Clin. Invest. *38:* 720–729, 1959.

Waddell, W. J. and Marlowe, C.: A hydraulic powered microtome in a commercial freezer: an improved cryostat for large sections. Stain Technol. *44:* 81–85, 1969.

Waddell, W. J., Ullberg, S., and Marlowe, C.: Localization of the bicarbonate and carbonate pools by whole-body autoradiography. Arch. Internatl. Physiol. Biochim. *77:* 1–9, 1969.

25

Application of Computers in Drug Metabolism Studies

THOMAS N. TOZER

I. INTRODUCTION

Two different approaches might be taken in discussing the application of computers in drug metabolism studies. One approach involves the use of a computer in data processing, including programming techniques and correlation of data. Another approach is that of the developing and testing of hypotheses or models. It would take more than one chapter to discuss the art and science of programming computers and the use of computers in data analysis; consequently, the second approach will be used in discussing the application of computers to drug metabolism.

In addition to quantitating the time course of the absorption, metabolism and general disposition of drugs, it is important to know how drugs pass membranes, how they are metabolized and the nature of the enzymatic reactions, how protein- or tissue-binding influences drug disposition, the nature of the excretion processes, the relationship between dose or concentration and the biological response, the nature and degree of contribution of biliary excretion, etc. Knowledge of these processes is often achieved by building and testing models. These models require a correlation of data, but more importantly they often provide a basis for prediction, help to identify areas of incomplete information, and suggest additional experiments. Computational methods involving model building and testing rather than data processing will be emphasized in this chapter.

II. METHODS OF COMPUTATION

A. Computation in Drug Metabolism Studies

The word *computation* conveys an impression of a numerical or discrete type of operation such as the addition, subtraction, multiplication and division of numbers. Computation may also be a continuous process, which is perhaps a more natural one. For example, unless one wants to count molecules, the processes of drug absorption, metabolism, distribution and excretion can best be thought of as continuous. Thus, there are two distinct methods of computation and two distinct types of computers as well. Numerical computation developed from an extension of the idea of finger counting. Consequently, devices for this purpose are called *digital* computers, simple adding machines as well as the complex electronic digital computers. Continuous computation is accomplished by the use of devices whose physical quantities are capable of being made analogous to the physical characteristics of a system under study. Analog computers include such devices as a slide rule, mechanical and hydraulic analogs as well as electronic analog computers.

The choice of a computational method is naturally going to depend on the nature of the problem to be solved. For determining the line of best fit of data or for statistical procedures in general, the digital computer has the greatest application. This is because the data are usually of the discrete type and, therefore, require numerical computation. However, the establishment of a model and the assessment of its consequences are best accomplished using analog computation.

Parts I and II of this book describe many complexities in drug absorption, distribution, metabolism and excretion that one might observe in the whole body following an oral or intravenous administration of a drug or in isolated systems. The analog computer offers certain unique advantages to solving these potentially complex problems in drug absorption and disposition and, therefore, will be the principal subject of this chapter.

B. Advantages and Disadvantages to the Use of Analog and Digital Computers

As stated before, the analog computer is essentially a continuous device, whereas the digital computer operates with discrete numbers. To solve certain problems by numerical methods involves approximation of continuous functions The use of compiler routines to aid in the solution of differential equations has made the digital computer competitive with the analog computer, particularly when the model is very complex. The principal disadvantages of digital computation are unit cost of a solution and the relatively slow speed of computation for some problems, limiting their use in real-time simulation. The unquestionable advantage of the digital computer is its high precision; another is its memory, i.e., storage of information. Analog devices leave something to be desired as precise computing aids. Accuracy in analog computation is seldom better than 0.2% of the maximum value of a variable. In drug metabolism studies this source of computation error is usually much smaller than assay and biological errors and is, therefore, of little significance.

The ability of the analog computer to rapidly provide a graphical plot of a problem solution on an X-Y recorder or to repetitively display the solution on an oscilloscope is of greatest advantage. Digital plotters provide a similar capability for the digital computer, but the cost of operation may be much greater and the operation is, of course, much slower. If a predetermined set of computer runs can be specified, the digital computer may be preferred. However, if human judgment is required in setting up parameters to be tried, the analog computer is the most economical tool to use. Such is the usual case in model building.

Many of the advantages of both the digital and analog computers have been combined in "hybrid" computers, a topic beyond the intended scope of this presentation. For further information see Bekey and Karplus (1969).

C. Capability of the Analog Computer

The analog computer can be used to solve mathematical problems or to construct a physical model of a system under study. In the latter case the machine variables are directly analogous to the variables of the physical (or biological or chemical) system. These two uses of the analog computer involve, in the first instance, the solution of mathematical models and, in the second, the use of the machine as a simulator. Herein, by the author's bias, lies the most useful application of the analog computer in drug metabolism.

The distinction between using the analog computer for simulation, i.e., development of a model or using it for solution of a mathematical model is most often a fine one. One person may formulate a complete mathematical model of his system and then solve it on the analog computer; another individual studying the same system may directly instrument the basic relationships known about his system without the intermediate steps of developing a mathematical model. Models obtained by simulating them on the analog computer are readily changed and tested. Thus, the analog computer is well-suited for fitting a model to a system.

III. DEVELOPMENT OF MODELS IN DRUG METABOLISM

The real world, particularly the biological world, is very complex. Quantitative information and understanding of the real world comes about primarily from studies of an isolated system. Prediction of the behavior of the system is usually best obtained by establishing a model which allows one to draw conclusions about reality. It does not directly prove reality, but when consistent with all established knowledge in reality, the model is termed valid and is very useful. The rule of thumb here is that the model should be only as complex as is necessary to be consistent with all observed behavior of the physical (or biological) system. There are many types of models; the three most common, as shown in Fig. 25.1, are: (1) symbolic model, (2) mathematical model, and (3) physical model.

The symbols in a symbolic model in drug metabolism studies might represent distinct chemical entities, the drug and its metabolites, or they might represent a given compound which behaves as though it were transferred between separate communicating compartments. The model represents a pictorial view of the system in a flow or block diagram. The reader is referred to the book by Riggs (1963) for a further insight into the meaning of compartments and for a general mathematical approach to biological problems.

The development of a mathematical model requires a reasonable facility with mathematics. This model is simply a collection of mathematical statements; it usually involves a set of simultaneous differential equations which describe the behavior and inter-relationships among variables in a system. In the mathematical model in Figure 25.1, the differential equations represent the relationships between rates of transfer (or metabolism) and the amounts of the drug and metabolites in various compartments. Testing of the model will determine whether the relationships and the basic model itself are adequate to quantitate and predict the real system.

Physical models are often used to simplify the real system or to scale down

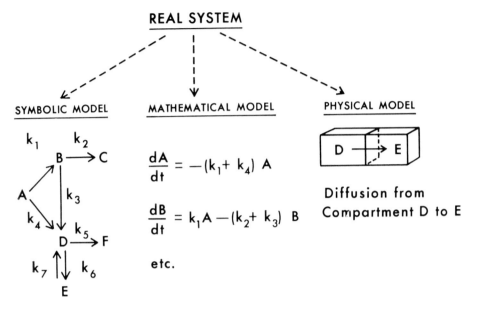

Fig. 25.1. Common models of a real system.

the real system for easy measurement. The use of synthetic membranes to simulate the passage of drugs across a biological membrane barrier is an example of the former type of physical model. Placing a small model airplane in a wind tunnel might be an example of the latter.

Establishing a pharmacokinetic model for the metabolism and disposition of a drug may be approached from two directions. An empirical approach is one in which experimental data are fitted by an empirical equation to describe a relationship between observed variables; nothing is implied about the underlying reasons for the relationship. For example, alcohol may be observed to disappear from the plasma by a constant rate, independent of the plasma concentration; however, the relationship does not indicate why this is so. The other approach is theoretical. It is not derived from experimental observations but rather from a hypothesis about the fundamental nature of a system. One might make the hypothesis for example that only the unbound (not protein bound) form of a drug in the plasma may undergo metabolism in the liver and thereby compute the effect of protein binding on drug disposition. The advantage of a theoretical approach is that, in addition to demonstrating the relationships between sets of data, this approach may explain why observed relationships exist. The theoretical approach to model building also often suggests a host of relationships to be tested.

It is important to realize that a model is not an end in itself. It serves as a basis to explain observations or to formulate a hypothesis. Every assumption and simplification that goes into the model should be stated explicitly. It was stated above that the simplest model is the best. This should be qualified in that there is a danger of oversimplification leading to easy mathematical analysis which may be so unrealistic as to be misleading of the real system. At the other extreme is a model which may be so hopelessly complex as to be incomprehensible or involve an inordinate amount of time for analysis.

IV. ANALOG COMPUTER COMPONENTS AND FUNCTIONS

Programming an electronic analog computer requires no special training in electronics. A minimal background in mathematics is, of course, necessary. A number of books are available on the use of analog computers (Johnson, 1964; Peterson, 1967; Jackson, 1960; Korn and Korn, 1964; Fifer, 1961). The applications given in these texts are primarily in the field of engineering. However, simulation crosses all fields of science; indeed, wherever a dynamic system is studied, the analog computer may be useful. There are only a relatively few major types of components in an electronic analog computer. The brief descriptions shown in Table 25.1 define the major operational components and show how they can be used to perform ordinary mathematical operations.

With these components essentially all mathematical operations can be accomplished. Differentiation may also be carried out. However, this is a "noise"-amplifying process, and since there are various sources of electronic noise, this procedure should be avoided. The real contribution of the analog computer in computation is in solving simultaneous differential equations.

V. SELECTED EXAMPLES OF THE APPLICATION OF ANALOG COMPUTATION TO DRUG METABOLISM STUDIES

The principal purpose of this section is to demonstrate the usefulness of analog computation in drug disposition studies, not to review or summarize the

TABLE 25.1
Analog computer components and function

Component	Symbol	Mathematical function	Comments
1. Inverter		Multiplication by -1 $x = -a$	For inversion of sign
2. Summer		Algebraic Addition $x = -(10a + 2b - c)$	Output is the algebraic sum of the inputs with sign reversal
3. Integrator		Integration $x = -\int a dt$	Input voltage is integrated with respect to time
4. Attenuator		Multiply by a constant $x = ka$	
5. Multiplier		Multiplication $x = -a.b$	Product of two variables
6. Divider		Division $x = -(a/b)$	Quotient of two variables
7. Function Generator		Square, square root, logarithm, exponential, sine, cosine, etc. $x = -f(a)$	Any function can be generated

applications of this computational method in the literature. A few other references have been selected to give the reader an idea of the types of problems related to drug metabolism that have been simulated by analog computation (Beckett *et al.*, 1968; Garrett *et al.*, 1960; Cohen *et al.*, 1965; Wagner and Alway, 1964; Garrett *et al.*, 1967; Schlender and Krüger-Thiemer, 1965; Garrett and Alway, 1964; Ballard and Goyan, 1966; Krüger-Thiemer *et al.*, 1964; Garrett *et al.*, 1963; Beckett and Tucker, 1968).

A. Kinetics of Metabolism, Distribution and Excretion of Acetylsalicylic Acid (ASA) and Salicylic Acid (SA)

Rowland and Riegelman (1968) studied the pharmacokinetics of ASA and SA following a single intravenous administration in man. On administering each drug the results could be adequately explained by proposing a two-compartmental open-system model for each drug. Such a model might symbolically be represented by Figure 25.2. Compartments 1 and 2 are respectively the central (where drug is administered and sampled) and tissue compartment; k_{12} and k_{21} are the transfer rate constants between the two compartments and k_{13} is the elimination rate constant.

Salicylic acid is essentially the only metabolite of ASA following its i.v. administration. ASA is very rapidly distributed into tissues and metabolized to SA; SA, on the other hand, is much more slowly eliminated from the plasma. The question arises as to how to interpret the kinetics of SA plasma levels following the intravenous administration of ASA. Several alternative models were proposed in which ASA hydrolysis to SA might occur in the "tissue" ASA compartment or in both central and tissue ASA compartments. A model was also proposed for a single SA compartment following ASA administration. Fitting the data to the computer curves allowed for only one of the models, *viz.*, that in which the drug and its metabolite are each distributed in two compartments and metabolism of ASA takes place only in the central compartment. Anatomically the compartments are undefined; the derived model, however, gives a much clearer understanding of the pharmacokinetics of ASA and SA in man. The authors give a word of caution, however; since the model was based on a single dose level of the drug, the model has not been completely tested. More information is needed before the model can be said to adequately describe the data for all dosage levels. Such a model immediately gives great insight into the distribution, metabolism and excretion of both ASA and SA.

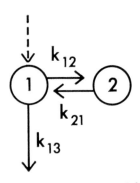

Fig. 25.2. I.V. administration of drug.

B. Vitamin B₁₂ Kinetics in Man

Another study showing the application of the analog computer is that of Reizenstein *et al.* (1966) on Vitamin B_{12} kinetics in man. Equations corresponding to the experimental data curves were obtained with an analog computer and the simplest compatible model was selected. Three compartments were required to fit the whole body and plasma clearance of intravenously injected radiocyanobalamin. One compartment was apparently intracellular and accounted for over 99% of body B_{12}. These kinetic studies have important implications on total-body B_{12}, human daily B_{12} requirements, and Vitamin B_{12} metabolism in disease.

C. Time- and Dose-Response Relationships of the Inhibition of 5-Hydroxyindoleacetic Acid Transport from the Brain by Probenecid

Dose-response relationships are commonly determined by measuring the response to various doses at a given time point; time-response by measuring the response at various times after a given dose. Thus, dose-response relationships are dependent on the time point chosen and time-response are dependent on the dose used. The following example is one on which the author is currently working (unpublished) and one which, it is believed, demonstrates the application of the analog computer in developing a model which can be used to correlate biological response with the tissue concentration of a drug *in vivo*. The correlation is unique in that it is independent of dose and time.

Previous studies (Neff and Tozer, 1968) have shown a number of compounds, including probenecid, to block the transport system for the elimination of 5-hydroxyindoleacetic acid (5HIAA) from the brain in rats. When essentially complete inhibition of the transport is maintained by repeated administration of large doses of probenecid. The levels of 5HIAA are observed to increase linearly with time at a rate equal to the rate of synthesis (Neff *et al.*, 1967). After a single dose of the inhibitor, the 5HIAA levels increase, reach a maximum value and then return to the normal steady-state value (time-response). With a larger dose the maximum level reached is higher and occurs at a later time, although the initial rate of increase is virtually the same for all large doses. In order to determine a dose-response relationship, the level of 5HIAA is determined at a given time following various doses. There is a maximum amount that can be accumulated in a given time, which rate is the synthesis rate. It immediately becomes apparent from the time-response that the determination of the dose of the inhibitor ID_{50} resulting in 50% of the maximum accumulation of 5HIAA is a function of the time chosen.

In order to quantitate the inhibition of transport with respect to time and dose, a tentative model was proposed. This model is primarily based on the hypothesis that the inhibitor competes for a carrier in the 5HIAA transport system by analogy to competitive enzyme inhibition kinetics. Furthermore, it is assumed that the uninhibited transport rate of 5HIAA is always proportional to the level of 5HIAA, i.e., the substrate level remains far below the level of saturation.

Using the hypotheses and assumptions above a symbolic model for the *in vivo* inhibition is established as shown in Fig. 25.3. The basic equations used in setting up a mathematical model (Fig. 25.3) are: (1) differential equation relat-

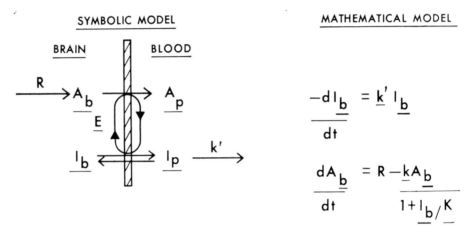

SYMBOLIC MODEL   MATHEMATICAL MODEL

Fig. 25.3. Model for inhibition of 5HIAA transport. Symbols: R, constant rate of synthesis; A_b, 5HIAA in brain; A_p, 5HIAA in blood; I_b, inhibitor in brain; I_p, inhibitor in plasma; E, the enzyme-like carrier involved; k^1, elimination rate constant for inhibitor; K, the inhibition equilibrium constant; k, rate constant for uninhibited transport of A_b.

ing the rate of disappearance of the inhibitor with the inhibitor concentration and (2) an equation of material balance which states that the rate of change of the 5HIAA level with time is a result of the net difference between the rate of synthesis and the rate of transport out of the brain. The rate of transport is assumed to be competitively dependent on the inhibitor concentration. The value of the rate constant k, for the disappearance of probenecid in brain is experimentally determined as well as the rate of synthesis R and the rate constant k for the uninhibited transport of 5HIAA.

The computer diagram (refer to Table 25.1 for the mathematical operations) for the model is shown in Fig. 25.4. The only unknown is that of the ratio of the initial inhibitor concentration I_b^0 to the inhibition equilibrium constant K. However, I_b^0 is also experimentally determined, leaving only K to be tested. The consequences of the model are readily observed for various values of the

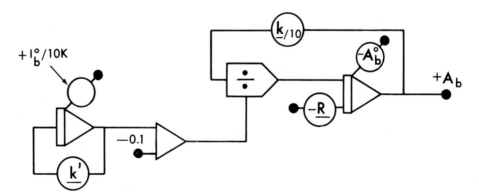

Fig. 25.4. Computer diagram for transport inhibition model. A_b^0 is the steady-state value of 5HIAA before giving inhibitor and $I_b^0/10K$ is an assigned value for the ratio of the initial inhibitor concentration to the inhibition equilibrium constant. Other symbols are defined in Fig. 25.3.

ratio. The only operation now required is to adjust the ratio so that the computer solution fits the experimental data.

At the present time the model has been tested for two doses of probenecid and the unpublished results indicate the validity of the model, both in terms of duplicating the 5HIAA levels with time after each of the doses and in obtaining the same value of K. Furthermore, the concentration of the inhibitor giving 50% of the maximum accumulation of 5HIAA at two hours is in good agreement with the K value from the computer solution.

One of the most interesting aspects of this model is that only a single dose is required to establish the K value for the inhibitor *in vivo* and, furthermore, in contrast to the usual method of determining dose response, the value of K (compared to the ID_{50}) is independent of time, i.e., does not depend on the rate of metabolism of the inhibitor nor on the time chosen to observe the net accumulation of 5HIAA.

VI. SELECTED REFERENCES TO THE APPLICATION OF DIGITAL COMPUTERS

Description of the capability and performance of both analog and digital computers without adequate attention to methodology and problem formulation presents an incomplete and unsatisfactory picture. Unfortunately such is the case in this chapter. Emphasis has been given to only one aspect of computer usage, *viz.*, that of model building and testing in drug metabolism studies. Digital computers offer a number of capabilities that have not been discussed here. For this reason a few selected references are given to the application of digital computers in biomedical and biological problems so that the reader may further pursue the topic. Problems related to drug metabolism are included as well as other problems using computational techniques also of value in drug metabolism studies. The selected references are: (1) Computers and Biomedical Research (Journal currently in Vol. *2*); (2) Symposium: Computers in Medicine, Journal of Chronic Diseases, *19:* No. 4, 1966; (3) Rochester Conference on Data Acquisition and Processing in Biology and Medicine, 1961-; (4) Proceedings of the San Diego Symposium for Biomedical Engineering, 1961-; and (5) Stacey, R. W. and Waxman, B. D.: *Computers in Biomedical Research*, Academic Press, New York, 1965.

In closing, it is hoped that this chapter has given the reader some appreciation of the application of both analog and digital computers in drug metabolism studies. Although emphasis has been placed on modeling for which the analog computer is well-suited, it should be reemphasized that analog methods must be placed in perspective to one's computational needs.

REFERENCES

Ballard, B. E. and Goyan, J. E.: Application of analog computer techniques to *in vivo* drug kinetic studies. Med. Biol. Engng. *4:* 483–490, 1966.

Beckett, A. H., Boyes, R. N., and Triggs, E. J.: Kinetics of buccal absorption of amphetamines. J. Pharm. Pharmac. *20:* 92–97, 1968.

Beckett, A. H. and Tucker, G. T.: Application of the analogue computer to pharmacokinetic and biopharmaceutical studies with amphetamine-type compounds. J. Pharm. Pharmac. *20:* 174–193, 1968.

Bekey, G. A. and Karplus, W. J.: *Hybrid Computation.* Wiley-Interscience, New York, 1969.

Cohen, E. N., Corbascio, A., and Fleischli, G.: The distribution and fate of *d*-tubocurarine. J. Pharmacol. Exp. Ther. *147:* 120–129, 1965.

Fifer, S.: *Analogue Computation: Theory, Techniques and Applications* (four vols.). McGraw-Hill, New York, 1961.

Garrett, E. R., Thomas, R. C., Wallach, D. P., and Alway, C. D.: Psicofuranine: kinetics and mechanisms *in vivo* with the application of the analog computer. J. Pharmacol. Exp. Ther. *130:* 106–118, 1960.

Garrett, E. R., Johnston, R. L., and Collins, E. J.: Kinetics of steroid effects on Ca⁴⁷ dynamics in dogs with the analog computer, II. J. Pharm. Sci. *52:* 668–678, 1963.

Garrett, E. R. and Alway, C. D.: Drug distribution and dosage: complex pharmacokinetic models and the analog computer. IIIrd International Congress of Chemotherapy, Stuttgart (1963) *2:* 1666–1686, 1964.

Garrett, E. R., Agren, A. J., and Lambert, H. J.: Pharmacokinetic analysis of receptor site models in multicompartmental systems. Int. J. Clin. Pharmacol. Ther. Tox. *1:* 1–14, 1967.

Jackson, A. S.: *Analog Computation.* McGraw-Hill, New York, 1960.

Johnson, C. L.: *Analog Computer Techniques* (2nd Ed.) McGraw-Hill, New York, 1964.

Korn, G. A. and Korn, T. M.: *Electronic Analog and Hybrid Computers.* McGraw-Hill, New York, 1964.

Krüger-Thiemer, E., Diller, W., Dettli, L., Bünger, P., and Seydel, J.: Demonstration des Einflusses der Eiweissbindung und der Ionisation auf die Pharmakokinetik am kombinierten gaskinetischen Modell nach van't Hoff und Langmuir. Antibiotica et Chemotherapia *12:* 171–193, 1964.

Neff, N. H., Tozer, T. N., and Brodie, B. B.: Application of steady-state kinetics to studies of the transfer of 5-hydroxyindoleacetic acid from brain to plasma. J. Pharmacol. Exp. Ther. *158:* 214–218, 1967.

Neff, N. H. and Tozer, T. N.: *In vivo* measurement of brain serotonin turnover. Adv. Pharmacol. *6A:* 97–109, 1968.

Peterson, G. R.: *Basic Analog Computation.* Macmillan, New York, 1967.

Reizenstein, P., Ek, G., and Matthews, C. M. E.: Vitamin B₁₂ kinetics in man. Implications on total-body-B₁₂-determinations, human requirements, and normal and pathological B₁₂ uptake. Phys. Med. Biol. *2:* 295–306, 1966.

Riggs, D. S.: *The Mathematical Approach to Physiological Problems,* Williams and Wilkins, Baltimore, 1963. (Reprinted by M. I. T. Press, 1970).

Rowland, M. and Riegelman, S.: Pharmacokinetics of acetylsalicylic acid and salicylic acid after intravenous administration in man. J. Pharm. Sci. *57:* 1313–1319, 1968.

Schlender, Von B. and Krüger-Thiemer, E.: Rechenautomaten und pharmakotherapie. Pharmakotherapie *2:* 1–30, 1965.

Tozer, T. N., Neff, N. H., and Brodie, B. B.: Application of steady-state kinetics to the synthesis rate and turnover time of serotonin in the brain of normal and reserpine-treated rats. J. Pharmacol. Exp. Ther. *153:* 177–182, 1966.

Wagner, J. G. and Alway, C. D.: Prediction of multiple dose serum levels of Lincocin from single dose serum levels when Lincocin (as the hydrochloride) was administered by constant rate of intravenous infusion. Nature *201:* 1101–1103, 1964.

Part Four

LABORATORY EXPERIMENTS
IN THE STUDY OF DRUG
METABOLISM AND DRUG
DISPOSITION

26

General Principles and Procedures for Drug Metabolism *In Vitro*

P. MAZEL

I. INTRODUCTION

The purpose of this section is to discuss both the physiological factors and the technical procedures which can affect *in vitro* hepatic microsomal enzyme activity. This section provides some necessary background for the laboratory experiments presented in Chapter 27. The present discussion is restricted to those drug metabolizing enzymes localized in the hepatic endoplasmic reticulum, and does not necessarily apply to the other tissues and systems.

Many of the physiological factors which ultimately affect the activity of microsomal enzymes have been reviewed (Gillette, 1963; Conney and Burns, 1962; Conney, 1967). The investigator, when designing drug metabolism experiments, must be cognizant of those factors and attempt to control them as far as possible.

However, the *in vitro* activity of microsomal enzymes is also affected by non-physiological factors, i.e., method of enzyme preparation, choice of buffers, cofactors, and other parameters related to methodology. Experience has shown that minor changes in methodology may markedly affect *in vitro* microsomal activity.

II. ESTABLISHMENT OF OPTIMAL CONDITIONS

A survey of the literature indicates wide variation in the incubation conditions utilized to measure microsomal enzyme activity. The same reaction has been studied utilizing varying concentrations of substrate, enzyme, cofactors, and incubation periods. Many authors have neglected to ascertain if the reaction measured was being carried out at optimal conditions. Thus, meaningful comparison between laboratories for the same reaction is often difficult. Therefore, it is *most important* that once the investigator has selected the substrate and the method of analysis, he standardize the preparation of the enzyme and incubation conditions in *his own laboratory*. Under standardized conditions, a high degree of precision should be obtained between experiments.

The enzymatic assay should be performed under conditions in which the concentration of substrate and cofactors are not rate-limiting, and product formation should be linear with time during the incubation period. Thus each of the various factors: enzyme, substrate, cofactors, and period of incubation must be evaluated to establish optimal conditions. After optimal conditions for the assay have been established, the investigator can proceed to study various experimental parameters which affect the rate of reaction.

III. FACTORS AFFECTING HEPATIC MICROSOMAL ENZYME ACTIVITY

A. Physiological Factors

When planning experiments in drug metabolism, particular attention must be paid to the choice of animals.

Sex: No detailed review of the literature on sex differences in metabolism will be presented, but it is important to point out the existence of sex differences in drug metabolism. The liver-microsomal fraction of male rats has a higher drug oxidizing activity than that from females toward a number of substrates. Thus males metabolize hexobarbital (Quinn et al., 1958), strychnine (Kato et al., 1962b), 3,4-benzpyrene, pentobarbital (Kuntzman et al., 1966), ethylmorphine (Davies et al., 1968), morphine, methadone and meperidine (Axelrod, 1956a), carisoprodol (Kato et al., 1962a), schradan (Davison, 1955), guthion and aminopyrine at a higher rate than females. Inscoe and Axelrod (1960) found a sex difference in the rate of glucuronide formation of aminophenol in vitro. Vesell (1968) found sex differences in the duration of action of hexobarbital in various strains of mice. Sex differences in mice have not been as extensively investigated as rats. However, no sex differences were found in the metabolism of aniline and zoxazolamine (Kato and Gillette, 1965).

In addition to differences in rate of metabolism, male and female rats responded differently to starvation, adrenalectomy and various drugs (Kato and Gillette, 1965). Sex-dependent differences of drug metabolism disappeared during starvation. Microsomal activity was increased in liver microsomes prepared from females and decreased in males.

Furthermore, there are differences in metabolism between sexually mature and immature animals. The four-day estrus cycle of the mature female rat may affect enzymatic activity.

In summary, the investigator should take into account the unusual sex differences in drug metabolism in the rat and expect to obtain less enzymatic activity toward many drug substrates if female rat microsomes are used. Furthermore, the response to various drugs, i.e., ACTH, epinephrine, thyroxine, alloxan will be different in males and females.

In view of the many factors that can effect female microsomal activity, the researcher should obtain animals of the same age and weight from the same supplier to standardize conditions and be able to compare results from different experiments.

Nutrition: The diet and nutritional status can markedly influence the activity of the hepatic microsomal drug metabolizing enzymes. Shargel and Mazel (1968) found that riboflavin deficiency decreased NADPH cytochrome c reductase, azoreductase, and benzpyrene hydroxylase levels whereas aminopyrine demethylase and cytochrome P-450 content were unaffected. McLean and McLean (1966) found a loss of hydroxylating enzyme activity from the liver microsomes when rats were placed on a protein-free diet for four days. Later, Seawright and McLean (1967) found that a protein-free diet depressed carbon tetrachloride metabolism. However, aminopyrine demethylase and carbon tetrachloride metabolism could be induced in these animals by the administration of DDT. Alvares *et al.* (1968) also observed that a protein-free diet decreased microsomal benzpyrene hydroxylase by 70%. However, pretreatment of deficient animals with 3-methylcholanthrene produced a 15-fold increase in benzpyrene hydroxylase activity. Shargel and Mazel (1968) found that phenobarbital induced microsomal azoreductase in flavin deficient rats, whereas 3-methylcholanthrene induction of azo-reductase was flavin dependent.

Dietary deficiencies do not always decrease microsomal drug metabolizing enzyme activity. Rubin *et al.* (1968) found that when rats were kept on a diet deficient in choline, casein, methionine and cysteine for 15 days there was an increase in microsomal aniline hydroxylase and nitroreductase.

Dixon *et al.* (1960) found that starvation decreased the rate of metabolism of hexobarbital, chlorpromazine, aminopyrine and acetanilide. Dingell *et al.* (1966) reported that a diet deficient in calcium impaired the oxidation of aminopyrine, hexobarbital and the reduction of p-nitrobenzoic acid. Starvation reduced oxidative pathways of male rats but had little effect on nitro and azoreductases.

Diurnal Variation: The circadian changes in the activities of several liver enzymes demonstrate the importance of the time as a variable in studying drug metabolism. Davis (1962) found a diurnal variation in response to pentobarbital by mice. Vesell (1968) using hexobarbital confirmed these findings and demonstrated that sleeping time was longer and hexobarbital oxidase activity lower during the light than the dark period. Thus, it is important to control the light cycle (12 hrs on–12 hrs off) in the animal room, and it is good practice to standardize the time at which animals are administered experimental compounds as well as the time they are removed from the animal room for sacrifice.

Species: It is well established that there are great differences in the metabolic fate of drugs in different animal species. The comparative patterns of drug metabolism have been reviewed by a number of authors (Williams, 1967; Parke, 1968; Gillette, 1963; Bousquet, 1962; Conney, 1967; Smith, 1968). Only a few examples will be cited here and the reader should consult the above references and Chapter 11 for additional details.

Amphetamine is mainly deaminated in rabbits, but is hydroxylated in dogs (Axelrod, 1954). Aniline is hydroxylated in the *para* position in the rabbit, but in the *ortho* position in the cat (Parke, 1968). Rats metabolize imipramine by demethylation but rabbit microsomes metabolize this drug mainly through hydroxyimipramine (Dingell, *et al.*, 1964). Quinn *et al.* (1958) found marked species differences in the metabolism of aminopyrine, aniline, and hexobarbital. Differences in hexobarbital metabolism correlated with the observed differences in duration of action of the barbiturate in various species. Thus, in planning microsomal drug metabolizing experiments the investigator must consider not only the species, but also the specific metabolic pathway that he intends to study.

An additional important aspect to be considered is species variation in enzyme induction. This area has been recently reviewed by Conney (1967). For example, DDT stimulated drug metabolism in the rat (Hart and Fouts, 1965a) but had no effect in the mouse. Phenylbutazone pretreatment stimulated 6β-, 7α- and 16α-hydroxylation of testosterone in rats but had no effect on the 7α-hydroxylation of testosterone in dogs (Conney and Schneidman, 1964).

Strain: In addition to species differences in metabolism, it is now well established that the activities of the drug-metabolizing enzymes differ among certain strains of the same species. Furthermore, there are strain differences in the inducibility of the hepatic drug metabolizing enzymes (Jay, 1955).

A large variation in hepatic microsomal hexobarbital oxidase was observed by Vesell (1968) in 11 strains of mice. Mitoma *et al.* (1967) observed similar differences in hexobarbital sleeping time and microsomal hexobarbital oxidase activity in various strains of rats. Strain differences were also noted in acetanilide, aminopyrine and o-nitroanisole metabolism. Page and Vesell (1969) found 2 to 3-fold differences in the metabolism of ethylmorphine and aniline in $9000 \times g$ supernatant fractions from liver homogenates obtained from 10 strains of Norway rats.

Strain differences in inducibility were demonstrated by Cram *et al.* (1965). They found that phenobarbital pretreatment increased hexobarbital and aminopyrine metabolism in some strains of rabbits whereas aminopyrine metabolism was not increased at all in one of the rabbit strains. Furthermore, phenobarbital pretreatment stimulated microsomal benzpyrene hydroxylase in only 2 of the 6 strains studied. Hexobarbital stimulation varied from 2-fold to 26-fold in the different strains.

In 10 inbred strains of rats, Page and Vesell (1969) found phenobarbital pretreatment elevated ethylmorphine metabolism 2.0 to 3.8-fold and aniline metabolism increased 1.5 to 3.5-fold.

Thus, in addition to selection of a particular species, the investigator must pay some attention to the selection of particular strain within that species. This may be important when studying a particular pathway of metabolism and the effects of drug pretreatment on the hepatic drug-metabolizing enzymes.

Age: Newborn animals have little or no ability to metabolize drugs (Jondorf *et al.*, 1959; Fouts and Adamson, 1959). However, treatment of newborn rabbits with phenobarbital enhances the activity of liver enzymes that metabolize drugs such as hexobarbital, aminopyrine and p-nitrobenzoic acid (Fouts and Hart, 1963).

Liver Pathology: The activities of hepatic drug metabolizing enzymes, such as pentobarbital oxidase, hexobarbital oxidase, aniline hydroxylase, aminopyrine demethylase, were decreased as much as 60% in tumor-bearing male and female rats (Kato *et al.*, 1968a, b). Furthermore, the components of the microsomal electron transport system were also decreased, i.e., NADPH-cytochrome c reductase, cytochrome P-450 and cytochrome b_5. Interestingly enough, phenobarbital pretreatment increased liver weight, protein and microsomal drug metabolizing activity in tumor bearing rats to a greater extent than in the normal rats.

Infection of mice with murine hepatitis virus reduced drug metabolizing activity of hepatic microsomes (Kato *et al.*, 1963). Hepatic microsomes from rabbits with obstructive jaundice show impaired metabolism of acetanilide and other drugs (McLuen and Fouts, 1961).

Recently it has been reported that the hepatic microsomes from rats bearing a pituitary mammotropic tumor showed a reduced ability to metabolize hexobarbital, aminopyrine and p-nitrobenzoic acid (Wilson, 1967; Wilson, 1968).

B. Environmental Factors

Animal Bedding: The choice of animal bedding may be significant in view of the finding that hexobarbital oxidase, aniline hydroxylase and ethyl-morphine

N-demethylase were increased in the liver microsomes of both rats and mice after three days on soft wood beddings (red cedar, white pine or ponderosa pine) (Ferguson, 1966). Hardwood or synthetic beddings did not cause enzyme induction (Vesell, 1968). The use of sheet metal floors increased the acute toxicity to respiratory depressant drugs compared to wire mesh floors (Winter and Flataker, 1962).

Stress: Adverse environmental conditions such as cold (stress) may alter microsomal enzyme activity. Stitzel and Furner (1967) found that the p-hydroxylation of aniline and the N-demethylation of ethylmorphine were increased when animals were maintained at 4°C for 4 days. In addition, Furner and Stitzel (1968) showed that exposure to cold decreased the metabolism of hexobarbital. Short term stress, hind limb ligation for 2.5 hours, decreased hexobarbital sleeping time and drug blood levels (Rupe *et al.*, 1963; Bosquet *et al.*, 1965). Inscoe and Axelrod (1960) found that cold exposure (3° for 12 days) increased acetanilide hydroxylase activity 87 % above controls, but N-demethylation of meperidine and methadon were depressed 50 %. They found glucuronyl transferase activity to be unaffected by cold exposure.

Insecticides: Some chlorinated hydrocarbon insecticides induce the synthesis of hepatic microsomal enzymes. Chlordane increased hexobarbital, aminopyrine and chlorpromazine metabolism (Hart *et al.*, 1963) and DDT stimulated hepatic microsomal enzyme activity in adult male rats (Hart and Fouts, 1963; Hart *et al.*, 1963; Kinoshita *et al.*, 1966; Hart and Fouts, 1965b).

These observations imply that the routine spraying of animal facilities with insecticides known to induce microsomal enzymes should be avoided, and it should be recognized that animal feeds may contain large amounts of pesticide residues.

Ambient Temperature and Cage Crowding: There are many examples in the literature which indicate that changes in room temperature markedly affect the response to a drug. The sleeping times induced by pentobarbital and thiopental are longer at lower temperatures (Borzelleca and Manthei, 1957). Setnikar and Temelcou (1962) found a difference in the acute toxicity of pentobarbital in rats kept at 30° and at 15°. A decrease of 5° in the temperature of the ambient atmosphere increased hexobarbital sleeping time, and this was reflected in a decreased activity of the hepatic (9,000 × g) hexobarbital oxidase (Vesell, 1968). He found that crowding of animals in a cage altered the sleeping time response to hexobarbital, presumably due to a change in the rate of its metabolism.

IV. PREPARATION OF TISSUE FRACTIONS

Sacrificing the Animal: For the sake of uniformity, animals should be given only water for 24 hours prior to sacrifice. Fasting decreases liver glycogen levels and prevents loss of microsomes during the centrifugal isolation procedure (Dallner, *et al.*, 1966). However, at times it may not be feasible to fast animals overnight, i.e., when using very young animals.

The animal is stunned and decapitated using either a guillotine, large knife or scissors, followed by exsanguination. If an anesthetic is used it should be established that it does not affect the liver microsomal enzyme activity. Once the liver has been removed, all operations must be carried out in the cold either with ice-buckets or in a cold room. Warming of the liver may result in autolysis.

Perfusion of the Liver: A number of investigators perfuse the liver prior to homogenization. The liver is perfused with ice-cold normal saline (0.9%) *in situ* through the hepatic portal vein or the thoracic aorta. The liver after perfusion is light tan in color and free of hemoglobin and red blood cells. Liver perfusion has been advocated by some investigators when microsomal spectra, i.e., cytochrome P-450 and drug binding are to be studied. However, some authors find that perfusion may result in losses in liver protein and cytochrome P-450. Furthermore, perfusion may increase liver size and weight by as much as 25%. This increase must be considered when preparing subcellular fractions or when studying enzyme induction. Liver perfusion may also decrease the activity of the 10,000 × g fraction. The microsomes may also be washed free of hemoglobin by resuspending them in isotonic KCl, followed by recentrifugation.

Choice of Homogenizing Media: Generally, isotonic sucrose (0.25M) or potassium chloride (1.15%) have been used to prepare the initial liver homogenate. When sucrose is used, the initial centrifugation should be somewhat higher than 10,000 × g in order to prevent mitochondrial contamination of the microsomal fraction. Microsomes isolated from sucrose solutions are appreciably less active than those isolated from isotonic KCl solutions (Roth and Bukovsky, 1961). When potassium chloride is used as the initial homogenizing media, there is agglutination of mitochondria and microsomes. Thus, mitochondrial contamination is avoided and 10,000 × g is sufficient for the initial centrifugation.

Increasing use has been made of media containing both sucrose and a buffer (0.25M sucrose–0.01M tris-HCl buffer pH 7.4) or KCl (1.15%)–phosphate buffer (0.01M), pH 7.4. These and similar combinations have been reported to increase the yield of microsomes.

Methods of Tissue Disruption: A number of techniques have been used to prepare tissue homogenates (Umbreit *et al.*, 1964). These include: (1) the Waring-Blendor, (2) the Potter-Elvehjem teflon pestle-glass tube homogenizer, and (3) the tissue press.

The Waring Blendor: The Waring-Blendor technique, in which the tissue is broken up by rotating knife blades, has been used by a number of investigators for preparing the initial homogenate (Hernandez *et al.*, 1967; Gillette, 1959; Silverman and Talalay, 1967).

The blendor method is very convenient if large amounts of tissue are to be processed, particularly to accumulate large quantities of a particular subcellular fraction for enzyme isolation and purification. Chunks of liver tissue are added to a blendor containing ice-cold homogenizing media and homogenized at top speed for 30–60 seconds. Excessive frothing and heating must be avoided. The homogenate is filtered through a double layer of gauze prior to differential centrifugation. The blendor method gives a low yield of broken cells, but it may produce broken mitochondria that contaminate the microsomal fraction (Schneider, 1964). As to enzymatic activity, Leadbeater and Davies (1964) found that the Waring-Blendor method resulted in a better yield and stability of microsomal demethylases than they obtained with the Potter-Elvehjem homogenizer.

The Potter-Elvehjem Homogenizer: The use of a teflon pestle and glass homogenizer tube is currently the most widely used method for tissue disruption (Fig. 26.1).

The steel rod of the teflon pestle is attached to the spindle of a special high-torque electric motor by means of a chuck. This allows the teflon pestle to be rapidly rotated while in the glass homogenizer tube. In addition, the homogenizer

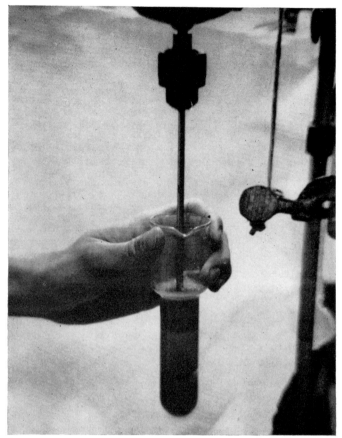

Fig. 26.1 Homogenization of rat liver utilizing a Potter-Elvehjem glass tube and teflon pestle.

tube is moved up and down relative to the stationary pestle through 6–8 excursions. Rapid rotation of the pestle and the vertical excursions causes disintegration of the tissue and disruption of the cells, yielding a homogenate consisting of diluted cell sap, intracellular particles (nuclei, mitochondria and microsomes) and some unbroken cells. The components may then be separated by fractional centrifugation.

The following points should be kept in mind:

a. The pestle should not fit so snugly that homogenization is difficult. A clearance of 0.10–0.15 mm is considered ideal.

b. It is much easier to homogenize well minced tissue than unminced tissue. Furthermore, it is easier and requires less time to homogenize small amounts of tissue. If too much tissue is used, the time for homogenization is prolonged and this may lead to overheating of the tube and enzyme destruction.

c. The homogenization should be done in a cold room, or the homogenizer tube must be immersed in an ice-bucket during the homogenization.

d. In addition to using optimal amounts of tissue, the investigator should limit and standardize the number of vertical excursions (6–8). This will avoid excessive destruction of tissue and overheating.

The Tissue Press: Von Jagow *et al.* (1965) found that the highest aniline hydroxylase activity per mg of microsomal protein was obtained in microsomes prepared from the pulp extracted by forcing liver through a 1–3 mm mesh screen. However, the diluted pulp contained less than half the total activity. These workers reported that the use of a rotating homogenizer increases inert protein, mitochondrial fragments and factors causing auto-inhibition.

In summary, when preparing a liver homogenate with a teflon-pestle and glass homogenizer it should be done as quickly as possible, in the cold, and the homogenate centrifuged at 10,000 × g as soon as possible.

V. STORAGE AND STABILITY OF MICROSOMAL PREPARATIONS

The investigator may desire to prepare large quantities of microsomal enzyme and store them for later use. As a general rule, it is good practice not to store microsomes unless absolutely necessary. Freshly prepared microsomes are preferred for spectral studies, i.e., cytochrome P-450, cytochrome b_5, drug binding and kinetic studies. If storage of microsomes is necessary, the investigator should determine the effect of storage on the particular reaction being studied, as storage has a profound effect on a number of metabolic pathways.

Microsomal enzyme preparations have been stored as: (1) a 10,000 × g supernatant at −15°, (2) a 10,000 × g lyophilized fraction (Leibman, 1965; Hernandez et al., 1969), (3) a microsomal pellet at −15° (Levin et al., 1969; Nakatsugawa et al., 1965), (4) a microsomal pellet under nitrogen at −20° (Imai and Sato, 1968), (5) a 25% suspension in glycerol at −15°, (6) freeze-dried washed microsomes (Leadbeater and Davies, 1964), (7) a microsomal suspension in buffer at −15° (Levin et al., 1969), and (8) a frozen intact liver at −20° (Chan and Terriere, 1969; Magnus and Fouts, 1967).

Storage of 10,000 × g Preparation: After storage of the 10,000 × g preparation or the microsomal suspension in buffer 0–2° for 24 hours, over 80% of codeine and aminopyrine demethylase activities were lost (Orrenius et al., 1964; Soyka, 1969). Chan and Terriere (1969) found that microsomal suspensions lost 40% of their aldrin epoxidase activity within 24 hours when stored at 4°. The loss could be reduced if the suspension contained 10^{-2}M cyanide. Levin et al. (1969) observed that microsomal suspensions kept at −15° for 20 days lost pentobarbital hydroxylase and ethylmorphine N-demethylase activity. The storage of the whole homogenate at 0° leads to losses in aminopyrine demethylase activity within a few hours. Since aminopyrine and codeine demethylase activities decreases rapidly even if the 10,000 × g preparation is stored in an ice-bucket, it is advisable to use the enzyme preparation for these substrates as soon as possible.

Leadbeater and Davies (1964) found that storage of the 10,000 × g supernatant fraction at 0° was very unsatisfactory. Enzymatic activities (codeine and morphine N-demethylases) were lost rapidly. These same workers found that microsomal preparations stored at −40° for 30 days retained full codeine and morphine N-demethylase activities. Under the same conditions codeine O-demethylase was unstable. The enzymes involved in the hydroxylation of acetanilide are stable when stored at −15° as the 10,000 × g supernatant fraction.

Lyophilized 10,000 × g supernatant fraction: Microsomal suspensions and the 10,000 × g fractions have been lyophilized in an effort to retain activity.

Leibman (1965) found that the lyophilized 10,000 × g fraction could be kept for 2 months or longer at −15° with negligible loss of activity (25%). The lyophilized preparation catalyzed the hydroxylation of acetanilide, dealkylation of aminopyrine, side chain oxidation of pentobarbital and the sulfoxidation of chlorpromazine. Hernandez *et al.* (1969) found negligible loss in activity toward a number of substrates when the 10,000 × g fraction was lyophilized and stored frozen for several months. Leadbeater and Davies (1964) observed losses of 10–25% after storage as a lyophilized preparation, and Levin *et al.* (1969) found that 16-α-testosterone hydroxylase activity also decreased when microsomes were stored as a lyophilized preparation for 20 days at −15°.

Microsomal Suspensions: The studies of a number of workers indicate that microsomes stored as a suspension in buffer at −15° or as lyophilized microsomes lost more activity than microsomes stored as a pellet (Levin *et al.*, 1969; Leadbeater and Davies, 1964). In contrast, Kashiwamata *et al.* (1966) observed that lyophilized microsomal preparations kept at −20° for several weeks had appreciable anthranilic hydroxylase activity.

Recently, Chan and Terriere (1969) reported that storage of the intact liver at −20° for 30 days led to little loss in NADPH-cytochrome c reductase, NADPH-neotetrazolium reductase and cytochrome P-450. Furthermore, microsomal suspensions from these livers showed higher aldrin epoxidase activity.

An interesting effect of storing microsomes was recently reported by Mannering (1969b). Storage of frozen microsomes for as little as one week resulted in the loss of Type I drug binding spectra characteristic of fresh microsomes.

In summary, the data available indicate that storage of microsomes as a pellet at −15° with 1.0 ml of buffer overlayed, provides a reasonably stable preparation of the drug metabolizing enzymes.

VI. COMPARISON OF POST-MITOCHONDRIAL SUPERNATANT (10,000 × G) AND ISOLATED MICROSOMES

The 10,000 × g supernatant fraction contains both the microsomal and soluble fractions. The soluble fraction has glucose-6-phosphate and isocitric dehydrogenases which, in the presence of NADP, generate the NADPH required for drug metabolism.

There are some reactions, i.e., S-demethylation of 6-methylmercaptopurine, which require soluble fraction in addition to microsomes and NADPH. For example:

$$\text{6-methylmercaptopurine} + \text{NADPH} \xrightarrow{\text{10,000} \times \text{g}} \text{R-SH} + \text{HCHO}$$

$$\text{6-methylmercaptopurine} + \text{NADPH} \xrightarrow{\text{microsomes}} \text{no formaldehyde formed}$$

For many studies there are advantages in using the 10,000 × g supernatant fraction rather than isolated microsomes. The 10,000 × g fraction is much easier to prepare, the reaction is linear for a longer period of time and the activity obtained is usually greater than that which can be achieved with microsomes plus a NADPH generating system. However, certain experimental conditions require the use of isolated microsomes, resuspended in buffer, as a source of enzyme. For example, when enzymatic activity is being followed spectrophotometrically, as in the demethylation of p-nitroanisole (Netter and Seidel, 1964) or the reduction of cytochrome c by NADPH-cytochrome c reductase, the $10,000 \times g$ supernatant fraction is generally too turbid to be used for these assays.

When studying the effect of drugs or other parameters on microsomal activity, it is often desirable to eliminate any possible effect of drug-soluble protein interactions. Furthermore, the drug used in pretreatment may be present in the soluble fraction of the cells and thus would be added to the incubation flask if the $10,000 \times g$ supernatant fraction were used. Pretreatment may also adversely affect the NADPH-generating system of the soluble fraction. In order to eliminate such possibilities, one can use isolated microsomes with either a NADPH generating system (glucose-6-phosphate plus glucose-6-phosphate dehydrogenase) or add a soluble fraction obtained from untreated animals. The effect of the drug on the soluble fraction may also be ascertained by doing a crossover experiment, using microsomes from controls and soluble fraction from pretreated animals and vice versa. The soluble fraction NADPH-generating activity is quite stable when stored at $-15°$ for several months and can be prepared in large quantities in advance.

Azo and nitro compounds are reduced non-enzymatically, to a small extent, by the soluble fraction. The activity contributed by the soluble fraction must be subtracted from the total activity (microsomes plus soluble fraction) in order to determine the true microsomal activity. Thus, for these particular assays, one must isolate microsomes.

When microsomes alone are used, the rate of metabolism may not continue at a linear rate nor be proportional to the protein concentration. This has been observed with benzpyrene hydroxylase (Alvares *et al.*, 1969) and for acetanilide hydroxylase. However, the reaction rates were proportional to enzyme concentration when the $10,000 \times g$ supernatant fraction was used. Alvares *et al.* (1969) obtained linearity with larger amounts of microsomes or when albumin was added to the incubation mixture. The latter also aided in solubilizing the substrate. These problems are of particular importance in kinetic studies with microsomal preparations in which variations are made in enzyme and substrate concentrations.

It should be mentioned that the difference in drug metabolism activity with microsomes plus the soluble fraction versus the microsomes plus NADPH or a NADPH generating system can not be eliminated by increasing the concentration of NADPH. Thus, there appears to be a factor or factors in the soluble fraction other than the NADPH generating system which accounts for maximal activity.

VII. PROBLEMS WITH NONPOLAR SUBSTRATES WITH THE MICROSOMAL SYSTEM

A wide variety of compounds with differing physico-chemical properties have been used as substrates in drug metabolism experiments. Water soluble compounds or compounds which readily form soluble salts can be added directly to the incubation mixture without difficulty. However, many substrates have very low solubility in water and must be added in a small volume of organic solvent. The addition of organic solvents may stimulate or inhibit the reaction under investigation. Furthermore, some solvents may affect the analytical procedures used in drug analysis directly or via their metabolites.

Substances which have been used to solubilize various substrates include methanol for p-nitrobenzoic acid (Fouts and Brodie, 1957), protonsil (Fouts *et al.*, 1957), and p-nitroanisole (Netter and Seidel, 1964). Ethanol has been used to solubilize benzpyrene (Silverman and Talalay, 1967), steroids (Tephley and Mannering, 1968) and dimethylbenzanthracene (DMBA) (Jellinck and Goudy, 1967). Propylene glycol has been used to solubilize steroids (Dao *et al.*, 1968) and the anesthetics, halothane and methoxyflurane (Van Dyke, 1966). Kinoshita *et al.* (1966) used ethanol (20%) plus propylene glycol (80%) to solubilize ethyl p-nitrophenyl-thiobenzene phosphonate. Other solvents used include dimethylsulfoxide for DMBA and 3-methylcholanthrene (3MC) (Dao *et al.*, 1968), ethylene glycol for naphthalene (Holtzman *et al.*, 1967), and acetone for DMBA (Conney and Levin, 1966).

In addition to organic solvents, water-insoluble compounds have been incubated in mixtures in which 1 mg of tween 80 per milliliter was employed as an emulsifying agent (Daly *et al.*, 1968). Trichloroethylene was presented to microsomes in an emulsion of cotton seed oil and tween 80. Alvares *et al.* (1969) have solubilized steroids and benzpyrene with albumin solutions.

Stable substrates may be added to the incubation flask dissolved in an organic solvent, i.e., methylene chloride, acetone and the solvent allowed to evaporate, leaving a thin film of substrate adhering to the glass. During the incubation, with good agitation, the lipids and proteins of the tissues will solubilize the substrate. Of course, this procedure should not be used for substances which adhere too strongly to the glass of the incubation flask.

Acetone in concentrations of 0.045–1.8M stimulated para-hydroxylation of aniline by hepatic microsomal fractions from rats, mice, rabbits and dogs. Acetone also stimulated hydroxylation of acetanilide and N-butylaniline (Anders, 1968). Aniline hydroxylase was also stimulated 54% by 2-pentanone (0.045M). Anders (1968) found that acetone produced no enhancement of N- and O-demethylation of a number of substrates and inhibited these reactions as the acetone concentration was increased. A number of solvents, i.e., ethanol, methyl cellulose and dimethylsulfoxide (DMSO), inhibited aniline hydroxylase. Dimethylsulfoxide when added to incubation mixtures in concentrations greater than 0.02% inhibited aniline hydroxylase (Stock, *et al.*, 1969).

Solvents such as propylene glycol and methanol are metabolized in part to formaldehyde. Thus, in demethylation studies, in which the extent of metabolism is measured by the production of formaldehyde, corrections must be made for any formaldehyde produced from the solvent.

VIII. METHODS TO EXPRESS ENZYMATIC ACTIVITY

The rate of an enzymatic reaction is usually determined by measuring the amount of product formed or the quantity of substrate that has disappeared per unit of time. Under optimal conditions, with saturating levels of substrate, determination of the quantity of product formed is preferred. The measurement of product, in the presence of large amounts of substrate, is a more accurate measurement than the disappearance of small amounts of substrate from a large reservoir. For the disappearance method one needs a highly sensitive and specific method.

The results are usually expressed as μg, μmole, mμmoles of product formed per mg or gram wet weight of liver (the amount of product formed from microsomes derived from an arbitrary number of mgs or a gram of liver, or the amount of product formed per mg of microsomal protein). Results should indicate the amount of product formed per unit of time. If an incubation is performed for 10 minutes it is not proper to multiply the results by 6 and report the data as the amount of product formed per hour. It is not valid to report results in such a manner, unless it is clearly stated to be an extrapolated value, or the reaction rate is known to be linear for one hour.

If the 10,000 $\times$ g supernatant fraction is used as the source of enzyme, one must isolate the microsomes by centrifuging at 100,000 $\times$ g and determine microsomal protein in order to calculate activity per mg of microsomal protein.

In our laboratory we express the activity as mμmoles of product formed per mg of microsomal protein per unit of time. One reason for this basis of calculation is that it is possible to have an increase in liver weight without a concomitant increase in microsomal protein under certain conditions. Generally, one finds that rat liver contains 20–35 mg of microsomal protein per gram of wet weight of liver.

IX. DETERMINATION OF MICROSOMAL PROTEIN

This method is based upon the colorimetric determination of protein by Lowry, et al. (J. Biol. Chem. *193*, 265 (1951) as modified by Miller (Anal. Chem. *31*, 964 (1959).

The colored complex formed is thought to be due to a complex between the alkaline copper-phenol reagent and the tyrosine and tryptophan residues of the protein. This complex formation is directly proportional to the protein concentration only in the range of 50 to 200 μg/ml.

Preparation of Microsomal Protein from 10,000 $\times$ g Liver Supernatant

1. Pipet 2.0 ml of each sample of 10,000 $\times$ g liver supernatant (corresponding to 333 mg of liver) into a small Spinco tube.
2. Add 10.5 ml of isotonic KCl-0.01M phosphate buffer solution, pH 7.4.
3. Place Spinco caps onto tubes. Be sure that tubes are full and that caps are fastened securely.
4. Centrifuge in the Spinco ultracentrifuge, size 40 rotor at 40,000 RPM for 1 hour or size 50 rotor at 50,000 RPM for $\frac{1}{2}$ hour.
5. Discard clear supernatant fluid.
6. Resuspend the pellet in distilled water using teflon pestle or 1.0 ml syringe. Dilute to a final volume of 100 ml in volumetric flask.
7. Use 1.0 ml of this dilution for protein determination.

Reagents

All reagents are freshly prepared from stock solutions.
1. *Folin-Phenol Reagent.* Dilute 5 ml of Folin-Phenol Reagent (Fisher Scientific) with 50 ml of distilled water.
2. *Copper Reagent* (from following stock solutions). 1 ml 1% copper sulfate; 1 ml 2% sodium/potassium tartrate; 20 ml 10% sodium carbonate in 0.5 M NaOH.

Preparation of Standard Protein Curve

1. Bovine serum albumin (BSA) used as the standard protein in concentrations of 50 to 200 $\mu g/ml$ of distilled water.

2. Prepare a solution of BSA containing 200 $\mu g/ml$. Dilute this solution with distilled water to obtain concentrations of 150 $\mu g/ml$, 100 $\mu g/ml$ and 50 $\mu g/ml$.

3. Do all determinations in duplicate. Use 1.0 ml of each BSA solution for the determination. Use 1 ml of distilled water as a reagent blank.

4. To 1 ml of each BSA solution and to 1 ml of the diluted microsomal sample (in duplicate) add 1 ml of the copper reagent. Mix, allow to stand 10 minutes at room temperature.

5. Add 3 ml of diluted folin-phenol reagent. Mix each tube immediately after addition of the reagent.

6. Heat tubes for 10 minutes at 50° in a water bath.

7. Read the optical density at 540 mμ in a colorimeter.

8. Prepare a standard curve by plotting optical density versus μg serum albumin per ml.

9. Calculate the amount of microsomal protein from the standard curve. If a 1:100 dilution was used the amount obtained from the standard curve must be multiplied by 100.

Note: If the microsomal sample reads off scale, one must further dilute the sample, i.e., 1:200, 1:250, and repeat the determination.

X. REQUIREMENTS FOR MICROSOMAL DRUG METABOLIZING ENZYMES

NADPH; NADPH-Generating Systems: Microsomal drug metabolizing enzymes require NADPH and oxygen. NADPH may be added directly or supplied by an auxiliary enzymatic reaction.

The soluble (100,000 × g) supernatant fraction of the liver contains glucose-6-phosphate dehydrogenase. Thus, in the presence of the substrate, the soluble fraction may be used to generate NADPH according to the following reactions:

$$\text{Glucose-6-Phosphate} + \text{NADPH} \xrightarrow[\text{Glucose-6-Phosphate Dehydrogenase}]{\text{Mg}++} \text{6-Phosphogluconolactone} + \text{NADPH}$$

Therefore, when the 10,000 × g supernatant fraction is used as the drug metabolism enzyme preparation only glucose-6-phosphate and NADP need be added as cofactors since glucose-6-phosphate dehydrogenase is present in this fraction.

In the absence of soluble fraction, NADPH must be added directly, or supplied through a NADPH-generating system. NADPH may be generated by adding glucose-6-phosphate dehydrogenase as previously described, or by isocitric dehydrogenase, according to the following reaction:

$$\text{D,L-Isocitric acid} + \text{NADP} \xrightarrow[\text{Isocitric Dehydrogenase}]{\text{Mg}++} \alpha\text{-Ketoglutaric acid} + \text{NADPH} + \text{H}^+ + \text{CO}_2$$

These systems are equally effective in generating NADPH and both enzymes are commercially available. If desired, one may use highly purified preparations of glucose-6-phosphate dehydrogenase, but Yeast-Type V-glucose-6-phosphate dehydrogenase (Sigma) has been adequate for most of our studies. Some workers prefer to use the isocitrate system rather than glucose-6-phosphate dehydrogenase because of the high content of microsomal glucose-6-phosphatase (Orrenius, 1965).

The auxiliary enzymes require magnesium as a cofactor and this cation must be included in the incubation mixture.

Regardless of which enzyme is used, a sufficient quantity must be added to effectively reduce the NADP. One unit of glucose-6-phosphate dehydrogenase will reduce one μmole of NADP per minute at pH 7.4 at 25°. One μmolar unit of isocitric dehydrogenase will convert 1 μmole isocitrate to α-ketoglutarate per minute at pH 7.4 at 37°.

NADPH may be added directly to the incubation vessel without the soluble fraction or a NADPH-generating system. NADPH is used directly in a number of assays, i.e., the spectrophotometric assay of NADPH-cytochrome c reductase. NADPH is not generally used for prolonged incubations because the quantity of NADPH should be added in divided portions every 5–10 minutes.

Magnesium: Mueller and Miller (1948) found that magnesium increased the demethylation of 4-dimethylamino azobenzene by hepatic homogenates. La Du et al. (1955) reported that aminopyrine demethylation was greater in the presence of magnesium. However, magnesium did not affect the rate of demethylation when NADPH was added directly. Probably, adequate amounts of magnesium were present in the microsomal pellet. Mazel et al. (1966) found the rate of puromycin demethylation to be identical in the presence or absence of magnesium. However, Trivus (1964) observed that magnesium was essential for hexobarbital oxidase and for the conversion of chlorpromazine to the corresponding sulfoxide. A requirement for magnesium was observed by Nebert and Gelboin (1968) for benzpyrene hydroxylase. Using NADPH directly, these workers showed that the magnesium effect was not due to stimulation of NADPH formation. Bogdanska et al. (1965) concluded from their studies that magnesium and/or calcium permitted a more rapid rate of NADPH oxidation or of electron transport from NADPH to various electron acceptors.

Nicotinamide: A number of investigators have reported that nicotinamide was an essential component of the *in vitro* incubation mixture. Nicotinamide has been used to prevent destruction of the pyridine nucleotide by tissue nucleosidases.

$$NAD \xrightarrow[\text{NADase}]{} \text{Nicotinamide} + \text{ADP-ribose}$$

La Du et al. (1955) found nicotinamide essential for aminopyrine demethylation. Roth and Bukovsky (1961) reported that it was necessary to add increased amounts of NADP or nicotinamide in order to obtain maximal N-demethylation of meperidine. Axelrod (1956b) found nicotinamide essential for maximal enzymatic cleavage of p-ethoxyacetanilide. Thus, nicotinamide has been used by most investigators as a component of the microsomal incubation mixture.

Recently Schenkman et al. (1967) reported that nicotinamide inhibited aminopyrine demethylase and aniline hydroxylase when the assay was conducted for short periods of time. These workers concluded that an accurate assay can be obtained in the absence of nicotinamide if the assay time is short, NADPH concentration is maintained at a high level, and concentration of microsomes in the media is kept low. Furthermore, Mannering (1969a) found nicotinamide did not affect the maximal velocity or the K_m of microsomal ethylmorphine demethylase.

Most workers avoid the use of nicotinamide, if possible, by increasing the concentrations of NADP and using short incubation times.

Choice of Gas Phase: The vast majority of *in vitro* microsomal enzyme incubations have been performed with air as the gaseous phase. When oxygen is used the rate of metabolism may be increased as much as 25%. The important criteria is the diffusion of the gas into the aqueous phase. Thus, it is important to increase the surface area of the incubate by shaking the incubation vessels. It may also be helpful to saturate the buffer mixture with oxygen prior to initiating the incubation (Netter and Seidel, 1964).

XI. INCUBATION PROCEDURES

A number of factors which affect microsomal enzyme activity have been discussed in the previous sections.

In order to minimize variation from one experiment to the next, the order of addition of the incubation components should be standardized. The incubation flask should be large enough to permit vigorous shaking without spilling. The enzyme preparation is usually added last, in order to minimize any possible interaction between the enzyme and substrate. Solutions of cofactors should be prepared just prior to starting an incubation. It is not good practice to store frozen solutions of NADP.

The rate of shaking, approximately 120 cycles per minute, should be adjusted in order to obtain maximum exposure of the enzyme and substrate to the gaseous phase.

Fouts and Waters (1969) observed that product formation was affected by the rate of shaking, the amount of protein in the incubate, the gas phase and diffusion of the gas into the aqueous phase. With high concentrations of microsomal protein, maximal activity was obtained when a glass marble was added to the incubation flask and the gas phase was oxygen rather than air. The marble, presumably, by increasing the surface area, increased diffusion of the gas into the aqueous phase and better exposure to the enzyme was obtained.

The rate of shaking becomes important when studying enzyme induction, as the concentration of protein in the incubation flask may be markedly increased.

XII. SUMMARY

Consideration has been given above to those factors which can ultimately affect the *in vitro* activity of the microsomal drug metabolizing enzymes. Only a few examples have been presented from the vast body of information that has accumulated in the area of drug metabolism. Particular attention has been given to the practical and technical procedures, rather than the physiological factors, which may affect enzyme activity.

The author has attempted to focus attention on the wide variation in incubation conditions, storage of microsomes and analytical procedures utilized from laboratory to laboratory. This has been done in an effort to demonstrate the importance of establishing optimal conditions for a particular assay by the investigator in his own laboratory.

REFERENCES

Alvares, A. P., Schilling, G. and Garbut, A.: Effect of albumin on the hydroxylation of 3,4-benzpyrene (BP) by rat liver microsomes. Fed. Proc. 28: 483, 1969.

Alvares, A. P., Schilling, G., Levin, W. and Kuntzman, R.: Alteration of the microsomal hemoprotein by 3-methylcholanthrene: Effects of ethionine and actinomycin D. J. Pharmacol. Exp. Ther. 163: 417–424, 1968.

Anders, M. W.: Acetone enhancement of microsomal aniline parahydroxylase activity. Arch. Biochem. Biophys. 126: 269–275, 1968.

Axelrod, J.: Studies on sympathomimetic amines, II. The biotransformation and physiological disposition of D-amphetamine, D-p hydroxyamphetamine and D-methamphetamine. J. Pharmacol. Exp. Ther. 110: 315–326, 1954.

Axelrod, J.: The enzymatic N-demethylation of narcotic drugs. J. Pharmacol. Exp. Ther. 117: 322–330, 1956a.

Axelrod, J.: The enzymatic cleavage of aromatic ethers. Biochem. J. 63: 634–639, 1956b.

Bogdanska, H. U., Kranch, L. and Johnson, B. C.: Effect of magnesium and calcium on the oxidation of reduced tri-phosphopyridine nucleotide by liver microsomes. Arch. Biochem. Biophys. 109: 248–258, 1965.

Borzelleca, J. F. and Manthei, R. W. Factors influencing pentobarbital sleeping times in mice. Arch. Int. Pharmacodyn. 111: 296–307, 1957.

Bousquet, W. F.: Pharmacology and biochemistry of drug metabolism. J. Pharm. Sci. 51: 297–309, 1962.

Bousquet, W., Rupe, B. D. and Miya, T. S. Endocrine modification of drug responses in the rat. J. Pharmacol. Exp. Ther. 147: 376–379, 1965.

Chan, T. and Terriere, L. C. Aldrin epoxidase activity of rat liver and rat liver microsomes under various conditions of storage. Biochem. Pharmacol. 18: 1061–1070, 1969.

Conney, A. H.: Pharmacological implications of microsomal enzyme induction. Pharmacol. Rev. 19: 317–366, 1967.

Conney, A. H. and Burns, J. J.: Factors influencing drug metabolism. Advan. Pharmacol. 1: 31–58, 1962.

Conney, A. H. and Levin, W.: Induction of hepatic 7,12-dimethylbenzanthracene metabolism by polycyclic aromatic hydrocarbons and aromatic azo derivatives. Life Sci. 5: 465–471, 1966.

Conney, A. H. and Schneidman, K.: Enhanced androgen hydroxylase activity in liver microsomes of rats and dogs treated with phenylbutazone. J. Pharmacol. Exp. Ther. 146: 225–235, 1964.

Cram, R. L., Jachau, M. R., and Fouts, J. R.: Difference in hepatic drug metabolism in various rabbit strains. Proc. Soc. Exp. Biol. Med. 118: 872–874, 1965.

Dallner, G., Siekevitz, P. and Palade, G. E.: Biogenesis of endoplasmic reticulum membranes. I. Structural and chemical differentiation in developing rat hepatocyte. J. Cell. Biol. 30: 73–96, 1966.

Daly, J., Jerina, D. and Witkop, B.: Migration of deuterium during hydroxylation of aromatic substrates by liver microsomes. I. Influence of ring substituents. Arch. Biochem. Biophys. 128: 517–527, 1968.

Dao, T. L., Omukai, Y., Libby, P. and Tominaga, T.: Effect of polycyclic hydrocarbons on steroid 11β-hydroxylase activity of the adrenal in rats. Cancer Res. 28: 559–563, 1968.

Davies, D., Gigon, P. and Gillette, J. R.: Sex differences in the kinetic constants for the N-demethylation of ethylmorphine by rat liver microsomes. Biochem. Pharmacol. 17: 1865–1872, 1968.

Davis, W. M.: Day-night periodicity in pentobarbital response of mice and the influence of socio-psychological conditions. Experientia 18: 235–237, 1962.

Davison, A. N.: The conversion of schradan (OMPA) and parathion into inhibitors of cholinesterase by mammalian liver. Biochem. J 61: 203–209, 1955.

Dingell, J. V., Joiner, P. D. and Hurwitz, L.: Impairment of hepatic drug metabolism in calcium deficiency. Biochem. Pharmacol. 15: 971–976, 1966.

Dingell, J. V., Sulser, F. and Gillette, J. R.: Species differences in the metabolism of imipramine and desmethyl imipramine (DMI). J. Pharmacol. Exp. Ther. 143: 14–22, 1964.

Dixon, R. L., Shultice, R. W. and Fouts, J. R.: Factors affecting drug metabolism by liver microsomes. IV. Starvation. Proc. Soc. Exp. Biol. Med. 103: 333–335, 1960.

Ferguson, H. C.: Effect of red cedar chip bedding on hexobarbital and pentobarbital sleep time. J. Pharm. Sci. 55: 1142, 1966.

Fouts, J. R. and Adamson, R. H.: Drug metabolism in the newborn rabbit. Science 129: 897–898, 1959.

Fouts, J. R. and Brodie, B. B.: The enzymatic reduction of chloramphenicol, p-nitrobenzoic acid and other aromatic nitro compounds in mammals. J. Pharmacol. Exp. Ther. *119:* 197–207, 1957

Fouts, J. R. and Hart, L. G.: Hepatic drug metabolism during the perinatal period. Ann. N.Y. Acad. Sci. *111:* 245–251, 1963.

Fouts, J. R., Kamm, J. J. and Brodie, B. B.: Enzymatic reduction of prontosil and other azo dyes. J. Pharmacol. Exp. Ther. *120:* 291–300, 1957.

Fouts, J. R. and Waters, L. R.: Too much protein, two slow shaking or using air instead of oxygen can minimize amount of hepatic microsomal drug-metabolizing enzyme induction measured in vitro. Toxicol. Appl. Pharmacol. *14:* 625–626, 1969.

Furner, R. L. and Stitzel, R. E.: Stress-induced alterations in microsomal drug metabolism in the adrenalectomized rat. Biochem. Pharmacol. *17:* 121–127, 1968.

Gillette, J. R.: Side chain oxidation of alkyl substituted ring compounds. I. Enzymatic oxidation of p-nitrotoluene. J. Biol. Chem. *234:* 139–143, 1959.

Gillette, J. R.: Metabolism of drugs and other foreign compounds by enzymatic mechanisms. Prog. Drug Res. *6:* 11–73, 1963.

Hart, L. G. and Fouts, J. R.: Effects of acute and chronic DDT administration on hepatic microsomal drug metabolism in the rat. Proc. Soc. Exp. Biol. Med. *114:* 388–392, 1963.

Hart, L. G. and Fouts, J. R.: Further studies on the stimulation of hepatic microsomal drug metabolizing enzymes by DDT and its analogs. Arch. Exp. Pathol. Pharmakol. *249:* 486–500, 1965a.

Hart, L. G. and Fouts, J. R.: Studies of the possible mechanisms by which chlordane stimulates hepatic microsomal drug metabolism in the rat. Biochem. Pharmacol. *14:* 263–272, 1965b.

Hart, L. G., Shultice, R. W. and Fouts, J. R.: Stimulatory effects of chlordane on hepatic microsomal drug metabolism in the rat. Toxicol. Appl. Pharmacol. *5:* 371–386, 1963.

Hernandez, P. H., Gillette, J. R. and Mazel, P.: Studies on the mechanism of action of mammalian hepatic azoreductase. I. Azoreductase activity of reduced nicotinamide adenine dinucleotide phosphate-cytochrome c reductase. Biochem. Pharmacol. *16:* 1855–1875, 1967.

Hernandez, P. H., Pittman, K. A. and Shargel, L.: Stabilization and preservation of hepatic drug-metabolizing systems. Pharmacologist *11:* 260, 1969.

Holtzman, J. L., Gillette, J. R. and Milne, G. W. A.: The incorporation of ^{18}O into naphthalene in the enzymatic formation of 1,2-dihydronaphthalene-1,2-diol. J. Biol. Chem. *242:* 4386–4387, 1967.

Imai, Y. and Sato, R.: Behavior of two states of the ethyl isocyanide compound of reduced P-450 in oxidation-reduction cycle. J. Biochem. *63:* 370–379, 1968.

Inscoe, J. K. and Axelrod, J.: Some factors affecting glucuronide formation *in vitro*. J. Pharmacol. Exp. Ther. *129:* 128–131, 1960.

Jay, G. E., Jr.: Variation in response of various mouse strains to hexobarbital (Evipal). Proc. Soc. Exp. Biol. Med. *90:* 378, 1955.

Jellinck, P. H. and Goudy, B.: Effect of pretreatment with polycyclic hydrocarbons on the metabolism of dimethylbenzanthracene-12-^{14}C by rat liver and other tissues. Biochem. Pharmacol. *16:* 131–141, 1967.

Jondorf, W. R., Maickel, R. P. and Brodie B. B.: Inability of newborn mice and guinea pigs to metabolize drugs. Biochem. Pharmacol. *1:* 353–355, 1959.

Kashiwamata, J., Nakashima, K. and Kotake, Y.: Anthranilic acid hydroxylation by rabbit-liver microsomes. Biochim. Biophys. Acta *114:* 244–254, 1966.

Kato, R., Chiesara, E. and Frontino, G.: Influence of sex difference on the pharmacological action and metabolism of some drugs. Biochem. Pharmacol. *11:* 221–227, 1962a.

Kato, R., Chiesara, E. and Vassanelli, P.: Metabolic differences of strychnine in the rat in relation to sex. Jap. J. Pharmacol. *12:* 26–33, 1962b.

Kato, R. and Gillette, J. R.: Sex differences in the effects of abnormal physiological states on the metabolism of drugs by rat liver microsomes. J. Pharmacol. Exp. Ther. *150:* 285–291, 1965.

Kato, R., Nakamura, Y. and Chiesara, E.: Enhanced phenobarbital induction of liver microsomal drug metabolizing enzymes in mice infected with murine hepatitus virus. Biochem. Pharmacol. *12:* 365–370, 1963.

Kato, R., Takanaka, A. and Oshima, T. Drug metabolism in tumor-bearing rats. II. *In vivo* metabolism and effects of drugs in tumor-bearing rats. Jap. J. Pharmacol. *18:* 245–254, 1968a.

Kato, R., Takanaka, A., Takahashi, A. and Onoda, K.: Drug metabolism in tumor-bearing rats. I. Activities of NADPH-linked electron transport and drug-metabolizing enzyme systems in liver microsomes of tumor-bearing rats. Jap. J. Pharmacol. *18:* 224–244, 1968b.

Kinoshita, F. K., Frawley, J. P., and Dubois, K. P.: Quantitative measurement of induction of hepatic microsomal enzymes by various dietary levels of DDT and toxaphene in rats. Toxicol. Appl. Pharmacol. *9:* 505–513, 1966.

Kuntzman, R., Mark, L. C., Brand, L., Jacobson, M., Levin, W. and Conney, A. H.: Metabolism of drugs and carcinogens by human liver enzymes. J. Pharmacol. Exp. Ther. *152:* 151–156, 1966.

La Du, B, N., Gaudette, L., Trousof, N. and Brodie, B. B.: Enzymatic dealkylation of aminopyrine (pyramidon) and other alkylamines. J. Biol. Chem. *214:* 741–752, 1955.

Leadbeater, L. and Davies, D. R.: The stability of the drug metabolizing enzymes of liver microsomal preparations. Biochem. Pharmacol. *13:* 1607–1617, 1964.

Leibman, K. C.: Metabolism of trichloroethylene in liver microsomes. Mol. Pharmacol. *1:* 239–246, 1965.

Levin, W., Alvares, A., Jacobson, M., and Kuntzman, R.: Effect of storage of frozen liver microsomal preparations on the hydroxylation of testosterone and pentobarbital and the N-demethylation of ethylmorphine. Biochem. Pharmacol. *18:* 883–889, 1969.

Lowry, O. H., Rosebrough, N. J., Farr, A. L. and Randall, R. J.: Protein measurement with the folin phenol reagent. J. Biol. Chem. *193:* 265–275, 1951.

Magnus, R. D. and Fouts, J. R.: Multiple action of 2'-diethylaminoethyl-2,2-diphenylpentanoate HCl (SKF 525-A) on rat liver tryptophan pyrrolase *in vivo.* Biochem. Pharmacol. *16:* 1323–1337, 1967.

Mannering, G. J.: Significance of stimulation and inhibition of drug metabolism in pharmacologic testing. In *Pharmacological Testing Methods,* ed. by A. Burger, Marcel Dekker, Inc., New York, 1969a.

Mannering, G. J.: Mechanisms of drug biotransformation. Pharmacol.-Toxicol. Program Symposium, Gaithersburg, Maryland, May, 1969b.

Mazel, P., Kwiatecki-Kerza, A. and Simanis, J.: Studies on the demethylation of puromycin and related compounds by liver microsomal enzymes. Biochim. Biophys. Acta *114:* 72–82, 1966.

McLean, A. E. M. and McLean, E. K.: The effect of diet and 11,1-trichloro-2,2-bis-(p-chlorophenyl) ethane (DDT) on microsomal hydroxylating enzymes and on sensitivity of rats to carbon tetrachloride poisoning. Biochem. J. *100:* 564–571, 1966.

McLuen, E. F. and Fouts, J. R.: The effect of obstructive jaundice on drug metabolism in rabbits. J. Pharmacol. Exp. Ther. *131:* 7–11, 1961.

Miller, G. L.: Protein determination for large numbers of samples. Anal. Chem. *31:* 964, 1959.

Mitoma, C., Neubauer, S. E., Badger, N. L., and Sorich, T. J.: Hepatic microsomal activities in rats with long and short sleeping times after hexobarbital: A comparison. Proc. Soc. Exp. Biol. Med. *125:* 284–288, 1967.

Mueller, E. C. and Miller, J. A.: The metab-

olism of 4-dimethylamino azobenzene by rat liver homogenates. J. Biol. Chem. *176:* 535–544, 1948.

Nakatsugawa, T., Ishida, M. and Dahm, P.: Microsomal epoxidation of cyclodiene insecticides. Biochem. Pharmacol. *14:* 1853–1865, 1965.

Nebert, D. W. and Gelboin, H. V.: Substrate-inducible microsomal aryl hydroxylase in mammalian cell culture. I. Assay and properties of induced enzyme. J. Biol. Chem. *243:* 6242–6249, 1968.

Netter, K. J. and Seidel, G.: An adaptively stimulated O-demethylating system in rat liver microsomes and its kinetic properties. J. Pharmacol. Exp. Ther. *146:* 61–65, 1964.

Orrenius, J.: On the mechanism of drug hydroxylation in rat liver microsomes. J. Cell Biol. *26:* 713–723, 1965.

Orrenius, S., Dallner, G. and Ernster, L.: Inhibition of the TPNH-linked lipid peroxidation of liver microsomes by drugs undergoing oxidative demethylation. Biochem. Biophys. Res. Commun. *14:* 329–334, 1964.

Page, J. G. and Vesell, E. J.: Hepatic drug metabolism in ten strains of Norway rat before and after pretreatment with phenobarbital. Proc. Soc. Exp. Biol. Med. *131:* 256–261, 1969.

Parke, D. V.: *The Biochemistry of Foreign Compounds.* Pergamon Press, N.Y., 1968.

Quinn, G. P., Axelrod, J. and Brodie, B. B.: Species, strain and sex differences in metabolism of hexobarbitone, amidopyrine, antipyrine and aniline. Biochem. Pharmacol. *1:* 152–159, 1958.

Roth, J. S. and Bukovsky, J.: Studies on an N-demethylating system in rat liver microsomes. J. Pharmacol. Exp. Ther. *131:* 275–281, 1961.

Rubin, E., Hutterer, F. and Lieber, C. S.: Ethanol increases hepatic smooth endoplasmic reticulum and drug metabolizing enzymes. Science *159:* 1469–1470, 1968.

Rupe, B. D., Bousquet, W. F. and Miya, T. S.: Stress modification of drug response. Science *141:* 1186–1187, 1963.

Schenckman, J. B., Ball, J. A. and Estabrook, R. W.: On the use of nicotinamide in assays for microsomal mixed-function oxidase activity. Biochem. Pharmacol. *16:* 1071–1081, 1967.

Schneider, W. C.: Methods for the isolation of particulate components of the cell. In *Manometric Techniques,* ed. by W. W. Umbreit, R. H. Burris and J. F. Stauffer, pp. 177–192, Burgess Publishing Co., Minneapolis, 1964.

Seawright, A. A. and McLean, A. E. M.: The effect of diet on carbon tetrachloride metabolism. Biochem. J. *105:* 1055–1060, 1967.

Setnikar, I. and Temelcou, O.: Effect of temperature on toxicity and distribution of pentobarbital and barbital in rats and dogs. J. Pharmacol. Exp. Ther. *135:* 213–222, 1962.

Shargel, L. and Mazel, P.: Phenobarbital and 3-methylcholanthrene induction of microsomal azoreductase in riboflavin deficient rats. Fed. Proc. *27:* 302, 1968.

Silverman, D. A. and Talalay, P.: Studies on the enzymic hydroxylation of 3,4-benzpyrene. Mol. Pharmacol. *3:* 90–101, 1967.

Smith, J. N.: The comparative metabolism of xenobiotics. In *Advances in Comparative Physiology and Biochemistry*, ed. by O. Lowenstein, Vol. 3, pp. 173–231, Academic Press, N.Y., 1968.

Soyka, L. F.: Determinants of hepatic aminopyrine demethylase activity. Biochem. Pharmacol. *18:* 1029–1038, 1969.

Stitzel, R. E. and Furner, R. L.: Stress-induced alterations in microsomal drug metabolism in the rat. Biochem. Pharmacol. *16:* 1489–1494, 1967.

Stock, B. H., Hansen, A. R. and Fouts, J. R.: Stimulation of hepatic aniline hydroxylase activity by dimethylsulfoxide administered to rats. Pharmacologist *11:* 285, 1969.

Tephly, T. R. and Mannering, G. J.: Inhibition of drug metabolism. V. Inhibition of drug metabolism by steroids. Mol. Pharmacol. *4:* 10–14, 1968.

Trivus, R. H.: Mg^{++}, a possible cofactor for some microsomal drug oxidations. Fed. Proc. *23:* 538, 1964.

Umbreit, W. W., Burris, R. H. and Stauffer, J. H.: *Manometric Techniques*, 4th ed., Burgess Publishing Co., Minneapolis, 1964.

Van Dyke, R. A.: Metabolism of volatile anesthetics. III. Induction of microsomal dechlorinating and ether-cleaving enzymes. J. Pharmacol. Exp. Ther. *154:* 364–369, 1966.

Vesell, E. S.: Genetic and environmental factors affecting hexobarbital metabolism in mice. Ann. N.Y. Acad. Sci. *151:* 900–912, 1968.

von Jagow, R., Kampffmeyer, H. and Kiese, M.: The preparation of microsomes. Arch. Exp. Pathol. Pharmakol. *251:* 73–87, 1965.

Williams, R. T.: Species comparative patterns of drug metabolism. Fed. Proc. *26:* 1029–1039, 1967.

Wilson, J. T.: Hepatic drug metabolism in rats bearing a manotropic tumor. Pharmacologist *9:* 202, 1967.

Wilson, J. T.: An investigation of the decrease in the metabolism of hexobarbital, aminopyrine and p-nitrobenzoic acid by liver from rats bearing a pituitary mammotropic tumor. J. Pharmacol. Exp. Ther. *160:* 179–188, 1968.

Winter, C. A. and Flataker, L.: Cage design as a factor influencing acute toxicity of respiratory depressant drugs in rats. Toxicol. Appl. Pharmacol. *4:* 650–655, 1962.

27

Experiments Illustrating Drug Metabolism *In Vitro*

P. MAZEL

The laboratory experiments have been designed to demonstrate many of the principles of drug metabolism which are presented throughout this text. Although methods are presented for the determination of microsomal activity toward a variety of substrates, the experiments have been, in the main, so designed that they may readily be adapted to study the *in vitro* metabolism of many other compounds.

Basic to all *in vitro* studies in drug metabolism is the establishment of optimum conditions. Thus, a number of experiments are concerned with: time-activity curves, determination of optimal enzyme and substrate concentrations, establishment of cofactor requirements, and subcellular localization of the enzyme and other factors.

Other types of experiments are concerned with various factors that affect microsomal enzyme activity. This group of experiments includes: the effect of compounds that stimulate the biosynthesis of liver microsomal drug metabolizing enzymes, e.g., phenobarbital, and the effect of compounds that inhibit these enzymes, e.g., β-diethylaminoethyldiphenylpropyl acetate (SKF-525A).

Another group of experiments is concerned with measuring some of the components involved in microsomal electron transfer. These include: the effect of phenobarbital pretreatment on cytochrome P-450, NADPH-cytochrome c reductase, and cytochrome b_5.

In addition, a number of experiments are given which deal with particular assays used in drug metabolism. These assays are similar since the enzyme source consists of the microsomal fraction of the liver, and the cofactor requirements include NADPH and oxygen or anaerobic conditions for certain microsomal reductases. These include assays for microsomal aminopyrine demethylase, ethylmorphine demethylase, p-nitroanisole demethylase, aniline hydroxylase, hexobarbital oxidase, azo and nitro reductase and neotetrazolium diaphorase.

I. DETERMINATION OF MICROSOMAL AMINOPYRINE DEMETHYLASE

A. Principles and Analytical Methods for Formaldehyde and 4-Aminoantipyrine

Many drugs are dealkylated by microsomal enzymes according to the following general equation.

$$R\text{—}\underset{H}{\underset{|}{N}}\text{—}CH_3 \xrightarrow[\text{NADPH} + O_2]{\text{microsomes}} R\text{—}NH_2 + HCHO$$

The rate of metabolism may be followed by either measuring the formation of the demethylated product or the quantity of formaldehyde formed or both.

The measurement of the metabolic conversion of aminopyrine is based on the following reaction:

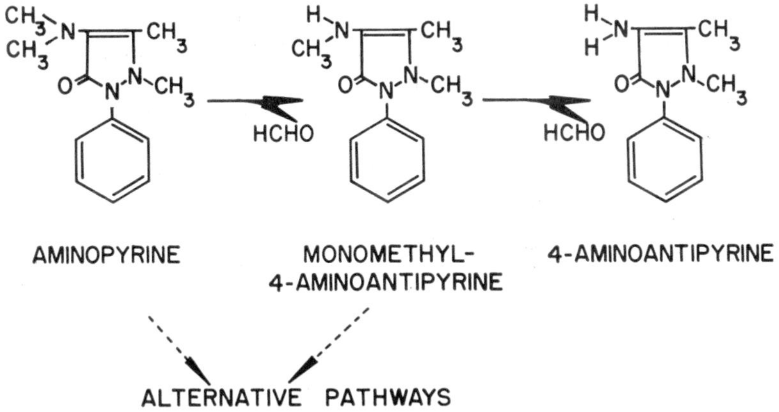

AMINOPYRINE   MONOMETHYL-4-AMINOANTIPYRINE   4-AMINOANTIPYRINE

ALTERNATIVE PATHWAYS

The above reaction indicates that dealkylation activity may be determined by measuring the formation of either formaldehyde or 4-aminoantipyrine. In the following experiments, methods to measure the formation of formaldehyde and 4-aminoantipyrine will be described. Theoretically, 2 moles of formaldehyde should be formed for each mole of 4-aminoantipyrine produced with aminopyrine as substrate.

The disappearance of aminopyrine or monomethyl-4-aminoantipyrine (MMAP) cannot be used as a measure of dealkylation, since appreciable amounts of these substrates have been found to disappear by alternate pathways.

Aminopyrine is a model substrate to study N-dealkylation of drugs, and the method described can be applied to a number of substrates which are demethylated by hepatic microsomal enzymes.

PREPARATION OF 10,000 × g RAT LIVER SUPERNATANT FRACTION

Fasted rats (overnight) are sacrificed followed by exsanguination. Their livers are removed and minced. All of the following operations are carried out in the cold. A 12.5 % (w/v) crude homogenate is prepared (1 gram of liver + 7 volumes of isotonic (1.15%) KCL-0.01 M Na+/K+ phosphate buffer, pH 7.4) by homogenizing the minced tissue in a glass Potter-Elvehjem homogenizer for 1 min. Centrifuge the crude homogenate at 10,000 × g for 10 minutes at 5° to remove nuclei and mitochondria. The 10,000 × g supernatant fraction contains microsomes and soluble proteins. 1.0 ml of the 10,000 × g supernatant fraction is equivalent to 125 mg of liver.

PREPARATION OF MICROSOMES FROM 10,000 × g RAT LIVER SUPERNATANT FRACTION

Pipette 10.0 ml samples of the 10,000 × g supernatant fraction into small Spinco tubes or equivalent. Be sure that the tubes are full and that the caps are fastened securely. Centrifuge in a Spinco or other ultra-centrifuge, size 40 rotor at 40,000 rpm for 1 hour. Discard the clear supernatant fluid. Resuspend the pellet in 10.0 ml of 0.05 M Na^+/K^+ phosphate buffer, pH 7.4.

1.0 ml of the microsomal suspension is equivalent to 125 mg of liver.

Incubation Procedure

Measure into a 25 ml erlenmeyer flask, immersed in ice, the following solutions in order:

1. Aminopyrine (5 μmoles) plus magnesium chloride (25 μmoles) in water. 1.0 ml
2. **Tissue Blanks:** To flasks which do not receive substrate add magnesium chloride (25 μmoles) in water. 1.0 ml
3. **Co-Factor Mixture:** To each flask add

3.0 ml of buffer solution containing the following:

NADP	0.65 μmole
Glucose-6-phosphate	10.0 μmoles
Nicotinamide	50.0 μmoles

(Preweighed and dissolved in 0.5 M Na^+/K^+ phosphate buffer pH 7.4 containing semicarbazide, 45 μmoles/3 ml)* 3.0 ml

4. Enzyme (10,000 $\times$ g supernatant fraction) containing microsomes equivalent to 250 mg of liver 2.0 ml

Total Volume 6.0 ml

5. Incubate with shaking for 30 minutes at 37°.

* Semicarbazide is included if formaldehyde is to be determined; it should be omitted if 4-aminoantipyrine will be measured.

DETERMINATION OF FORMALDEHYDE

Procedure

1. At the end of 30 min of incubation remove the flasks and stop the reaction by adding 2.0 ml of zinc sulfate (15 %) to each flask. Mix each flask well and wait 5 min.
2. Add 2.0 ml of saturated barium hydroxide to each flask. Mix well and wait 5 min.

Note: It is important to use proper concentrations of barium and zinc.

Saturated Barium Hydroxide: Barium hydroxide is much more soluble in boiling water. Therefore, add barium hydroxide to boiling water until the solution is well saturated. Filter the hot solution and note crystal growth on cooling.

3. Pour the entire contents of the incubaflask into a heavy duty centrifuge tube and centrifuge for 10 min. Use a speed high enough to completely settle the precipitate.
4. Transfer 5.0 ml of the supernatant to a test tube. Add 2.0 ml of **Nash Reagent,** mix well and place in water bath (60°) for 30 min. (See below for preparation

of the Nash Reagent and its use in the determination of HCHO.)

5. If solutions are cloudy, filter into a test tube using Whatman No. 1 filter paper (7.0 cm) and a small funnel.
6. Measure the absorbance at 415 mμ in a colorimeter with the tissue blank set at 0 absorbance. There is usually a small amount of endogenous formaldehyde formed by the tissue blanks. This must be subtracted from the total amount of formaldehyde formed and thus the necessity of setting the tissue blanks to 0 absorbance. The tissue blank may vary from day to day depending on experimental conditions.
7. Determine the quantity of formaldehyde formed from the standard curve. Multiply this amount by 2.0 to obtain the total amount of formaldehyde in the flask. The total amount of formaldehyde formed multiplied by 4 and divided by the molecular weight of formaldehyde (30) gives the μmoles of formaldehyde formed per gram of tissue per 30 min.

Note: To report the data as μmoles per mg

of protein one must centrifuge the 10,000 × g in an ultracentrifuge at 100,000 × g. Resuspend the micro-somes and determine the amount of protein per incubate. See Protein Method, Chapter 26, p. 538.

The Nash Reaction and the Determination of Formaldehyde

The Nash reaction has been widely used; it is simple, fast and accurate. Formaldehyde formed during the incubation is trapped as the semicarbazone (by semicarbazide in the incubation mixture) and measured by the colorimetric procedure of Nash, based on the Hantzsch reaction (Nash, 1953; Cochin and Axelrod, 1959).

The Hantzsch reaction requires a β-diketone (acetylacetone), an aldehyde (formaldehyde) and an amine (NH_3 from ammonium acetate) as shown in the equation below. With the indicated reactants, the product formed is 3,5-diacetyl-1,4-dihydrolutidine (DDL) which can be determined by its absorption at 415 mμ.

2 ACETYLACETONE + AMMONIA + FORMALDEHYDE ⟶ 3,5-DIACETYL-1,4-DIHYDROLUTIDINE + 3 H_2O

Comments on the Hantzsch reaction

The optimal pH for the reaction is from 5.5 to 6.5. Acetaldehyde also reacts to yield diacetylhydrocollidine, which has an absorption peak at 388 mμ. Large amounts of acetaldehyde interfere with the measurement of formaldehyde but at the molar concentration of formaldehyde, acetaldehyde produces only 1% inter-ference. It should be mentioned that de-ethylation of drugs to acetaldehyde would be a source of the latter aldehyde under certain experimental conditions. Acetone, chloral and glucose do not interfere, but microsomes and soluble frac-tions obtained in sucrose solutions yield lower values of formaldehyde. Amines such as methylamine and ethylenediamine compete with ammonia in the reac-tion, sulfites (0.001M) inhibit the reaction, and periodate destroys the colored product.

The reaction product is relatively stable, but is affected by prolonged exposure to light and oxidizing agents. Although the color development is faster at 60° (10–20 min) than at 37° (60 min), the lower temperature has been recommended for the determination of low concentrations of formaldehyde by fluorometry.

Preparation of Standard Formaldehyde Curve

A standard formaldehyde curve may be prepared using formaldehyde solution (40%). Although formaldehyde solution contains 12% methanol the final dilu-tions are such that methanol does not interfere in the reaction. Some investiga-tors prefer to use solid compounds for preparation of the standard formaldehyde curve. Thus, one can use paraformaldehyde or 1-hydroxymethyl, 5,5-dimethyl hydantoin (Matheson Co.). One μmole of the hydantoin compound has been shown to yield one μmole of formaldehyde.

Procedure

1. Dilute the formaldehyde solution in water so as to obtain the following concentrations: 4, 2, 1, 0.5 μg/ml. Analyze each concentration in duplicate.
2. Pipette 5.0 ml portions of each concentration into a test tube.
3. Use 5.0 ml of water as a **blank.**
4. Add 2.0 ml of Nash Reagent to each tube and mix well.

Nash Reagent:

Ammonium Acetate	30.0 g
Acetyl Acetone	0.4 ml
Distilled Water to	100.0 ml

The Nash Reagent is quite stable and may be kept in the refrigerator for many weeks.

Freshly prepared, the reagent is colorless. If the reagent turns yellow or the acetyl acetone used is yellow the reagent should be discarded.

5. Place the tubes in a 60° water bath for 30 minutes and allow the color to develop.
6. Determine the absorbance of each concentration in a colorimeter at 415 mμ with the water blank set to 0 absorbance.
7. Plot on graph paper the average optical density found for each concentration versus the amount of formaldehyde present in 5.0 ml of the standard solutions (2.5, 5, 10 and 20 μg). To convert μg of formaldehyde to μmoles, divide the μg in each tube by the molecular weight of formaldehyde (30).

DETERMINATION OF 4-AMINOANTIPYRINE

Principle

The analysis of 4-aminoantipyrine involves diazotization followed by coupling with α-naphthol to yield a colored product which can be measured directly at 540 mμ after acidification, or the colored complex can be extracted into a small volume of isoamyl alcohol for higher sensitivity (Brodie and Axelrod, 1950).

Procedure*

1. At the end of incubation period add 5.0 ml of 10 % trichloroacetic acid. The precipitated protein is removed by centrifugation.
2. To 5.0 ml of TCA supernatant add 1.0 ml of 0.2 % sodium nitrite. Cool for 10 min.
3. Add 1.0 ml of 1 % ammonium sulfamate. Mix by shaking and wait 5 min.
4. Add 0.2 ml of a 5 % ethanol solution of resublimed α-naphthol.

*See incubation Procedure (p. 548), and note that semicarbazide should be omitted from the flasks if 4-aminoantipyrine is to be determined.

5. Add 2.0 ml of 4 N sodium hydroxide. Allow to stand 10 min.
6. Add 1.0 ml of concentrated hydrochloric acid followed by 3.0 ml of isoamyl alcohol. Shake well and centrifuge.
7. Draw off the isoamyl alcohol and read in a colorimeter 10 min later at 540 mμ.
8. *Blanks:* Carry incubates through the same procedure which did not receive substrate.
9. Determine the quantity of 4-aminoantipyrine formed from a previously prepared curve of 4-aminoantipyrine (0.5–4 μg/ml) in 5 % TCA or carried through the tissue incubates.

REFERENCES

Brodie, B. B. and Axelrod, J.: The fate of aminopyrine (Pyramidon) in man and methods for the estimation of aminopyrine and its metabolites in biological material. J. Pharmacol. Exp. Ther. *99:* 171–184, 1950.

Cochin, J. and Axelrod, J.: Biochemical and pharmacological changes in the rat following chronic administration of morphine, nalorphine, and normorphine. J. Pharmacol. Exp. Ther. *125:* 105–115, 1959.

Gilbert, D. and Goldberg, L.: Liver response tests. III. Liver enlargement and stimulation of microsomal processing activity. Fd. Cosmet. Toxicol. *3:* 417–432, 1965.

La Du, B. N., Gaudette, L., Trousof, N. and Brodie, B. B.: Enzymatic dealkylation of aminoyprine (Pyramidon) and other alkylamines. J. Biol. Chem. *214:* 741–752, 1955.

Nash, T.: The colorimetric estimation of formaldehyde by means of the Hantzsch reaction. J. Biol. Chem. *55:* 416–412, 1953.

B. Subcellular Localization of Aminopyrine Demethylase

The purpose of this experiment is to separate a homogenate of rat liver into the major subcellular fractions (nuclei-debris, mitochondrial, microsomal and soluble) by the technique of differential centrifugation, and to determine the localization of aminopyrine demethylase.

The intracellular localization of various enzymes in cell organelles is a matter of considerable importance in the organization, function, and control of metabolic cycles and drug metabolism. In addition, it is frequently desirable to prepare large quantities of mitochondria, microsomes, etc., for isolation of a specific enzyme associated with such organelles. Differential centrifugation methods for the quantitative separation of cell components have been devised. Successful separation depends on the gradients produced in the centrifuge tube by layers of sucrose solution of varying densities and the use of progressively greater centrifugal forces to bring about the separation of the major cell components. Furthermore, the use of sucrose solutions avoids osmotic changes in the mitochondria. The force of centrifugation is expressed in gravitational units (g). The number of g's is directly related to the distance from the center of rotation and the speed of the centrifuge squared.

Centrifugal force is calculated by the equation:

$$F = S^2r/89500$$

where F is the centrifugal force (in gravitational units, g), r is the radial distance in cm from the center of rotation, and S is the speed in revolutions per min.

The accompanying nomogram (Fig. 27.1) is provided in order to make inter-conversions from the stated centrifugal force values ($\times$ g) to revolutions per minute (rpm) for the specific centrifuge that is employed. The rotor radius (cm) must first be determined. This is conveniently done by constructing a cross-section diagram of the rotor. Determine the depth and diameter of the rotor cup, the distance from the axis to the lip of the cup, and the angle of the cup relative to the axis. The angle, which sometimes varies from that specified by the manufacturer, is determined by cutting a filing card so that one edge can rest on top of the rotor and extend into the cup opening in such a way that a corner of the card is directly below the outer rim of the cup. The points representing the axis and the inner and outer rims are marked on the card, which is then used to mark the corresponding points on the scale drawing. The drawing is then completed for angle measurement and radius determination.

To use the nomogram extend a line from the appropriate point on the radius scale through the stated G value (B)−, in this case 9000 $\times$ g, and the rpm scale (C). Thus for a rotor with a centrifugal radius of 7.0 cm, the centrifuge should be set for 11,000 rpm in order to obtain a centrifugal force of 9000 $\times$ g.

Centrifuge speeds and g values are calculated for a specified point in the tube, usually for the center or bottom of the tube.

a. Fractionation of Liver Cell Components. The characterization of various subcellular fractions can be carried out by biochemical and cytological means. The enzyme distribution in subcellular fractions can be ascertained by determining the activities of each fraction with selected substrates (Schneider,

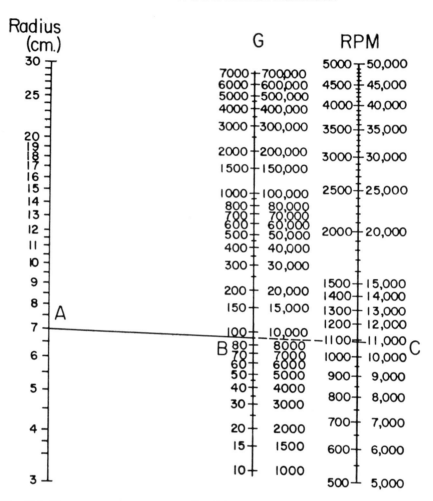

Fig. 27.1. Nomogram to convert centrifugal force values (× g) to revolutions per minute (rpm).

1964). For example, cytochrome oxidase and succinic dehydrogenase serve as marker enzymes for mitochondria. Glucose-6-phosphatase is useful as a marker for the microsomal particles (Harper, 1963; Swanson, 1955).

Procedure

1. In order to minimize autolytic processes during centrifugal fractionation of tissues, it is necessary to carry out all steps at *as low* a temperature as possible. The tissue and tissue fractions must be kept cold (in ice water) or the separation performed in a cold room.
2. Quickly stun and decapitate two male rats (200–250 g), which have been fasted overnight, and rapidly excise the livers.

3. Rinse the livers free of excess blood by immersing in a beaker of ice-cold 0.25M sucrose (reagent grade). Gently blot the livers with gauze in order to remove adhering fat and fibrous tissues. Weight the livers.
4. Prepare a 25% whole liver homogenate using 3 ml of ice-cold sucrose solution (0.25M) for each gram of liver.
5. Mince the livers into fine pieces with scissors while immersed in a measured volume of ice-cold sucrose.

6. Pour an aliquot of the liver mince into a Potter-Elvehjem homogenizing tube. Homogenize quickly, approximately 1 min, with 5–8 downward strokes of the pestle. Pour the homogenate into a beaker immersed in ice. Continue homogenizing aliquots of the liver in the sucrose solution. Gently mix the total homogenate with a glass stirring rod.

7. Transfer 8.0 ml of the homogenate to a tube labeled *whole homogenate*, immersed in ice.

8. Centrifuge the remaining homogenate in plastic or corex glass centrifuge tubes at 24,000 × g in a refrigerated centrifuge for 10 min. This procedure sediments nuclei, unbroken liver cells, red blood cells and mitochondria. Carefully transfer the supernatant, which contains the microsomes and soluble fraction, to another tube.

9. *Isolation of nuclear-debris fraction:* Gently resuspend the sediment obtained in the first centrifugation with the aid of a stirring rod and a small volume of 0.25M ice-cold sucrose solution. Add sufficient sucrose solution to reconstitute the original volume of the initial homogenate.

10. Layer this solution over an equal volume of cold 0.34M sucrose. (The 0.34M sucrose may be introduced *under* the 0.25M sucrose tissue suspension with a syringe.) Centrifuge for 10 min at 700 × g in a refrigerated centrifuge. Slow acceleration and deceleration prevents any disturbance of the gradient.

11. Withdraw as much of the supernatant fluid as possible without disturbing the loosely sedimented nuclei-debris fraction. The supernatant is layered over an equal volume of 0.34M sucrose, and the centrifugation procedure repeated.

12. Resuspend the pellets in 0.25M sucrose and recentrifuge at 700 × g. This is the *nuclear-debris* fraction. **Note:** A series of washings and recentrifugations of the fractions serves to ensure a clean preparation, but the above method must be somewhat modified for the isolation of pure nuclei. Resuspend the nuclear-debris fraction in isotonic KCl (1.15%) to the original volume of the homogenate and keep in ice-bucket.

13. *Isolation of mitochondria:* The supernatant fluid from the separation of nuclei-debris is centrifuged for 10 min at 5000 × g. The opalescent supernatant fraction is drawn off, including as much of the pink "fluffy" layer as possible. Be careful not to remove appreciable amounts of the brownish *mitochondrial* pellet. The microchondria are washed by redispersion in 0.25M cold sucrose solution followed by centrifugation of 5000 × g. The *mitochondrial pellet* is resuspended in isotonic KCl to the original volume of the homogenate.

14. *Isolation of microsomes:* The supernatant suspension obtained in the first centrifugation at 24,000 × g (step 8) and the supernatant fractions after centrifugation of mitochondria (step 13) are transferred to a lusteroid tube and centrifuged for 60 min at 100,000 × g in a preparative ultracentrifuge.

15. Gently remove and discard the small fatty material at the top of the tube. Remove the clean supernatant (*soluble fraction*) to another tube and make up to 20.0 ml, if necessary, with isotonic KCl.

16. The microsomal pellet is washed once by resuspending in isotonic KCl and recentrifuging at 100,000 × g for 60 min. The *microsomal fraction* is resuspended in isotonic KCl to the same volume as the original homogenate.

A summary of the procedure is presented in Figure 27.2. However, all washes and recombing of fractions are not shown.

b. Subcellular Localization of Aminopyrine Demethylase Activity. Incubation protocol.

Set up 20, 25–30 ml incubation flasks, in duplicate, as shown in Table 27.1.

Incubation Procedure

1. *Incubation mixture:* Pipette into the incubation flasks the following solutions in the order given:

   a. Aminopyrine (5 μmoles) + magnesium chloride (25 μmoles)   1.0 ml

OR

Magnesium chloride (25 μmoles) in those flasks not getting substrate   1.0 ml

b. Cofactor—buffer mixture:

NADP   0.65 μmoles
Glucose-6-phosphate   10.0 μmoles

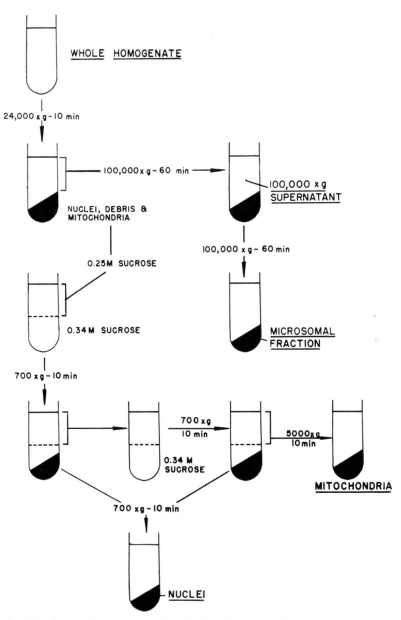

Fig. 27.2. Schematic representation for fractionation of liver cell components.

TABLE 27.1

Cell fraction	Flask no.	Mg++ + Amino-pyrine 1 ml	Mg++ alone 1 ml	Buffer + cofactors 2 ml	100,000 g supernatant 1 ml	Cell fraction 2 ml
Whole homogenate Blank	1 2	−	+	+	+	+
Drug	3 4	+	−	+	+	+
Nuclei-debris Blank	5 6	−	+	+	+	+
Drug	7 8	+	−	+	+	+
Mitochondria Blank	9 10	−	+	+	+	+
Drug	11 12	+	−	+	+	+
Microsomes Blank	13 14	−	+	+	+	+
Drug	15 16	+	−	+	+	+
100,000 × g supernatant Blank	17 18	−	+	+	+	+
Drug	19 20	+	−	+	+	+

Nicotinamide 50.0 μmoles
   (preweighed and dissolved in 0.5M Na+/K+ phosphate buffer pH 7.4 containing semicarbazide (45 μmoles/2 ml) 2.0 ml
c. 100,000 × g supernatant fraction (to provide glucose-6-phosphate dehydrogenase for generating NADPH). 1.0 ml
d. Cell fraction equivalent to 500 mg liver 2.0 ml

Total volume 6.0 ml
   Incubate with shaking for 30 min at 37°.
2. At the end of the incubation period, add 2.0 ml of 15% zinc sulfate to each flask. Mix well and wait 5 min.
3. Add 2.0 ml of saturated barium hydroxide to each flask. Mix well and wait 5 min. Centrifuge the tubes.
4. Add 2.0 ml of Nash reagent to 5.0 ml aliquots of each tube and heat in a water bath for 30 min at 60°. Determine the amount of formaldehyde formed from a

standard curve as described on p. 548. Subtract the average O.D. of the blanks from the average O.D. of the test flasks prior to calculating the total quantity of formaldehyde formed. Multiply by 2.0 to obtain the total quantity of HCHO.

5. The data may be reported as mμmoles of formaldehyde formed per cell fraction equivalent to 500 mg of liver wet weight per 30 min.

6. *Protein determination:* The data may also be reported as mμmoles of formaldehyde formed/30 min/mg protein. For protein determination, use 1.0 ml (in duplicate) of each of the following:
   a. Whole homogenate diluted 1 to 1000.
   b. Nuclear fraction diluted 1 to 500.
   c. Mitochondrial fraction diluted 1 to 100.
   d. Microsomal fraction dilute 1 to 100.
   e. 100,000 $\times$ g supernatant fraction diluted 1 to 250.

Proceed as outlined in section on Determination of Microsomal Protein (p. 538).

7. Complete summary Table 27.2.

TABLE 27.2

Fraction	Protein		Enzyme Activity		Specific Activity mμmoles HCHO formed/ 30/min/mg protein
	To-tal[1]	% Recov-ery[2]	To-tal[3]	% Recov-ery[4]	
Whole homogenate	100		100		
Nuclei-debris					
Mitochondria					
100,000 $\times$ g Supernatant					
Microsomes					

[1] Total protein = mg protein/ml $\times$ total volume of fractions (i.e., 100 ml)

[2] % Recovery (Protein) =
$$\frac{\text{Total protein in each fraction}}{\text{Total protein in whole homogenate}} \times 100$$

[3] Total activity = mμmoles HCHO formed/30 min/ml $\times$ total volume of fraction (i.e., 100 ml).

[4] % Recovery (Activity) =
$$\frac{\text{Total activity in each fraction}}{\text{Total activity in whole homogenate}} \times 100$$

REFERENCES

Harper, A. E.: Glucose-6-Phosphatase. In *Methods of Enzymatic Analysis*, ed. by H. V. Bergmeyer, pp. 788–792, Academic Press, Inc., New York, 1963.

Hogeboom, G. H.: Fractionation of cell components of animal tissues. In *Methods in Enzymology*, ed. by S. P. Colowick and N. O. Kaplan, Vol. 1, pp. 16–19, Academic Press, Inc., New York, 1955.

Mahler, H. R. and Cordes, E. H.: *Biological Chemistry*, Harper and Row, New York, 1966.

Roodyn, D. B.: *Enzyme Cytology*, Academic Press, Inc., New York, 1967.

Schneider, W. C.: Methods for the isolation of particulate components of the cell. In *Manometric Techniques*, ed. by W. W. Umbreit, R. H. Burris, and J. F. Stauffer, pp. 177–192, Burgess Publishing Co., Minneapolis, 1964.

Swanson, M. A.: Glucose-6-Phosphatase from liver tissue. In *Methods in Enzymology*, ed. by S. P. Colowick and N. O. Kaplan, pp. 541–543, Academic Press, Inc., New York, 1955.

C. Cofactor Requirements for Hepatic Drug Metabolizing Enzymes

The cofactor requirements for microsomal aminopyrine demethylase will be determined by measuring enzymatic activity in the presence and absence of various cofactor combinations and selective deletion of these agents.

The drug metabolizing enzymes have been shown to require oxygen and NADPH. Thus, when studying the metabolism of a compound one should ascertain whether the drug is metabolized by a system similar or different from the previously described microsomal enzymes.

The effect of the following cofactors on microsomal demethylation of aminopyrine will be demonstrated:

Oxygen: The oxidative demethylation of aminopyrine requires an atom of oxygen which is derived from molecular oxygen. Therefore, in an atmosphere of nitrogen or 100% carbon monoxide the demethylation of aminopyrine should be inhibited.

NADPH: On the conversion of NADP to its reduced form (NADPH), it functions as the direct donor of reducing equivalents for the oxidative demethylation of aminopyrine.

Nicotinamide: Prevents the destruction of NADP by NADPase which is present in microsomal preparations.

Glucose-6-Phosphate: Its oxidation by the NADP-linked enzyme glucose-6-phosphate dehydrogenase serves to generate NADPH.

Mg^{++}: This divalent cation is an essential cofactor for the activity of glucose-6-phosphate dehydrogenase.

Substitution of NAD for NADP: This procedure is used to demonstrate the pyridine nucleotide specificity for microsomal demethylation.

Adding NADPH Directly: NADPH may be used directly in place of glucose-6-phosphate, NADP and dialyzed 100,000 × g supernatant. Thus, one can demonstrate that glucose-6-phosphate, NADP and supernatant (which contains glucose-6-phosphate dehydrogenase) serve only as a means of generating NADPH.

Substitution of Glucose-6-Phosphate Dehydrogenase for Dialyzed 100,000 × g Supernatant: This procedure will further demonstrate that the supernatant serves only as a source of glucose-6-phosphate dehydrogenase.

Procedure

1. *Note:* This experiment requires the use of dialyzed 100,000 × g liver supernatant fraction which must be prepared a day before performing the enzymatic assays. The microsomal fraction may be prepared at the same time and stored as a pellet overnight in the deep freeze (−15°).

2. Fast 3 male rats (125–150 g) overnight. Prepare a pooled liver homogenate (1 gram of liver + 3 volumes of isotonic KCl .01M Na$^+$/K$^+$ phosphate buffer pH 7.4) as described on p. 531. *Note:* This homogenate is 25% (w/v).

3. Centrifuge the whole homogenate for 15 min at 10,000 × g followed by centrifugation of the 10,000 × g supernatant at 100,000 × g in the ultracentrifuge. Carefully transfer the 100,000 × g supernatant fraction to a container immersed in an ice bucket.

Layer 1.0 ml of 0.05M phosphate buffer pH 7.4 over the microsomal pellet. Stopper the lusteroid tube and place in the deep freeze (−15°) overnight.

5. *Preparation of Dialyzed 100,000 × g:* Pipette 25 ml of the 100,000 × g supernatant fraction into a strip of dialysis tubing (Union Carbide Corp.) which has been previously soaked in .01M phosphate buffer pH 7.4 overnight in the cold room. The bottom and top of the tubing should be tied securely with string. Suspend the tube (attached to a glass stirring rod) in a beaker containing 4 liters of ice-cold 0.01M phosphate buffer pH 7.4. Be certain that the entire 100,000 × g is covered by the buffer. Mix the buffer gently with a magnetic stirrer and dialyze the preparation for 18–20 hours in the cold room.

6. On the morning of the experiment, prepare and immerse in an ice-bucket the following solutions in 0.5M phosphate buffer pH 7.4 containing neutralized semicarbazide (15 μmoles/ml). Magnesium chloride should be dissolved in water.

NADP	2 μmoles/ml
Nicotinamide (Nico)	80 μmoles/ml
Glucose-6-Phosphate (G-6-P)	4 μmoles/ml

Magnesium Chloride
(Mg^{++}) in water   500 μmoles/ml
NAD   2 μmoles/ml
NADPH   10 μmoles/ml
Glucose-6-Phosphate De-
hydrogenase (G-6-PD)   20 units/ml
Dialyzed 100,000 × g
(Dial-Super)
Enzyme (microsomes re-
suspended in .05M Phos-
phate Buffer 1.0 ml =
250 mg liver wet weight)
Aminopyrine   5 μmoles/ml
0.5M Na$^+$/K$^+$ Phosphate
Buffer 7.4 containing 15
μmoles/ml neutralized
semicarbazide

7. Pipet into an incubation flask, immersed in ice, the previously prepared solutions in the amounts indicated, and in the order given on the protocol.

Note: In the flask where nitrogen is replaced with oxygen, it is important to *thoroughly* gas the incubation mixture, while on ice, and to stopper the flasks securely during the period of incubation. The NADPH solution should be added in 0.1 ml aliquots at 0 time and at 5, 10, 15, 20 and 25 min after beginning the incubation.

8. Incubate the flasks with shaking for 30 min at 37°.

9. At the end of 30 min stop the reaction with zinc sulfate and barium hydroxide and determine the quantity of formalde-

hyde formed as described on p. 548. *Be sure to correct the readings with the appropriate blank* (see Table 27.4).

10. Calculate the mμmoles of formaldehyde formed per 30 min/microsomes equivalent to 250 mg liver wet weight or per mg of microsomal protein. Determine the mg of microsomal protein using the General Procedure for Protein Determination p. 538.

11. Complete Table 27.3.

TABLE 27.3

Data Summary

	mμmoles Formaldehyde/30 min/mg protein	% of control
COMPLETE SYSTEM (Control)		100
Under Nitrogen		
−NADP		
−Nicotinamide		
−Glucose-6-Phosphate		
−Magnesium		
+NAD −NADP		
+NADPH		
+ Yeast G-6-PD		

Comments. Although glucose-6-phosphate and glucose-6-phosphate dehydrogenase were used in conjunction with NADP to generate NADPH one can use, if desired, NADP + sodium DL-isocitrate + isocitric dehydrogenase to generate NADPH.

The activity obtained with microsomes plus a NADPH-generating system or with microsome plus NADPH may be somewhat less than that obtained with the soluble fraction.

La Du *et al.* (1955) found that magnesium increased activity.

REFERENCES

La Du, B. N., Gaudette, L., Trousof, N. and Brodie, B. B.: Enzymatic dealkylation of aminopyrine (pyramidon) and other alkylamines. J. Biol. Chem. *214*(2): 741–752, 1955.

TABLE 27.4

Protocol: Cofactor Requirements for Aminopyrine Demethylase

Check off each added component

	Flask no.	Buffer	NADP	Nico.	G-6-P	Mg++	NAD	NADPH	G-6-PD	Dal. super.	Enz.	Amino-pyrine
Blank	1 + 2	2.0	.50	.50	.50	.50	—	—	—	1.0	1.0	—
+Aminopy-rine	3 + 4	1.5	.50	.50	.50	.50	—	—	—	1.0	1.0	.50
+N₂ −O₂	5 + 6	1.5	.50	.50	.50	.50	—	—	—	1.0	1.0	.50
−NADP	7 + 8	2.0	—	.50	.50	.50	—	—	—	1.0	1.0	.50
−Nicotina-mide	9 + 10	2.0	.50	—	.50	.50	—	—	—	1.0	1.0	.50
−G-6-P	11 + 12	2.0	.50	.50	—	.50	—	—	—	1.0	1.0	.50
−Mg++	13 + 14	2.0	.50	.50	.50	—	—	—	—	1.0	1.0	.50
+NAD −NADP	15 + 16	1.5	—	.50	.50	.50	.50	—	—	1.0	1.0	.50
Blank +NADPH	17 + 18	3.4	—	.50	—	.50	—	0.1*	—	—	1.0	—
Aminop. +NADPH	19 + 20	2.9	—	.50	—	.50	—	0.1*	—	—	1.0	.50
Blank +G-6-PD	21 + 22	2.5	.50	.50	.50	.50	—	—	0.5	—	1.0	—
Aminop. +G-6-PD	23 + 24	2.0	.50	.50	.50	.50	—	—	0.5	—	1.0	.50

* Repeat addition at 5, 10, 15, 20, and 25 min.

D. The Effect of Enzyme Concentration on Aminopyrine Demethylation

In this experiment the cofactors, substrate, and incubation period are kept constant while the quantity of microsomal enzyme is varied. This will demonstrate the relationship between enzyme concentration and aminopyrine demethylase activity.

Procedure

Prepare a liver homogenate (1 g liver + 3 volumes isotonic KCl—0.01M phosphate buffer, pH 7.4 from male rats previously fasted overnight.

Isolate the microsomal fraction (p. 547) so that each tube contains the microsomes from 3 grams of liver. *Note:* The micro-

somes are prepared from a 25% whole homogenate (w/v).

3. Remove and save (in ice-bucket) the 100,000 × g supernatant.

4. Resuspend all the microsomal pellets so that each ml of isotonic KCl—0.01M phosphate buffer, pH 7.4, contains the microsomes equivalent to 1 gram of liver

wet weight. Set aside 6.0 ml of this suspension (1 g/ml).

5. Dilute the remaining microsomal suspension (1 g/ml) with KCl—0.01M phosphate buffer so as to obtain 6.0 ml of the following concentrations: 750 mg/ml, 500 mg/ml, 250 mg/ml and 125 mg/ml.

6. Prepare to incubate 4 flasks at each enzyme concentration; duplicate flasks with substrate, and duplicate tissue blanks (no substrate) at each enzyme concentration.

7. Measure into incubation flasks, immersed in ice, the following solutions in order:

a) Aminopyrine (5 μmoles) plus magnesium chloride (25 μmoles) in water   1.0 ml

OR

b) *Tissue Blanks:* To flasks which do not receive substrate add magnesium chloride (25 μmoles) in water   1.0 ml

c) *Cofactor Mixture*

NADP	.65 μmoles
Glucose-6-phosphate	10.0 μmoles
Nicotinamide	50.0 μmoles

Preweighed and dissolved in 0.5M Na$^+$/K$^+$ phosphate buffer pH 7.4 containing semicarbazide, 45 μmoles/3 ml   3.0 ml

d) Enzyme suspension (varying concentrations)   1.0 ml

e) 100,000 $\times$ g supernatant fraction   1.0 ml

Total volume   6.0 ml

8. Incubate with shaking for 30 min at 37

9. At the end of 30 min, remove the flask and stop the reaction with zinc sulfat and barium hydroxide as described o p. 548.

10. Determine the mμmoles of formaldehyd formed for the various amounts of enzym used (p. 548). After correction for tissu blanks.

11. Determine the mg of microsomal pro tein (p. 538) in each flask. Dilute th various enzyme concentrations with wate as follows:

Microsomal suspension equivalent to

1g/ml	dilute	1:400
750/ml	"	1:300
500/ml	"	1:200
250/ml	"	1:100

Calculate the mg of protein from standar curve and correct for the dilution factor.

12. Calculate the mμmoles of formaldehyd formed per mg of protein/30 min.

13. Plot on graph paper:

a) mμmoles of formaldehyde versus mg microsomal protein, and

b) mμmoles of formaldehyde forme versus microsomes equivalent to th mg of liver tissue (wet weight).

14. How do the two curves compare? De termine the optimal amount of enzym protein for this assay. At what concentr tions of enzyme is the reaction linear?

E. Kinetics of Aminopyrine Demethylase

Phenobarbital pretreatment has been shown to increase hepatic microsomal aminopyrine demethylase activity. The effect of phenobarbital on the initial velocity and the specific activity of the microsomal enzyme will be studied by comparing control liver microsomes with those prepared from rats pretreated with phenobarbital.

Procedure

1. Inject 3 male rats (125–150 gm) with sodium phenobarbital (90 mg/kg) once daily i.p. in 0.3 ml normal saline for 3 days. Controls receive 0.3 ml saline.

2. Fast the animals overnight and sacrifice

the animals on the morning of the fourt day. Pool the livers of each group. Pr pare a liver homogenate (1 gram of liv + 7 volumes of isotonic KCl—0.01 Na$^+$/K$^+$ phosphate buffer pH 7.4) described on p. 532.

3. Centrifuge the homogenate at 10,000 × g in a refrigerated centrifuge for 10 min. Carefully remove the 10,000 × g supernatant fraction, which will serve as the enzyme preparation.

4. Pipette 2.0 ml of the 10,000 × g supernatant fractions of the control and phenobarbital homogenates in separate cellulose nitrate 12.0 ml Spinco tubes. Add 10.0 ml of KCl—.01M phosphate buffer to each, and centrifuge in the ultracentrifuge at 100,000 × g for 60 min. These tubes are to be used for the determination of the microsomal protein.

5. Prepare to assay for microsomal aminopyrine demethylase in the control and phenobarbital 10,000 × g supernatant fractions according to the following protocol.

Group	Flasks	Additions				
		Aminopyrine + Mg⁺⁺	Mg⁺⁺ Alone	Buffer + Cofactors	10,000 × /g supernatant Control	10,000 × /g supernatant Phenobarb.
1 Tissue blank-control	1–10	—	1.0	3.0	2.0	—
2 Substrate-control	11–20	1.0	—	3.0	2.0	—
3 Tissue blank-phenobarbital	21–30	—	1.0	3.0	—	2.0
4 Substrate-phenobarbital	31–40	1.0	—	3.0	—	2.0

2 flasks from each of the 4 groups (8 flasks) re to be removed at zero time and after 15, 0, 45 and 60 min for duplicate analyses of ach set at the 5 time periods.

. Measure into an incubation flask, immersed in ice, the following solutions in order:

Aminopyrine (5 μmoles) plus magnesium chloride (25 μmoles) in water.   1.0 ml

OR

Tissue Blanks: To flasks which do not receive substrate add magnesium chloride (25 μmoles) in water   1.0 ml

Co-Factor Mixture: To each flask add 3.0 ml of buffer solution containing the following:

NADP   0.65 μmoles
Glucose-6-phosphate   10.0 μmoles
Nicotinamide   50.0 μmoles
(Preweighed and dissolved in 0.5M Na⁺/K⁺ phosphate buffer pH 7.4 containing semicarbazide, 45 μmoles/3 ml)   3.0 ml
Enzyme (10,000 × g supernatant fraction) Microsomes equivalent to 250 mg of liver   2.0 ml

Total Volume   6.0 ml

Incubate with shaking for 30 min at 37°.

7. After all the components have been added to the flasks, remove 2 zero-time flasks of the 4 groups. Add 2.0 ml of 15% zinc sulfate to these flasks and mix.

8. Place the remaining 32 flasks in the shaker-incubator and set a timer for 15 min.

9. Add 2.0 ml of saturated barium hydroxide to the flasks removed at 0-time (containing zinc sulfate). Mix well and set aside.

10. At the end of 15 min remove another 8 flasks for that time period and add the zinc sulfate and barium hydroxide as previously described (p. 548). Repeat the procedures at 30, 45 and 60 min.

11. Pour the contents of each flask into a 15 ml heavy duty centrifuge tube and centrifuge at a speed sufficient to settle the precipitate.

12. Remove 5.0 ml from each tube. Add 2.0 ml of Nash Reagent. Heat in a water bath (60°) for 30 min, filter, if necessary, and read in a colorimeter at 415 mμ against a water blank.

13. Subtract the average optical density of blanks from the average optical density of the test flasks for the corresponding time periods.

14. Determine the amount of formaldehyde formed from the previously prepared

standard curve. Multiply by 2.0 to obtain the total amount of formaldehyde contained in the incubate. (See 12, above; 5.0 ml of 10.0 ml were analyzed.)

15. Resuspend the microsomal pellet (step 4) in 100 ml of water. Determine the mg of microsomal protein contained in the incubation flask for both control and the phenobarbital pretreated homogenates. (See Protein Procedure, p. 538.)

16. Determine the mμmoles of formaldehyde formed/30 min/mg protein for control

and the phenobarbital homogenates for each time period.

17. Calculate the effect of phenobarbital pretreatment as % of control with respect to formaldehyde formed at each time period. Calculate the mg of microsomal protein per gram of liver for both control and phenobarbital and the % increase in microsomal protein produced by phenobarbital pretreatment.

18. Plot on graph paper the mμmoles formaldehyde formed/mg protein versus time for both liver homogenates.

II. INHIBITION OF THE N-DEMETHYLATION OF ETHYLMORPHINE BY 2-DIETHYLAMINOETHYL 2,2-DIPHENYLVALERATE HCl (SKF 525A)

Purpose

To determine: (1) the apparent K_m (Michaelis constant) for microsomal ethylmorphine demethylase, (2) the kinetics of the inhibition of ethylmorphine demethylase by SKF-525A, and (3) the K_I (inhibition constant) of SKF-525A for ethylmorphine demethylase.

Introduction

One determination that is usually made when an enzyme is being characterized is the Michaelis constant (K_m). This is the substrate concentration at half-maximum velocity of the reaction. The magnitude of the K_m gives a measure of the affinity of an enzyme for its substrate, low values of K_m indicate that the enzyme binds the substrate strongly, whereas high values indicate a low affinity of enzyme for the substrate. *Quantitative* interpretation of K_m values of microsomal drug metabolizing enzymes is fraught with difficulties as one is dealing with an impure enzyme. However, the qualitative aspects of microsomal kinetics have provided important information on the mechanism and characteristics of these enzymes.

Ethylmorphine is an ideal substrate for kinetic studies since it is metabolized *in vitro* only by dealkylation. The small amount of acetaldehyde formed by deethylation does not interfere with the formaldehyde determination by the Nash

ETHYLMORPHINE HYDROCHLORIDE

N-Demethylation of Ethylmorphine

reaction. N-methylbarbital would be a good substrate since it only undergoes demethylation. However, its rate of demethylation in non-induced animals is so slow that it is impractical.

SKF-525A has been extensively utilized in drug metabolism studies. It inhibits the metabolism of a number of substrates both *in vivo* and *in vitro*. These include:

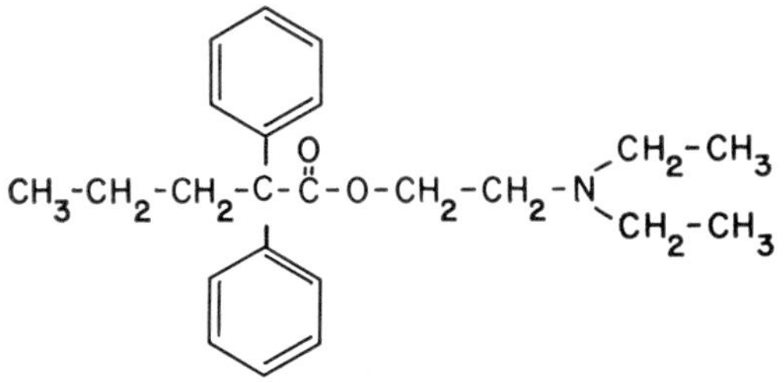

β-DIETHYLAMINOETHYL-DIPHENYL PROPYLACETATE (SKF-525A)

(1) N- and O-demethylation, (2) deamination, (3) side chain oxidation of barbiturates, (4) hydrolysis of procaine, and (5) the formation of morphine glucuronide.

The metabolism of a number of compounds, however, are not inhibited by SKF-525A. These include the N-dealkylation of N-methylaniline, O-dealkylation of phenacetin, sulfoxidation of chlorpromazine and the reduction of aromatic nitro compounds and azo-dyes (Mannering, 1969).

The inhibitory effect of SKF-525A is readily demonstrable utilizing three techniques: (1) measuring the duration of action and the half-life of a compound after administration of SKF-525A (25 mg/kg) intraperitoneally, (2) by measuring the activity *in vitro* of microsomes isolated from rats previously administered SKF-525A, and (3) by adding SKF-525A directly to an incubation flask containing microsomes from animals which have *not* been injected with SKF-525A.

Procedure

1. Microsomes plus a NADPH-generating system will be used as the enzyme preparation.
2. Sacrifice 2–3 male rats (150 g) after fasting overnight. Prepare a 25% liver homogenate in isotonic KCl 0.01 M phosphate buffer as described on p. 532.
3. Centrifuge the 10,000 × g supernatant at 100,000 × g and isolate the microsomal fraction. Resuspend the microsomes in 0.05 M phosphate buffer so that each ml is equivalent to the microsomes from 250 mg of liver wet weight.
4. Prepare to incubate 34 flasks using varying concentrations of ethylmorphine and SKF-525A according to the protocol herewith.

PROTOCOL

	Ethylmorphine Concentration (mg/6.0 ml)				
	Tissue Blanks	4.60	2.30	1.52	1.16
Controls	1	3	5	7	9
	2	4	6	8	10
SKF 525 Concentration, μg/6 ml					
1. 9.5	11	13	15	17	—
	12	14	16	18	—
2. 23.8	19	21	23	25	—
	20	22	24	26	—
3. 59.5	27	29	31	33	—
	28	30	32	34	—

The data obtained from flasks 1–10 will be used to calculate the apparent K_m of ethylmorphine demethylase. Use the average value from duplicate flasks, minus the tissue blanks, to calculate the quantity of formaldehyde formed.

The effect of 3 concentrations of SKF-525A will be tested on only 3 concentrations of ethylmorphine. The protocol will permit one to plot and calculate the results by a number of differing methods.

5. Prepare solutions of SKF-525A in water containing 9.5 μg/ml (flasks 11–18), 23.8 μg/ml (flasks 19–26) and 59.5 μg/ml (flasks 27–34).

6. Add 1.0 ml of microsomal enzyme suspension (equivalent to 250 mg liver) to all flasks. Gently swirl the flasks containing SKF-525A for a few sec.

7. Add 1.0 ml of magnesium chloride solution (25 μmoles/ml) to flasks 1, 2, 11, 12, 19, 20, 27 and 28.

8. Add 1.0 ml of 0.05 M phosphate buffer pH 7.4 to flasks 1 and 2.

9. To all flasks (1–34) add 3.0 ml of buffer cofactor mixture which contains per 3.0 ml of 0.5 M phosphate buffer pH 7.4 (neutralized semicarbazide 15 μmoles/ml) the following:

NADP	2.0 μmoles
Nicotinamide	20.0 μmoles
Glucose-6-Phosphate	10.0 μmoles
Glucose-6-Phosphate Dehydrogenase	2.0 units

10. Prepare solutions of ethylmorphine in the magnesium chloride solution (25 μmoles/ml) containing ethylmorphine 4.60 mg/ml (flasks 3, 4, 13, 14, 21, 22, 29, 30), 2.30 mg/ml (flasks 5, 6, 15, 16, 23, 24, 31, 32), 1.52 mg/ml (flasks 7, 8, 17, 18, 25, 26, 33, 34) and 1.16 mg/ml to flasks 9 and 10 only.

11. Incubate the flasks with shaking for 10 min at 37°.

12. Stop the reaction with zinc sulfate and barium hydroxide as described under the general protocol for aminopyrine demethylase (p. 548).

13. Add 2.0 ml of Nash reagent to a 5.0 ml aliquot of each tube and determine the quantity of formaldehyde formed from the previously prepared standard curve. Multiply by 2.0 to obtain the total quantity of formaldehyde formed.

14. **Treatment of Data**

a. *Determination of apparent Michaelis constant (K_m) for Ethylmorphine Demethylase.*

The K_m is obtained from the values of the relative velocities at different substrate concentrations in the absence of inhibitor by plotting 1/S against 1/v (v = mμmoles of formaldehyde formed per ten min).

1). Complete the following table:

Substrate	(S)	1/S	v	1/v
4.60 mg =	2× 10^{-3} M	0.5× 10^3 M		
2.30 mg =	1× 10^{-3} M	1.0× 10^3 M		
1.52 mg =	.67× 10^{-3} M	1.5× 10^3 M		
1.16 mg =	.50× 10^{-3} M	2.0× 10^3 M		

2). Plot 1/S against 1/v as shown in Figure 27.3.

3). Note that in Figure 27.3 the intercept on the X-axis (abscissa) is at −1.0. Then −1/K_m = −1.0 and therefore K_m = 1.0 × 10^{-3}M

b. *Determination of Type of Inhibition Exhibited by SKF-525A.*

1). Complete the following table:

Ethylmorphine Concentration	SKF-525A Concentration					
	4 μM		10 μM		25 μM	
1/S	v	1/v	v	1/v	v	1/v
0.5 × 10^3 M						
1.0 × 10^3 M						
1.5 × 10^3 M						
2.0 × 10^3 M						

Note: SKF-525A 9.5 μg/6.0 ml = 4 ×

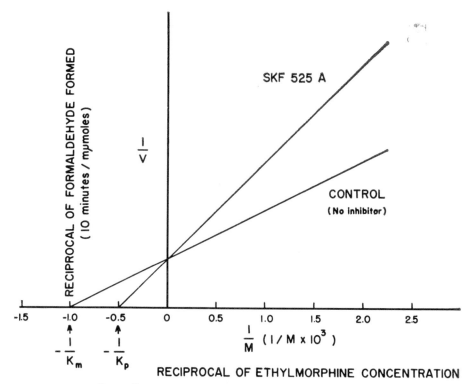

Fig. 27.3. Plot of 1/v against 1/S for the determination of K_m and for competitive inhibition.

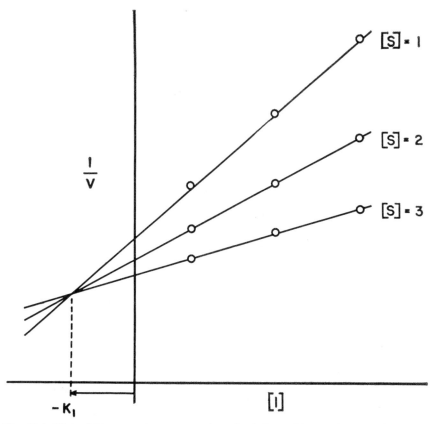

Fig. 27.4. Plot of 1/v at each concentration of ethylmorphine against varying concentrations of inhibitor, SKF-525A.

10^{-6}M, 23.8 μg/6.0 ml = 10 $\times$ 10^{-6}M, 59.5 μg/6.0 ml = 25 $\times$ 10^{-6}M.

2). Plot 1/S vs 1/v where the substrate concentration is varied and the concentration of inhibitor is constant. With a competitive inhibitor the graph will appear as shown in Figure 27.3. Observe that there is an increase in slope and no significant change in intercept.

c. *Calculation of K_i (Inhibition Constant).*

The inhibition constant may be calculated from the data in Figure 27.4. Note that in the presence of inhibitor the line intersects on the abscissa at a point $-1/K_p$. K_p is calculated in the same manner as K_m. Thus the K_i may be calculated from the expression

$$K_i = \frac{[I]}{\dfrac{K_p}{K_m} - 1}$$

where [I] = concentration of inhibitor i.e., 10 μM versus varying concentration of substrate.

d. *Graphical Determination of K_i*

Using the data of the table on p. 564 plot 1/v at each concentration of ethyl morphine against varying concentration of SKF-525A [I]. With a competitive inhibitor the lines intersect to the left of the ordinate axis. The value $-K_i$ can be read directly from the graph. An example of the type of graph one should obtain is shown in Figure 27.4.

REFERENCES

Anders, M. W. and Mannering, G. J.: Kinetics of the inhibition of the N-demethylation of ethylmorphine by 2-diethylaminoethyl 2,2-diphenylvalerate HCl (SKF-552A) and related compounds. Mol. Pharmacol. *2*: 319–327, 1966.

Dixon, M. and Webb, E. C.: *Enzymes.* Academic Press, New York, 1964.

Mannering, G. J.: Significance of stimulation and inhibition of drug metabolism in pharmacologic testing. In *Pharmacologic Testing Methods*, ed. by A. Bergen. Marcel Dekker, Inc., New York, 1969.

Sasame, H. A.: Mechanism of Inhibition of NADPH-Dependent Enzymes in Liver Microsomes. Ph.D. Thesis, George Washington University, 1968.

III. MICROSOMAL p-NITROANISOLE O-DEMETHYLASE

Contributed by Vincent G. Zannoni

The microsomal O-demethylation of p-nitroanisole can be used to study the overall liver microsomal drug metabolizing system. The substrate is an excellent "model drug" since its demethylated product, p-nitrophenol, absorbs light at 420 mμ at pH 7.8 and the demethylation reaction can be followed continuously in an incubation mixture. The formation of p-nitrophenol is based on the following reaction:

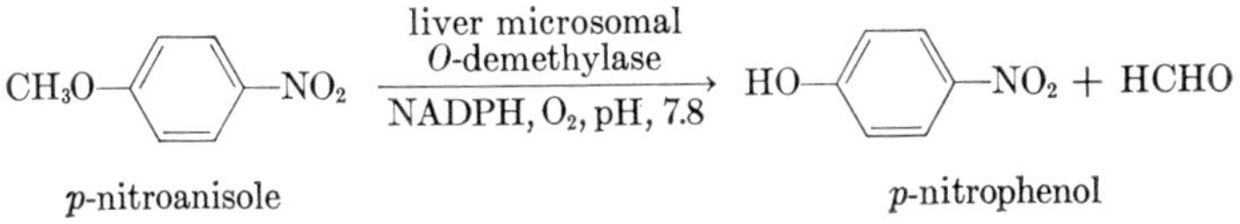

$$CH_3O-\bigcirc-NO_2 \xrightarrow[\text{NADPH, O}_2, \text{pH, 7.8}]{\substack{\text{liver microsomal} \\ \text{O-demethylase}}} HO-\bigcirc-NO_2 + HCHO$$

p-nitroanisole   p-nitrophenol

A. Experimental Procedure

The following method may be used to measure O-demethylase activity with either the 15,000 $\times$ g rat liver supernatant fraction, or a preparation of rat liver microsomes.

Preparation of reagents

1. $NaH_2PO_4 \cdot H_2O$ buffer—0.07 M, pH 7.8. The buffer solution is oxygenated by bubbling through oxygen for 5 min prior to the experiment.

2. Nicotinamide·HCl: A stock solution of 0.12 M is made up in 0.07 M sodium phosphate buffer, pH, 7.8 and readjusted with drops of 1.0 N NaOH to pH 7.8.
3. MgCl₂·6H₂O: A stock solution of 0.30 M is made up in distilled water.
4. Glucose-6-phosphate·Na₂·3H₂O: A stock solution of 0.30 M is made up in 0.07 M sodium phosphate buffer, pH 7.8.
5. p-Nitroanisole: A stock solution of 2.0×10^{-3}M is made up in 0.07 M sodium phosphate buffer, pH 7.8. The compound is dissolved by heating the solution to 45° in a water bath. The solution is kept at 27° and is stable for at least 8 hours.
6. Glucose-6-phosphate dehydrogenase (Sigma grade II): The stock solution containing 300 μg per ml is made up in 0.07 M sodium phosphate buffer, pH 7.8. The solution is kept at 5° and is stable for at least 8 hours.
7. a) Rat liver supernatant fraction (15,000 × g): A 20% rat liver (w/v) homogenate is prepared in ice cold reagent grade sucrose (0.25M). Prior to homogenization in a glass Potter-Elvehjem homogenizing tube for 1 min, rinse the livers in ice cold sucrose solution and gently blot to remove the excess blood. Centrifuge the crude homogenate at 15,000 × g for 30 min at 5° to remove nuclei and mitochondria. The 15,000 × g supernatant fraction contains the microsomes and soluble proteins, and it has a protein concentration of about 25 mg per ml. This enzyme preparation is stable at 5° for at least 8 hours.

b) Rat liver microsomes: Portions of the 15,000 × g supernatant fraction are centrifuged at 100,000 × g for 1 hour. The supernatant fraction is removed, and the microsomal pellet of each tube is resuspended gently in ice cold sucrose and centrifuged at 100,000 × g for 30 min. The microsomes are made up in ice cold sucrose to one-half the volume of the original 15,000 × g supernatant fraction. The final microsomal preparation has a protein concentration of approximately 8 mg per ml and is stable at 5° for at least 8 hours.
8. NADP·Na·2H₂O: A stock solution of 3.0×10^{-3}M is made up in 0.07 M sodium phosphate buffer, pH 7.8 and is stable at 5° for at least 8 hours.

O-Demethylase Assay

Pipette the following solutions into 3.0 ml Coleman cuvettes (10 × 75 mm) in the following order:

	C	E	C	E
1. PO₄ buffer (0.07M, pH 7.8)	0.55	0.45	0.65	0.55
2. Nicotinamide (6.0 μmoles)	0.05	0.05	0.05	0.05
3. MgCl₂ (15 μmoles)	0.05	0.05	0.05	0.05
4. Glucose-6-PO₄ (15 μmoles)	0.05	0.05	0.05	0.05
5. p-Nitroanisole (3.0 μmoles)	1.50	1.50	1.50	1.50
6. Glucose-6-PO₄ dehydrogenase (30 μg)	—	—	0.10	0.10
7. Rat liver supernatant fraction (15,000 × g)	0.30	0.30	—	—
Rat Liver microsomes (100,000 × g)	—	—	0.10	0.10
8. NADP (0.3 μmole)	—	0.10	—	0.10

The total fluid volume of the reaction mixture is 2.50 ml and the concentration of p-nitroanisole is 1.2×10^{-3}M.
9. After the addition of NADP, mix the cuvettes and set the colorimeter at zero absorbance at 420 mμ with the C (control) cuvette and record the absorbance

of the E (experimental) cuvette in O.D. units. After recording the zero time absorbance, incubate the C and E cuvettes at 37° in a water bath. Measure the optical density in the E cuvette at 3 min intervals for 24 min, resetting the colorimeter at zero absorbance with the C cuvette each time.

Calculations

1.0 μg product, p-nitrophenol (M.W. = 139) under the conditions of the assay (total reaction volume of 2.5 ml) gives an optical density reading of 0.021.

The specific activity of O-demethylase is defined as μmoles of p-nitrophenol formed/hour/100 mg of protein at 37°.

Formula for calculations of specific activity of O-demethylase in 15,000 × g supernatant fraction:

$$\frac{\text{O.D.}(420 \text{ m}\mu)/\text{min} \times 60 \text{ min} \times 100}{0.021 \times 139 \times 7.5^*} = \mu\text{moles p-nitrophenol}$$

formed/hr/100 mg protein

* Protein in 15,000 × g supernatant fraction = 25 mg/ml reaction mixture contains 0.3 ml of this fraction.

B. Determination of the Michaelis-Menten constant (Km) of p-nitroanisole

Phenobarbital pretreatment of rats has been shown to induce liver microsomal p-nitroanisole O-demethylase activity. The purpose of this experiment is to determine the K_m value of p-nitroanisole with non-induced (control) and induced rat liver microsomes. A comparison of the calculated K_m values will be made to see if there is an alteration in the apparent affinity of the substrate under conditions of microsomal induction.

Phenobarbital induction of liver microsomal p-nitroanisole O-demethylase

Inject (i.p.) male rats weighing 125–150 grams with sodium phenobarbital 120 mg/Kg/day, for 3 days. Give the drug in two injections of 0.5 ml of saline per day, at 9:00 A.M. and 4:00 P.M. Control animals receive 0.5 ml of saline (i.p.) 2 times daily. Sacrifice the animals on the morning of the fourth day and prepare control and induced microsomes from a 20% (w/v) crude homogenate as described in Experimental Procedure, p. 547.

Km Determinations

The assay of p-nitroanisole O-demethylase activity in control and induced microsomes should be followed as described in section A procedure except for the following modifications.
1. Activity will be determined at different substrate concentrations; the range should include the following concentrations of substrate in the incubation mixture; 1.2×10^{-3}M, 6.0×10^{-4}M, 3.0×10^{-4}M, 1.5×10^{-4}M and 7.5×10^{-5}M. Appropriate dilutions of the p-nitroanisole stock solution with 0.07 M sodium phosphate buffer, pH 7.8 are used.
2. In these experiments, 0.2 ml of control microsomes should be used throughout the substrate range in order to ensure an adequate rate of O-demethylation,

especially at the lower substrate concentrations; 0.1 ml of the induced microsomal preparation should prove adequate for the determination of the various rates of O-demethylation over the substrate range.

Calculations

The data should be plotted by a variety of methods in order to determine and compare the Km in control and induced microsomes; various types of plots are shown as follows:

	Ordinate	Abscissa	Ordinate	Abscissa	Ordinate	Abscissa
plot	$1/v$	$1/S$	v	v/S	S/v	S
intercept	$1/V$	$-1/Km$	V	V/Km	Km/V	$-Km$
slope		Km/V		$-Km$		$1/V$

S = molar concentration of p-nitroanisole.

v = μmoles of p-nitrophenol formed per unit time (this should be an estimate of the initial velocity).

V = maximum velocity (theoretical value, to be calculated at infinite substrate concentration from the above plots).

Comments

The above assay for O-demethylation has been designed for the Coleman Colorimeter, but it may be adapted to a Beckman DU Spectrophotometer with the following minor modifications:

1. The reaction is carried out in a 1.5 ml quartz cuvette (10 mm light path) with a reaction mixture having a total volume of 1.1 ml. The formation of product, p-nitrophenol is followed at 420 mμ. Under these conditions, 1.0 μg of p-nitrophenol gives a reading of 0.096.

2. Additions of 0.07 M sodium phosphate buffer, pH 7.8, nicotinamide, MgCl₂, glucose-6-phosphate and p-nitroanisole are adjusted so that the final concentration of each reagent in the 1.1 ml of reaction mixture is the same as that described for the assay using a Coleman Colorimeter (reaction mixture volume of 2.5 ml). However, it is not necessary to reduce the amounts of glucose-6-phosphate dehydrogenase or NADP.

3. The enzyme may be assayed in the 15,000 × g supernatant fraction using 0.1 or 0.2 ml per incubation, or microsomes (0.1 ml) may be used. The reaction may be followed at 27° or 37°.

REFERENCES

Conney, A. H. and Burns, J. J.: Factors influencing drug metabolism. Advan. Pharmacol. *1:* 31–58, 1962.

Conney, A. H.: Pharmacological implications of microsomal enzyme induction. Pharmacol. Rev. *19:* 317–366, 1967.

Netter, K. J. and Seidel, G.: An adaptively stimulated O-demethylating system in rat liver microsomes and its kinetic properties. J. Pharmacol. Exp. Ther. *146:* 61–65, 1964.

IV. DETERMINATION OF MICROSOMAL ANILINE HYDROXYLASE

The rate of aniline metabolism *in vitro* may be determined by measuring the quantity of p-aminophenol formed according to the following reaction:

ANILINE   p-AMINOPHENOL

In general, two procedures have been used for the quantitative determination of p-aminophenol (PAP) formed by aniline hydroxylation. One method involves extraction of p-aminophenol from the incubation mixture. Phenol is then added to form the blue phenol-indophenol complex which is measured at 640 mµ. In the second procedure trichloroacetic acid is used to precipitate the protein and the quantity of p-aminophenol is determined in an aliquot of the trichloroacetic acid (TCA) supernatant fraction.

METHOD 1

A. *Incubation Conditions*

Into a series of flasks, immersed in ice, add the following components.

Aniline hydrochloride (5 µmoles in
    water)   1.0 ml
Co-factor mixture:
    NADP   0.5 µmole
    Glucose-6-phosphate   10.0 µmoles
    Nicotinamide   50.0 µmoles
    Magnesium chloride   25.0 µmoles
Dissolved in Na+/K+ phosphate 2.0 ml
    buffer (0.1M), pH 7.4
Enzyme: 10,000 × g supernatant 1.0 ml
    fraction containing microsomes
    equivalent to 250 mg of liver, wet
    weight.
Total Incubation Volume   4.0 ml
Incubate the flasks with rapid
    shaking for 20 min at 37°.

B. *Analytical Procedure*

1. Transfer 2.0 ml of the incubation mixture to a 50 ml glass-stoppered centrifuge tube containing 0.8 g of sodium chloride and 25.0 ml of peroxide-free ether.
2. Shake the tubes for 10 min. Separate the phases by centrifugation.
3. Transfer 20.0 ml of the ether phase to a second 50 ml glass-stoppered centrifuge tube. Add 1.0 ml of 1.6% phenol followed by 1.0 ml of 0.5 M tribasic sodium phosphate (Na₃PO₄). Shake well for five min and centrifuge.
4. Carefully remove the ether layer and allow the color to develp for 20–30 min.
5. Add 2.0 ml of water and read the

absorbance of the blue color in a colo imeter at 640 mµ.

6. The quantity of p-aminophenol forme is determined from a previously pr pared standard curve. The amount p-aminophenol formed (from the grap) must be multiplied by 2.0 to corre for the total incubation volume. Th value obtained must be multiplied b 5/4 to correct for the total volume ether (20 of 25 ml). Since a 1 + homogenate was used as enzym multiply by 4.0 to obtain the tot amount of p-aminophenol formed p gram of tissue. The amount of p-am nophenol (µg) formed divided by 14 (M.W. of p-aminophenol HCl) yiel µmoles of p-aminophenol.

7. *Calculations:*

$$\frac{\mu\text{g p-aminophenol (from standard curve)} \times 2 \times 5/4}{146} \times$$

or µg p-aminophenol × .068 = µmol p-aminophenol formed/gram of tissue 20 min.

C. *Preparation of Standard p-aminophen Curve*

1. Prepare a series of tubes containing aminophenol hydrochloride in water the following concentrations: 8 µg/m 4 µg/ml, 2 µg/ml and 1 µg/ml.
2. To 2.0 ml of each concentration (duplicate) add 1.0 ml of 1.6% phen followed by 1.0 ml of 0.5 M Na₃PC Allow color to develop for 20–30 min.
3. *Blanks:* Use 2.0 ml of water (no drug)

4. Determine the absorbance at 640 mμ.
5. A plot is then made of optical density (ordinate) versus μg of p-aminophenol (abscissa). *Note:* a constant for the determination may be made by dividing the quantity of p-aminophenol indicated at any convenient point on the line by the corresponding optical density. This figure multiplied by the optical density of an unknown gives the amount of p-aminophenol in the unknown.

METHOD 2

A. *Determination of Microsomal Aniline Hydroxylase*

1. Incubation conditions are the same as described for Method 1.
2. At the end of the incubation period add 2.0 ml of 20 % trichloroacetic acid (TCA) to the incubation flasks. Mix well.
3. Pour the contents of the incubation flasks into heavy duty 15 ml centrifuge tubes and centrifuge well.
4. To a 2.0 ml aliquot of the TCA supernatant add 1.0 ml of 10 % Na$_2$CO$_3$ and mix well.
5. Add 2.0 ml of 2 % phenol in 0.2N NaOH and allow the color to develop for 30 min at 37°. Read the absorbance in a colorimeter at 640 mμ.
6. Determine the quantity of p-aminophenol formed from a previously prepared standard curve. Multiply this number by 3.0 to obtain the total amount of p-aminophenol in the incubation flask. This number is multiplied by 4 to obtain the μg of p-aminophenol formed/gram of tissue/20 min.

B. *Preparation of Standard p-aminophenol Curve*

1. Prepare a series of tubes containing p-aminophenol HCl (1–4 μg/ml) in 6.67 % trichloroacetic acid (2.0 ml) as this is the final concentration of TCA after adding 20 % TCA to the incubate.
2. To 2.0 ml of each concentration in TCA (in duplicate) add 1.0 ml of 10 % Na$_2$CO$_3$ followed by 2.0 ml of 2 % phenol in 0.2N NaOH. Allow color to develop and read at 640 mμ. Plot a standard curve as described under Method 1.

General Comments

The procedures described for the determination of microsomal aniline hydroxylase activity are both simple and sensitive. A number of modifications have been made. For example, by increasing the concentration of NADP and decreasing the time of incubation to ten min, nicotinamide may be eliminated from the incubation mixture. Using Method 1, the solid sodium chloride can be replaced with 2.0 ml of a saturated solution of sodium chloride.

The methods described permit one to have a final volume adequate for a colorimeter tube. If desired, the sensitivity may be increased by reducing the final volume (Method 1) to 2.0 ml and reading the optical density in a cuvette.

With Method 1 it is important to use peroxide-free ether. If necessary, peroxide-free ether may be prepared by washing ether with 1/5 volume of a nearly saturated FeSO$_4$ (1 %) solution followed by a number of water washes.

The aniline hydroxylase assay is suitable for isolated microsomes with a NADPH-generating system. Some investigators also add 2 units of glucose-6-phosphate dehydrogenase to the co-factor mixture and pre-incubate briefly prior to adding enzyme and substrate. Others use 1 % ortho-cresol in 0.1N NaOH in place of phenol to form the blue color complex.

It should be mentioned that if p-aminophenol alone is incubated with the

10,000 × g for as long as 30 min, it disappears from the incubation flask. The rate of p-aminophenol disappearance is much less in the presence of aniline. These observations point out the necessity for keeping the incubation period as short as possible. The investigator should establish the optimum conditions in his laboratory.

REFERENCES

Kato, R. and Gillette, J. R.: Effect of starvation on NADPH-dependent enzymes in liver microsomes of male and female rats. J. Pharmacol. Exp. Ther. *150:* 279–284, 1965.

Imai, Y., Ito, A. and Sato, R.: Evidence for biochemically different types of vesicles in the hepatic microsomal fraction. J. Biochem. (Japan) *60:* 417–428, 1966.

V. DETERMINATION OF MICROSOMAL HEXOBARBITAL OXIDASE

The decrease in sleeping time response to hexobarbital has been used as an indicator of increased hepatic microsomal metabolism activity. Hexobarbital metabolism may also be followed *in vitro* by measuring the rate of *disappearance* of hexobarbital from an incubation mixture containing microsomes.

Procedure

1. Into flasks, immersed in the ice, add the following:

   Co-factor mixture: 0.1M phosphate buffer, pH 7.4 containing the following per 3.0 ml:

NADP	.65 μmoles	
Nicotinamide	50.0 μmoles	
Glucose-6-phosphate	10.0 μmoles	
Magnesium chloride	25.0 μmoles	3.0 ml
Sodium hexobarbital in water 1.0 mg/ml.	1.0	1.0 ml
Enzyme: 10,000 × g supernatant fraction, containing microsomes from 250 mg liver.		1.0 ml
Total Volume		5.0 ml

2. Incubate at 37° for 30 min.
3. *At zero time,* transfer 0.5 ml of the incubation mixture to a glass-stoppered centrifuge tube containing 1.0 ml of 0.5 citrate buffer (pH 5.5) saturated with sodium chloride + 15.0 ml of heptane containing 1.5 % isoamyl alcohol. Shake well for 10 min and centrifuge. Remove the citrate buffer layer and discard.
4. Wash the heptane phase by adding fresh citrate buffer (1.5 ml). Shake and centrifuge then discard aqueous layer.
5. Remove 10.0 ml of the heptane layer to a clean glass-stoppered centrifuge tube containing 2.5 ml of 0.8M phosphate buffer pH 11.0. Shake and centrifuge. Discard heptane layer.
6. *Blanks:* Incubates containing no drug should be extracted as described.
7. Read the aqueous layer in a spectrophotometer at 245 and 280 mμ against an extracted tissue blank.

8. Calculate from a previously prepared standard curve (hexobarbital 1–20 $\mu g/ml$ in 0.8M phosphate buffer pH 11.0) the optical density differences 245 mμ minus 280 mμ and thus the amount of hexobarbital which has disappeared from the difference in the amount extracted at ZERO TIME (unincubated) versus the experimental flasks (incubated).

9. *Note:* Hexobarbital is not very stable at high pH and the readings should be carried out as soon as possible (30 min) after transferring the barbiturate into the pH 11.0 buffer.

REFERENCES

Cooper, J. R. and Brodie, B. B.: The enzymatic metabolism of hexobarbital. J. Pharmacol. Exp. Ther. *114:* 409–417, 1955.

VI. THE EFFECT OF PHENOBARBITAL PRETREATMENT ON MICROSOMAL CYTOCHROME P-450 AND CYTOCHROME b₅

This experiment illustrates how to compare cytochrome P-450 and cytochrome b$_5$ of liver microsomes from control and phenobarbital pretreated rats.

Determination of Cytochrome P-450

Cytochrome P-450 (carbon monoxide-binding pigment) is a hemoprotein found in liver microsomes and in the mitochondrial fraction of the adrenal cortex. P-450 has been implicated as a terminal oxidase in microsomal drug metabolism. The reduced form of the pigment readily combines with carbon monoxide to form a complex having an absorption maximum at 450 mμ and a minimum at 405 mμ. Thus, its presence in microsomes can be detected spectrophotometrically only as a difference-spectrum in its carbon monoxide derivative form (Fig. 27.5).

Procedure

Male rats (150–200 g) are given single daily intraperitoneal injections of 100 mg/kg of sodium phenobarbital in normal saline for 3 days. Control animals receive an equal volume of normal saline. The rats are starved overnight and sacrificed on the 4th day (24 hours after the last injection of phenobarbital).

1. Prepare a 25% liver homogenate in isotonic KCl-0.01M phosphate buffer as described on page 531 and isolate the microsomal fraction.

2. Wash the microsomes by resuspending the pellet in ice-cold 1.15% KCl. Recentrifuge at 100,000 × g for 30 min. The washing procedure removes most of the hemoglobin. If the liver has been perfused as described in the general introduction, the washing step may be eliminated.

3. The microsomes isolated from 500 mg of liver (wet weight) are resuspended in 6.0 ml of 0.05M phosphate buffer, pH 7.6 (EDTA 10^{-3}M). The protein concentration of this suspension is approximately 2 mg per ml.

4. All subsequent procedures may be done at room temperature.

5. Two ml of the suspension is placed into each of two matched cuvettes with either teflon or glass stoppers.

6. A baseline is determined using the recording spectrophotometer (Beckman DB) by scanning from 510 to 400 mμ.

7. Carbon monoxide is bubbled gently into the sample cuvette for 20 sec. Add a few milligrams of solid sodium dithionite ($Na_2S_2O_4$). Invert the cuvette and gas the sample cuvette again with carbon monoxide for an additional 20 sec. Place the cap on securely.

8. The reference cuvette is treated only with a few milligrams of sodium dithionite. Mix well.

9. Record the spectrum from 510 mμ to 400 mμ.

10. The quantity of cytochrome P-450 is

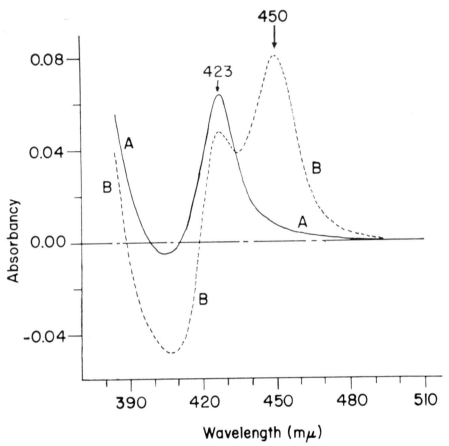

Fig. 27.5. Spectrophotometric determination of cytochrome b_5 and microsomal cytochrome P-450 of beef adrenocortical microsomes.

A. Difference-spectrum between reduced and oxidized cytochrome b_5 (reduced with NADPH).

B. Difference-spectrum for the carbon monoxide-binding pigment. Reference treated with NADPH. Sample treated with NADPH and carbon monoxide (from Estabrook *et al*, 1963).

calculated from the optical density difference (450–480 mμ) and the molar extinction coefficient of 91 mM^{-1}cm^{-1}.

11. *Example Calculation*

Optical density difference, 450–480 mμ
$$= 0.11$$

Mg of protein in cuvette $= 2.5$

$$\frac{0.11 \times 1000}{91 \times 2.5} = 0.48 \text{ m}\mu\text{moles of}$$

cytochrome P-450 per mg of protein

Determination of Cytochrome b_5

Cytochrome b_5, a component of the endoplasmic reticulum, is largely responsible for the intense red color of the microsomal pellet. Cytochrome b_5 is reduced by NADH through *NADH-cytochrome b_5 reductase*, a specific flavoprotein. Reduced cytochrome b_5 can reduce cytochrome c by a direct cytochrome to cytochrome transfer. However, NADH cytochrome b_5 reductase is not able to reduce cytochrome c in the absence of cytochrome b_5. Microsomal cytochrome b_5 content is increased by pretreatment with phenobarbital.

Procedure

1. A microsomal suspension is prepared similar to that prepared for the determination of cytochrome P-450.

2. Two ml of the microsomal suspension is placed into each of two matched cuvettes and a baseline is recorded with the spectrophotometer from 500 mμ to 400 mμ.

3. A few milligrams of powdered sodium dithionite (Na$_2$S$_2$O$_4$) is added to the *sample* cuvette only.

4. The difference spectrum of the reduced cytochrome is determined by recording the absorbance from 500 mμ to 400 mμ in the spectrophotometer.

5. The quantity of cytochrome b$_5$ is calculated from the optical density difference (423 mμ–500 mμ) and the molar extinction coefficient of 171,000 (171 cm^{-1}mM^{-1}) as follows:

$$\frac{\text{optical density difference}}{171 \times \text{mg protein}} \times 1000$$

$$= \frac{\text{m}\mu\text{moles cytochrome b}_5}{\text{mg protein}}$$

REFERENCES

Estabrook, R. W., Cooper, D. Y. and Rosenthal, O.: The light reversible carbon monoxide inhibition of the steroid C$_{21}$-hydroxylase system of the adrenal cortex. Biochem. Z. *338:* 741–755, 1963.

Omura, T. and Sato, R.: The carbon monoxide binding pigment of liver microsomes. J. Biol. Chem. *239:* 2370–2378, 1964.

Strittmatter, P. and Velick, S. F.: The isolation and properties of microsomal cytochrome. J. Biol. Chem. *221:* 253–264, 1956.

VII. COMPARISON OF MICROSOMES FROM CONTROL AND PHENOBARBITAL PRETREATED RATS AS TO NADPH-CYTOCHROME C REDUCTASE ACTIVITY

This experiment illustrates how to determine NADPH-cytochrome c reductase activity from control and phenobarbital pretreated rats.

The microsomal flavoprotein enzyme, NADPH-cytochrome c reductase, has been implicated as one of the enzymes involved in microsomal electron transport and thus is an important component of the drug-metabolizing system. The enzyme has been solubilized and purified and shown to catalyze the reduction of a number of compounds. These include: cytochrome c (1-electron acceptor), menadione (2-electron acceptor), neotetrazolium and azo-dyes (4-electron acceptors). The equations for the reactions are as follows:

$$\text{NADPH} + \text{H}^+ + 2 \text{ cytochrome c}^{3+} \rightarrow \text{NADP}^+ + 2 \text{ cytochrome c}^{2+} + 2\text{H}^+$$

$$\text{NADPH} + \text{H}^+ + \text{dye} \rightarrow \text{reduced dye} + \text{NADP}^+$$

Microsomal NADPH-cytochrome c reductase is induced by pretreatment with phenobarbital but not by 3-methylcholanthrene pretreatment.

Principle of the Analytical Method

One of the assays for enzyme activity depends upon measurement of the rate of cytochrome c reduction. Cytochrome c has a characteristic absorption spectrum in the oxidized state and an equally definite absorbance in the reduced state (Fig. 27.6). The reduced form has a pronounced maximum at 550 mμ which is absent in the oxidized spectrum. Thus, one follows the rate of reduction of cytochrome c by observing the increase in optical density at 550 mμ with time.

Procedure

1. *Reagents:*
   Solution I
   NADPH   5.7 mg

KCN   9.75 mg
Nicotinamide   366 mg
Dissolve the above in 100 ml of 0.05M Na$^+$/K$^+$ phosphate buffer pH 7.6 containing 10^{-3}M EDTA.

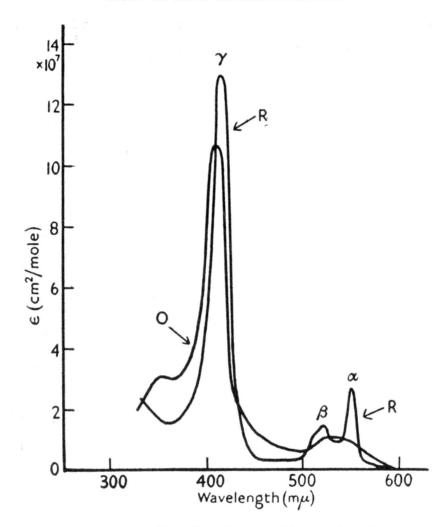

Fig. 27.6. Spectra of oxidized (O) and reduced (R) forms of cytochrome c.

Solution II

Cytochrome c (3.68 mg/ml in water) (Sigma type III or VI)

Solution III

KCN   9.75 mg
Nicotinamide   366 mg

Dissolve the above in 100 ml of 0.05M Na^+/K^+ phosphate buffer pH 7.6 containing $10^{-3}M$ EDTA.

2. In a small test tube incubate 2.0 ml of Solution I and in another tube 2.0 ml of Solution III at 25° for eight min. (*Note:* Solution III contains no NADPH and will serve as the reference (blank).)

3. At the end of eight min add 0.5 ml of

Solution II (cytochrome c) to each tube and incubate an additional two min.

4. Add 0.5 ml of enzyme suspension (microsomes from 10–20 mg of liver in buffer) to each tube. Mix rapidly and pour the contents into 1 cm light path cuvettes.

5. Place the cuvettes into the compartment of a recording spectrophotometer maintained at 25° by a circulating water bath, and record the change in optical density at 550 mμ between the blank and sample cuvette during the first 3 or 4 min when the reaction rate is linear.

6. *Calculations*

One unit of NADPH-cytochrome c re

ductase is defined as the amount of enzyme which produces a change in optical density of 1.0 at 550 mμ in one min. The micromoles of cytochrome c reduced per min are calculated from the molar extinction coefficient of 19.1×10^6 cm² × mole⁻¹ for the difference between reduced and oxidized cytochrome c.

Example

Total volume	= 3.0 ml
Change in O.D. for 1 min	= 0.55
Amount of protein	= 1.0 mg

$$\frac{0.55 \times 3.0 \text{ (volume)}}{19.1 \times 1.0 \text{ (mg protein)}} \times 1000$$

$$= 86.0 \text{ m}\mu\text{moles of cytochrome c}$$
$$\text{reduced/min/mg protein}$$

In the absence of a recorder, a stopwatch or other timer may be used. The change in optical density per minute is recorded for 3–4 min. One plots optical density versus time and calculates the activity as described above.

7. *Calibration of instrument (wavelength)*

On occasion, it may be necessary to calibrate the instrument being used for the assay. This is carried out by checking the wavelength for maximum absorption of cytochrome c as follows:

a. Set the spectrophotometer and recorder to zero using matched cuvettes containing 2.5 ml of Solution III (blank) and 0.5 ml of Solution II (cytochrome c).

b. Add a very small amount of powdered sodium dithionite to the sample cuvette. Mix gently by inversion.

c. Set the instrument on SCAN and record the spectrum from 600 mμ to 500 mμ. The wavelength which gives maximum absorbance for the reduced cytochrome is to be used for the assay.

REFERENCES

Phillips, A. V. and Langdon, R. G.: Hepatic triphosphopyridine nucleotide-cytochrome c reductase: Isolation, characterization and kinetic studies. J. Biol. Chem. *237*: 2652–2660, 1962.

Masters, B. S. S., Williams, Jr., C. H. and Kamin, H.: The preparation and properties of microsomal TPNH-cytochrome c reductase from pig liver. *In Methods in Enzymology*, Vol. X, pp. 565–573, ed. by Estabrook, R. W. and Pullman, M. E., Academic Press, New York, 1967.

Umbreit, W. W., Burris, R. H. and Stauffer, J. H.: *Manometric Techniques*, 4th Ed., Burgess Publishing Co., Minneapolis, 1964.

Dixon, M. and Webb, E. C.: *Enzymes*, p. 383, Academic Press, New York, 1964.

VIII. DETERMINATION OF MICROSOMAL NEOTETRAZOLIUM DIAPHORASE ACTIVITY

The reduction of neotetrazolium salts leads to the formation of highly colored water insoluble formazan derivatives. The reaction will proceed in an atmosphere of either nitrogen or oxygen. The formazan is solubilized by the use of Triton-X mixture and the quantity of formazan formed measured spectrophotometrically

NEOTETRAZOLIUM   NEOTETRAZOLIUM FORMAZAN

Procedure:

Incubation mixture

1. Into flasks, immersed in the ice, add the following:

NADP	0.3 μmoles
Nicotinamide	1.2 μmoles
Glucose-6-Phosphate	1.5 μmoles

(The above in 0.2 ml of .05M phosphate buffer pH 7.6 with EDTA 10⁻³M)   0 2 ml

2. Glucose-6-Phosphate Dehydro-

genase 1.8 units or 0.2 ml of 100,000 × g supernatant (1 ml = soluble fraction from 250 mg liver)   0.2 ml

3. Neotetrazolium Chloride (0.15 μmoles) (MW = 668)   0.2 ml

4. Preincubate the above for five minutes at 37°. Remove the flasks from the incubator and immerse in ice.

5. Add the enzyme. Microsomal suspension equivalent to approximately 3 mg of liver in 0.4 ml of buffer.   0.2 ml

6. Incubate for an additional 10 minutes at 37°.

7. Stop the reaction by the addition of 3.0 ml of the following mixture:

Water	40 ml
10 % Triton X-100	3.6 ml
Formalin 40 %	5.0 ml
Formate Buffer (1M)	10.0 ml

8. *Blanks:* Add Triton-X mixture to complete incubation mixture at 0 time.

9. Read the absorbance in a colorimeter at 500 mμ. Determine the amount of formazan formed from the molar extinction coefficient of 14 cm^{-1} × mM.

10. *Calculations:*

$$\frac{\text{Optical Density (500 m}\mu)}{14 \times \text{mg Protein}} \times 1000$$

$$= \text{m}\mu\text{moles formazan}$$
$$\text{formed/10 min/mg protein}$$

REFERENCES

Lester, R. L. and Smith, A. L.: Studies on the electron transport system. XXVIII. The mode of reduction of tetrazolium salts by beef heart mitochondria; role of coenzyme Q and other lipids. Biochim. Biophys. Acta *47:* 475–496, 1961.

Williams, C. H. and Kiamin, H.: Microsomal triphosphopyridine nucleotide cytochrome c reductase of liver. J. Biol. Chem. *237:* 587–595, 1962.

IX. DETERMINATION OF MICROSOMAL AZO AND NITRO-REDUCTASE ACTIVITIES

A number of azo-dyes are reductively cleaved *in vitro* by hepatic microsomal enzymes. For example, the reduction of prontosil and neoprontosil yields sulfanilamide which can be determined by the method of Bratton and Marshall (1939).

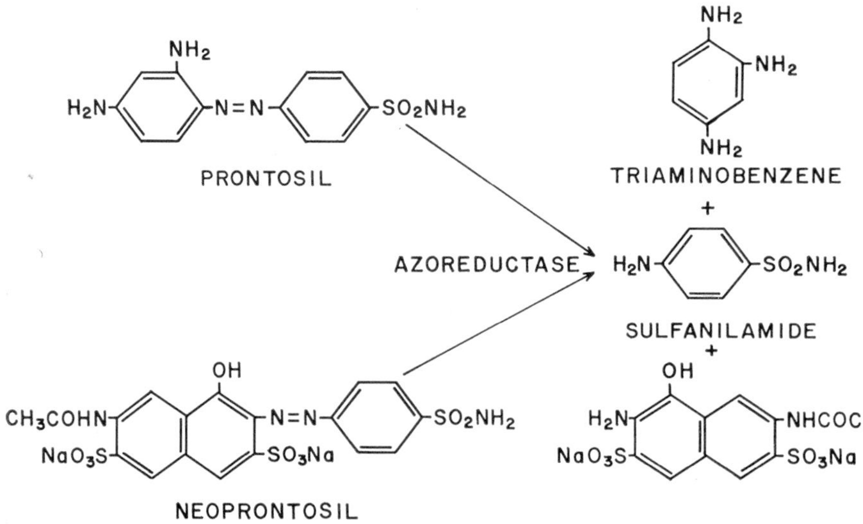

Microsomal nitro-reductase activity can be determined by measuring the quantity of p-aminobenzoic acid (PABA) formed from the reduction of p-nitrobenzoic acid (PNB).

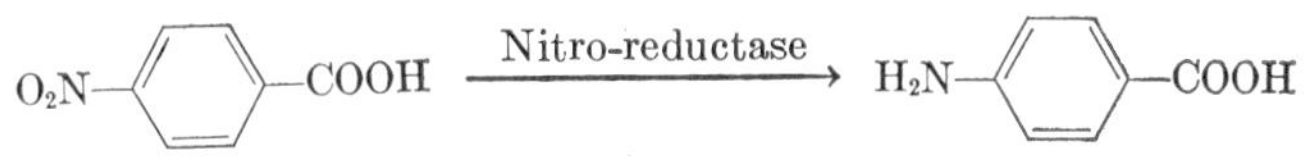

$$O_2N-\!\!\bigcirc\!\!-COOH \xrightarrow{\text{Nitro-reductase}} H_2N-\!\!\bigcirc\!\!-COOH$$

Both nitro and azo-reductase are sensitive to oxygen and therefore the assay must be done in a nitrogen atmosphere. Furthermore, azo and nitro compounds are reduced by the soluble fraction, non-enzymatically, to a small extent, and thus requires separation of the microsomes from the soluble fraction. The non-enzymatic activity is subtracted from the total activity to obtain the enzymatic activity due to the microsomal fraction.

When prontosil or neoprontosil are used as substrates for azo reductase the highly colored substrate must be separated from the product (sulfanilamide) prior to the determination of the sulfanilamide. A separation method is described below. However, the azo-dye, 1,2-dimethyl-4-(p-carboxyphenylazo)5-hydroxy-benzene(CPA) (Nutritional Biochemicals Corp.), does not form a highly colored solution in acid (Smith and van Loon, 1969; Shargel *et al.*, 1969) and therefore one can measure the reduced product (p-aminobenzoic acid) in the presence of the parent compound.

One can use the azo dye CPA to study azo-reductase or p-nitrobenzoic acid (PNB) to study nitro-reductase using a similar incubation and analytical procedure to measure the formation of p-aminobenzoic acid (PNB).

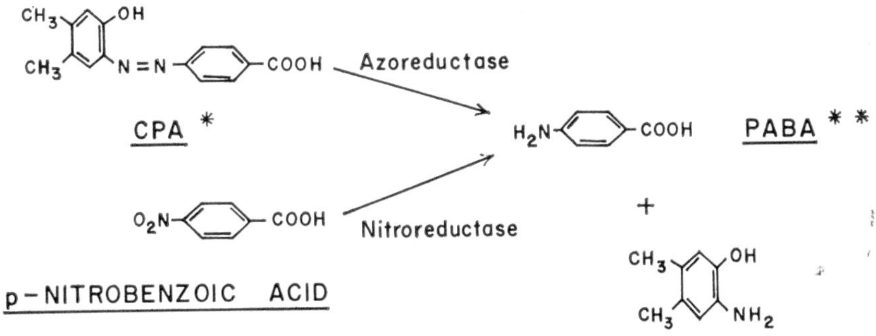

* 1,2-DIMETHYL-4-(p-CARBOXYPHENYLAZO)-5-HYDROXYBENZENE

** p-AMINOBENZOIC ACID

A. Reduction of Nitro and Azo Compounds by Microsomal Reductases

Procedure

1. Anaerobic conditions are required and the incubation must be carried out with a nitrogen atmosphere. Thunberg tubes can be used for this experiment.
2. Pipette into the incubation flasks, while on ice, 6.0 μmoles of p-nitrobenzoic acid (in 0.1 ml methanol) or 10.0 μmoles of the CPA azo dye. The CPA is soluble in methanol or may be added as the

sodium salt. Sodium-CPA solutions have a pH of approximately 8.5.

3. To each flask add 3.0 ml of .05M Na+/K+ phosphate buffer solution (10^{-3}M EDTA) containing 0.5 μmoles NADP, 100 μmoles nicotinamide and 50 μmoles of glucose-6-phosphate.
4. Add 1.0 ml of soluble fraction (100,000 × g) equivalent to 250 mg liver/wet weight to each flask.
5. Add 1.0 ml of 0.05M phosphate buffer

(10^{-3}M EDTA) to those flasks which *do not receive the enzyme.*

6. Add 1.0 ml of enzyme (microsomes obtained from 250 mg of liver) resuspended in 0.05M Na^+/K^+ phosphate buffer. DO NOT ADD TO NON-ENZYMATIC FLASKS.

7. While on ice, flush the stoppered flasks with nitrogen, which is passed through a deoxygenizer mixture (0.5% sodium dithionite + .05% 2-anthroquinone sodium sulfonate in 0.1N NaOH) for 5 min.

8. Incubate the flasks at 37° for 30 min.

9. At the end of the incubation period add 5.0 ml of 10% trichloroacetic acid solution to each flask. Mix well and centrifuge.

10. An aliquot (5.0 ml) of the TCA supernatant is removed and used for the assay of p-aminobenzoic acid (PABA).

11. To 5.0 ml of the TCA supernatant add 1.0 ml of 0.1% sodium nitrite. Mix well and wait 3 min.

12. Add 1.0 ml of 0.5% ammonium sulfamate solution, Mix well. Wait 3 min.

13. Add 1.0 ml of 0.1% solution of N-(1 naphthyl)ethylene diamine HCl. Mix well.

14. Read the absorbance in a colorimeter a 540 mμ and determine the quantity o PABA formed from a previously pre pared standard curve (1–4 μg/ml o PABA in 5% TCA).

15. *Calculations:*

$$\frac{\mu g \text{ (from standard curve)} \times 2 \times 4}{137 \text{ (M.W. PABA)}}$$

$$= \mu \text{moles PABA formed/gm of tissue/30 mi}$$

Note: If a Thunberg tube is used for th above assays, the tube should be alter nately evacuated and flushed with oxygen free nitrogen. The reaction should be initiated by tipping in the substrate from the side arm.

Principle of the Analytical Method

The principle is that any primary arylamine will, under certain conditions react with nitrous acid to form a diazonium salt. The diazonium salt will "couple" with another aromatic amine to form a dye. The amount of dye color is a measure of the amount of arylamine originally present.

Diazotization of the sulfonamide. The sulfonamide reacts with nitrous acid to form a diazonium salt.

(1) $H_3\overset{+}{N}$—⟨benzene⟩—SO_2–$\overset{H}{\underset{|}{N}}$–R + HONO ⟶ $N\equiv\overset{+}{N}$—⟨benzene⟩—SO_2–$\overset{H}{\underset{|}{N}}$–R + 2 H_2O

Destruction of excess nitrite. If nitrous acid were not eliminated at this point, it would react with both amino groups of the coupling reagent. It is the relatively strongly basic primary aliphatic amino group of the coupling reagent that gives a dye highly ionized and thus soluble, at the pH of the reaction mixture. Sulfamate reacts with nitrous acid in this way:

(2) H_2N-SO_3^- + HONO ⟶ N_2 + $SO_4^=$ + H^+ + H_2O

Coupling. The diazonium salt reacts with the coupling reagent to form an azo dye.

(3)

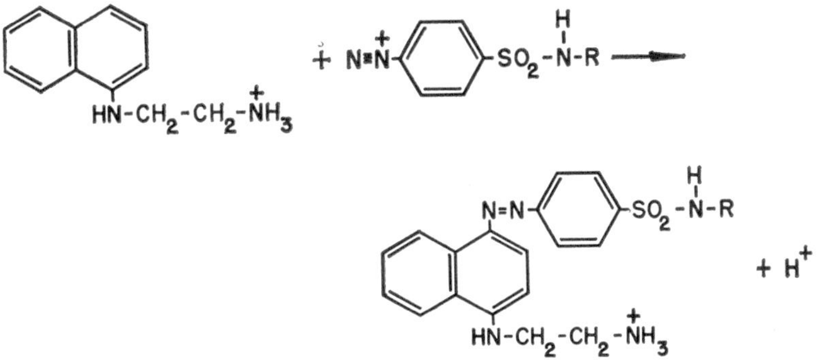

B. Reduction of Neoprontosil by Azo-reductase

Procedure

The incubation conditions are the same as described for the azo-dye CPA (p. 579) except that 10 μmoles of neoprontosil in water (0.1 ml) is used as substrate. The incubation is done under nitrogen for 30 min. Correction must be made for the non-enzymatic activity of the 100,000 × g supernatant. Therefore, flasks containing 100,000 × g fraction and no microsomal enzyme must be included. At the end of 30 min, place incubation tray back into ice and stop reaction with 15 ml of 6.67 % trichloroacetic acid solution (TCA). Centrifuge the mixture for 10 min. An aliquot of the TCA supernatant will be analyzed for sulfanilamide.

Separation of sulfanilamide from neoprontosil

Neoprontosil is separated from sulfanilamide in the TCA supernatant by the use of Dowex 50-x8 (200 to 400 mesh).
a) Prepare column by placing an aliquot of a slurry of Dowex 50-x8 in water in a small glass column (1.0 × 13 cm), stopped by a pellet of glass wool.
b) The final 1.0 × 2.0 cm resin bed is washed with distilled water.
c) A 5 ml aliquot of the TCA supernatant is placed on the column.
d) The column is then washed with about 5 ml of water until no red neoprontosil is left in the resin and the eluent is colorless.

e) Sulfanilamide is eluted off the column with two successive portions of 10 ml of 3 N HCl and mixed.
6. *Determination of sulfanilamide*
a) 5 ml of the 3 N HCl eluent containing the sulfanilamide is neutralized to pH 1–2 using 4.0 ml of 2 M K_3PO_4 solution.
b) 1 ml of 0.1 % NaNO$_2$ solution is added and mixed.
c) Wait 5 min.
d) Add 1 ml of 0.5 % ammonium sulfamate.
e) Mix and wait 5 min.
f) Add 1 ml of 0.1 % of N-(1-Naphthyl)-ethylenediamine HCl solution.
g) Read O.D. at 545 mμ in a colorimeter.
h) Calculate μmoles of sulfanilamide from standard curve (standards made from sulfanilamide 1 to 4 μg/ml in 3N HCl).
i) *Note:* In order to determine the total amount of sulfanilamide formed in the incubate, corrections must be made for the aliquot of TCA used (5 of 20 ml) and for the 3N HCl (5 of 20 ml). The total amount of sulfanilamide (μg) divided by the M.W. of sulfanilamide (172) × 1000 yield mμmoles of sulfanilamide formed. Therefore:

$$\frac{\text{Total } \mu g \text{ (in 3N HCl)} \times 4 \times 4}{172}$$

= mμmoles sulfanilamide formed/30 min/mg protein*

* From microsomal protein determination (p. 538).

REFERENCES

Bratton, A. C. and Marshall, E. K., Jr.: A new coupling component for sulfanila-mide determine. J. Biol. Chem. *128:* 537–550, 1939.

Fouts, J. R. and Brodie, B. B.: The enzymatic reduction of chloramphenicol p-nitrobenzoic acid and other aromatic nitro compounds in mammals. J. Pharmacol. Exp. Ther. *119:* 197–207, 1957.

Fouts, J. R., Kamm, J. J. and Brodie, B. B.: Enzymatic reduction of prontosil and other azo dyes. J. Pharmacol. Exp. Ther. *120:* 291–300, 1957.

Hernandez, P. H., Gillette, J. R. and Mazel, P.: Studies on the mechanism of action of mammalian hepatic azoreductase. I. Azoreductase activity of reduced nicotinamide adenine dinucleotide phosphate-cytochrome c reductase. Biochem. Pharmacol. *16:* 1859–1875 (1967).

Shargel, L., Akov, S. and Mazel, P.: The reduction of nitro and azo compounds by housefly microsomes. J. Toxicol. Appl. Pharmacol. *14:* 645, 1969.

Smith, E. J. and Van Loom, E. J.: Anal. Biochem. *31:* 315 320, 1969.

28

Experiments Illustrating Drug Distribution and Excretion

V. G. ZANNONI

I. INTRODUCTION

To cause a therapeutic effect, a drug must reach its site of action in effective concentrations and remain at these sites for a sufficient length of time. The tissue concentration of a drug depends upon several factors; one of the most important, is its concentration in the blood. The concentration of drug in the blood is determined by the amount of drug administered, its rate of absorption, the rate and extent of its distribution, and the rate at which the drug and its metabolites are excreted. Drug absorption, distribution within the body, and drug excretion depend to a large extent on the lipoid-nature of the particular cellular boundaaries the drug must penetrate, and the intrinsic lipophilic properties of the drug. The latter properties will be determined by the chemical structure of the drug and relative amount of unionized species (U) of the drug present in the physiological fluids. In order to determine the ratio of unionized form present in a physiological fluid or tissue, the degree of ionization of the drug must be determined. For this calculation, the pKa or pKb of the drug and the hydrogen ion concentration of the fluid or tissue must be considered. The relationship between environmental pH and the fraction of drug in the unionized form can be mathematically expressed by the Henderson-Hasselbalch equation since most drugs are weak organic acids or weak organic bases. For a drug which is a weak organic acid; $pH = pKa + \log (I)/(U)$ and for a drug which is a weak organic base; $pH = pKa$ (base) $+ \log (U)/(I)$. Knowledge of the degree of ionization of a drug at a particular physiological pH will allow a reasonable prediction of its tissue distribution and its renal excretion or reabsorption.

This experiment is a quantitative study of the distribution and excretion of an unknown sulfonamide (one of the six listed in Table 28.1). The list includes analogues of sulfanilamide that vary in their pKa values from 5.4 to 10.4. After intravenous injection of a carefully measured amount of the unknown sulfonamide in a female dog weighing 10–14 kg, samples of blood, urine, saliva and cerebrospinal fluid are collected during the following 60 minutes. The concentration of the sulfonamide will be determined in these biological fluids by the Bratton-Marshall diazotization reaction. In addition, the total amount of sulfonamide excreted in saliva and urine for the 60 min experimental period will be measured. Furthermore, the extent of binding of the particular sulfon-

TABLE 28.1

Distribution and excretion of sulfonamides in the dog

		Sulfa(a)acetamide	Diazine	Thiazole	Merazine	Pyridine	Nilamide
pKa		5.4	6.5	7.1	7.1	8.4	10.4
% bound*	Av.	11	20	57	31	28	15
	Range	(10–13)	(17–21)	(56–62)	(28–34)	(26–31)	(13–16)
ER	Av.	1.3	0.34	1.3	0.28	0.37	0.61
	Range	(1.2–1.4)	(0.28–0.41)	(1.2–1.6)	(0.22–0.38)	(0.32–0.49)	(0.55–0.78)
VdR	Av.	0.62	0.52	1.6	0.72	1.2	1.0
	Range	(0.60–0.68)	(0.50–0.65)	(1.4–1.9)	(0.62–0.78)	(1.1–1.5)	(0.92–1.2)
Rcsf†	Av.	0.07	0.31	0.20	0.62	0.96	0.65
	Range	(0.06–0.08)	(0.28–0.34)	(0.16–0.25)	(0.55–0.70)	(0.84–1.1)	(0.58–0.72)

Average value = mean of 14 individual classroom experiments.

* When total concentration in plasma (free + bound) = 5 mg/100 ml.

† Not necessarily an equilibrium value; data obtained at 60 min.

amide to dog plasma protein will be determined prior to the *in vivo* administration of the drug to the animal by an *in vitro* equilibrium dialysis experiment.

These data will be used to calculate certain constants which characterize the tissue distribution and excretion behavior of the unknown sulfonamide. These constants include: the per cent of sulfonamide bound to plasma protein, the excretion ratio (ER), the apparent volume of distribution ratio (VdR) and the relative concentration of the sulfonamide in the cerebral spinal fluid to that in plasma (Rcsf). By comparing the derived constants with those given in Table 28.1, it should be possible to identify which unknown sulfonamide was given.

II. MATERIALS AND REAGENTS

The following materials and reagents are needed for each dog experiment.

Materials for Part I

1 dog board and ropes
1 pelvic board
1 infusion buret (100 ml.)
1 urethral catheter
1 bowl for saliva
1 lamp
1 tracheal cannula
1 long arm clamp
1 screw clamp

1 cannula tubing ⚡190
1 cotton cord (2 feet)
1 table top clinical centrifuge
1 dialysis tubing (1 inch flat width × 4 inches)
1 magnetic stirrer

2 test tube racks
15 test tubes, heavy wall, 14 × 100 mm
5 test tubes, 18 × 150 mm
3 erlenmeyer flasks (500 ml)
2 graduate cylinders (100 ml)
2 beakers (250 ml)
2 syringes (5 ml)
3 syringes (10 ml)
6—1 inch needles (22 gauge)
1—2 inch needle (18 gauge)
1 speculum
1—2 inch spinal tap needle (Quincke ⚡22)
1 dissecting kit (scissors, forceps, hemostats, scapels)

Also, cotton thread, adhesive tape, parafilm, gauze, paper tape, china marker, Kleenex.

Reagents for Part I

All reagents are made up in distilled H_2O and are stable for at least one week at 5°.

10% $Na_2SO_4 \cdot 10H_2O$ (250 ml)		0.1% Pilocarpine·HCl (15 ml)
0.9% NaCl (500 ml)		0.9% KCl, pH 7.4 (1000 ml)
20% $K_2C_2O_4 \cdot H_2O$ (15 ml)		dog plasma (10 ml)

Sulfonamides. Stock solutions are prepared for each sulfonamide containing 100 mg/ml.

	pKa	
sulfacetamide	5.4	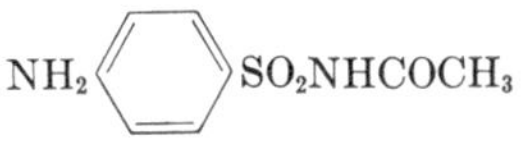 NH_2⟨benzene⟩$SO_2NHCOCH_3$
sulfadiazine	6.5	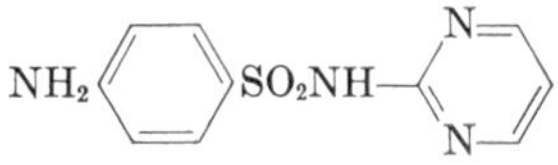 NH_2⟨benzene⟩SO_2NH—⟨pyrimidine⟩
sulfathiazole	7.1	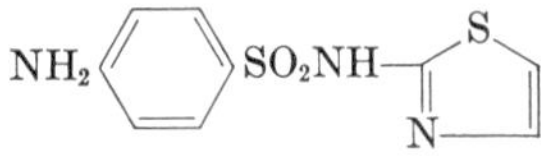 NH_2⟨benzene⟩SO_2NH—⟨thiazole⟩
sulfamerazine	7.1	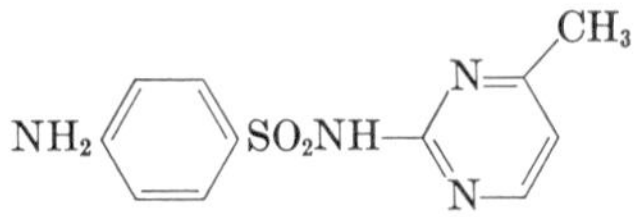 NH_2⟨benzene⟩SO_2NH—⟨methylpyrimidine, CH_3⟩
sulfapyridine	8.4	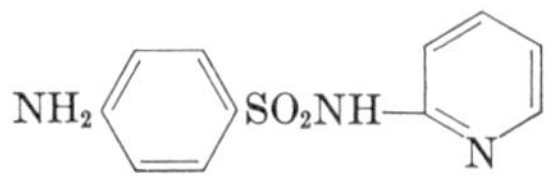 NH_2⟨benzene⟩SO_2NH—⟨pyridine⟩
sulfanilamide	10.4	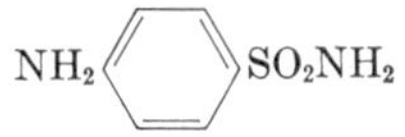 NH_2⟨benzene⟩SO_2NH_2

Each stock solution is prepared by suspending 5 grams of sulfonamide in 25 ml of distilled water in a 50 ml volumetric flask, followed by the addition of pellets of NaOH until the drug is dissolved. Additional distilled water is added to 50 ml. The stock solution is kept at 25° and is stable for at least 2 weeks. Appropriate dilution of this stock solution should be made for the *in vitro* equilibrium dialysis experiment.

Materials for Part II (Chemical Analysis)

2 test tube racks
24 cuvettes (19 × 105 mm) (Coleman)
2 graduates (50 ml)
24 erlenmeyer flasks (125 ml)
12 short stem funnels (65 × 65 mm)
24 pipettes, Mohr measuring (1.0 ml)
6 pipettes, Mohr measuring (5.0 ml)
20 pipettes, Mohr measuring (10.0 ml)
1 box filter paper, #1, (11 cm)
1 Coleman colorimeter
China marker, kleenex, parafilm

Reagents for Part II

All reagents are made up in distilled H_2O and are stable for at least one week at 5°.

0.1% N-(1-naphthyl)ethylenediamine·2HCl (50 ml)
0.5% Ammonium sulfate (50 ml)

0.1 % NaNO₂ (50 ml)

0.1 % $NaNO_2$ (50 ml)

15 % Trichloroacetic acid (250 ml)

Distilled H_2O (1000 ml)

III. EXPERIMENTAL PROCEDURE

A. Part I

1. Sulfonamide Binding to Plasma Protein by Equilibrium Dialysis.
An equilibrium dialysis experiment to determine the per cent binding of the
sulfonamide to dog plasma protein is performed one day prior to the administration of the unknown sulfonamide to the animal

Procedure

10 ml of dog plasma is dialysed at 5°
against 1 liter of 0.9 % KCl, pH 7.4, containing the sulfonamide at a concentration
of 0.05 mg/ml. The dialysis is carried out for
16 hours with constant stirring, at which

time equilibrium should be reached. An
change in plasma volume is recorded and
dilution factor is incorporated into the calcu
lation of the per cent of bound drug. 5 m
samples of plasma and dialysate are remove
and saved for chemical analysis (Part II).

2. In Vivo Administration of Sulfonamide

Procedure

1. A female dog is provided, previously
   anesthetized with pentobarbital (33
   mg/kg body weight). It is important
   that the level of anesthesia is adequate
   before starting the surgical procedure.
2. Insert a urethral catheter and tie it in
   place.
3. Insert a tracheal cannula and tie it in
   place.
4. Insert the polyethylene tubing into an
   exposed jugular vein and connect it to
   an infusion buret. Start the infusion of a
   mixture of equal parts of 10 % Na_2SO_4
   and 0.9 % NaCl at a rate of 3 ml/min in
   order to ensure adequate diuresis during
   the experiment. Continue the infusion
   for the remainder of the experiment and
   adjust the rate, as necessary, to obtain
   approximately 200 ml of urine during
   the experimental hour.
5. Start collecting the control urine sample
   through the urethral catheter immediately after the infusion is started. Save
   approximately 10 ml of a *control urine*
   sample.
6. Expose one femoral vein and use this

vessel for removing blood sample
Carefully label all blood and urin
samples.
7. Withdraw approximately 8 ml as
   control blood sample from the femora
   vein using a ⌗20 gauge needle and a 1
   ml syringe containing 2 drops of potas
   sium oxalate (20 %) and mix thoroughly
   Place approximately 6 ml of the blood i
   a heavy-walled test tube containing
   drops of potassium oxalate. Balance th
   tubes and centrifuge the samples for 1
   min. Pipet off the *control plasma* sampl
   and save for chemical analysis.
8. Inject 2.5 ml of pilocarpine·HCl (0.1 %
   via the polyethylene tubing into th
   jugular vein. Pilocarpine is a cholinomi
   metic alkaloid which stimulates salivar
   glands. Place the dog's head on the sid
   with its tongue hanging down above th
   saliva bowl. Collect and save approxi
   mately 5 ml of *control saliva*. Collec
   the saliva for the 60 minute experimenta
   period starting from time zero (adminis
   tration of unknown sulfonamide). Meas
   ure the total volume of saliva excrete
   during the 60 min period.

9. At zero time, slowly inject (i.v.) (up to 1 min) the sulfonamide at a dosage of 50 mg/kg body weight via the poly ethylene tubing into the jugular vein. To avoid contamination do not use this syringe for subsequent sampling.

0. At zero time, replace the flask containing control urine with a clean collection flask and collect the subsequent urine for 60 min. Measure the total volume of urine voided during the 60 min experimental period.

1. At 20, 40 and 60 min after zero time, take 8 ml blood samples from the femoral vein as described above, in step 7.

2. After taking the last blood sample turn the dog on its abdomen and perform a cisternal puncture. Withdraw from 3 to 5 ml of cerebrospinal fluid avoiding contamination with blood. (Ask Instructor, if assistance is needed.)

13. Sacrifice the animal by injecting 10 ml of chloroform (i.v.) through the jugular vein cannula.

There are a total of 11 samples for chemical analysis (Part II).

Samples					
	Con- trol	20 min	40 min	60 min	
Binding					
Plasma	X	—	—	—	record dilu- tion
Dialysate	X	—	—	—	
In vivo					
Plasma	X	X	X	X	
Saliva	X	—	—	X	record total volume
Urine	X	—	—	X	record total volume
CSF	—	—	—	X	

B. Part II. Chemical Analysis

1. Preparation of trichloroacetic acid filtrates

Plasma: Pipet 1.0 ml of plasma (control, 20, 40 and 60 min samples) into a 125 ml erlenmeyer flask containing 31 ml of distilled water. Add 8.0 ml of 15% trichloroacetic acid, mix and allow 10 min for the denaturation of the plasma proteins. Filter and pipet two 10 ml aliquots of each acidified filtrate into cuvettes and save for chemical analysis.

Saliva and Cerebrospinal fluid: Carry out the procedure as for plasma using 1.0 ml of each secretion (control and 60 min saliva sample; 60 min CSF sample). Filtration may be omitted if the solution remains clear after the addition of trichloroacetic acid. Pipet 2-10 ml aliquots of each acidified filtrate into cuvettes and save for chemical analysis.

Urine: Dilute the urine (control and 60 min sample) 1 to 4 with 3 parts of distilled water. Pipet 1.0 ml of the diluted urine into a 125 ml erlenmeyer flask and carry out the procedure as for plasma. Filter if the solution is not clear after addition of trichloroacetic acid. Pipet 2-10 ml aliquots of each acidified sample into cuvettes and save for chemical analysis.

Equilibrium Dialysis Samples: Pipet 1.0 ml samples of the plasma and the dialysate into 125 ml erlenmeyer flasks and carry out the procedure as for plasma. Filtration may be omitted with the dialysate sample. Pipet 2-10 ml aliquots of each acidified filtrate into cuvettes and save for chemical analysis.

Reagent Blank: A reagent blank should be prepared to set the colorimeter at zero absorbance. Add 8 ml of 15% trichloroacetic acid to a 125 ml erlenmeyer flask containing 32 ml of distilled water. Pipet 1-10 ml aliquot of this solution into a cuvette and save for the addition of the analytical reagents.

2. Chemical Analysis of Sulfonamide

Diazotization Reaction

1. Formation of diazonium salt with sulfonamide and nitrous acid:

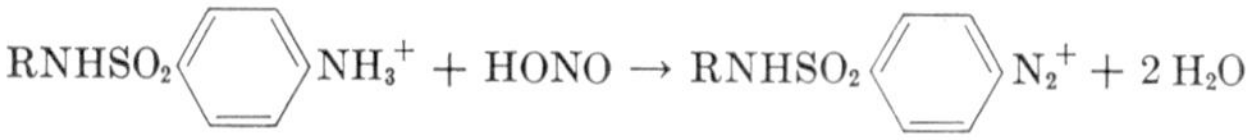

2. Destruction of excess nitrous acid with ammonium sulfamate:

$$HONO + H_2NSO_3^- \rightarrow N_2 + SO_4^= + H^+ + H_2O$$

3. Coupling of diazonium salt with N-(1-naphthyl)ethylenediamine to form azo dye:

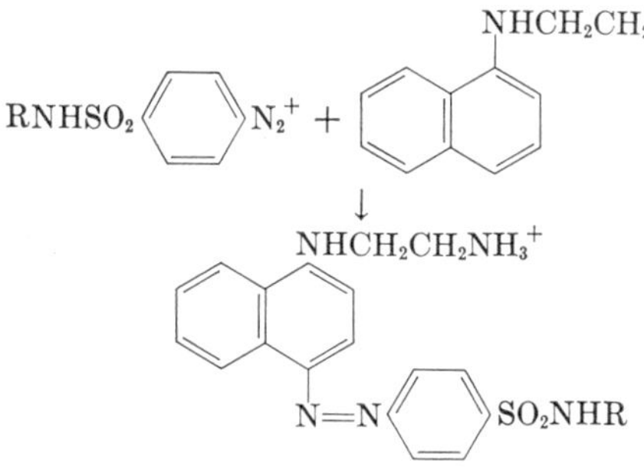

azo dye, maximum absorption at 540 mμ.

Procedure

To each cuvette containing 10 ml of the acidified filtrates (22 samples plus 1 reagent blank), pipet 1.0 ml of 0.1% sodium nitrite and shake thoroughly. After 5 min, add 1.0 ml of 0.5% ammonium sulfamate and shake. After 5 min, add 1.0 ml of 0.1% N-(1-naphthyl) ethylene-diamine·2HCl and shake. *This order of addition of reagents must be followed.* Allow color development for 15 min. The resulting chromagen is stable for at least 2 hours at room temperature. All samples are read against the reagent blank at 540 mμ. Dilution of the chromagen with distilled water may be necessary if the color in any of the cuvettes is too intense (readings above 0.800 O.D.).

Standard Curve

Standard curve of each sulfonamide listed in Table 28.1 has been prepared previously (5.0 μg to 30 μg of sulfonamide in a total reagent volume of 13 ml) and the proper one should be used to determine the quantity of sulfonamide present in each sample. For example, 1.0 μg of sulfacetamide gives a reading of 0.021 O.D. unit, and 1.0 μg of sulfathiazine gives a reading of 0.0182 O.D. unit.

Sample Calculation:

Sulfacetamide in plasma, saliva, CSF and dialysate

$$\frac{O.D.(540 \text{ m}\mu) \times 4}{0.021 \times 1000} = \text{mg sulfacetamide/ml plasma}$$

Sulfacetamide in urine

$$\frac{\text{O.D.}(540 \text{ m}\mu) \times 16}{0.021 \times 1000} = \text{mg sulfacetamide/ml urine}$$

IV. DEFINITIONS AND CALCULATIONS

1. Weight of dog   ____Kg
2. Total amount of sulfonamide given   ____mg
      dose of sulfonamide = 50 mg/Kg body weight
      50 mg/Kg × weight of animal (Kg) = total amount
3. Total amount of sulfonamide excreted (urine + saliva)   ____mg
      mg of sulfonamide/ml of urine × ml of urine in 60 min   ____mg
      mg of sulfonamide/ml of saliva × ml of saliva in 60 min   ____mg
4. Sulfonamide remaining in dog at the end of the 60 min experimental
      period
      Total amount of sulfonamide given − total amount of sulfona-
      mide excreted   ____mg
5. Per cent of free sulfonamide calculated from plasma binding equi-
      librium dialysis   ____%
      Sulfonamide in plasma (in dialysis bag) in mg/ml = bound + free drug
      Sulfonamide in dialysate (outside dialysis bag) in mg/ml = free drug

% Bound to plasma =

$$\frac{[(\text{sulfonamide})_{\text{plasma}} - (\text{sulfonamide})_{\text{dialysate}} \times \text{dilution factor}] \times 100}{(\text{sulfonamide})_{\text{plasma}}}$$

$$\text{dilution factor} = \frac{\text{final plasma volume}}{\text{initial plasma volume}}$$

$$= \text{fractional increase in plasma volume during dialysis}$$

The dilution factor should be less than 1.1 and would be an inappropriate
correction for a very large change in volume.

6. Plasma concentration of sulfonamide during 60 min experimental
      period   ____mg/ml
      average of 20, 40 and 60 min plasma levels (free + bound drug)
7. Plasma concentration of free sulfonamide during 60 min experi-
      mental period   ____mg/ml
      average plasma concentration in mg/ml × % free sulfonamide
8. Excretion ratio (ER)
      The excretion ratio is an index of how the drug is handled by the kidney,
      i.e.; mainly through reabsorption, filtration or secretion.

$$\frac{\text{rate of sulfonamide excreted in urine (mg/min)}}{\text{rate of free sulfonamide filtered by kidney (mg/ml)}}$$

$$\text{rate of sulfonamide excreted} = \frac{\text{total amount in urine after 60 min (mg)}}{60 \text{ min}}$$

rate of free sulfonamide filtered =

$$\text{glomerular filtration rate (ml/min)} \times \text{average free drug}$$
$$\text{plasma concentration (mg/ml)}$$

The glomerular filtration rate in a female dog weighing 10–14
Kg is approximately 40 ml/min
The average free drug plasma concentration = average of 20, 40, and
60 min plasma levels (mg/ml) × % free

9. Apparent volume of distribution (Vd)   ____liters
   The volume of distribution of the sulfonamide is the space in liters in
   which the drug is apparently dissolved. It is assumed that the drug has
   a uniform concentration throughout this space and this is equal to the
   concentration of *free* drug in the plasma.

$$Vd = \frac{\text{total amount of drug in animal at 60 min (mg)}}{\text{free drug plasma concentration (mg/liter) at 60 min}}$$

10. Volume of distribution ratio (VdR)   _____
    The volume of distribution ratio is equal to the apparent volume of dis-
    tribution (Vd) divided by the weight of the animal. This ratio represents
    the fraction of body weight which apparently contains the drug. For
    example, a ratio of 0.65 suggests that the drug is uniformly distributed in
    total body water.

$$VdR = \frac{Vd \text{ liters}}{\text{Weight of animal (Kg)}}$$

Body weight in Kg and volume in Liters are used for this calculation
since the density of the tissues is assumed to be 1.

11. Rcsf   _____
    The relative concentration of the sulfonamide in the cerebrospinal fluid
    compared to the plasma concentration of free drug is an index of the
    ability of the drug to penetrate the blood-brain barrier.

$$Rcsf = \frac{\text{concentration of sulfonamide in csf (mg/ml)}}{\text{free drug plasma concentration (mg/ml)}}$$

The free drug plasma concentration = the 60 min plasma level
(mg/ml) × % free drug

GENERAL REFERENCES

Bratton, A. C. and Marshall, E. K., Jr.: A new coupling component for sulfanilamide determination. J. Biol. Chem. *128:* 537–550, 1939.

Brodie, B. B.: Physico-chemical factors in Drug Absorption. In *Absorption and Distribution of Drugs*, ed. by T. B. Binns, p. 16–47, The Williams and Wilkins Company, Baltimore, 1964.

Brodie, B. B., Kurz, H. and Schanker, L. S.: The importance of dissociation constant and lipid solubility in influencing the passage of drugs into cerebrospinal fluid. J. Pharmacol. Exp. Ther. *130:* 20, 1960.

Davis, B. D.: The binding of sulfonamide drugs by plasma proteins. A factor in determining the distribution of drugs in the body. J. Clin. Invest. *22:* 753–762, 1943.

Despopoulos, A. and Callahan, P. X.: Molecular feature of sulfonamide transport in renal excretory processes. Am. J. Physiol. *203:* 19–26, 1962.

Fisher, S. H., Troast, L., Waterhouse, A. and Shannon, J. A.: The relation between chemical structure and physiological disposition of a series of substances allied to sulfanilamide. J. Pharmacol. Exp. Ther. *79:* 373–391, 1943.

Goldstein, A., Aronow, L. and Kalman, S. M.: In *Principles of Drug Action, The Basis of Pharmacology*, Chap. 2, The absorption, distribution and elimination of drugs. Harper and Row, Publishers, N.Y. p. 106–205, 1968.

Klotz, I. M. and Walker, F. M.: The binding of some sulfonamides by bovine serum albumin. J. Am. Chem. Soc. *70:* 943–946, 1947.

Schanker, L. S.: Mechanisms of drug absorption and distribution. Ann. Rev. Pharmacol. *1:* 29, 1961.

Shannon, J. A.: The relationship between chemical structure and physiological disposition of a series of substances allied to sulfanilamide. Annals of N.Y. Acad. Sci. *44:* 455–476, 1943.

29

Correlation of Drug Disposition with Pharmacologic Actions

A. TREVOR

I. INTRODUCTION

The following experiments were designed to introduce participants at the Third Workshop on Drug Metabolism to some of the methods used in drug metabolism studies and to illustrate many of the principles presented in formal lectures. In the present context they serve primarily a teaching function at the level of predoctoral education, since they represent a simple experimental illustration of a primary objective of drug metabolism investigations—namely the relationship of biotransformation processes to pharmacological action.

The duration and intensity of action of many drugs is critically influenced by the rate of their metabolism. The activities of the microsomal drug-metabolizing enzyme systems vary markedly depending upon sex, age, nutrition and other factors. These activities can also be changed by the prior treatment of animals with various compounds some of which may be structurally unrelated to the drug metabolized.

The present experiments demonstrate the effects of administration of compounds that either stimulate liver drug-metabolizing enzymes (phenobarbital and benzpyrene) or that inhibit these enzymes (SKF 525-A) on:

1. The duration of action of the paralyzing drug zoxazolamine.
2. The half-life of zoxazolamine in the rat.
3. The activity of liver microsomal enzymes as indicated by the *in vitro* hydroxylation of zoxazolamine.

The 3 experiments involve the action of the paralyzing drug zoxazolamine (2 amino-5-chlorobenzoxazole; McNeil Laboratories). Zoxazolamine appears to have a central action in causing muscle relaxation by inhibiting reflex pathways within the spinal cord (Kamijo and Koelle (1955); Geiger *et al.* (1958)), but its precise mechanism of action is not understood. The agent also possesses uricosuric properties (Burns *et al.* (1958)) but this aspect of its action is not examined in the present experiments.

The metabolic fate of zoxazolamine in man has been investigated by Conney *et al.* (1960). It is metabolized principally by hydroxylation to 6-hydroxy zoxazolamine which is excreted as the glucuronide and to a minor extent to chlorzoxazone (fig. 29.1). The 6-hydroxy derivative has marginal muscle relaxant properties similar to the parent drug but has no uricosuric action. Although rat liver microsomal preparations actively metabolize zoxazolamine, the extent to which 6-hydroxylation occurs in the rat has not been reported although

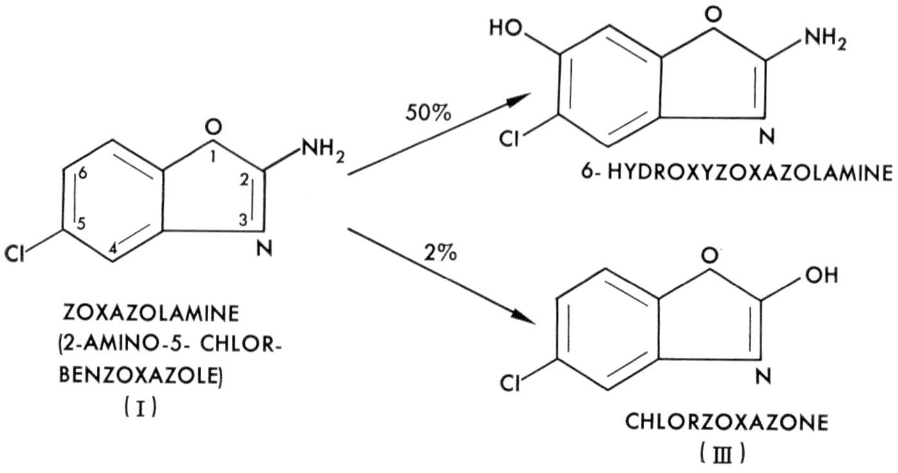

Fig. 29.1. Metabolism of zoxazolamine in man.

Conney *et al.* (1960) have indicated 6-hydroxyzoxazolamine is a major metabolite of the drug in the Wistar strain. While the drug is no longer used therapeutically, it is a convenient compound to use for illustrative purposes because its disposition and pharmacologic actions can be easily determined.

II. GENERAL PROCEDURES

A. Analytical Methodology for Zoxazolamine

Introduction: In the development and use of any analytical procedures for the determination of a drug present in biological fluids or tissue extracts, it is necessary that certain facts concerning the procedure be known. These are usually determined during the logical development of the methodology and include:

1. The potentials and limitations of the technique chosen.

2. Construction of an absolute calibration curve to determine the characteristics (linearity) of the measuring instrument.

3. Determination of a calibration curve for the total procedure by extraction from aqueous drug solutions to give "aqueous recovery" value.

4. Determination of calibration curve for the total procedure by extraction from biological fluid/extract drug solutions (plasma, urine, tissue "recovery" values).

5. Determination of specificity.
    a. Biological fluid/extract "blank."
    b. Drug metabolites.

6. Estimation of precision and accuracy of the method.

Methods for estimation of zoxazolamine from biological fluids and tissues have all been based on the procedure developed by Burns *et al.* (1958). Zoxazolamine is isolated from the alkalinized biological material by extraction with a suitable organic solvent (ethylene dichloride, chloroform, heptane). The drug is then back-extracted from the organic solution into HCl and measured spectrophotometrically at 278 mμ where it exhibits a pronounced peak.

Nicotinamide, sometimes present in fortified tissue dispersions, interferes with the assay. Buffer washing (0.3M sodium borate, 0.1M sodium acetate, pH 5.6) of the organic solution prior to acid extraction removes the nicotinamide, but only negligible amounts of zoxazolamine. Chlorzoxazone, 6-hydroxy-zoxazolamine and 6-hydroxy-chlorzoxazone do not interfere with this method for the estimation of zoxazolamine.

Absolute UV calibration curve for zoxazolamine in acid:

Standard solutions of zoxazolamine in 0.1N HCl should be provided.

1. Commencing with the lowest concentration, measure the absorbance of the standard solutions A-F at 278 mµ.

2. Use 0.1N HCl as the reference sample.

3. Rinse the silica cells with distilled water and dry with acetone between determinations.

4. Construct a Beer-Lambert plot and determine the molar extinction value of zoxazolamine.

Standard Solution	Concentration µg/ml	Absorbance	Corrected Absorbance
0.1N HCl	0		
A	1.0		
B	2.5		
C	5.0		
D	10.0		
E	20.0		
F	30.0		

Wavelength:—

Slit width:—

Solvent:—

Reference sample:—

Path length:—

Molecular weight of zoxazolamine = 168.59

$\epsilon = E/C \times L$ where E = absorbance
C = gm. moles/liter
L = path length (cm.)

Calibration curve for zoxazolamine from rat total body homogenate: Reagents: Standard zoxazolamine solutions in 0.1N HCl (10–100 µg/mg).

0.1N HCl.

Chloroform (reagent grade).

1N NaOH.

10 % (w/v.) rat total body homogenate in 0.1N HCl.

Procedure:

Prepare 6 screw-capped 20 ml culture tubes as detailed in table below.

	1	2	3	4	5	6
Rat Homogenate (2 ml)	+	+	+	+	+	+
Standard Zoxazolamine (1 ml)	−	D	F	G	H	I
1N NaOH (0.5 ml)	+	+	+	+	+	+
Chloroform (12.5 ml)	+	+	+	+	+	+
0.1N HCl (1 ml)	+					
Zoxazolamine (µg/ ml homogenate)	0	5	15	25	37.5	50
Absorbance (278 mµ)						
Corrected absorbance	0.00					

2. Cap tubes and shake on mechanical shaker for 15 min at pre-set speed.

3. Centrifuge tubes for 15 min then discard upper aqueous phase.

4. Transfer 10 ml of chloroform layer to fresh tube containing 4 ml 0.1N HCl. Shake for 5 min.

5. Centrifuge for 5 min to separate phases. Take acid phase and measure absorbance at 278 mµ. Use disposable pasteur pipets for transferring acid. Clean and dry cuvettes between each determination.

6. Correct readings for homogenate "blank."

7. Construct a calibration curve and from this calculate average percentage recovery corrected for aliquot loss.

% extraction =

$$\frac{\text{corrected reading} \times 12.5/10 \times 4/2 \times 100}{\text{corrected absolute reading at same conc.}}$$

Response factor =

$$\frac{\text{Any arbitrary concentration (50 } \mu\text{g/n}}{\text{corresponding absorbance}}$$

8. Calculate the "response" factor for the total procedure.

B. Preparation of Microsomal-Supernatant Fraction from Rat Liver

Animals are sacrificed by decapitation and the livers removed and placed in a weighed beaker containing ice-cold 1.15% KCl solution. The beaker is re-weighed and the tissue then minced with scissors and homogenized in 2 volumes of the cold KCl solution using a Potter-Elvehjem homogenizer (Teflon pestle). A high torque electric motor is used to rotate the pestle in the glass homogenizer tube which is moved up and down through 8–10 complete excursions. Care is taken to keep the tissue cold during these operations. The rapid rotation of the pestle coupled with the vertical movements disintegrates the tissue and disrupts the cells to produce a diluted suspension of cell sap, intracellular components (nuclei, mitochondria and microsomes) and some unbroken cells. These components can then be separated by differential centrifugation.

The larger components including the cell debris, nuclei and mitochondria are sedimented by centrifugation at 9000 g (av) for 30 min at 1°–3° in a refrigerated centrifuge. The supernatant fluid is removed from the tube using a pasteur pipette, care being taken to avoid the fatty layer present on the surface. Samples of the supernatant fraction, which contains microsomal components as well as diluted cell cytoplasm, are taken for analysis of protein and drug-metabolizing enzyme activity. In the present experiments isolated microsomal fragments are not essential for estimating zoxazolamine hydroxylating activity. Such methods are detailed in the laboratory experiments of Chapter 27.

C. Determination of Tissue Protein

The following method for protein determination in tissue samples, based on that of Lowry et al. (1951), is simple and readily reproducible.

1. Reagent A: 2% Na_2CO_3 in 0.1N NaOH.
2. Reagent B: 0.5% $CuSO_4$, 1% NaK tartrate in deionized water.
3. Reagent C: 50 ml. of reagent A and 1 ml. B made fresh daily.
4. Reagent E: Folin-Ciocalteau phenol reagent adjusted to 0.1 N (store in amber bottle).

Preparation of standards: Standard solution of bovine serum albumin (200 μg/ml) should be provided and the range between 10–60 μg should be determined. Unknown proteins are read from the standard curve, since determinations are not strictly linear over the entire range.

Take duplicate samples of protein standard solution, 50λ, 100λ, 200λ and 300λ and dilute to 1.5 ml. with deionized water. Reagent blank should contain water only. To each tube add 1 ml. reagent C and stir. After 10 min add 100λ of reagent E, stirring each tube *immediately* after addition. Wait 30 min for color to develop and read optical densities immediately at 750 mμ against reagent blank. Construct a standard curve of O.D. against protein concentration.

Determination of protein: Dilute a 100λ sample of the microsomal-supernatant fraction to 2 ml. with deionized water and take 50λ samples (duplicates) of the diluted solution for assay. Add 1.45 ml. of water to each tube and repeat procedure outlined for standards starting with the addition of reagent C. Estimate protein concentrations from standard curve and calculate the amount in the microsomal-supernatant fraction.

Results:

Standard protein	OD$_{750}$ 1.	2.	Microsomal Protein μg/ml
10 μg			
20 μg			
40 μg			
60 μg			
Microsomal protein			
A			
B			
C			
D			

D. Pretreatment Schedules

The following pretreatment schedules were used in the Drug Metabolism Workshop Laboratory. Male Sprague-Dawley rats (50–70 g weight) were pretreated in *one* of the following ways:

Group A Phenobarbital (intra-peritoneal) 30 mg/kg in saline 2× daily for 4 days. Last injection 24 hours before laboratory experiments.

Group B. 3–4 Benzypyrene (intra-peritoneal) 20 mg/kg in corn oil, single injection 24 hours before laboratory experiments.

Group C. Phenobarbital treatment as for Group A. Single injection of SKF-525A (diethylamine ethyl diphenyl propyl acetate) 100 mg/kg. Sixty min prior to injection of zoxazolamine.

Group D. Control animals injected intra-peritoneally with isotonic saline, 2× daily for 4 days prior to laboratory experiment.

III. DURATION OF ZOXAZOLAMINE PARALYSIS

Groups should be provided with 6 young (30-day old) male Sprague-Dawley rats (weight 50–70 g) which have been pretreated according to the schedules A–D.

Procedure:

Weigh each animal and inject intraperitoneally with zoxazolamine (100 mg/kg) using the solution provided (20 mg/kg in 0.2N HCl)

Observe onset and character of the induced paralysis, noting the time at which each animal loses its righting reflex. Separate any animals which fail to become paralyzed (inform staff member).

3. Record the times of recovery of righting reflex. If the animal is able to right itself twice in succession, consider this to be the end-point of the test.
4. Since some animals will remain paralyzed for a number of hours, arrange to make observations at frequent intervals until all are recovered.
5. Calculate the mean paralysis time and standard deviation (S.D.), using the data sheet provided below.

Duration of Zoxazolamine Paralysis

Pretreatment schedule:

Rat No.	Time of start of paralysis	Time of Recovery	Duration of paralysis (min) Pi	Pi − Pm	(Pi − Pm)²
1					
2					
3					
4					
5					
6					

Mean duration of paralysis (Pm) $=$

$$\epsilon(Pi - Pm)^2 =$$

Standard deviation (S.D.) $=$

$$\sqrt{\frac{\epsilon(Pi - Pm)^2}{n-1}}$$

$$=$$

Where n $=$ number of animals paralyzed

IV. INFLUENCE OF PRETREATMENT WITH VARIOUS DRUGS ON THE BIOLOGICAL HALF LIFE OF ZOXAZOLAMINE IN THE RAT

In the previous experiment the influence of certain drugs on the duration of paralysis induced by zoxazolamine was determined. The mechanism of drug interactions and the effect of these on the intensity and duration of pharmacological responses are not always clear. However, mechanisms affecting drng response include changes in absorption, metabolism, excretion, protein binding, distribution and drug-receptor interaction.

In this experiment, the effects of pretreatment of rats with phenobarbital, benzypyrene and phenobarbital plus SKF 525A on *in vivo* drug metabolism will be examined. Changes produced in the elimination of zoxazolamine from the rat will be determined as total body decay curves for the drug. An attempt will be made to determine if there is any correlation between the *in vivo* elimination of the drug and the duration of paralysis.

Procedure:

Each group will be provided with 6 rats which have been pretreated as detailed above.

1. Inject 5 rats with 100 mg/kg zoxazolamine (IP injection: 0.1 ml of 10 mg/ml per 10 g body weight). *Note time of injections.* The sixth rat is not injected but used to determine "blank" body zoxazolamine level.

2. At the indicated time intervals after injection (depending on pretreatment schedule) kill the rat by a sharp blow to the head.

3. Place animal in Waring blendor containing 9 volumes of 0.1N HCl (assume 1 g rat weight = 1 ml). Blend 2 min and allow to stand 5 min.

4. Take 12 ml homogenate and centrifuge for 5 min (wash, rinse and dry blendor).

5. Pipet 2 ml of clear homogenate into cu ture tube containing 1 ml 0.1N HC Add 0.5 ml N NaOH and 12.5 ml chlore form. Continue extraction procedure a described previously (calibration curve)

6. Using the previously determined "re sponse-factor" calculate from the absorb ance data, the concentration and tota amount of zoxazolamine in the homog nate.

7. Calculate zoxazolamine present per gra rat body weight (μg/g). Correct for blan using the uninjected rat value. Constru a semi-log plot of body level/time assum ing that at zero time the level is 100 μg/

8. Fit the best "by eye" line to the data an calculate the half-life for the decay curv From the curve determine the body lev of zoxazolamine at the "paralysis time S.D." obtained previously.

Note: After removal of 2 ml homogenate sample reserve the remaining homogenate until the experiment is complete in case of accidental loss.

Do not start the extraction procedures until the 6 samples have been collected. The samples are then treated as a batch.

Sampling Intervals. Times of sacrifice after injection.

Group A (phenobarbital treated): 15 min, 30 min, 1 hr, 1½ hr, 2 hrs plus uninjected animal.

Group B (benzpyrene treated): 5 min, 10 min, 20 min, 30 min, 45 min, plus uninjected animal.

Group C (phenobarbital + SKF 525A): 30 min, 1 hr, 2 hr, 3 hr, 4 hr, plus uninjected animal.

Group D (saline): 30 min, 1 hr, 2 hr, 3 hr, 4 hr, plus uninjected animal.

RESULTS

Pretreatment schedule:

Rat No.	Weight (g)	Zoxazol- amine injected (ml)	In- jected time	Sacri- fice time	×9 volume	Total volume (ml)
1						
2						
3						
4						
5						
6						

Rat No.	Absor- bance	Conc. (µg/ml)	Total µg	µg/g	Corrected µg/g	Dupli- cated µg/g
1						
2						
3						
4						
5						
6						

Biological half life =

Body level at "paralysis time" =

V. MICROSOMAL HYDROXYLATION OF ZOXAZOLAMINE

The capacity of rat liver microsomal/supernatant fractions to hydroxylate zoxazolamine aerobically in a fortified system capable of NADPH generation will be examined. Measurement of hydroxylation depends on the fact that zoxazolamine is completely extractable into chloroform from basic aqueous solution whereas the ionized phenolic metabolite is retained in the aqueous phase under these conditions.

Reagents:

Sodium phosphate buffer (0.1M, pH 7.35).

Sodium phosphate buffer containing glucose-6-phosphate (10 mg/ml), nicotin-amide (30.5 mg/ml) and magnesium sulfate (6.2 mg/ml).

NADP (2 mg/ml).

Sodium acetate buffer (0.1M, pH 5.6).

Zoxazolamine (1 mg/ml).

Sodium hydroxide (1N).

Chloroform.

HCl (0.1N).

Procedure:

Each group will be provided with 4 rats which have been pretreated according to one of the schedules A–D.

1. Prepare liver microsomal/supernatant fraction by the method detailed above.
2. Set up the 6 reaction vessels to contain the solutions as shown in the protocol below. Add each component of the reac-

tion mixture in the order shown, the substrate (zoxazolamine) being the last addition.

3. Place the vessels in a metabolic shaker at 37° and stop the reaction in 3 of these by addition of 0.5 ml 1N NaOH (zero time). Incubate for 60 min then terminate the reaction in the remaining vessels by adding NaOH.

4. Transfer 1 ml of the reaction mixture to the 20 ml culture tubes which contain 12.5 ml chloroform and 0.5 ml 1N NaOH. Cap tightly and shake for 15 min on the mechanical shaker.

5. Centrifuge to separate the layers and discard the upper (aqueous) layer. Add 3.5 ml of acetate buffer and shake for 10 min. Recentrifuge and again discard the aqueous layer.

6. Transfer 10 ml of the chloroform layer to fresh tubes containing 4 ml 0.1N HCl. Shake for 5 min then centrifuge to separate layers. Take acid extract and measure absorbance at 278 mμ.

7. Estimate the concentration of zoxazolamine from the previously determined calibration curve. The difference between zero time and 60 min zoxazolamine levels represents the extent of metabolism of

the drug by the microsomal/supernatant fraction.

8. Calculate the activity of the liver fractions in terms of mμ moles zoxazolamine converted/mg protein/hr, using the data from your protein determination (molecular weight zoxazolamine 168.6).

Protocol

Ingredient	Tube Number					
	1	2	3	4	5	6
Phosphate buffer (1.15 ml)	+	+	+	+	+	+
Buffer containing G-6-P, nicotinamide, MgSO$_4$ (0.5 ml)	+	+	+	+	+	+
Liver microsomal/supernatant Fraction (0.5 ml)	+	+	+	+	+	+
NADP (0.1 ml)			+	+	+	+
Zoxazolamine (0.25 ml)			+	+	+	+
1 N NaOH (0.5 ml)						
Added at time zero	+		+		+	
Added after incubation		+		+		+
Absorbance at 278 mμ						

Change in absorbance = mean absorbance (zero time) − mean absorbance (60 min)

=

Results

The following data pertaining to the above experiments was obtained by a heterogenous group of Workshop participants during a single day's experimentation. Table 29.1 is a summary sheet which demonstrates a reasonable correlation between duration of paralysis, whole body zoxazolamine decay (T$\frac{1}{2}$), drug concentration at recovery and liver microsomal hydroxylation ac-

TABLE 29.1

Summary data—drug metabolism experiments

Experiment	Saline Treated	Phenobarbital Treated	Benzpyrene Treated	Phenobarbital and SKF
Paralysis Time (mins)	137 ± 15	62 ± 21	20 ± 12	151 ± 27
Whole Body Decay T ½ (min)	102	38	12	125
Drug Concentration at recovery (μg/g)	38	38	34	43
Zoxazolamine Metabolism (mμmoles/mg protein/hr)	3.4	14	15.3	6.1

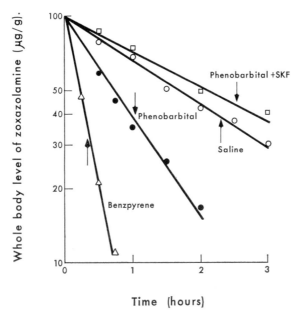

Fig. 29.2. Whole body decay of zoxazolamine in rats following pretreatment.

tivity, for 3 of the experimental groups examined. The paralysis times for the phenobarbital treated and benzpyrene treated animals were significantly different from each other (p < .05) and from the control animals (p < .01) when the data was analyzed by the student "t" test. The data for the group of animals pretreated both with phenobarbital and SKF 252A is less amenable to attempts at correlation, but is included for the sake of completeness. Fig. 29.2 is a semilog. plot of zoxazolamine body level/time from which $T\frac{1}{2}$ values were estimated.

Acknowledgements

The author wishes to express his appreciation to the following members of the Pharmacology Department, University of California, San Francisco Medical Center, for their assistance in the design and execution of these experiments: Drs. Grant Wilkinson, Barry Berkowitz, Horace Loh, Richard Howland, and E. L. Way.

REFERENCES

Burns, J. J., Yu, T. F., Berger, L., and Gutman, A. B.: Zoxazolamine. Amer. J. Med. 25: 401 (1958).

Conney, A. H., Trousof, N. and Burns, J. J.: The metabolic fate of zoxazolamine in man. J. Pharm. Exp. Therap. 128: 335 (1960).

Geiger, L. E., Cervoni, P., Bertino, J. R. and Monteleone, F.: Action of zoxazolamine on spinal segmental reflexes. J. Pharm. Exp. Therap. 123: 164 (1958).

Juchau, M. R., Cram, R. L., Plaa, G. L. and Fouts, J. R.: The induction of benzpyrene hydroxylase in the isolated perfused rat liver. Biochem. Pharmacol. 14: 473 (1965).

Kamijo, K. and Koelle, G. B.: 2-amino-5-chlorobenzoxazole, A long acting spinal cord depressant. Proc. Soc. Exp. Biol. Med. 88: 565 (1955).

Lowry, D. H., Rosebrough, N. J., Farr, A. L. and Randall, J.: Protein measurement with the Folin phenol reagent. J. Biol. Chem. 193: 265 (1951).

Index

36
LH